HEMATOLOGY:
Principles and Procedures

Contributors to Chapter 6

Rouette C. Hunter, M.T. (ASCP)
Assistant Supervisor, Hematology
Tufts New England Medical Center Hospital
Boston, Massachusetts

Alison M. O'Hare, M.T. (ASCP)
Section Leader, Hematology
Tufts New England Medical Center Hospital
Boston, Massachusetts

HEMATOLOGY:
Principles and Procedures

Barbara A. Brown, B.A., M.T. (ASCP), M.S.

Supervisor, Hematology Section, Clinical Pathology Department,
Tufts New England Medical Center Hospital
Boston, Massachusetts

FIFTH EDITION

1988

Lea & Febiger   Philadelphia

Lea & Febiger
600 Washington Square
Philadelphia, PA 19106-4198
U.S.A.
(215) 922-1330

First Edition, 1973
    Reprinted, 1974
Second Edition, 1976
    Reprinted, 1977, 1978, 1979
Third Edition, 1980
    Reprinted, 1981, 1982 (Twice)
Fourth Edition, 1984
    Reprinted, 1985 (Twice)
Fifth Edition, 1988

Library of Congress Cataloging-in-Publication Data
Brown, Barbara A.
    Hematology: principles and procedures.
    Bibliography: p.
    Includes index.
    1. Blood—Examination. 2. Hematology—Technique.
I. Title. [DNLM: 1. Hematologic Diseases—diagnosis—
laboratory manuals. 2. Hematology—instrumentation—laboratory manuals. WH 25 B877h]
RB45.B76   1988   616.1′5   87-21394
ISBN 0-8121-1125-7

PRINTED IN THE UNITED STATES OF AMERICA

Print Number   4   3   2   1

Foreword

It is a deep personal honor and privilege to have been invited to write this foreword for the 5th Edition of Hematology: Principles and Procedures, by Barbara A. Brown.

The major concept and purpose of the text remain the same: to acquaint the reader with a basic knowledge of hematology. In addition, this basic hematology text serves as an excellent mode of continuing education for re-entry medical technologists, as well as other health related professionals in today's cost-minded environment.

Photomicrographs have been utilized to demonstrate more nuclear and cytoplasmic detail. Special stain procedures and appropriate instrumentation review have been strengthened throughout this edition. The author has shared her own skills and techniques which greatly contribute to learning with a personal touch. What the bench laboratory professional needs to know, or at least to understand, can be readily acquired from skill- and theory-focused methodology.

This textbook was originally developed to be a starting point as a principle that informs the reader of essential needs to perform cost-effective and quality health care service and/or research. It is the culmination of the author's graduate degree thesis which was completed at the State University of New York's Health Science Center (previously Upstate Medical Center) in Syracuse, New York in 1970. Through the years, the initial work has been fine tuned with both structure and strategy which makes this, in my considered opinion, an excellent text. It covers those areas of concern with which all bench laboratorians can expect to deal on a day-to-day basis. This includes both principles and practices necessary to accomplish appropriate laboratory tasks.

This text, then, is not just a starting point, but rather a travel down the path that leads to a special destination of interest in Hematology. This is both a comprehensive and highly selective book prepared by an extremely bright, dedicated, and competent clinical laboratory professional for the modern-day laboratory professional.

I would like to dedicate this foreword to Barbara A. Brown whose thirst for knowledge and quest for quality educational material are evident in this new 5th Edition.

Bettina G. Martin, MS, MBA

Preface

I am very gratified by the opportunity to write this fifth edition. The purpose of this edition, as previous ones, is to give the undergraduate medical technology student a fundamental knowledge of hematology. It is written as a first step for the hematology student in preparation for studying and understanding the advanced hematology texts. In addition to students in hematology, the book may also be helpful to technologists needing a review of theory and principles after having been away from the field for a period of time, teachers of hematology, and as a procedural reference for supervisors and technologists working in the hematology laboratory. Workers in the allied health professions may find the book helpful to them in the area of hematology.

The basic format of the book remains unchanged with two exceptions: Chapter 2 has been changed back to Hematopoiesis and Chapter 3 is now Routine Hematology Procedures. These changes were made as a result of suggestions from a number of people using the previous edition. The subject matter in each chapter essentially remains the same. All areas have been updated where applicable. In Chapter 1, Basic Laboratory Technology, a short section on Centrifugation has been added. Chapter 2, Hematopoiesis, has been completely updated. Routine Hematology Procedures, Chapter 3, has been updated where applicable. A color plate of special stains has been added to illustrate the special stain procedures described in Chapter 4. Several of the special hematology procedures have been changed in favor of more improved techniques. Procedures for hemoglobin A_2, hemoglobin H, and the Sucrose Hemolysis test have been added. In Chapter 5, Coagulation, the basic theory of hemostasis, coagulation, and fibrinolysis has been updated. As in the previous chapter, a number of procedures have been changed and modified to improve techniques. The Reptilase Time, von Willebrand Factor Assay, Platelet Neutralization Procedure, Antithrombin III, Heparin Assay, Plasminogen Assay, and Platelet Aggregation tests have been added. Chapter 6, Diseases, has again been expanded, with a more lengthy discussion of the Leukemias. Automation, Chapter 7, has been greatly expanded, with the following instruments added: Sysmex™ E-5000, Ortho ELT-1500 Hematology Analyzer, Coulter Counter Models VI and STKR, Miniprep^R Automatic Blood Smearing Instrument, Hematrak^R Differential Counter, Coag-A-Mate XC, MLA 800, and The KoaguLabs 40-A and 16-S.

I am most appreciative of the help from Alison M. O'Hare, M.T. (ASCP), and Rouette C. Hunter, M.T. (ASCP), who, together, reviewed, revised, and updated Chapter 6, Diseases. Betsy Fitch, M.T. (ASCP), spent many hours drawing all of the new illustrations, including the color plate of malarial parasites. I am appreciative of her efforts and high quality work. Sonia Alexander was helpful in taking the photomicrographs for the special stains color plate and the photographs of the malaria illustrations. I also wish to gratefully acknowledge the many long hours of help Theresa Kuszaj has contributed through the tedious job of proofreading (all five editions).

For this new edition, I greatly appreciate the suggestions and material that I received from Bio/Data Corporation (Roberta A. Bowen), Technicon Instruments Corporation (Lou Ann Page), American Scientific Products (Beth Peterson and Con-

vii

nie DuBois), Coulter Electronics, Inc. (Sandy Piepho), Ortho Diagnostic Systems, Inc. (Susan J. Singer and Cathy Okrepky), BBL Microbiology Systems (David A. Power), Organon Teknika (Jane G. Lenahan), Miles Laboratories, Inc. (Thomas R. Hens), Medical Laboratory Automation, Inc. (Richard L. Minnihan), and Becton Dickinson (Joan D. Wiseman).

The fifth edition of this book has been built from previous editions which were made possible with the help of a number of other people whom I wish to acknowledge and thank again: Beth Conley (photomicrographs), Arianne Graddick, Steven Halpern (photomicrographs), Bettina Martin, Douglas A. Nelson, M.D., Kathleen Yount, and James J. Bonner (art work).

For this and all previous editions I wish to thank the Copy Editing Department and all others at Lea & Febiger for their valuable assistance with the manuscript and for helping to make this book successful.

Randolph, Mass.   Barbara A. Brown

Contents

5. Coagulation   195

6. Diseases

1

Basic Laboratory Techniques

Hematology is defined as the study of blood. This textbook deals primarily with the formed elements of the blood and with those components of the plasma which are necessary for the coagulation (clotting) of blood.

COMPOSITION OF BLOOD

The total blood volume in an adult is 5 to 6 liters, or 7 to 8% of the body weight. Approximately 45% of the blood is composed of formed elements: *red blood cells, white blood cells,* and *platelets.* The red cells contain hemoglobin, the white blood cells defend the body against foreign substances such as infections, and the platelets primarily function in the stoppage of bleeding. The remaining 55% of the blood is the fluid portion, termed *plasma,* of which approximately 90% is water. The remaining 10% is composed of proteins (albumin, globulin, and fibrinogen), carbohydrates, vitamins, hormones, enzymes, lipids, and salts.

When coagulation is prevented by the use of anticoagulants, the liquid portion of the blood is termed plasma and contains the protein fibrinogen. If a blood specimen is allowed to clot, the liquid portion released from the clot is called *serum* and does not contain any fibrinogen due to the fact that the fibrinogen was utilized to form the fibrin threads of the blood clot.

The blood may be thought of as a transportation system. As it circulates through-out the body, oxygen is transported from the lungs to the tissues, products of digestion are absorbed in the intestine and carried to the various tissues of the body, and substances produced in various organs are transferred to other tissues for use. Cellular elements of the blood may also be transported to fight infection or aid in blood coagulation. At the same time, waste products from the tissues are picked up by the blood to be excreted through the skin, kidneys and lungs.

COLLECTION OF BLOOD

The medical technologist most often comes in contact with a patient during the process of blood collection or bone marrow aspiration. The patient in a hospital is anxious, fearful, and in ill health. He is anxious about his physical condition; he fears because he does not know what will happen next; and he is physically uncomfortable as a result of his sickness or injury. He is also separated from his known surroundings and family. For these reasons, a person's mental attitude is often at its worst when he is in the hospital as a patient. It is important, therefore, for the medical technologist to show the patient, at all times, the kindness and understanding that can mean so much.

When the technologist is dealing with a child, his approach is doubly important. This may be the first time the child has had a blood test. If it turns out to be a

1

horrendous experience, it will be remembered and feared by the child for many years. Therefore, it is important to gain the child's confidence before proceeding with blood collection. The child should be informed of what is going to happen. If the child is told that the puncture will not hurt, the child's confidence will be lost because this statement is generally not true. A routine venipuncture may be compared to a bee sting, while the fingerstick may be described as a mother pricking her finger with a needle or pin while sewing.

The techniques used in obtaining blood are not learned overnight. They are an art that must be developed by study, observation, and practice, until the technologist has the necessary skill and self confidence.

Skill, patience, understanding—these are the qualities of a good phlebotomist.

Microsample Technique

Microsampling refers to blood collection by skin puncture and is frequently used on the following types of patients:

1. *Infants less than 6 months* of age generally do not have a large blood supply, and it is dangerous to remove the volume of blood involved in venipuncture.
2. In *young children,* if only a small amount of blood is needed, the tip of the third or fourth finger may be used to obtain blood.
3. When an *adult* has poor veins, when the veins cannot be used because of intravenous (I.V.) infusions, or in the case of a severely burned patient, the third or fourth finger may be used to obtain blood.

REAGENTS AND EQUIPMENT

1. Isopropyl alcohol, 70% (v/v), or prepared alcohol prep pads.
2. Sterile gauze pads.
3. Sterile blood lancet (Fig. 1).
4. Appropriate capillary tubes (Figs. 2, 3, and 4), Microtainers (Fig. 5), Un-

opette (Fig. 6), and/or pipets and diluting fluids.

PROCEDURE

1. *Location of phlebotomy site.* When obtaining blood from infants less than 1 year of age, blood is generally obtained from the foot. The site cho-

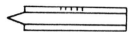

Fig. 1.   Blood lancet.

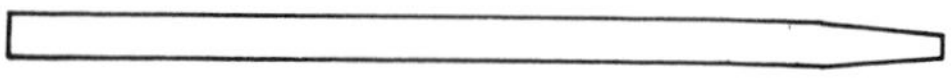

Fig. 2.   Caraway pipet.

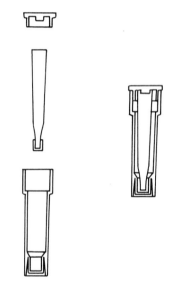

Fig. 3.   Sarstedt 300 μL capillary blood collection system.

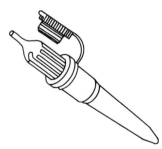

Fig. 4.   Sarstedt 1 mL capillary blood collection system.

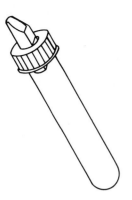

Fig. 5. Becton Dickinson Microtainer.

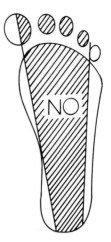

Fig. 7. Acceptable/unacceptable puncture sites on the foot.

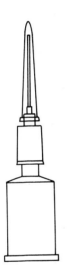

Fig. 6. Unopette.

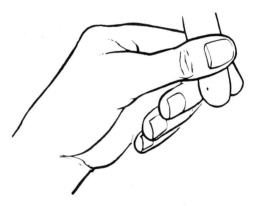

Fig. 8. Site of fingertip puncture.

sen should be on the inside. (medial) or outside (lateral) portions of the sole (plantar surface) of the foot by drawing an imaginary line from the middle of the large toe to the heel, and a line from between the fourth and fifth toes to the heel (Fig. 7). The heel area is the recommended site. At no time should the back curvature of the heel be used. The depth of the puncture must be no greater than 2.4 mm. Because the blood vessels of an infant's heel are located between 0.35 and 1.6 mm below the surface of the skin, the puncture need not be any deeper than 1.6 mm. When the finger is used to obtain a blood specimen, the distal portion should be used. Perform the puncture on the palmar surface, slightly off-center, but not on the side or tip of the finger (Fig. 8). The puncture should be no deeper than 3.1 mm in this area since the distance between the skin surface and bone will vary from 3.1 to 10.9 mm. The distance to the bone is only 1.2 to 2.2 mm in infants, so the finger should never be used on this age group of children. The puncture site should contain no swelling and have no previous puncture sites.

2. *Preparation of the puncture site.*
   a. Make certain the puncture site is

warm. If it is not, use a *warm* (not hot) moist cloth and cover the site for 3 to 5 minutes.

   b. Clean the site with 70% isopropanol (v/v). (Betadine should not be used since this will cause some chemistry values to be erroneously high.)

   c. Thoroughly dry the site with a sterile gauze. (Any alcohol left on the puncture site may cause the blood to hemolyze.)

3. Using the appropriate blood lancet, puncture the site, inserting the lancet as far down as it will go. A superficial puncture will yield a good blood flow, and makes it unnecessary to repeat the procedure. With a good single puncture, ½ to 1 ml of blood may be obtained.

4. Using a dry gauze, wipe away the first drop of blood, making certain the area is completely dry.

5. Apply moderate pressure, approximately 1 cm behind the site of the puncture to obtain a drop of blood.

6. Release this pressure immediately to allow recirculation of the blood.

7. Hold the collection tube (or pipet) in a horizontal to slightly downward position. When the tube comes in contact with the drop of blood, the blood should flow freely into the collection tube.

8. Repeat steps 5, 6, and 7 until enough blood has been collected.

9. When blood collection is complete, the foot may be elevated above the body (the finger may be held in an upward position) and a sterile gauze pad pressed against the puncture site until bleeding stops. A band-aid may be applied, but it should be kept in mind that adhesive can be irritating on the skin of young infants.

DISCUSSION

1. The puncture site should not be squeezed too tightly. This will cause the tissue juice to mix with and dilute the blood.

2. When collecting blood for hematology tests, the finger must be wiped dry after each test. (Platelets clump immediately in the blood at the puncture site.) Because of platelet adhesiveness and aggregation at the site of puncture, it is advisable to collect the platelet count and blood smears (if requested) first when samples for a number of tests are to be obtained.

3. An automatic lancet for microsampling techniques is available. This device, the Autolet (Fig. 9), is manufactured by Owen Mumford Ltd., Woodstock, Oxfordshire, England, and is available through most hospital laboratory distributors in this country. The Autolet is a small, portable device that rapidly and automatically makes a standardized, usually painless incision in the finger or heel. The disposable, sterile Monolet lancet (manufactured by Sherwood Medical, Inc.) is used in the Autolet.

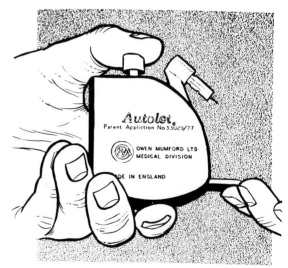

Fig. 9. Autolet.

Venipuncture

A venipuncture must be performed with care. The veins of a patient are the main source of blood for testing and the entry point for medications, intravenous solutions, and blood transfusions. Because there are only a limited number of easily accessible veins in a patient, it is important that everything be done to preserve their good condition and availability. Part of this responsibility lies with the medical technologist.

The ideal procedure is to have the patient lie down. If this is not possible, he should sit in a sturdy, comfortable chair with his arm firmly supported on a table or chair arm and easily accessible to the technologist. A patient should never stand or sit on a high stool during any process of blood collection. The technologist must be ready for the occasional patient who faints during this procedure; however, this rarely occurs with hospital inpatients who are lying flat in bed.

REAGENTS AND EQUIPMENT

1. Isopropyl alcohol, 70% (v/v), or prepared 70% alcohol prep pads.
2. Sterile gauze pads.
3. Tourniquet.
4. Appropriate test tubes for tests ordered.
5. Vacutainer holder (Fig. 10) or syringe (Fig. 11). The vacutainer system is the most widely used since it allows the blood to pass directly from the vein into the test tube.
6. Needle. The choice of needle depends on the size of the vein. The most commonly used needle is the 20-gauge. The higher the gauge number, the smaller the diameter, or bore, of the needle. For small veins, a 21- or 22-gauge needle is recommended. The length of needle used is chosen by the individual technologist. The two most widely used needle lengths are 1 inch and 1½ inches. Blood may be obtained from most deep veins with a 1-inch needle. If the vacutainer system is used, a special vacutainer needle (Fig. 10) is used. The hypodermic needle (Fig. 12) is employed with use of the syringe technique.
7. Band-aid.

PROCEDURE

1. *Make certain you have ACCURATELY IDENTIFIED the patient.* For inpatients, this may be done by checking the wristband. When collecting blood from an outpatient, ask him his name. (A tube of blood mislabeled for a blood transfusion can end in a patient's death.)
2. Prepare the vacutainer assembly if this method is to be used. Insert the shorter end of the vacutainer needle into the holder. (The end of the needle is generally covered by a rubber like sleeve to prevent blood leaking from the needle when collecting more than 1 tube of blood.) Insert the first tube into the vacutainer holder until the top is even with the line on the holder. Do *not* puncture the top of the tube with the inside needle.

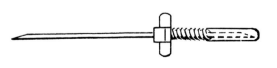
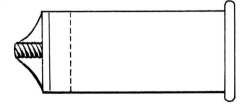
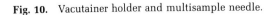

Fig. 10. Vacutainer holder and multisample needle.

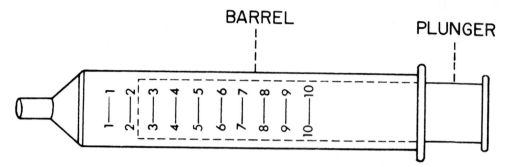

Fig. 11. Syringe.

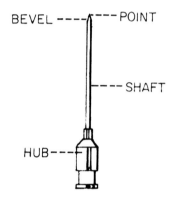

Fig. 12. Hypodermic needle.

Each tube contains a vacuum which is responsible for drawing the appropriate amount of blood into the tube. Puncturing the top causes loss of this vacuum.

3. When using a syringe to draw blood, move the plunger up and down in the barrel once or twice to make sure it does not stick. Expel all air from the syringe. Place the needle on the syringe (while keeping the cap on the shaft of the needle) and twist it to make certain it fits securely.

4. Apply the tourniquet several inches above the bend of the elbow, as shown in Figures 13 and 14, just tightly enough to be uncomfortable to the patient.

5. Ask to patient to make a tight fist. This makes the vein more easily palpable.

6. Select a suitable vein for puncture

(Fig. 15). The three main veins of the arm, which are the sites of the majority of venipunctures, are the accessory cephalic, median cephalic, and median cubital. Generally, the median cephalic is the vein of choice because it is generally well anchored in tissue and does not roll when the vein is punctured. The median cubital vein, at the inner portion of the arm, tends to roll in many patients. The accessory cephalic vein is located on the edge of the outer part of the arm where the outside skin tends to be a little tougher.

7. Using the index finger of the left hand, palpate the arm until the best vein has been found. It should feel similar to an elastic tube. (A frequent error made is the failure to find the best vein because of carelessness or haste.) If the vein is not readily palpable, one of several techniques may be used to help locate the vein: (1) Force blood into the veins by massaging the arm from the wrist to the elbow, (2) tap sharply on the vein site with the index and third finger to cause the vein to dilate, (3) apply a warm, moist cloth to the vein site, or, (4) allow the arm to hang in a vertical position so that the veins will fill to capacity with blood.

8. When the vein has been chosen, cleanse the puncture site with 70% alcohol. Allow the area to dry in or-

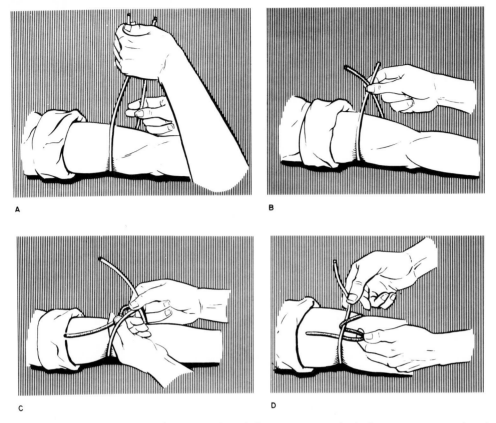

Fig. 13. Method of tourniquet application. A. Stretch the tourniquet to obtain the correct amount of tension. B. Grasp both sides of the tourniquet with the right hand while continuing to maintain the proper tension. C. With the left hand, reach through the loop and grasp the left side of the tourniquet. D. With the left hand, pull the tourniquet halfway through the loop. Release hands carefully.

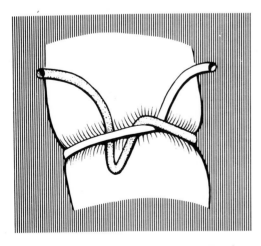

Fig. 14. Front view of tourniquet on arm. To release the tourniquet, carefully pull the end of the tourniquet on the left (shaded end).

der to prevent hemolysis of the blood and also a burning sensation to the patient. Once the area has been cleaned, do not touch the puncture site with any unsterile object or fingers.

9. Grasp the patient's arm 1 to 2 inches below the puncture site, pulling the skin tight with your thumb.

10. Hold the vacutainer assembly, or syringe, with the opposite hand, between the thumb and last three fingers. Rest the index finger against the hub of the needle to serve as a guide.

11. The needle should be in the bevel up position (needle opening facing upward), point in the same direction as the vein, and should make an approximately 15° angle with the arm.

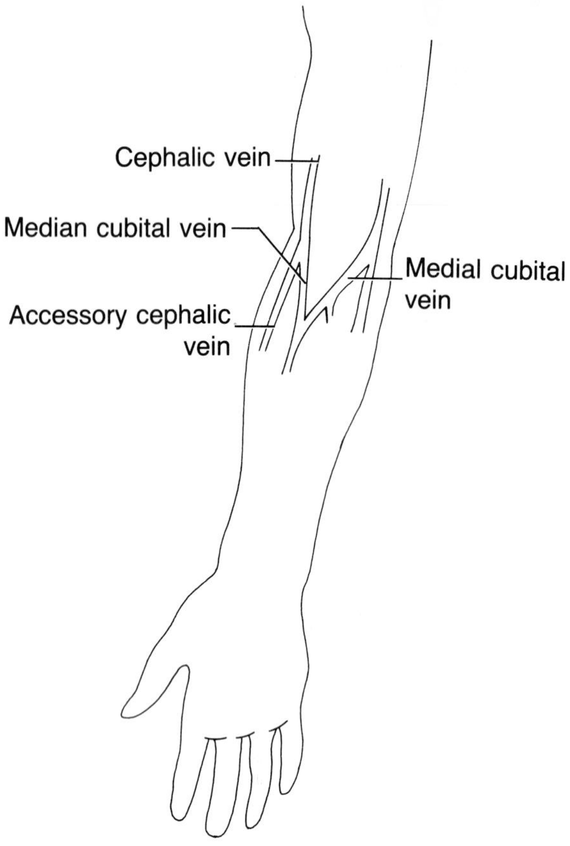

Fig. 15. Major veins of the arm.

12. The vein should be entered slightly below the area where it can be seen. In this way, there is tissue available to serve as a an anchor for the needle.

13. A prominent vein may be entered quickly with a one-step puncture of the skin and vein. When the veins are deeper or the entry more difficult, a two-step procedure may be followed. First, the skin is punctured, and then, if need be, the left index finger may be used to palpate above the puncture site to confirm the exact location of the vein. The second step is to puncture the vein.

14. As the needle enters the vein slightly less resistance will be felt.

15. If the vacutainer assembly is being used, as soon as the needle is in the vein, push the tube firmly but carefully in as far as it will go, ensuring that the needle is kept steady.

16. If a syringe is used, a small amount of blood will flow into the neck of the syringe as the needle enters the vein. Care should be taken when pulling back on the plunger. Do not pull back with too much force since this may cause the blood to hemolyze, the force may pull the wall of the vein down on top of the bevel of the needle causing the blood flow to stop, or, the needle may inadvertently be pulled out of the vein.

17. The tourniquet may be loosened as soon as the blood enters the tube or syringe, or it may be left on until the process is complete. It should be noted, however, that the tourniquet should not be left on longer than 1 minute, or the blood in the area will have an increased concentration of cells (hemoconcentration). (If desired, the patient may open his fist as soon as the blood begins to flow.)

18. Release the tourniquet as soon as the

blood specimen has been obtained, before the needle is removed from the vein.

19. Apply a sterile, dry gauze to the puncture site and quickly and smoothly withdraw the needle from the patient's arm.

20. Have the patient apply gentle pressure to the site of puncture for several minutes until the bleeding has stopped. Apply a bandaid if desired. The patient may also keep his arm raised in a vertical position for several minutes to decrease pressure in the blood vessel.

21. If a syringe is employed, remove the needle before expelling the blood into the appropriate tubes. This process should be accomplished quickly before the blood begins to clot.

DISCUSSION

1. When the vacutainer system is being used to obtain several tubes of blood, collect a nonanticoagulated tube first. As soon as a tube containing anticoagulant is filled, invert the tube for mixing about 10 times while the next tube is filling with blood. If an anticoagulated tube is the only, or last specimen, mix the tube immediately. It is advisable not to collect specimens for coagulation testing first.

2. In the event that you have been unable to puncture the vein immediately, use your free index finger to locate the vein. It may be that the needle has not gone deeply enough, or perhaps it is slightly to the left or right of the vein. Do not attempt to puncture the vein from that location. This is painful to the patient and may cause tissue damage. Withdraw the needle until the point is almost to the surface of the skin and then redirect the needle. This procedure is acceptable if the needle is close to the vein, but care should be taken that the patient is not caused too much pain. Sometimes a second venipuncture is necessary.

3. If a patient is receiving intravenous infusions in both arms, it is acceptable to puncture the vein 3 to 4 inches below the site of the I.V. device.

4. A technologist or student should not stick a patient more than 2 to 3 times. If the blood sample has not been obtained after the second attempt, it is usually advisable to call another technologist. By this time, both you and the patient have lost confidence.

5. It is important that pressure be applied to the site of the venipuncture. Failure to follow this procedure leads to a hematoma (bleeding into the tissues).

6. If the area surrounding the puncture site begins to swell while blood is being withdrawn, this usually indicates that the needle has gone through the vein or the bevel of the needle is halfway out of the vein and blood is leaking into the tissues. The tourniquet should be released and the needle withdrawn immediately, with pressure applied to the site.

7. In some instances, it is almost impossible to locate a vein in the arm. In such a case, the veins of the lower arm, wrist, or hand may be used. The student should gain a reasonable amount of skill and confidence before attempting a venipuncture in these areas.

8. When a venipuncture must be carried out on a small child, it may be necessary to release the tourniquet when the blood starts to enter the syringe. Children's veins are small and collapse quickly because blood is removed from the vein faster than it enters it. Therefore, release the tourniquet carefully to improve the blood circulation.

9. When performing a venipuncture in

the lower arm or hand, on small children, or on a patient with poor or small veins, a syringe or pediatric (small) vacutainer assembly and tubes is generally used. The use of standard sized vacutainer tubes tends to collapse these veins.

10. When disposing of used needles, they should be placed in a specially prepared container provided for this purpose. Never throw them directly into the wastebasket.

11. Regardless of the disease the patient has, be careful not to stick yourself with the needle. If this happens, report it to the supervisor immediately.

Isolation Techniques

Isolation techniques are used for 2 primary reasons: (1) When a patient has an infectious or communicable disease, certain safeguards must be followed to prevent further spread of the infection to hospital personnel or to other patients, and (2) special techniques are also needed to shield or protect infection-prone patients from pathogens.

To ensure optimal care of the patients and hospital personnel, the medical technologist should follow isolation procedures. Examples are given below and may vary slightly between hospitals.

1. Strict isolation is used in cases of active tuberculosis, meningococcal meningitis, rabies, diphtheria, viral encephalitis, polio, and certain infectious diseases such as measles, smallpox, and mumps. A gown, mask, and gloves are generally worn by the technologist.

2. Enteric and wound isolation techniques are used when coming in contact with patients who have dysentery and other disorders which spread through direct contact with a wound or discharge. The technologist is generally required to wear a gown and gloves.

3. In respiratory isolation, the patient has infections which are transmitted via droplets or by an airborne route. In these cases the technologist should always wear a mask.

4. Protective isolation requires the technologist to protect the patient from infection. These are patients with leukemia, severe burns, body radiation, kidney transplants, and plastic surgery. The technologist is usually required to wear a gown, mask, gloves, and sometimes shoe coverings.

DISCUSSION

1. When drawing blood from a patient in isolation, it is especially important that technologists wash their hands before and after working with each patient. (This should also be done when working with non-isolation patients.) It is also important that a minimum of equipment be taken into the patient's room.

2. When the technologist has completed the venipuncture all disposable equipment should be placed in appropriate receptacles in the patient's room (in all types of isolation except protective isolation).

3. If a patient has a disease which may be transmitted through body fluids, all specimen tubes should be labeled appropriately (e.g., Precaution). (It should be noted, however, that all specimens a technologist deals with should be considered as potentially capable of transmitting infectious diseases.)

ANTICOAGULANTS

Most hematology procedures must be performed on whole blood or plasma. Therefore, as soon as the blood is withdrawn from the patient, it is mixed with an anticoagulant to prevent coagulation. Three anticoagulants are most commonly used for hematologic procedures.

1. *EDTA* (sequestrene or versene) is the

disodium or dipotassium salt of ethylene-diaminetetraacetic acid. It is the most widely used anticoagulant for hematologic procedures. The dipotassium salt is more soluble than the disodium salt and is used in concentrations of 1.5 ($\pm$0.25) mg/mL. EDTA prevents coagulation by its chelating effect on (combination with) the calcium in the blood. (Calcium is required for blood coagulation.) This anticoagulant also prevents formation of artifacts and may be used for the preparation of blood films for 2 hours after blood collection. Excessive concentrations of EDTA causes shrinkage of the red blood cells leading to a decreased spun hematocrit, an increased MCHC, and a falsely low erythrocyte sedimentation rate. The hemoglobin, however, should not be affected. Increased concentrations also cause degenerative changes in the white cells, and the platelets will swell and break up thus causing increased platelet counts due to the broken fragments. Blood may be stored at 4°C for 24 hours without any evidence of change in the hemoglobin, hematocrit, white blood count, or red blood count. Blood stored at room temperature for 24 hours shows an elevated hematotocrit reading and may show a slightly decreased platelet count. EDTA is an excellent anticoagulant for the prevention of platelet clumping.

2. *Sodium citrate* is the anticoagulant of choice for coagulation studies. It is used in a concentration of 1 part 0.109 M sodium citrate to 9 parts whole blood. It prevents coagulation by binding the calcium of the blood in a soluble complex. It helps to maintain the stability of some of the coagulation factors, most notably factors V and VIII. It also helps the platelets to retain their functional capabilities.

3. *Heparin* may be used in a concentration of 15 ($\pm$2.5) IU/mL of whole blood. Coagulation is prevented for a period of approximately 24 hours by the inactivation of the activated forms of factors X and II. The use of heparin as an anticoagulant may cause clumping of the white cells and platelets. It is, therefore, of limited use in hematology and is the anticoagulant of choice for only a few special hematology procedures (e.g., osmotic fragility test) where the addition of salts to the blood may affect the test results.

THE MICROSCOPE

The microscope used in the routine hematology laboratory is, in simple terms, a magnifying glass. It is termed a *compound light microscope* because it contains two separate lens systems, the objective and the ocular. This microscope generally consists of an *eyepiece, objective,* a *mechanical stage,* a *substage condenser* system with an *iris diaphragm,* and a *light source* (Fig. 16).

EYEPIECE LENS

The conventional eyepiece lens, or ocular, has a magnification of 10$\times$. ($\times$ is used to designate the units of magnification, know as diameters. If a lens has a magnification of 10$\times$, this does not mean that it magnifies an object to 10 times its original size [area], but rather that the diameter of the object is magnified 10 times it original size.) A monocular microscope consists of one eyepiece; a binocular microscope, the most commonly used today, contains two eyepieces.

OBJECTIVE LENS

Most light microscopes contain three objectives lenses, each with different powers of magnification. The most commonly employed objectives are 10$\times$ (low power), 40$\times$ (high dry), and 100$\times$ (oil immersion). A fourth lens, 50$\times$ (low oil immersion), may be utilized by experienced technologists for performing a differential cell count.

OPTICAL TUBE

The optical tube length is the distance between the eyepiece and objective lenses and is generally 160 mm.

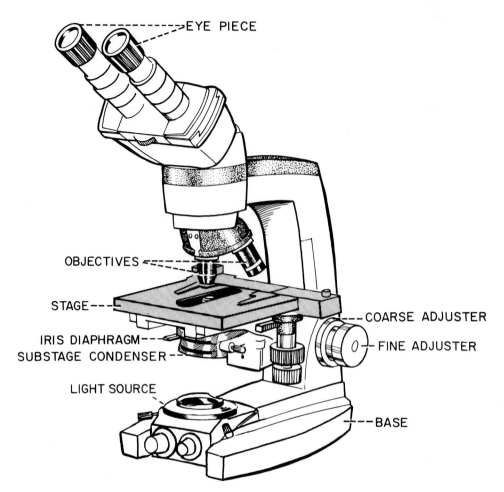

Fig. 16.   Binocular microscope.

STAGE

The stage holds the slide that is being examined and contains a moveable assembly to facilitate the study of different parts of the slide.

SUBSTAGE CONDENSER

The most commonly used substage condenser is the Abbe condenser which directs the beam of light from a source onto the specimen. It consists of two lenses (Fig. 17). The light is focused on the object or specimen by raising or lowering the condenser system. Lack of a substage condenser causes fuzzy rings and haloes around the object being studied.

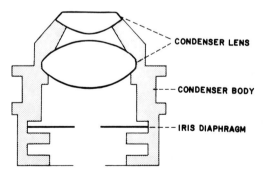

Fig. 17.   Substage condenser and iris diaphragm.

IRIS DIAPHRAGM

The iris diaphragm contains a number of leaves that are opened or closed to increase or decrease the amount of light illuminating the object (Fig. 17).

LIGHT SOURCE

There are two different types of light sources which may be employed. The older and less commonly used illuminator consists of an outside light source. This microscope is equipped with a mirror, in front of which is placed a substage lamp or special microscope light. The mirror is then adjusted so that the rays of light from the lamp are projected upward into the condenser system. The newer microscopes contain a built-in light source at the base of the microscope. This type of light source may or may not contain a built-in transformer to adjust the light intensity. There is also a swing-in neutral density filter present in this light source. Centering screws enable the viewer to center the light passing up through the condenser. A field iris diaphragm is also present in the light source. It may be opened or closed and is used in focusing the light which passes up through the condenser.

TOTAL MAGNIFICATION AND IMAGE

Total magnification is equal to the magnification of the eyepiece times the magnification of the objective lens. For example, using a 10× eyepiece and the 40× objective lens, the total magnification is 400×. The magnification of each system is printed on each of the appropriate parts. The image seen by the eye through a compound microscope, the virtual image, is upside down and reversed. The right side is seen as the left side and vice versa; therefore, movement of the slide is also reversed.

NUMERICAL APERTURE

The numerical aperture is a designation of the amount of light entering the objective from the microscopic field (or, as in the condenser, the amount of light entering the substage condenser from the light source). It may be thought of as a method for expressing the fraction of the wave front admitted by a lens (Fig. 18). The numerical aperture is constant for any single lens and is dependent on the radius of the lens (AC) and the focal length of the lens (PC).

$$\text{Numerical aperture} = R \times \sin \mu$$

μ = The angle made by the one ray passing through the edge of the lens, with the other ray passing through the center of the lens

R = The refractive index of the medium between the object and the objective lens

The numerical aperture of the objective should be the same as the numerical aperture of the substage condenser. If these numerical apertures are not similar, interference effects occur.

REFRACTIVE INDEX

The refractive index of a substance is calculated as the speed with which light travels in air divided by the speed with which light travels through the substance. (Since light travels more slowly through immersion oil, the numerical aperture is increased by placing oil between the oil immersion objective and the object.)

RESOLVING POWER

Resolving power is the useful limit of magnification. It is the ability of the mi-

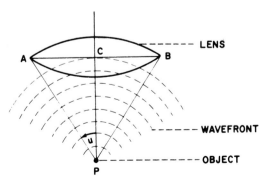

Fig. 18.   Numerical aperture.

croscope, at a specific magnification, to distinguish two separate objects situated close to one another and the ability of the lens to reveal fine detail. The smaller the distance between the two specific objects that can be distinguished apart, the greater the resolving power of the microscope.

$$\begin{matrix} \text{Minimal distance} \\ \text{between two objects} \\ \text{(resolvable distance)} \end{matrix} = \frac{0.612 \times \lambda}{\text{Numerical aperture}}$$

λ = The wavelength of the light

The resolving power is, therefore, dependent on the wavelength of light and the numerical aperture. The light source remains constant and so, in routine work, may be ignored. The larger the numerical aperture, the smaller the resolvable distance, and hence, the more efficient the resolving power.

DEPTH OF FIELD

Depth of field is the capacity of the objective lens to focus in different planes at the same time. This is largely dependent on the numerical aperture. The greater the numerical aperture, the smaller the depth of field. It is possible to increase the depth of field slightly by closing the iris diaphragm (thus decreasing the numerical aperture).

ABERRATIONS

Different wavelengths of light are not bent in the same way as they pass through the lens and, therefore, are not brought to the same focus. These are called *chromatic aberrations* (Fig. 19).

With *spherical aberrations,* the light

waves, as they travel through the lens, are bent differently, depending on which part of the lens they pass through. Rays passing through the peripheral portions of the lens are brought to a shorter focal point than those rays passing through the thicker part of the lens (Fig. 20).

LENSES

To compensate for aberrations, *achromatic* and *apochromatic lenses* are employed. The achromatic lens is the most commonly used lens for color correction. It brings rays of two colors to a common focus and obtains a reasonable compromise for the remaining colors. Apochromatic lenses are the finest lenses produced and correct for chromatic and spherical aberrations. This lens brings three colors (blue, yellow, and red) to a common focus. A factor that must be taken into consideration for the most effective use of the microscope lens is the medium between the objective and the object being studied. The low power ($10\times$) and high dry objective lenses ($40\times$) use air. When oil immersion lenses are employed, a drop of oil should be used; otherwise, bending of the light waves occurs (Fig. 21).

Operating Procedures

1. With the $10\times$ objective in position, place the object to be studied (slide or counting chamber) on the microscope stage.
2. If you are using a binocular microscope, adjust the distance between the eyepieces as necessary.
3. Focus the object, using the coarse ad-

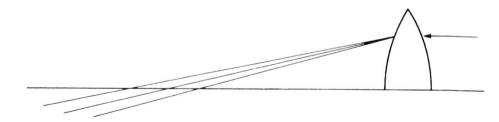

Fig. 19. Chromatic aberration.

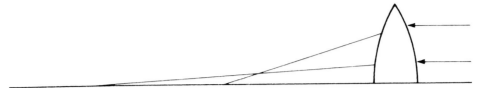

Fig. 20.   Spherical aberration.

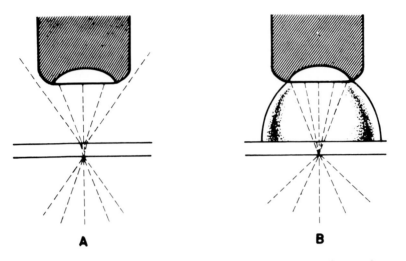

Fig. 21.   Light path through the high dry objective lens (A) and oil immersion objective lens (B).

justment knob. Bring the object into sharp focus with the fine adjustment knob.

4. While looking through the microscope, close the field diaphragm on the light source so that the image of the leaves of the diaphragm may be seen in the field of view.

5. Focus the condenser by raising or lowering it until the leaves of the iris diaphragm are in sharp focus. The condenser should now be left in this position for use with all like objects to be studied.

6. Center the light source by using the two centering screws (on the light source) so that the image of the field diaphragm in the field of view is in the center. Open the field diaphragm until the iris leaves just disappear from view.

7. Remove one eyepiece and, while looking through the microscope

(without the eyepiece), close the condenser diaphragm. Reopen the diaphragm until the diaphragm leaves just disappear from view. (Further closing of the condenser diaphragm may increase contrast and depth of focus, depending on the specimen.) This procedure allows you to obtain the best resolving power for the microscope. Replace the eyepiece.

8. Generally, as you increase the magnification of the microscope (change objectives), the condenser diaphragm must be opened while the field diaphragm (light source) is further closed. The condenser and field diaphragms should not be used to control light intensity. This is generally done by adjusting the transformer setting on the light source or by using filters.

DISCUSSION

1. When employing the high-dry or oil

immersion objectives, a suitable field for study should be found and focused using the low power objective (10×). A drop of oil may then be placed on the slide and the oil immersion objective swung into place. Never use oil with the high-dry objective.

2. To clean the lenses, only lens paper should be used. The paper is designed for this purpose and will not scratch the lenses, which other, more harsh paper or material might do.

3. The oil must be removed from the oil immersion lens (with lens paper) whenever it is not in use to prevent oil seepage to the inside of the lens.

4. If xylene or lens cleanser is used to remove oil and clean the lenses, the structures holding the objective lenses may loosen in time because of the solvent qualities of these solutions.

5. If the field of study is dirty, the cause may be dirt on the eyepiece. Revolve the eyepiece as you are looking through the microscope. If the dirt also revolves, the eyepiece needs cleaning.

Phase Microscopy

Phase microscopy is employed in hematology for the counting of platelets. Performing this procedure on a light microscope is tedious and more liable to error because the platelets are unstained and small. Phase microscopy enables the viewer to see platelets and various structures in larger cells while they are still alive, due to differences in the refractive index, shape, and absorption characteristics of the cells and cellular components.

Light travels in waves. If two sets of light waves in phase are allowed to travel through the same medium, they remain in phase (Fig. 22), and the brightness of the light is the sum of the two amplitudes (height of the peaks). If one of the two light waves (which were originally in phase)

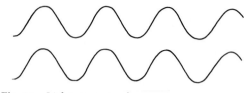

Fig. 22.   Light waves in phase.

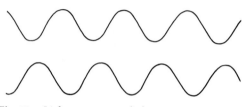

Fig. 23.   Light waves out of phase.

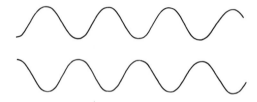

Fig. 24.   Light waves out of phase.

passes through an object, it is slowed down; the two waves are then out of phase (Fig. 23), and the light is diminished.

If the two light waves are out of phase by a half of a wavelength, there will be no light because the peak of one wave is cancelled by the trough of the other light wave (Fig. 24).

When rays of light pass through a slide containing cells, platelets, or living unstained organisms, those rays which pass through the cells may be retarded or slowed down but not diffracted from their pathway. These are termed direct rays. Other light waves may be retarded and, at the same time, diffracted. The amount of retardation of the light wave is dependent on the optical density, refractive index, and shape of the cell or cellular component.

For maximum contrast between the cell and its surroundings, the light wave should be retarded by a quarter of a wavelength. Cells and cellular components,

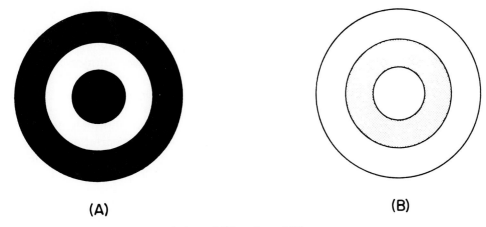

(A)   **(B)**

Fig. 25.   Annular diaphragm (A) and phase-shifting element (B).

however, are not able to retard the wavelength to this great a degree. Therefore, two additional parts are added to the light microscope to increase the small wave changes by about a quarter of a wavelength. This then becomes the phase microscope. An annular diaphragm is placed below, or in the substage condenser, and a phase shifting element is situated in the rear focal plane of the objective. The light passes up from its source, through the clear circular area of the annular diaphragm (Fig. 25), and through the specimen. The phase shifting element is constructed so that light waves pass quickly through the clear areas (Fig. 25) but are retarded by a quarter of a wavelength when going through the shaded circular area. These two components are so situated that the diffracted rays pass directly through the clear area of the phase shifting element. All light waves that are undiffracted pass through the treated (shaded) areas of the phase shifting element and are, therefore, slowed by an additional quarter of a wavelength. These alterations in the phases of the rays increase the contrast and enable the viewer to get a more highly visible picture of the cells and their components.

Electron Microscopy

Magnifications greater than 1500× are not practical with the light microscope due to a decreased efficiency in resolving power. For this reason, the electron microscope has come into use, where magnifications of 50,000× may be obtained with a high degree of resolving power. The electron microscope employs a stream of electrons moving at a high velocity in place of a beam of light of short wavelength. The image is produced when the electrons hit a phosphorescent screen which then emits photons visible to the human eye. (This is similar to a television picture tube.)

SPECTROPHOTOMETRY

If a substance can be converted into a soluble, colored material, its concentration can then be determined by the amount of color present in the solution. The filter photometer and spectrophotometer are widely used in today's laboratory as the main instruments for this type of measurement. There are relatively few tests in the hematology laboratory which employ spectrophotometry, unlike chemistry, in which spectrophotometry is much more widely used. This section gives the student a basic outline of this tool.

In both the filter photometer and spectrophotometer, a photoelectric cell is used to measure color intensity. This is done by measuring the amount of light from a source which passes through the colored solution. To obtain the greatest or optimal sensitivity, the light permitted to pass through the solution is of a particular wavelength. If a filter is used to determine the wavelength, the colorimeter is termed a *filter photometer*. In the *spectrophotometer,* the wavelength is selected by a prism, or diffraction grating.

As shown in Figure 26, the light source (1) passes through a filter, prism, or diffraction grating (2). Only light of the preset wavelength can pass from the filter through the cuvet (3) containing the material to be measured. The amount of light passing through the solution (those light waves not absorbed by the material) comes in contact with the photoelectric cell (4), where the light energy is converted into electric energy. This electric energy is proportionally increased by the amplifier (5) and measured by the galvanometer (6). A scale located on the galvanometer is generally calibrated to read optical density (O.D.) or percent transmittance (%T). Optical density, or absorbance, measures the amount of light absorbed by the solution. The percent transmittance measures the amount of light allowed to pass through the solution. All colors which make up light have a wavelength of a specific length measured in nanometers (nm) (Fig. 27). A blue solution is blue because all colors except blue have been absorbed by the so-

lution. In other words, the blue color wavelength passes through the solution.

The principle of photometry is based on the Lambert-Bouger-Bunsen-Roscoe-Beer laws, which have been combined to give what is commonly known as *Beer's law.* According to this law, the absorbance (optical density) of a solution is directly proportional to the concentration of the solute (material in solution being tested for) and the length of the light path through this solution. Since the predetermined wavelength is the same and cuvets with a given, constant diameter are employed, the length of the light path through the solution is set, and the optical density is, therefore, directly proportional to the concentration of the solute. If the optical density and concentration of a standard are known, the unknown concentration may be calculated if its optical density is known.

$$\frac{\text{Concentration of unknown}}{\text{Concentration of standard}}$$
$$= \frac{\text{Optical density of unknown}}{\text{Optical density of standard}}$$

OPTICAL DENSITY VS. % TRANSMITTANCE

If L represents the light energy entering the solute and Lo is the light energy leav-

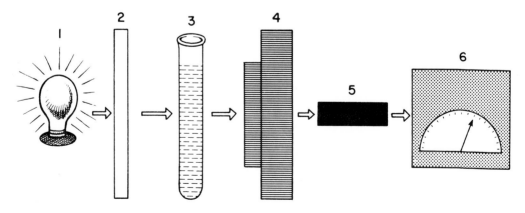

Fig. 26.   Principle of a filter photometer or spectrophotometer.

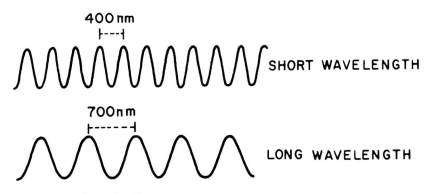

Fig. 27. Measurement of wavelengths.

ing the solute (that light hitting the photoelectric cell), then $\dfrac{Lo}{L}$ equals the transmittance (T) of the solute. If the energy leaving the solute is the same as the energy entering the solute, then $\dfrac{Lo}{L} = 1$ and, $1 \times 100 = 100\%$ transmittance, and the solution does not contain any of the material for which it is being tested. Optical density and % transmittance are related logarithmically to each other:

$$O.D. = -\log T$$

When plotting a curve using optical density, regular graph paper is used. In plotting percent transmittance, semilog paper is employed. If solutions of varying concentrations are used, a straight line curve will be obtained if the test follows Beer's law. Not all solutions, however, follow Beer's law, in which case a curved line results.

DETERMINATION OF THE WAVELENGTH

To determine the optimal wavelength to be used for a specific test, an absorbance curve, reading optical density, should be plotted against the wavelength, as shown in Figure 28. Using a single concentration of the solution and the appropriate blank, take optical density readings at a series of different wavelengths. Plot the results on graph paper. Where the absorbance is at a

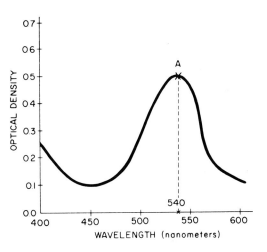

Fig. 28. Determination of wavelength.

maximum (point A), there should be maximum sensitivity, and this will, therefore, be the wavelength chosen for this test (540 nm). Care should be taken that (1) the solution follows Beer's law in the wavelength chosen, (2) the sensitivity is not so great as to give too many readings at the extreme ends of the scale (for the greatest accuracy, readings should be taken between 20% transmittance and 90% transmittance), and (3) interfering substances are not picked up at this wavelength.

PREPARATION OF A CURVE

To construct a curve for a specific test, various known concentrations of the substance must be used. A graph is made, plotting the concentration of the substance (on the X axis, or abscissa) against the optical density or % transmittance readings (on the Y axis, or ordinate). All unknown readings from this curve should then fall in between the highest and lowest standards used in setting up the curve. The graph should be checked daily, using known controls. When new reagents or new bulbs are used, a new curve should be made up. Graphs and tables supplied with a new instrument by the manufacturer should not be used, for the obvious reason that reagents and conditions in your laboratory are not the same as those found in the manufacturer's laboratory.

Discussion

1. Reagent blanks should generally be used with all tests and must contain all the reagents used in the unknown, with the exception of the unknown specimen.
2. Care must be taken to ensure that the cuvets used are not scratched. It is advisable to use the same cuvet for each sample. Rinsing the cuvet between samples is unnecessary if drainage is efficient, except in cases where the unknown is much more diluted or concentrated than the previous sample. In this instance, rinse the cuvet with a small amount of the mixture to be read next.
3. The cuvet should be placed in the spectrophotometer facing in exactly the same direction for each reading. If the cuvet is turned around slightly, there may be a significant difference in the reading.
4. Spectrophotometers must be allowed to warm up when they are first turned on. See the manufacturer's directions for the amount of time required.
5. Any turbidity present in the sample will cause erroneous results to be obtained unless the procedure used is measuring only for turbidity.
6. When taking readings on more than

one sample, it may be necessary to reset the reagent blank in between unknowns. This will depend on the stability of the instrument. It may be possible to read numerous samples without resetting the reagent blank.

CENTRIFUGATION

A centrifuge is used to sediment particles suspended in a liquid and separate different densities of a mixture. A wide variety of centrifuges may be used in the hematology and coagulation laboratory, from small table top models to larger floor-type centrifuges. Refrigerated centrifuges are also available for use in the special coagulation laboratory.

Most centrifuges are capable of using two different types of centrifuge heads:

1. The specimen cups in the *horizontal centrifuge heads* are in a vertical position when the centrifuge is at rest. During centrifugation, the cups are in a horizontal position. These centrifuge heads are capable of speeds up to about 3000 revolutions per minute (RPM). Higher speeds than this will generally cause excessive heat buildup developed by air friction. Using this head, as the specimen is centrifuged, the particles being sedimented, travel down through the liquid to the bottom of the tube. When the centrifuge stops and the tubes swing to a vertical position there may be some remixing of the sediment with the supernatant liquid.
2. *Angle centrifuge heads* are capable of higher speeds and contain drilled holes which hold the tubes at a fixed angle (at about a 52° angle with the center shaft around which they rotate). There is much less heat developed during centrifugation due to very low friction with the air. During centrifugation, the particles travel across the column of liquid to the side of the tube where they clump

together and then rapidly move to the bottom of the tube.

Centrifuges generally contain an *on/off switch* for turning the electrical power on and off, a *timer* which automatically turns the centrifuge off after a preset time, and a *tachometer* or *dial* for setting the speed (RMP) of the centrifuge (a few centrifuges will not contain this dial and can only be used at maximum speed). A *braking device* for rapidly stopping (de-acceleration) the centrifuge may also be present.

Specimens must be centrifuged for a specific time and at a certain speed depending upon the type and purpose of the specimen. This information should be included in all laboratory procedures, and may be critical for accurate test results. The speed of a centrifuge is termed the *relative centrifugal force (RCF)* and is expressed as the number x gravity (or, the number x g, or, the number g). The RCF is calculated from the RPM (revolutions/minute), the radius (distance, in centimeters, from the center shaft to the middle of the centrifuge tube), and the constant, 1.118×10^{-5}, according to the following formula:

$$RCF = 1.118 \times 10^{-5} \times r \times N^2$$
Where: r = radius   N = RPM

Most centrifuge instruction manuals will contain what is termed a nomogram, which is a chart for automatically determining the RCF when the radius and RPM are known. In coagulation, specimens should be centrifuged for 10 to 15 minutes at 150 to 200 g in order to obtain platelet rich plasma and at 1200 to 1500 g for 15 minutes to obtain platelet poor plasma.

It is important, when centrifuging, that the weights of the tubes and carriers be exactly balanced. Similar carriers should be placed opposite one another and the specimen tubes placed across from another should be of equal weight. Alternatively, the carriers and tubes may also be placed in the centrifuge in a geometrically symmetrical arrangement. Use water filled tubes for balancing when necessary.

Centrifuges should have maintenance performed on a regular schedule: the timer should be checked for accuracy and the RPM should be measured. A strobe light or a mechanical or elecronic tachometer (available from most laboratory distributors) should be used to check the routinely used speeds on the centrifuge. The temperature of refrigerated centrifuges should also be closely monitored.

STATISTICAL TOOLS IN THE EVALUATION OF LABORATORY RESULTS

In hematology, as in other departments of the laboratory, statistical tools are used to identify and define the normal values for a test, and to validate test results.

REPRODUCIBILITY VS. ACCURACY

Regardless of how good a technologist's technique is, there is a certain amount of error in all tests. This is unavoidable. An *accurate* method is one which gives values, or results, which agree closely with the known value. On the other hand, a *reproducible* method is one which gives closely similar results when multiple tests are made on the same specimen. All laboratory procedures should be both accurate and reproducible.

Determination of Normal Values

The purpose of laboratory testing is to determine whether a patient's blood contains a normal, low, or elevated amount of the substance for which it is being tested. To determine this, a normal range must be determined for each procedure so that the abnormal patient may be identified. The normal range for a test depends on several factors. Two such factors are (1) the method used by a particular laboratory and (2) the geographic location of the patients being tested.

For most laboratory procedures there are several different methods. Each of these methods may have different sensitivities. That is, method #1 may be only sensitive enough to react with 90% of the substance being tested for, whereas method #2 can pick up 99% of the substance but also reacts with 5% of interfering substances present in the specimen. Therefore, a specific normal range must be determined for each method of a laboratory procedure.

Certain components in the blood vary in different geographic locations. For example, a healthy person living in mountainous regions normally has a higher hemoglobin level than a person living in lower altitudes. (There is a decreased oxygen concentration at high altitudes. To compensate for this, the blood must contain more red blood cells so that the tissues continue to receive the proper amount of oxygen.) In such a case, a normal range must be determined for this particular locale.

METHOD FOR DETERMINING NORMAL VALUES

1. Select a large number (50 to 100) of normal, healthy individuals.
2. Determine and record the test value for each individual.
3. Construct a graph, placing the number of subjects on the abscissa (vertical axis) and the test values received for the subjects on the ordinate (horizontal axis).
4. Plot the test values on the graph. A normal frequency distribution curve is shown in Figure 29.
5. Point A, or the central point, is the mean or average value for this series of tests and is contained within the *mode* (the most frequently occurring value in a frequency distribution). The curve is now described in terms of distances from the mean, using standard deviation as the unit to measure this distance. The central area of this curve from −1 standard deviation to +1 standard deviation contains 68% of the values received. Within ±2 standard deviations, 95% of the values are found, and 99.7% of the test values are contained within ±3 standard deviations. There will be 0.3% of the values outside of ±3 standard deviations. The normal range for the particular test will be those values which fall within ±2 standard deviations of the mean and

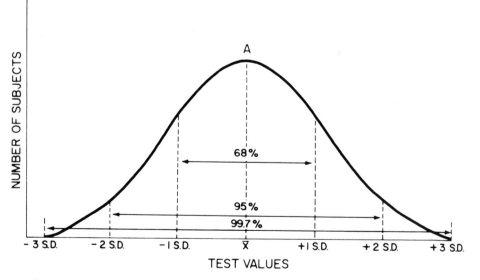

Fig. 29. Gaussian curve (normal frequency distribution curve).

will contain 95% of the normal population. An individual's test value which falls outside of the ± 3 standard deviation limit is said to be abnormal. If the test value falls between the second and third standard deviation limit, this may or may not be considered abnormal. The frequency distribution is termed the *gaussian curve* (Fig. 29). (Note: If the population being tested does not show a normal frequency distribution, the resulting curve will be skewed and not gaussian in character. In this instance, the standard deviation is not applicable because it is valid only when the freqeuncy distribution curve is normal.)

Validation of Test Results

Standard deviation is also used to determine the validity of test results. For example, if certain reagents are contaminated, if the equipment used is not working well, or if the technologist performing the test has made an error in the procedure, inaccuracies will appear in the results. Calculation of the standard deviation is based on the test results received from known control plasma, serum, or whole blood. The specimens must be from the same pool, if pooled blood is used, or from the same lot number, if a commercial control is employed.

Procedure for Determining the Standard Deviation

1. Perform the test on the control specimen each day for a minimum of 30 days (or, perform the test several times a day until 25 to 30 control values have been obtained). Determination of the standard deviation for hemoglobin will be used as an example. (See Table 1 for the calculations used in this procedure.)
2. Calculate the average, or mean ($\overline{X}$), by determining the sum of all the test

TABLE 1. HEMOGLOBIN CONTROL VALUES FOR SEPTEMBER (AND DETERMINATION OF THE STANDARD DEVIATION)

DATE	HGB IN G/DL	$(\overline{X} - X)$	$(\overline{X} - X)^2$
9/1	13.8	0.2	0.04
9/2	13.9	0.1	0.01
9/3	14.1	0.1	0.01
9/4	14.1	0.1	0.01
9/5	13.6	0.4	0.16
9/6	14.0	0.0	0.00
9/7	14.2	0.2	0.04
9/8	14.0	0.0	0.00
9/9	13.9	0.1	0.01
9/10	13.9	0.1	0.01
9/11	14.2	0.2	0.04
9/12	13.9	0.1	0.01
9/13	14.0	0.0	0.00
9/14	14.1	0.1	0.01
9/15	14.0	0.0	0.00
9/16	13.8	0.2	0.04
9/17	14.1	0.1	0.01
9/18	14.0	0.0	0.00
9/19	14.0	0.0	0.00
9/20	13.9	0.1	0.01
9/21	14.0	0.0	0.00
9/22	13.8	0.2	0.04
9/23	14.0	0.0	0.00
9/24	14.0	0.0	0.00
9/25	14.1	0.1	0.01
9/26	13.9	0.1	0.01
9/27	14.2	0.2	0.04
9/28	13.8	0.2	0.04
9/29	14.2	0.2	0.04
9/30	14.1	0.1	0.01
	420.0		0.60

results (Σ), and dividing by the number of tests run (N).

$$\overline{X} = \frac{\Sigma}{N}$$

$$\overline{X} = \frac{420 \text{ g/dl}}{30}$$

$$\overline{X} = 14.0 \text{ g/dL}$$

3. Determine the difference from the mean for each of the control results $(\overline{X} - X)$ and then square this difference $(\overline{X} - X)^2$. (The individual control result is represented by X.)
4. Add the squared differences and divide by one less than the number of test results (N − 1). (Σ = the sum of.)

$$\frac{\Sigma\ (\overline{X} - X)^2}{N - 1} = \frac{0.60}{29} = 0.0206896 \text{ or } 0.0207$$

5. Determine the standard deviation (S.D.) by calculating the square root of the preceding result. (For a review of square root calculation, see the end of this chapter.)

$$\text{S.D.} = \sqrt{0.0207} = 0.1438 \text{ or } 0.14 \text{ g/dL}$$

That is, 1 S.D. = 0.14 g/dL

$$2 \text{ S.D.} = 2 \times 0.14 \text{ g/dL}$$
$$= 0.28 \text{ g/dL}$$
$$3 \text{ S.D.} = 3 \times 0.14 \text{ g/dL}$$
$$= 0.42 \text{ g/dL}$$

The formula for standard deviation is:

$$\text{S.D.} = \sqrt{\frac{\Sigma\ (\overline{X} - X)^2}{N - 1}}$$

COEFFICIENT OF VARIATION (C.V.)

The coefficient of variation is the standard deviation expressed as a percent of the mean (average). Using the previous figures from the hemoglobin calculations, the percent of variation of one standard deviation from the mean (C.V.) would be:

$$\text{C.V.} = \frac{\text{S.D.}}{\overline{X}} \times 100$$

$$\text{C.V.} = \frac{0.14}{14.0} \times 100 = 1.0\%$$

One standard deviation is then regarded as being 1% of the mean value.

DISCUSSION

1. Standard deviation, as it refers to frequency distribution, should not be confused with standard deviation as it relates to error in measurement. The standard deviation of a frequency distribution curve is calculated from single test values made on different individuals. The standard deviation used to indicate errors in measurement is calculated from multiple test values made on the same sample or specimen. Mathematically, however, standard deviation, as it refers to frequency distribution, is calculated in the same way as the standard deviation that relates to errors in measurement.

2. Of the values determining the standard deviation (in error of measurement), 68% should fall within ± 1 S.D., 95% within ± 2 S.D., and 99% of the values should lie within ± 3 S.D.

Quality Control Charts

STANDARD DEVIATION

A control blood or serum should be run each time a test is performed on patient specimens. A quality control chart is prepared for each procedure, and the control results are plotted daily. The values for these controls should fall within ± 2 S.D. from the mean. For example, using the previous figures for a hemoglobin control, the control value received each day should be 14.0 g/dL, ± 0.28 g/dL. The test, therefore, has an acceptable range of 13.7 g/dL to 14.3 g/dL (Fig. 30). When interpreting this graph, attention must be given to several details: (1) As stated previously, 68% of the control values obtained will fall within ± 1 S.D., 95% within ± 2 S.D., and the remaining 5% outside the S.D. limit. Therefore, one might expect to receive a control value outside the 2 S.D. limit 5% of the time or on 1 of every 20 samples. Since this occurs by chance, it must be interpreted along with the preceding values. If the control is repeated at this time, the value should then fall within ± 2 S.D. If it does not, the chances are that the test is out of control. (2) If the control value consistently falls above (below, or on) the median for 5 or 6 successive days, an out of control situation is most likely present, and investigative work should be performed to determine the cause, even though these values fall within ± 2 S.D.

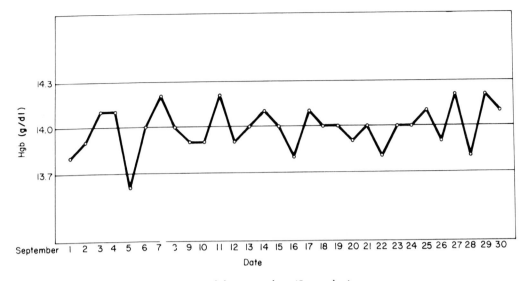

Fig. 30. Quality control graph for hemoglobin procedure (September).

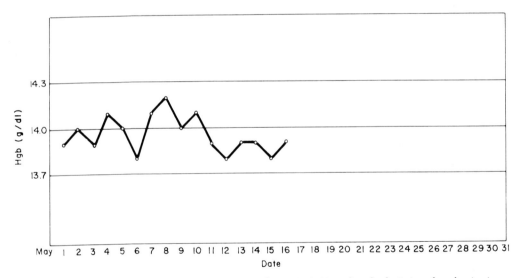

Fig. 31. Quality control graph for hemoglobin procedure (May). Note that the last six values beginning on May 11 are all below the mean. By May 15 there should be concern about these values and investigation made as to their cause.

(Fig. 31). (3) There should be an equal scattering of values above and below the mean (Fig. 32, June 1 through 12).

Several possible sources of error and/or reasons why control values fall outside of the allowable ±2 S.D. limit: dirty or contaminated glassware, technical error, improper calibration of equipment, use of the wrong or deteriorated reagents or controls, or improperly working equipment.

TWIN PLOT CHART

When two control samples (normal and abnormal) are run, the twin plot graph of Youden, modified by D.B. Tonks, may be utilized. This same graph may also be employed using two control values by the same method or one control value from each of 2 separate methods.

The graph is prepared by drawing on the vertical axis the mean +2 S.D. and the

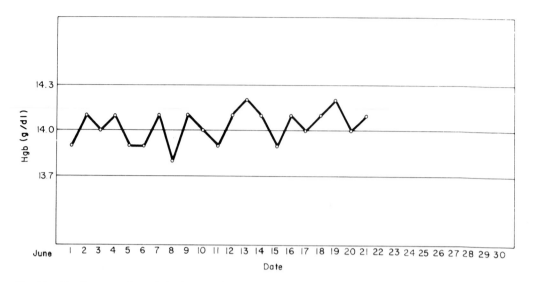

Fig. 32. Quality control graph for hemoglobin procedure (June). Beginning on June 12 there appears to be an upward trend in the control values. Even though five or six successive plots are not above the mean, the cause for this shift should be found.

mean − 2 S.D. limits for the abnormal control, or control #2. On the horizontal axis, mark off the mean + 2 S.D. and the mean − 2 S.D. limits for the normal control or control #1. Draw a square field in the middle of the graph connecting the 2 S.D. limits (Fig. 33). The cross in the middle of the square denotes the mean for both control samples. The line drawn connecting the bottom left corner with the top right corner denotes the line of normal distribution. Each day the control value is plotted with regard to both control results. As an example, the following results were obtained on the dates indicated and plotted as shown (Fig. 34).

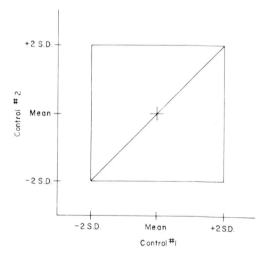

Fig. 33. Twin-plot graph.

When interpreting this graph, several details should be noted: (1) Under normal conditions, when the test procedure is in control, the plotted control values should fall along the diagonal line of normal distribution, as seen in Figure 34 for July 1 through July 7. (2) If one of the controls is high and the other control is low, something is probably wrong. Both control samples were not affected in the same manner in the procedure, and patient values may

Date	Normal Hgb Control (g/dL)	Abnl Hgb Control (g/dL)
July 1	14.0	7.9
2	13.8	7.9
3	14.1	8.1
4	14.3	8.2
5	13.9	8.0
6	14.0	8.0
7	14.1	8.1
8	14.3	7.8
9	14.2	8.1
10	14.4	8.3
11	14.0	8.1
12	14.2	8.2
13	14.1	8.1
14	14.3	8.2

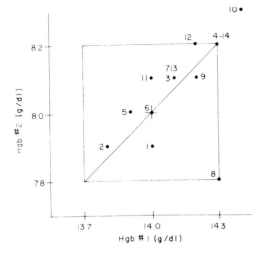

Fig. 34. Twin-plot chart for normal and abnormal hemoglobin results (July).

be erratic. This condition shows up in the chart by the appearance of the plotted point in the lower right or upper left corner of the square, as shown in Figure 34 for July 8. (3) The plotted values should fall along the diagonal line from the lower left corner to the top right corner. An uneven distribution in one of the two corners indicates an upward or downward shift, and, therefore, an out of control situation. Note that beginning with July 9, all values are in the upper right corner, indicating an upward trend (Fig. 34). (4) If, at any time, both control values fall outside the ± 2 S.D. limit, something is wrong with the procedure and the cause for these results should be found. In Figure 34, the control values for July 10 were both outside of normal limits.

THE CUMULATIVE SUM (CUSUM) GRAPH

The CUSUM graph is a third method for charting control results. In this method, after the mean for the control is determined, this result is subtracted from each control result as it is obtained. The resulting value is added to the total of the previous days to give a cumulative difference from the mean. Each day the control is run, the cumulative difference is plotted on the graph.

The CUSUM graph consists of a single line representing the mean. Negative cumulative differences are plotted below the mean line and positive differences are plotted above the line (Fig. 35). As an example, the following hemoglobin control results were obtained in the month of August, at which time the mean hemoglobin was 14.0 g/dL.

Date		Hgb Result g/dL	Difference from Mean	Cumulative Difference
Aug.	1	13.8	−0.2	−0.2
	2	14.1	+0.1	−0.1
	3	13.9	−0.1	−0.2
	4	14.2	+0.2	0.0
	5	14.2	+0.2	+0.2
	6	13.9	−0.1	+0.1
	7	13.8	−0.2	−0.1
	8	14.2	+0.2	+0.1
	9	13.8	−0.2	−0.1
	10	14.1	+0.1	0.0
	11	14.2	+0.2	+0.2
	12	13.8	−0.2	0.0
	13	13.9	−0.1	−0.1
	14	13.9	−0.1	−0.2
	15	14.0	0.0	−0.2
	16	13.9	−0.1	−0.3
	17	14.0	0.0	−0.3
	18	13.9	−0.1	−0.4
	19	14.1	+0.1	−0.3
	20	13.9	−0.1	−0.4
	21	14.0	0.0	−0.4

When the test procedure is in control, the plotted graph should show a line moving back and forth close to and above and below the 0 line (Fig. 35, Aug. 1 through Aug. 12). If the graph begins to show a trend upward or downward, this indicates a trend toward high or low control results, respectively. Beginning on Aug. 12, there is a downward trend of the control. Any time five or six successive plots go down or up on this graph, it is an indication that the test is out of control.

Calculation of Square Root

To determine the square root of 691.503:
1. Separate the numbers into pairs beginning at the decimal point and working to the left

$$\sqrt{691.5030}$$

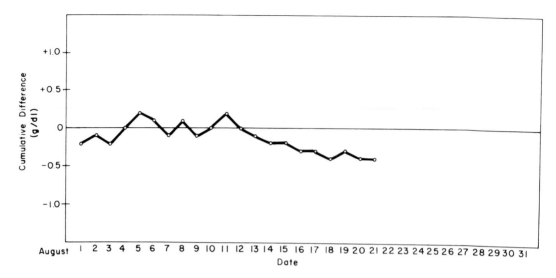

Fig. 35.   Cumulative difference graph for hemoglobin (August).

and/or right. (The answer will contain one number for each of the paired numbers.) If the number on the far left has only one number, as shown (the 6), use this number by itself. When there is a single number to the far right, add a 0. Place the decimal point directly above the one under the square root sign.

2. Using the first number or pair of numbers on the far left, find the largest perfect square number which is smaller than this number and place it above

$$\sqrt{691.5030}\ \ \overset{2\quad .}{\phantom{\sqrt{691.5030}}}$$

the number, as shown.

3. Square this number (2) and place it beneath the 6. Subtract and bring down the next pair of numbers.

$$\begin{array}{r}2\\ \sqrt{691.5030}\\ 4\\ \hline 291\end{array}$$

4. Double the partial answer above the square root sign and place it on the left.

$$\begin{array}{r}2\\ \sqrt{691.5030}\\ 4\\ \hline 4\quad 291\end{array}$$

5. Select a number which, when placed on the right of the 4, will give the closest result to 291 (must be less than 291) when this number (46) is multiplied by the number selected (6). Place this number above the square

$$\begin{array}{r}2\ 6.\\ \sqrt{691.5030}\\ 4\\ \hline 46\ \ 276\\ \hline\end{array}$$

root sign over the number 91.

6. Subtract this number from the number above and bring down the next pair of numbers.

```
    2 6.
√ 691.5030
  4
  291
46 276
   15 50
```

7. Double the partial answer, as in step 4, and bring it down to the left.

```
     2 6.
√ 691.5030
  4
  291
46 276
   15 50
52
```

8. Select a number which, when placed on the right of 52, will give the closest result to 1550 when this number (522) is multiplied by the number selected (2).

```
     2 6. 2
√ 691.5030
  4
  291
46 276
   15 50
522  10 44
      5 0630
```

9. Double the partial answer, as in step 4, and bring it down to the left. Select a number which, when placed on the right of 524, will give the closest result to 50630

```
      2 6. 2 9
√ 691.5030
  4
  291
46 276
   15 50
522  10 44
      5 0630
5249  4 7241
      3389
```

when this number (5249) is multiplied by the number selected (9).

10. This procedure may be continued to a third or fourth decimal place by adding one pair of zeros for each decimal place desired when the answer does not come out to an even number. In such cases, calculations should be carried out to one more decimal place than is needed. The number is rounded off to the desired decimal point.

```
      2 6. 2 9
√ 691.503000
  4
  291
46 276
   15 50
522  10 44
      5 0630
5249  4 7241
        338900
```

If it is necessary to find the square root to one decimal point, the result received (26.29) would be rounded off to 26.3. The number of significant decimal places used in laboratory calculations depends on the procedure involved. Calculations rarely have to be carried out beyond two decimal places.

2

Hematopoiesis

There are three types of cellular elements present in the blood: red blood cells (erythrocytes), white blood cells (leukocytes), and platelets (thrombocytes) (Fig. 36). (The platelet is not considered to be a true cell in that it does not contain a nucleus.) Each of these cells has its own function, differs morphologically from the others, and has a life span characteristic for that particular cell type. In health, the destruction and production of cells is balanced, and, therefore, the number of cells present in the blood at any particular time is relatively constant. *Hematopoiesis* is a term used to signify the production of blood cells.

In the same way that a person goes through various stages until he becomes an adult, the blood cells must also go through certain stages before they mature and are able to carry out their intended functions. In a healthy person, only the mature adult cells are found in the blood, whereas in many diseases, the immature and abnormal forms of the cells may be present. For this reason, it is imperative

that the student of medical technology be able to identify the immature and abnormal cell forms.

In the fetus, hematopoiesis takes place at various intervals in the liver, spleen, thymus, bone marrow, and lymph nodes (Fig. 37). Within 2 weeks of embryonic life, primitive red blood cells are produced. By the second month, granulocytes and megakaryocytes begin to appear. Lymphocyte production starts at approximately the fourth month, and monocytes are produced by the fifth month.

At birth, and continuing into adulthood, major blood cell production is confined to the bone marrow. In the child, hematopoietic bone marrow (red marrow) is located in the flat bones of the skull, clavicle, sternum, ribs, vertebrae, and pelvis and also in the long bones of the arms and legs. By 18 years of age and for the remainder of the adult life, the red marrow is normally confined to the flat bones only (skull, clavicle, sternum, ribs, vertebrae, pelvis, and the proximal ends of the long bones [femur and humerus]). The remain-

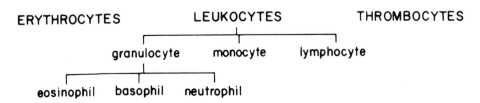

ERYTHROCYTES   LEUKOCYTES   THROMBOCYTES

granulocyte   monocyte   lymphocyte

eosinophil   basophil   neutrophil

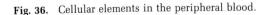

Fig. 36. Cellular elements in the peripheral blood.

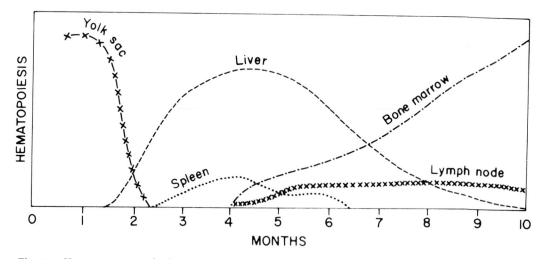

Fig. 37. Hematopoiesis in the fetus. (Modified from Wintrobe, M.M: *Clinical Hematology,* 8th Ed., Lea & Febiger, Philadelphia, 1981.)

ing marrow space is occupied by fat cells which can be replaced by hematopoietic cells under certain situations of intensive stimulation.

ORIGIN AND INTERRELATIONSHIP OF BLOOD CELLS

One of the more perplexing and controversial problems in hematology has concerned the origin of the blood cells and their relationship to one another. Today, as shown in Figure 38, it is believed that an uncommitted pluripotential (or multipotential) stem cell gives rise to: (1) the lymphoid stem cell, and, (2) the myeloid or hematopoietic stem cell. (Stem cells have the ability to reproduce themselves and to differentiate. They are not morphologically identifiable and are thought to look very similar to the small or intermediate sized lymphocyte.) The hematopoietic stem cell is thought to be the common precursor for red cells, granulocytes, monocytes, and megakaryocytes (platelets) and gives rise to the committed stem cells through stimulation by various environmental factors within the body.

Existence of the stem cells has been shown by various culture techniques. The uncommitted stem cell has been given the designation CFU-S (colony forming unit-

spleen), while those stem cells committed to forming blood cells are termed CFU-C (colony forming unit-culture) and require CSF (colony stimulating factor).

The relationship of the lymphocyte to the CFU-S has not been firmly established. The CFU-S gives rise to the CFU-C but may not directly give rise to the lymphocyte. The lymphocyte precursor (CFU-L) and CFU-S may have a more primitive stem cell in common which may give rise to both the CFU-S and the lymphocyte.

The primitive red blood cells have been termed burst forming units—erythroid (BFU-E), which, in turn, give rise to colony forming units—erythroid (CFU-E) as a response to erythropoietin. The primitive eosinophils (colony forming unit—eosinophil [CFU-Eo]) give rise to eosinophils in response to a substance (Eo-CSF) produced by stimulated lymphocytes. CFU-M is the primitive megakaryocytic line which gives rise to the megakaryocyte and ultimately the platelets, in response to Mg-CSF and thrombopoietin. CFU-G,M give rise to the monocytes and neutrophils. Colony forming units for basophils probably also exist. Due to their limited number little research has been done in this area.

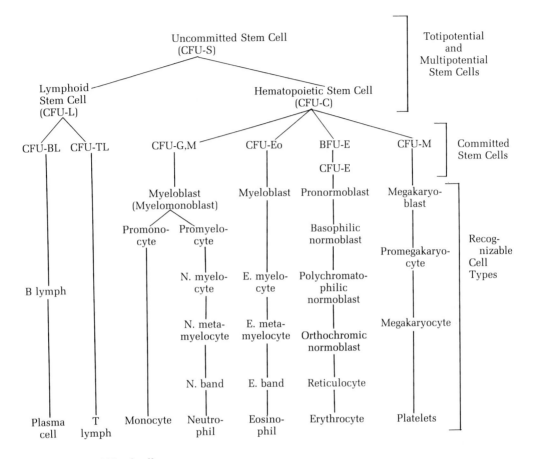

Fig. 38.   Origin of blood cells.

CELL STRUCTURE

As an aid in the proper identification of cells, it is important to know their basic structure and composition. One should also have a basic understanding of the function of these cellular components.

The *plasma membrane* surrounds the outer limits of the cell and is composed of three distinct layers: a middle lipid layer located between two layers of protein (Fig. 39). The "head" of the phospholipid molecules (adjacent to each protein layer) is the water-soluble portion and is positively charged. The inner ends of the lipids, or "feet," repel water (are water insoluble). Also present in the cell membrane are small pores through which substances may pass.

The *cytoplasm* of the cell is contained within the plasma membrane and is composed of a variety of organelles (Fig. 40). Among these organelles are the *mitochondria*, which are rod-shaped structures. Their membrane wall is composed of two layers. The inner layer juts out into the cavity and forms projections within the structure. The mitochondria supply a

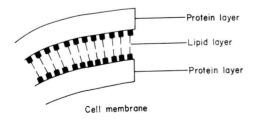

Protein layer

Lipid layer

Protein layer

Cell membrane

Fig. 39.   Hypothetical diagram of a portion of a cell membrane.

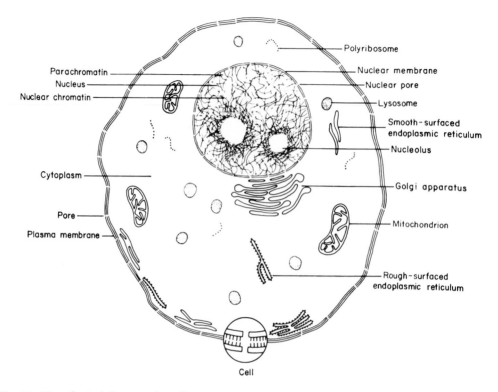

Fig. 40. Hypothetical diagram of a cell.

large portion of the cell's respiration and energy requirements. These structures do not stain with Wright's stain.

The *Golgi apparatus* is located in the cytoplasm of the cell near the nucleus. It is here that the cytoplasmic granules of the monocyte and granulocyte are formed. From studies performed on rabbits, it was found that azurophilic granule formation takes place on the inner Golgi membranes (closest to the nucleus). These granules contain enzymes and are also termed lysosomes. The specific granules are formed on the outer membranes (near the cytoplasm) of the Golgi apparatus. The enzymes formed within the Golgi membranes become concentrated at the ends and ultimately pinch off from the membrane and form granules. These granules then move off and scatter throughout the cytoplasm.

The *endoplasmic reticulum* is composed of tubules contained within a membrane. One system of tubules is termed *rough-surfaced endoplasmic reticulum* and possesses *ribosomes* adhering to the membrane. The *smooth-surfaced endoplasmic reticulum* contains none of these ribosome granules. The ribosomes contain ribonucleic acid (RNA) and are active in protein synthesis. There are also small groups of RNA molecules in the cytoplasm which form *polyribosomes.* The RNA present in the cytoplasm stains blue with Wright's stain.

The *nucleus* of the cell consists primarily of deoxyribonucleic acid (DNA). This chromosomal material stains a dark purple color with Wright's stain and is called the *nuclear chromatin.* Light or unstained areas within the nucleus are termed the *parachromatin.* Located within the nucleus (of generally immature cells) is the *nucleolus.* (There may be more than one nucleolus present in a nucleus.) The nucleolus stains a bluish color with Wright's stain and is composed of RNA. There is a double nuclear membrane separating the nucleus from the cytoplasm. This membrane contains small holes, or pores, through which the RNA of the nucleolus is thought to carry messages from the DNA template to the cytoplasm.

NORMAL CELL MATURATION

Blood cells go through several stages of development. On the following pages the maturation of the cells is described and illustrated. Progression from one stage to the next is not abrupt. It is important to keep this fact in mind because many times the cell being studied may be in between the two stages described here. (When this occurs, the cell is generally given the name of the more mature stage.) As a cell is transformed from the primitive blast stage to the mature form found in the blood, there are changes in the cytoplasm, nucleus, and cell size. Normally, all three of these changes occur gradually and at the same time. In some disease states, these changes may take place at different rates. For example, the cytoplasm may mature more quickly than the nucleus. This occurrence is termed *asynchronism.* For convenience, these cellular changes are described individually.

Cytoplasmic Maturation

The immature cytoplasm generally stains a deep blue color (basophilic) because of the high content of RNA present. As the cell matures, there is a gradual loss of cytoplasmic RNA and, therefore, a lessening of the blue color. In certain of the cells (for example, the myeloid cells), granules appear in the cytoplasm as the cell matures. At first, these granules are few and relatively nonspecific. As the cell matures further, these granules increase in number and take on specific characteristics and functions. The amount of cytoplasm in relationship to the rest of the cell usually increases as the cell matures.

Nuclear Maturation

The nucleus of the immature cell is round or oval and is large in proportion to the rest of the cell. As the cell matures, the nucleus decreases in relative size and may or may not take on various shapes (depending on the cell type). The nuclear chromatin transforms from a fine, delicate pattern to become more coarse and clumped in the mature form, and the staining properties change from a reddish purple to a bluish purple. Nucleoli present in early stages of cell development usually disappear gradually as the cell ages.

Cell Size

As a cell matures, it usually becomes smaller in size. (For the new student, this change may be difficult to detect. The normal mature red blood cells or small lymphocytes are generally of relatively constant size and may be used as a guide for comparison.) The student should know the relative size of each cell type.

Identification of Cells

In identifying a cell, the technologist should think in the following terms:
1. What is the size of the cell?
   a. Small.
   b. Medium.
   c. Large.
2. What are the characteristics of the nucleus?
   a. Shape.
   b. Relative size.
   c. Chromatin pattern: smooth or coarse.
   d. Presence of nucleoli.
3. What are the characteristics of the cytoplasm?
   a. Granular or nongranular; specific or nonspecific granules.
   b. Color (staining properties).
   c. Relative amount.

When attempting to identify a cell, it is important to note the degree to which the cells take up the stain. For example, if all cells seem bluer than normal, the staining technique may be poor, and cell identification must be made accordingly.

Unless otherwise stated, all cells in this text are described as they appear in Wright-stained smears.

RED BLOOD CELLS

The red blood cells are produced in the bone marrow.

Pronormoblast (Rubriblast) (Fig. 41).

Size: 14 to 20 μm in diameter.

Cytoplasm: Deeply basophilic.
Relatively small amount, appearing as a band around the nucleus.
May show a lighter staining area around the nucleus (perinuclear halo).
Non-granular.

Nucleus: Relatively large.
Round or slightly oval.
Reddish purple in color.
Fine chromatin pattern.
Usually 1 to 2 nucleoli.
Nucleoli are larger than those found in the myeloblast and may stain with a slightly bluish tint.

Basophilic Normoblast (Prorubricyte) (Fig. 42).

Size: 12 to 17 μm in diameter.

Cytoplasm: Intensely basophilic.
At times there is only a small increase in the relative amount of cytoplasm from the previous stage (pronormoblast).
Non-granular.

Nucleus: Relatively large.
Round or slightly oval.
Chromatin pattern is slightly coarser than in the previous stage.
Nucleoli are usually not visible if present.

Polychromatophilic Normoblast (Rubricyte) (Fig. 43).

Size: 10 to 15 μm in diameter.

Cytoplasm: Blue-gray to pink-gray (shows a large range in color) due

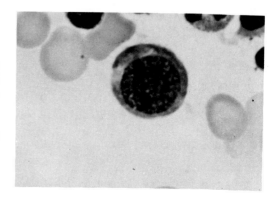

Fig. 42.   Basophilic normoblast (center).

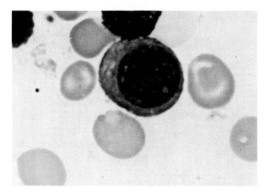

Fig. 41.   Pronormoblast (center).

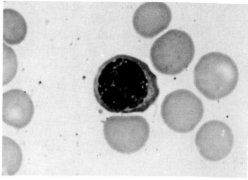

Fig. 43.   Polychromatophilic normoblast.

to the start of hemoglobin production in the cell.

A slight increase in relative amount.

Non-granular.

Nucleus: Round.

Smaller than previous stage.

More condensed. The chromatin pattern is coarse and clumped. Stains a deeper blue-purple.

Orthochromic Normoblast (Metarubricyte) (Fig. 44).

Size: 7 to 12 μm in diameter.

Cytoplasm: Pinker than previous stage. Increased in amount compared to previous stage. Non-granular.

Nucleus: Pyknotic nucleus (a homogeneous blue-black mass with no structure). This is a primary difference between the rubricyte and the metarubricyte.

Reticulocyte

Size: 7 to 10 μm in diameter. (Approximately the same size or slightly larger than the mature red blood cell.)

Cytoplasm: Pink to a slight pinkish gray.

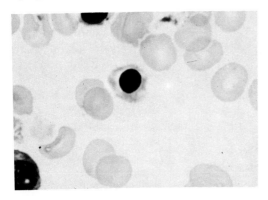

Fig. 44. Orthochromic normoblast (small cell in center).

Contains a fine basophilic reticulum of RNA, which only stains with supravital stain (see the section entitled Reticulocyte Count in Chapter 3).

Nucleus: None present.

Mature Red Blood Cell

Size: 6 to 8 μm in diameter.

Cytoplasm: Pink in color.

The mature red blood cell is a non-nucleated, round, biconcave cell (Fig. 45).

Erythropoiesis

Normally, the rate of production of red blood cells determines the hemoglobin level (or red blood cell count) in the peripheral blood and shows little variation among normal individuals.

During maturation of the erythroid cell, three to four mitotic divisions occur between the pronormoblast and the polychromatophilic normoblast stages. Thus, up to sixteen erythrocytes may be produced from each pronormoblast. It takes approximately 3 days for the pronormoblast to develop into the orthochromic normoblast. When the cell reaches the orthochromic normoblast stage, the nucleus is extremely condensed and the cell is incapable of further mitosis. After approximately 1 more day, the nucleus is extruded and the cell becomes a reticulocyte. The reticulocyte is slightly larger than the normal mature red blood cell and is slightly adhesive (sticky), appearing to be coated with a globulin, part of which may be transferrin. This characteristic may be responsible for keeping it in the bone mar-

Fig. 45.   Cross section of the mature red blood cell.

row for an additional 2 to 3 days before it is released into the peripheral blood as a more mature reticulocyte. The reticulocytes in the peripheral blood are slightly fewer in number than the marrow reticulocytes. The red blood cells of the circulating blood have a life span of approximately 120 days, ± 20 days.

Production of red blood cells (erythropoiesis) is initiated by a hormone, called erythropoietin, which is produced mainly by the kidney and found in the plasma. When a person's hemoglobin level is below normal, the oxygen tension in the kidneys is reduced. This condition stimulates the kidneys to increase their production of erythropoietin, which activates the stem cells of the bone marrow to differerentiate into pronormoblasts. An increased number of red blood cells are then produced. In addition, the rate of mitosis is increased and the maturation process of the red blood cells in the bone marrow is shortened. Hemoglobin is manufactured more quickly, and the reticulocytes are not delayed as long before they are released into the peripheral blood. As a result, the immature reticulocytes prematurely released may appear somewhat larger than the normal circulating red blood cells (generally 20 to 25% larger) and are polychromatophilic (staining gray to blue-gray in color). These cells are frequently termed *shift cells* and may be indicative of increased red blood cell production.

Various substances are required for the production of new red cells and hemoglobin. Iron is required for both the proliferation and maturation of the red blood cell. Folic acid and vitamin B_{12} are necessary for normal DNA replication and cell division. Manganese, cobalt, and vitamins C, E, B_6, thiamine, riboflavin, and pantothenic acid are also needed for normal erythropoiesis, along with the hormones, erythropoietin, thyroxine, and androgens.

Hemoglobin Structure and Synthesis

The primary function of the red blood cell is to carry hemoglobin, which, in turn, transports oxygen to the tissues and carbon dioxide from the tissues to the lungs. The hemoglobin molecule is composed of heme and the protein, globin. The synthesis of heme begins in the mitochondria with the formation of delta-aminolevulinic acid from glycine and succinyl-coenzyme A in the presence of pyridoxal phosphate (vitamin B_6) and delta-aminolevulinic acid synthetase (Fig. 46). The process continues in the cytoplasm of the cell, where two molecules of delta-aminolevulinic acid combine in the presence of delta-aminolevulinic acid dehydrase to form porphobilinogen. Four molecules of porphobilinogen combine to form uro-phyrinogen III in the presence of uroporphyrinogen I synthetase and uroporphyrinogen III cosynthetase. Coproporphyrinogen III is then formed by the action of uroporphyrinogen decarboxylase, which removes four carboxyl groups from the acetic acid side chains. Heme is then produced in the mitochondria, where protoporphyrinogen IX is formed by the action of coproporphyrinogen oxidase. Protoporphyrin IX is formed in the presence of protoporphyrinogen oxidase, and ferrous iron is incorporated into the molecule in the presence of the enzyme ferrochelatase (also termed heme synthetase) to form the heme molecule (Fig. 47). The atom of iron is located in the center of the structure. In the ferrous state (Fe^{++}), it binds oxygen.

Iron is delivered to the red blood cell by a specific transport protein, *transferrin* (also termed *siderophilin*). The transferrin attaches to receptors on the red blood cell membrane. This causes the red cell membrane to invaginate, forming an intracellular vacuole. The iron is then released and the transferrin-receptor complex returns to the cell membrane. The major portion of this iron is utilized in heme synthesis. Upon insertion into the red blood cell, it proceeds to the mitochondria, where it enters the protoporphyrin molecule. Some of the iron not used for heme

Succinyl coenzyme A + Glycine

Pyridoxal phosphate $\quad\Big|\quad$ delta-Aminolevulinic acid synthetase

delta-Aminolevulinic acid

$\Big|$ delta-Aminolevulinic acid dehydrase

Porphobilinogen

$\Big|$ Uroporphyrinogen III cosynthetase

Uroporphyrinogen III

$\Big|$ Uroporphyrinogen decarboxylase

Coproporphyrinogen III

$\Big|$ Coproporphyrinogen oxidase

Protoporphyrinogen IX

$\Big|$ Protoporphyrinogen oxidase

Protoporphyrin IX

Ferrochelatase $\quad\Big|\quad$ Fe^{++}

Heme molecule

Fig. 46. Biosynthesis of heme.

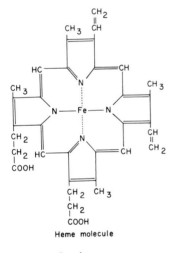

Heme molecule

Fig. 47. Heme molecule.

production may accumulate in the cytoplasm of the red blood cell as ferritin aggregates. (This may be demonstrated by the Prussian blue stain.)

While the heme molecule is being synthesized, the globin portion of hemoglobin is produced on specific ribosomes in the cytoplasm of the red blood cells. The globin portion of each hemoglobin molecule consists of four polypeptide chains which determine the type of hemoglobin formed. (In the normal adult, three hemoglobin types are present: hemoglobins A, F, and A_2, with hemoglobin A having a concentration of approximately 96 to 97%.) The polypeptide chains are composed of amino acids arranged in a specific sequence. Each chain is bent and coiled and forms a three-dimensional structure. The type and number of amino acids and their sequence are dependent on the type of chain being formed and are determined by the DNA molecules in the nucleus of the cell. This information in the nucleus of the cell is transferred to the cytoplasmic ribosomes by messenger RNA. Once the ribosome receives this information, it can function, without further messages from the nucleus, to synthesize the polypeptide chains. Hemoglobin A is composed of four polypeptide chains, two alpha (α) and two beta (β) chains. Hemoglobin F is made up of two α and two gamma (γ) chains, whereas hemoglobin A_2 is composed of two α and two delta (δ) chains. (The amounts of hemoglobin A and F are significant in that they will show increased levels in certain disorders of globin synthesis.)

Using hemoglobin A as an example, when the individual α and β chains are produced, one α and one β chain combine to form a dimer. These dimers are then free in the cytoplasm of the cell, where they combine with the heme molecule and form the tetrad hemoglobin molecule consisting of two α chains, two β chains, and four heme groups. One heme group is attached to each polypeptide chain by a linkage from the iron in the heme group, to a specific amino acid (histidine) in each α and β chain. When globin production is decreased (as is found in certain disorders of impaired synthesis of protoporphyrin III or porphyrin), there is no corresponding decrease in iron uptake by the red blood cell. As a result, the excess iron may accumulate in the cytoplasm of the red blood cell as ferritin aggregates or may build up in the mitochondria and may be seen around the nucleus of the immature red blood cell *(ringed sideroblast)*.

The production of heme and globin begins in the polychromatophilic normoblast stage and ends in the reticulocyte. The reticulocyte is able to synthesize hemoglobin for approximately 2 days after the cell has been lost its nucleus. No hemoglobin synthesis takes place in the mature red blood cell.

Function of Hemoglobin

The red blood cell functions primarily to supply oxygen to the tissues and remove carbon dioxide. It is the hemoglobin molecule within the red blood cell that is responsible for supplying the tissues with oxygen. The normal hemoglobin molecule has an attraction (affinity) for oxygen (which binds to the iron). As soon as one atom of iron binds oxygen, the remaining three atoms of iron more readily bind oxygen. In other words, the affinity of hemo-

globin for oxygen increases as the molecule binds more oxygen. This characteristic has been termed *heme-heme interaction.*

The amount of oxygen which the hemoglobin molecule binds varies in relationship to the amount of oxygen in the blood. For example, when the oxygen tension in arterial blood is high (about 95 mm Hg), the hemoglobin molecule is about 95% saturated with oxygen. In the veins and tissues, the oxygen tension is lower. The hemoglobin molecule picks up and binds oxygen while in the capillary system of the lungs. As this hemoglobin travels through the tissue capillaries, in which the oxygen concentration is decreased, it releases this oxygen to the tissues.

The affinity of hemoglobin for oxygen is represented graphically by the *oxygen dissociation curve* (Fig. 48), in which pO_2 represents the partial pressure of oxygen in the lungs. P_{50} represents hemoglobin's affinity for oxygen and is used to designate the partial pressure of oxygen at which the hemoglobin molecule is 50% saturated with oxygen. (Normally, the partial pressure of oxygen is 26.6 mm Hg when the hemoglobin is half saturated with oxygen.) The normal oxygen dissociation curve is sigmoidal in shape and shows its steepest

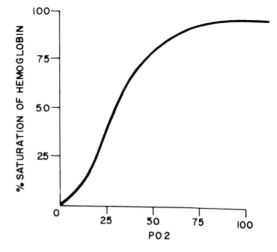

Fig. 48.   Oxygen dissociation curve of hemoglobin.

slope at the pO_2 levels that are generally found in the tissues. In this area of the curve, hemoglobin gives up and binds oxygen with relatively small changes in pO_2. A decreased affinity of the hemoglobin molecule for oxygen shifts this curve to the right, and hemoglobin then gives up oxygen readily. If this curve shifts to the left, hemoglobin has an increased affinity for oxygen, that is, it binds oxygen readily but does not release it to the tissues easily. The P_{50} therefore, increases as the curve shifts to the right and decreases with a shift to the left. The normal position of the oxygen dissociation curve is dependent on carbon dioxide, hydrogen ions, and 2,3 DPG, and on the structure of the hemoglobin molecule.

Hemoglobin's affinity for oxygen is also influenced by the pH. This has been termed the *Bohr effect.* As the pH becomes more acid, hemoglobin's affinity for oxygen decreases. In the tissues, due to the presence of carbon dioxide, the pH is more acid, and hemoglobin is further influenced to release oxygen to the tissues. The organic phosphate 2,3 DPG also affects hemoglobin's affinity for oxygen. When the hemoglobin molecule releases oxygen, the beta chains move apart allowing 2,3 DPG to enter. The 2,3 DPG binds with the deoxygenated hemoglobin, thereby having an inhibitory effect on hemoglobin binding with oxygen. Hemoglobin gives up more oxygen to the tissues with increased concentrations of 2,3 DPG in the blood, and the oxygen dissociation curve is shifted to the right.

The major portion of carbon dioxide is transported from the tissues by the red blood cell. Carbon dioxide reacts with water to form carbonic acid (H_2CO_3). Hydrogen ions, liberated from the H_2CO_3 (leaving $H_2CO_3^-$), are free to combine with deoxygenated hemoglobin, further decreasing the affinity of the hemoglobin molecule for oxygen. (Deoxygenated hemoglobin has more affinity for hydrogen ions because oxygenated hemoglobin

is the stronger acid.) (The enzyme, carbonic anhydrase catalyzes the conversion of carbon dioxide to bicarbonate in the red cell, and then also catalyzes the release of carbon dioxide from the bicarbonate when the red cell is in the capillaries of the lungs.) Some of the carbon dioxide remaining in the tissues combines with the amino acid groups of deoxygenated hemoglobin to form carbaminohemoglobin. Also, a small amount of carbon dioxide is removed from the tissues by the plasma in solution.

Erythrocyte Membrane

The normal, mature red blood cell may be described as a 'biconcave disk'. This distinctive shape allows the red blood cell to have maximum membrane surface area for its size, which facilitates the transfer of gases in and out of the cell. In addition, it enables the red blood cell to easily undergo the changes in shape necessary for its travel through such areas as the microvasculature.

The red blood cell membrane is composed of protein (50%), lipid (40%), and a small amount of carbohydrate (10%) and can be penetrated by most solutes. The membrane is two molecules thick and contains tightly packed phospholipids. The polar surfaces of the phospholipids face the inside and the outside of the cell, with the nonpolar groups at the center of the membrane. The external surface of the membrane is rich in phosphatidylcholine, glycolipid, and sphingomyelin, while the internal surface contains phosphatidylethanolamine, phosphatidylinositol, and phosphatidylserine. The cholesterol content of the membrane depends upon the concentration of the plasma cholesterol, bile acids, and the activity of the enzyme, lecithin:cholesterol acyltransferase.

There are two classes of proteins in the membrane: integral and peripheral (Fig. 49). The integral proteins, primarily glycophorin A and component a, are in contact with both the inner and outer surfaces

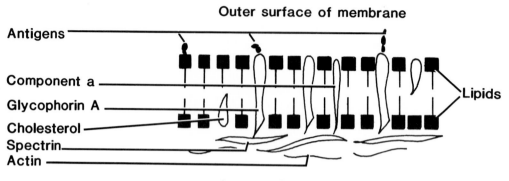

Fig. 49. Diagrammatic illustration of the red blood cell membrane.

of the membrane. Glycophorin A is probably responsible for the negative charge of the red blood cell surface. Spectrin and actin are peripheral proteins which are present on the inner portion of the membrane and probably create the framework for the cell and thus determine the shape of the red blood cell. They are attached to the inner ends of the integral proteins.

The integral membrane proteins carry various antigens on the membrane surface, while some antigens are also attached to the lipid portions of the membrane surface. Over 300 red blood cell antigens have been identified of which most are intrinsic components appearing on the membrane during early development of the red cell.

Changes in the shape of the red blood cell may result from alterations in the plasma lipids. Increases in cholesterol and phospholipid may be one cause of target cells. With increased concentrations of membrane cholesterol, the red cell has ex-

cess membrane which then makes the red cell appear as a target or spiculated red blood cell. Acanthocytes (in patients who lack beta lipoprotein) is a result of abnormalities in the ratios of membrane lecithins and sphingomyelins. An abnormality in the peripheral proteins may be responsible for the shape of the red blood cell in hereditary elliptocytosis and spherocytosis. Cells which lack the Rh antigens are termed Rh null cells, appear as stomatocytes on the peripheral smear, and have a shortened life span.

Metabolism of the Red Blood Cell

The mature red blood cell consists primarily of hemoglobin (about 90% of the dry weight). The membrane is composed of lipids and proteins. In addition, there are numerous enzymes present which are necessary for oxygen transport and cell viability. The red blood cell derives its energy from the breakdown of glucose.

About 90% of the glycolysis in the red blood cell follows the Embden-Meyerhof pathway (Fig. 50). In this way, two moles of adenosine triphosphate (ATP) are generated for every glucose molecule broken down to lactic acid. ATP is used to control the flow of sodium and potassium into and out of the red blood cell, maintain the biconcave shape of the cell, and protect the membrane lipids.

The methemoglobin reductase pathway (Fig. 50) maintains the iron present in the hemoglobin molecule in a functional state (Fe^{++}).

The Rapoport-Leubering pathway allows for the production of 2,3 diphosphoglycerate (2,3 DPG), which affects the affinity of the hemoglobin molecule for oxygen. The 2,3 DPG combines reversibly with the deoxygenated hemoglobin, decreasing the affinity of hemoglobin for oxygen. DNA and RNA present in the early stages of the maturing red blood cell are absent in the mature cell.

The remaining 10% of the glucose molecules follow the hexose monophosphate shunt (pentose phosphate pathway) (Fig. 50), where reduced glutathione is made available to prevent oxidative denaturation of hemoglobin. When the red blood cell is exposed to an oxidant drug, the activity of the pentose phosphate pathway increases in order to maintain the hemoglobin molecule in its reduced state. Decreased activity of an enzyme in this pathway, results in oxidized hemoglobin, which denatures and precipitates as *Heinz bodies*.

Breakdown of the Red Blood Cell

As a red blood cell ages, there is a decrease in its enzymes, a decrease in ATP, a decrease in size, and an increase in density. Approximately 1% of the red blood cells leave the circulation each day and are broken down by the reticuloendothelial system. This may be termed extravascular destruction and most commonly occurs in the spleen. (Severely damaged red cells may be removed by the liver, while some completely damaged red cells will be destroyed as they circulate through the vascular system [intravascular destruction].)

When the red cell has been removed from the circulation, the membrane is disrupted and the hemoglobin is broken down within the macrophages of the reticuloendothelial system by the action of the enzyme, heme oxygenase. The iron returns to the plasma transferrin and is carried back to the erythroid bone marrow for reuse by new red blood cells, or, the iron may be stored within the reticuloendothelial cells as ferritin and hemosiderin. The amino acids from the globin are returned to the amino acid pool. The protoporphyrin ring is broken at one of the methene bridges, yielding biliverdin and carbon monoxide. The biliverdin is reduced to bilirubin in the reticuloendothelial cells and is then carried by the plasma albumin to the liver for eventual excretion (Fig. 51). The carbon monoxide appears in the blood attached to hemoglobin and is exhaled.

If hemoglobin is released directly into the blood, it dissociates into alpha-beta dimers and becomes attached to *haptoglobin* (a plasma globulin), taken to the reticuloendothelial cell, and processed in the normal way. If the plasma haptoglobin becomes depleted, the hemoglobin (dimers) are converted to *hemosiderin* or are excreted as free hemoglobin or methemoglobin in the urine. If free hemoglobin is present in the blood, it may be oxidized to *methemoglobin.* If this occurs, the heme groups dissociate and are bound to another transport protein, *hemopexin,* leave the circulation via the liver, and are catabolized. If all hemopexin is used up, the excess heme groups will combine with albumin to form *methemalbumin* until hemopexin becomes available for transfer to the liver.

MEGALOBLASTIC ERYTHROPOIESIS

A nuclear maturation defect occurs in vitamin B_{12} and folic acid deficiencies. As

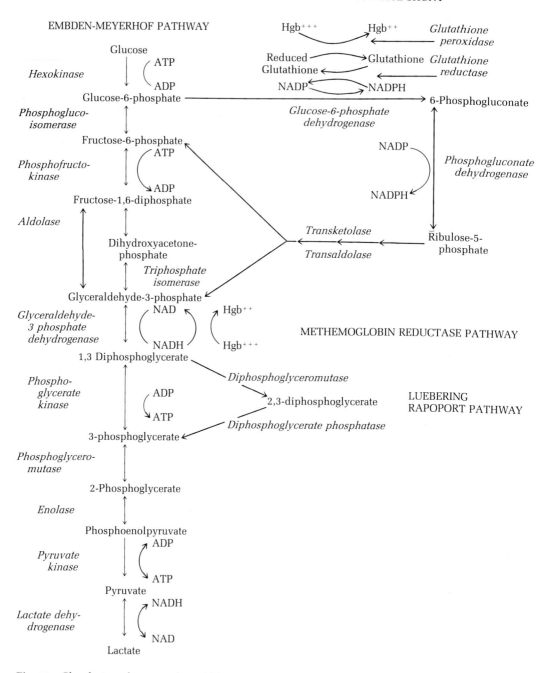

Fig. 50.   Glycolytic pathways in the red blood cell.

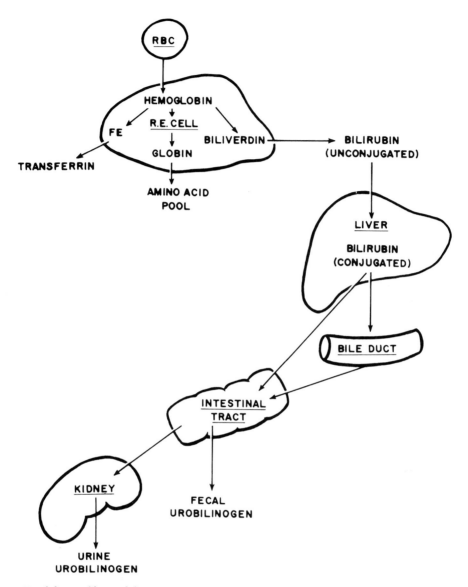

Fig. 51. Breakdown of hemoglobin.

a result, the red blood cell and its precursors are much larger in sizer than normal. Thus, the term *megaloblast* is used, 'megalo' meaning large. The maturation of the megaloblast proceeds through the same stages of development as the normal red blood cell. Because of the defect in nuclear development (abnormal DNA synthesis), maturation of the nucleus takes longer than the cytoplasm, which matures at a more normal rate. Cell division is delayed because of the nuclear defect, whereas development of the cytoplasm continues. As a result, the cytoplasm appears to have matured to one stage, whereas the nucleus appears much more immature (asynchronism). The nuclear chromatin in these cells shows a much more open pattern with increased or prominent parachromatin.

Promegaloblast (Fig. 52).

Size: 19 to 28 µm in diameter.

Cytoplasm: More abundant than in the pronormoblast.
Deeply basophilic.
Non-granular.

Nucleus: Fine chromatin pattern.
Chromatin pattern is more open than in the pronormoblast.
3 to 5 nucleoli.

Basophilic Megaloblast (Fig. 53).

Size: 17 to 24 µm in diameter.

Cytoplasm: Deeply basophilic.
Non-granular.

Nucleus: No nucleoli visible.
Chromatin pattern is more open than in the basophilic normoblast.

Polychromatophilic Megaloblast (Fig. 54).

Size: 15 to 20 µm in diameter.

Cytoplasm: Blue-gray to pinkish-gray.
May contain *Howell-Jolly bodies* (nuclear fragments).

Nucleus: Chromatin pattern is more open than in the polychromatophilic normoblast.
There may be a breaking up of the nucleus *(karyorrhexis)*.

Orthochromic Megaloblast (Fig. 55).

Size: 10 to 15 µm in diameter.

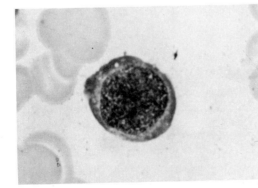

Fig. 52.   Promegaloblast (large cell in center).

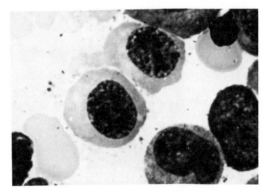

Fig. 54.   Polychromatophilic megaloblast (large cell in center).

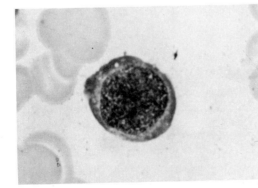

Fig. 53.   Basophilic megaloblast.

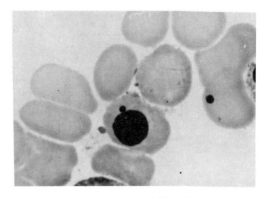

Fig. 55.   Orthochromic megaloblast (center).

Cytoplasm: Almost pink in color.
More abundant than is found in the orthochromic normoblast.

Nucleus: Chromatin may be clumped but is much less condensed than the normal orthochromic normoblast.

Macrocyte

Size: 9 to 12 μm in diameter.

The macrocyte may appear oval on the stained blood smear.

RED BLOOD CELL MORPHOLOGY

In anemias and other diseases, the mature red blood cells of the peripheral blood may show certain significant changes. The terms applied to each of these abnormalities are defined and illustrated on the following pages.

Normal red blood cells (discocytes), Figures 56 and 64, are round, have a small area of central pallor, and show only a slight variation in size. (As the relative amount of hemoglobin in the red cell decreases [or increases], the area of central pallor will increase [or decrease] accordingly.)

Microcytic red blood cells, Figure 57, show a decrease in size and are found in thalassemia and a variety of anemias.

Macrocytic red blood cells, Figure 58,

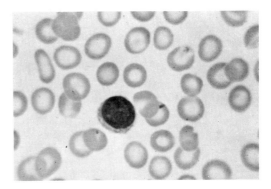

Fig. 57. Microcytes (compare red blood cell size with the size of the lymphocyte nucleus). (Magnification ×1000)

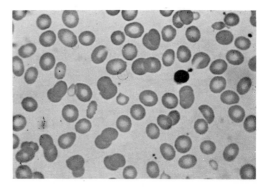

Fig. 58. Macrocytes, oval. (Compare red blood cell size with the size of the lymphocyte nucleus.) (Magnification ×500)

show an increase in size. These cells may be found in liver disease. When associated with vitamin B_{12} or folic acid deficiency, the macrocytes may appear slightly oval in shape.

Anisocytosis, Figure 59, indicates a variation in the size of the red blood cells.

Hypochromia, Figure 60, denotes red blood cells with a large area of central pallor and is due to a decreased concentration of hemoglobin in the cell. Hypochromia is characteristically present in iron deficiency anemia but is also present in other forms of anemia.

Polychromatophilia indicates young red blood cells which contain residual RNA. These cells are generally larger than normal and stain a pinkish gray to pinkish

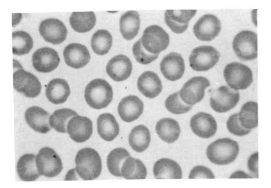

Fig. 56. Normal red blood cells. (Magnification ×1000)

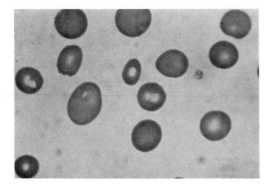

Fig. 59.   Red blood cells showing anisocytosis. (Magnification ×1000)

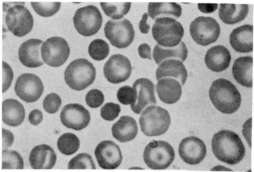

Fig. 61.   Spherocytes. (Note the group of three spherocytes in the center of the illustration that show no area of central pallor. There are several more spherocytes also present.) (Magnification ×1000)

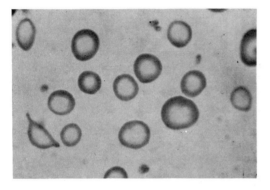

Fig. 60.   Hypochromic red blood cells. (Magnification ×1000)

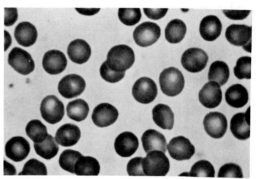

Fig. 62.   Spheroidocytes. (Note the red blood cells showing only a small off-center area of pallor.) (Magnification ×1000)

blue color (Plate VJ). These cells show up as reticulocytes when stained supravitally with brilliant cresyl blue.

Spherocytic red blood cells, Figures 61 and 64, are almost spherical in shape. They are not biconcave like a normal red blood cell and do not have the central area of pallor which a normal red cell shows. The spherocyte has a smaller surface area for the cell size. These cells are associated with hemolytic anemia and hereditary spherocytosis. In some hereditary red cell enzyme deficiencies, the spherocytes may have many fine needle-like projections on the surface of the cell.

Spheroidocytes, Figures 62 and 64, are thicker than normal red blood cells, have higher than normal concentrations of hemoglobin, and show a small area of pallor that is usually off center.

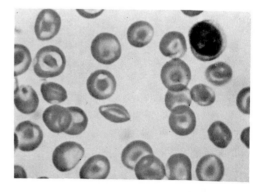

Fig. 63.   Target cells. Note the *pocketbook-shaped* red blood cell located near the center of the illustration. (Magnification ×1000)

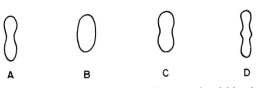

Fig. 64. Cross section of A, the normal red blood cell; B, the spherocyte; C, the spheroidocyte; and D, the target cell.

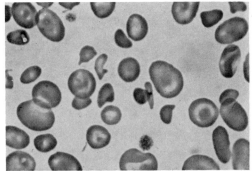

Fig. 66. Poikilocytosis of the red blood cells. Small red blood cell fragments, or schistocytes, are also present. (Magnification ×1000)

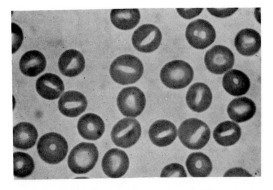

Fig. 65. Stomatocytes. (Note the oval-shaped area of central pallor in the red blood cells as compared to the round area in normal red blood cells. (Magnification ×1000)

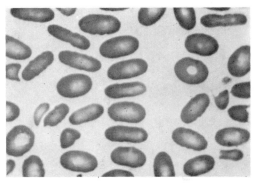

Fig. 67. Numerous ovalocytes and elliptocytes. (Magnification ×1000)

Target cells (leptocytes), Figures 63 and 64, show a centrally stained area and are associated with liver disease and certain hemoglobinopathies (abnormal hemoglobins): hemoglobin SC disease, hemoglobin C disease, and sickle cell anemia.

Stomatocytes, Figure 65, show an oval or rectangular area of central pallor. These cells have lost the indentation on one side and may be found in liver disease, electrolyte imbalance, and hereditary stomatocytosis.

Poikilocytosis, Figure 66, indicates a variation in the shape of the red blood cells.

Ovalocytes, Figures 67 and 68, are oval-shaped red blood cells. *Elliptocytes,* more oval than ovalocytes, are cigar-shaped. Both of these cells are found in hereditary elliptocytosis in large numbers. They are also present in various anemias but at a much lower concentration, no more than 6 to 10% of the mature red blood cell pop-

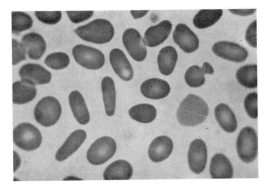

Fig. 68. Ovalocytes and elliptocytes. Note the *pincer cell* (red blood cell, shown in the upper right, which appears as if it has been pinched). (Magnification ×1000)

ulation. (These cells show normal shape in the nucleated and reticulocyte stages.)

Teardrop shaped red blood cells, Figure 69, are found most notably in myelofibrosis, pernicious anemia, myeloid metaplasia, thalassemia, and some hemolytic anemias.

Crenated red blood cells (echinocytes), Figure 70, have blunt spicules evenly distributed over the surface of the red blood cell and are usually due to faulty drying of the blood smear, or, may be a result of hyperosmolarity.

Burr cells, Figures 71 and 72, are red blood cells with uniformly spaced, pointed projections on their outer edges. These cells occur in uremia, acute blood

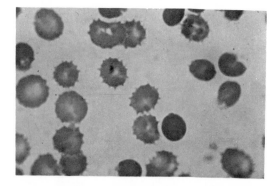

Fig. 71.   Burr cells. (Magnification × 1000)

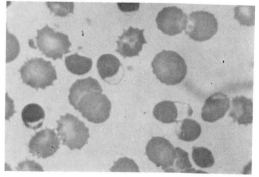

Fig. 72.   *Blister cells* and burr cells. (Magnification × 1000)

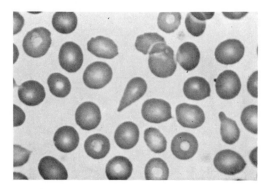

Fig. 69.   Teardrop-shaped red blood cell (center of illustration). (Magnification × 1000)

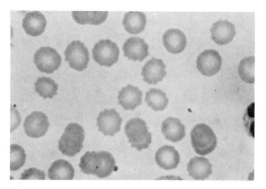

Fig. 70.   Crenated red blood cells. (Note that the projections on the surface of the red blood cells are rounded, not pointed as in the burr cell.) (Magnification × 1000)

loss, cancer of the stomach, and pyruvate kinase deficiency.

Schistocytes, Figure 66, are red blood cell fragments and may occur in microangiopathic hemolytic anemia, uremia, severe burns, and hemolytic anemias caused by physical agents, as in disseminated intravascular coagulation (DIC).

Acanthocytes, Figure 73, are red blood cells with irregularly spaced projections. These spicules vary in width but usually contain a bulbous, rounded end. These cells have a decreased survival time and are found in abetalipoproteinemia and certain liver disorders.

Sickle cells (drepanocytes), Figure 74, are red blood cells in the shape of a sickle or crescent. To be considered as sickle cells, they must come to a point at one end. These cells are associated with hemoglo-

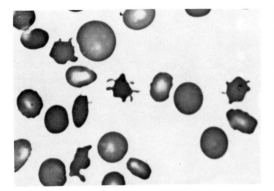

Fig. 73. Acanthocyte (center). (Magnification ×1000)

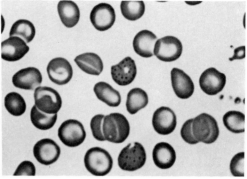

Fig. 75. Basophilic stippling (note the stippling in the red blood cell having a flattened side). (Magnification ×1000)

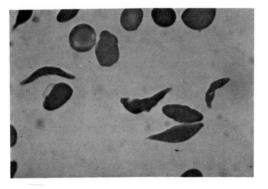

Fig. 74. Sickled red blood cells. (Magnification ×1000)

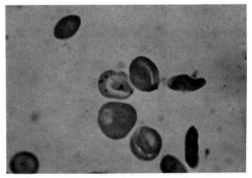

Fig. 76. Pappenheimer bodies (present in the red blood cell located in the middle of the illustration). (Magnification ×1000)

bin S and are found in sickle cell anemia and hemoglobin SC disease.

Basophilic stippling, Figure 75, is present as many coarse or fine, purple-staining granules in the red blood cell. The granules result from aggregation of ribosomes and are found in lead poisoning, anemias with impaired hemoglobin synthesis, alcoholism, and megaloblastic anemias.

Siderocytes are deposits of iron in the red blood cell. They are generally seen near the periphery of the cell and may appear as a single granule or as multiple granules. When present on a Wright-stained smear, the granules appear less vividly stained than Howell-Jolly bodies and are termed *Pappenheimer bodies* (Fig. 76). In contrast, when the iron deposits are stained only by iron stains, as in the Prussian blue reaction, the cells are termed *sid-erocytes.* These iron staining granules are present in sideroblastic and megaloblastic anemias, alcoholism, following splenectomy, and in some hemoglobinopathies.

Howell-Jolly bodies, Figure 77, are round, purple staining nuclear fragments in the red blood cell. They generally appear singly in hemolytic anemia and following splenectomy. Multiple Howell-Jolly bodies in a red blood cell occur in megaloblastic anemia and in other forms of nuclear maturation defects.

Hemoglobin C crystals, Figures 78 and 79, may be found in patients with homozygous hemoglobin C disease and characteristically in patients with hemoglobin SC disease.

Cabot rings, Figure 80, are purple stain-

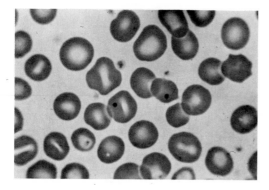

Fig. 77. Howell-Jolly bodies (one Howell-Jolly body is located in each of the two red blood cells shown in the center of the illustration). (Magnification ×1000)

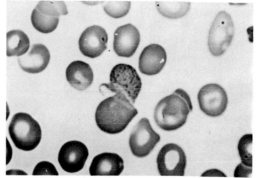

Fig. 80. Cabot ring. (Note the red blood cell in the center containing basophilic stippling and partially covered by another red blood cell. The cabot ring appears as a faintly stained circle within the red blood cell.) (Magnification ×1000)

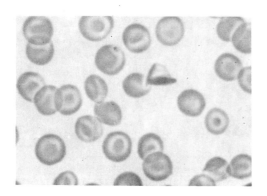

Fig. 78. Hemoglobin C crystal. Target cells are also present. (Magnification ×1000)

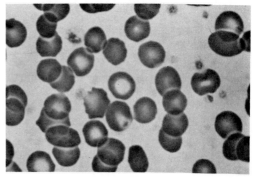

Fig. 81. Note the platelet on top of the red blood cell. When seen, there is generally a halo or clear-staining area in the red blood cell surrounding the platelet. (Magnification ×1000)

ing threadlike filaments in the shape of a ring or figure 8 in the red blood cell. They are thought to be microtubules from a mitotic spindle and are seen rarely in pernicious anemia and lead poisoning. They probably indicate abnormal erythropoiesis.

Platelets on top of red blood cells, Figure 81, should not be confused with a red blood cell inclusion body. Compare the platelet with platelets in the surrounding field. Also, there is generally a nonstaining halo surrounding the platelet when it is positioned on top of the red blood cell.

Rouleaux formation, Figures 82 and 83, represents erythrocytes arranged in rolls

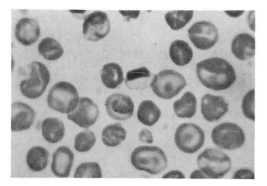

Fig. 79. Hemoglobin C crystal. Target cells are also present. (Magnification ×1000)

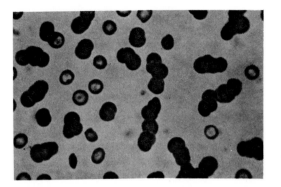

Fig. 82. Rouleaux formation of the red blood cells. (Magnification ×500)

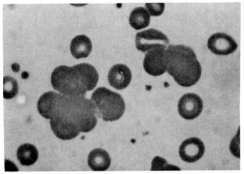

Fig. 84. Agglutination of the red blood cells. (Magnification ×1000)

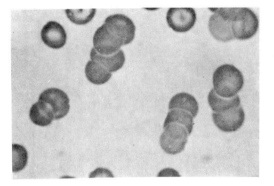

Fig. 83. Rouleaux formation of the red blood cells. (Magnification ×1000)

or stacks. This may be due to an artifact (as a result of not preparing the blood smear soon enough after placing the blood on the slide) or, may be due to the presence of high concentrations of abnormal globulins or fibrinogen. This formation of the red blood cells is found in multiple myeloma and macroglobulinemia.

Agglutination of the red blood cells, Figure 84, is found in patients who have a cold agglutinin (antibody), or autoimmune hemolytic anemia. Note the clumping of the red blood cells rather than the stacking as found in rouleaux formation. When agglutination of the red blood cells is seen on a blood smear, routine automated methods of red blood cell counting and sizing should not be utilized.

Crescent bodies are faintly staining bod-

ies in the shape of a quarter moon. They are probably ruptured red blood cells.

When examining a blood smear, any of the preceding red blood cell changes should be noted. An occasional crescent body, however, may be ignored. Whenever possible, a red blood cell abnormality should be described in as much detail as possible. For example, when poikilocytosis is present, the type(s) of irregularly shaped cells should be noted. The generally accepted methods of reporting red blood cell irregularities include commenting on the degree of variability (slight, moderate, marked, or 1 +, 2 +, 3 +) present. Regardless of the method chosen, it should be used consistently in each laboratory. Because the reporting of red blood cell morphology may vary among technologists, it is also helpful for each laboratory to have a uniform grading system. For example, using the 1 +, 2 +, 3 + system, the presence of 1 to 5 spherocytes (or poikilocytic red blood cells) per oil immersion field may constitute a rank of 1 + spherocytosis, 6 to 15 spherocytes, a 2 +, and greater than 15 spherocytes, a 3 +. The grading will depend upon the abnormality present. For red blood cell inclusions, 1 to 2 per oil immersion field may represent 1 +, 3 to 5 per field, a 2 +, and greater than 5 per field, a 3 +. It is important to select the proper area of the smear when determining red blood cell morphology. Using wedge or coverslip smears, the areas of the smear in which some red blood cells begin to overlap is generally used to determine red blood cell morphology.

WHITE BLOOD CELLS

Granulocytic Cells

There are three types of mature granulocytes: the neutrophil, eosinophil, and basophil. These three cell types are distinguishable from each other by the presence of specific granules that appear in the myelocyte stage.

The committed stem cell for the neutrophils (and monocytes), CFU-G,M, gives rise to the myeloblast. The eosinophil, however, is thought to have its own committed stem cell, CFU-Eo, which gives rise to the myeloblast for further maturation to the eosinophil. The committed stem cell from which the basophil ultimately develops has not yet been identified. Because the maturation of the neutrophil, eosinophil, and basophil are very similar, and because these three cell types are granulocytic, their development is described simultaneously on the following pages.

Myeloblast (Figs. 85 and 93).

Size: 15 to 20 μm in diameter.

Cytoplasm: Small amount in relation to the rest of the cell.
Usually a moderate blue in color.

Texture is smooth and usually nongranular.

Nucleus: Round or slightly oval.
Occupies about four-fifths of the cell.
Extremely fine chromatin pattern.
Reddish purple in color.
Contains two to three nucleoli.

Promyelocyte (Figs. 86 and 93).

Size: 15 to 21 μm in diameter. This cell is normally slightly larger than the myeloblast.

Cytoplasm: Pale blue.
Contains a few to many, blue to purple-staining nonspecific granules.

Nucleus: Occupies half or more of the cell.
Oval or round.
Chromatin pattern may become a little coarser, although it will still be relatively fine.
Two or three nucleoli present.

Myelocyte (Figs. 87 and 93). This is the last stage capable of cell division.

Size: 12 to 18 μm in diameter.

Cytoplasm: Moderate amount.

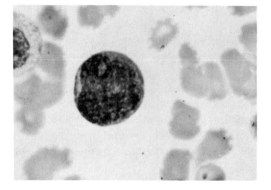

Fig. 85.   Myeloblast (center).

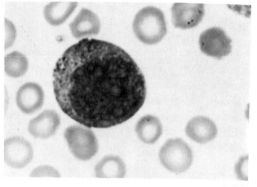

Fig. 86.   Promyelocyte (center).

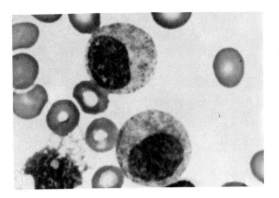

Fig. 87.   Myelocytes, two.

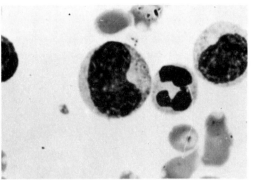

Fig. 88.   Metamyelocyte and neutrophil.

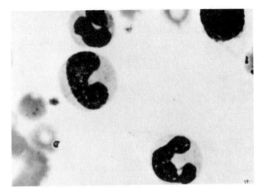

Fig. 89.   Neutrophilic band.

May contain a few patches of blue.

Few to moderate number of nonspecific granules.

Specific granules begin to appear in this stage.

Neutrophil myelocyte: the pink specific granules may be seen as pinkish or lighter staining areas in the cytoplasm, usually appearing near the nucleus first.

Eosinophil myelocyte: the specific granules first appear as dirty orange to blue. These granules are larger than the nonspecific granules and are larger than the specific granules of the neutrophil.

Basophil myelocyte: the specific granules are few, large, and stain a dark blue-purple.

Nucleus: Oval or round.

Chromatin pattern becomes coarser.

Generally shows no nucleoli.

Nucleus may be centrally located or eccentric.

Metamyelocyte (Figs. 88 and 93).

Size: 10 to 15 μm in diameter.

Cytoplasm: Moderate   to   abundant amount.

A few nonspecific granules.

Full complement of specific granules.

Neutrophil metamyelocyte: the granules are pinker and more numerous.

Eosinophil metamyelocyte: the granules are a brighter orange-red and more numerous.

Basophil metamyelocyte: the dark purple granules are more numerous.

Nucleus: Indented or kidney-shaped.

Chromatin pattern is coarse and clumped.

Band (Figs. 89 and 93).

Size: 9 to 15 μm in diameter.

Cytoplasm: Same as the metamyelocyte.

Nucleus: Rod or band shaped.
Thinner than in the metamyelocyte.
Chromatin pattern is coarse
and clumped.

Segmented Neutrophil (Figs. 88, 90, and 93).

Size: 9 to 15 μm in diameter.

Cytoplasm: Full complement of pink to
rose-violet specific gran-
ules.
Abundant amount.
Few nonspecific granules are
present.

Nucleus: Normally two to five lobes.
Coarse, clumped chromatin
pattern.

Eosinophil (Fig. 91).

Size: 9 to 15 μm in diameter.

Cytoplasm: Contains the full complement
of large, reddish-orange
granules.

Nucleus: Usually has two lobes.
Coarse, clumped chromatin
pattern.

Basophil (Fig. 92).

Size: 10 to 16 μm in diameter.

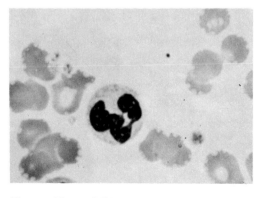

Fig. 90.   Neutrophil (center).

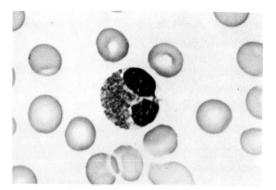

Fig. 91.   Eosinophil.

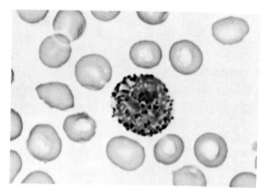

Fig. 92.   Basophil.

Cytoplasm: Stains slightly pink to colorless.
Contains specific dark purple
granules.
There are fewer granules present than are found in the
eosinophil. The granules
are water-soluble and tend
to wash out when stained.

Nucleus: Does not appear as coarse as
in the neutrophil or eosin-
ophil.
Generally has two to four
lobes.

When differentiating white blood cells,
it should be noted that, except in unusual
circumstances, the different stages of the
eosinophil or basophil are not identified.
The cells are denoted merely as eosinophils or basophils. The neutrophil stages

are always differentiated. Identification of the neutrophil band varies from one laboratory to another. In this text, a neutrophil is considered to be mature if the nucleus is indented by greater than one half of its diameter.

With present staining techniques, it is often impossible to differentiate the various types of blast cells. Many times, the cell is merely termed a 'blast' cell. Otherwise, the cell is identified by the company it keeps, that is, by placing it in the same family of cells as the identifiable ones in the area surrounding the blast cell.

Neutrophilic Granulocytes

Neutrophil production and maturation occur in the bone marrow. The mature neutrophil moves into the peripheral blood and then into the tissues where it carries out its major functions of ingesting and killing invading microorganisms.

Neutrophil Kinetics

As the myeloblast develops into the mature segmented neutrophil, the myeloblast, promyelocyte, and myelocyte undergo cell division. These cells consti-

tute the mitotic pool (Fig. 94) and will generally undergo a total of three to five cell divisions over a period of 6 to 7 days. During the promyelocyte stage the cell produces primary (azurophilic) granules. The number of granules per cell will decrease with each cell division. At the myelocyte stage the cell produces secondary (specific) granules. (Synthesis of primary granules stops when the cell begins secondary granule production.)

Once the cell reaches the metamyelocyte stage it is no longer capable of mitosis. It spends the next 7 to 8 days in the storage pool during which time it matures into the segmented neutrophil. The number of bands and segmented neutrophils in the storage pool is about 15 times the number in the peripheral blood and the mitotic pool is approximately one-third the size of the storage pool.

When the neutrophilic cells are mature, they are ready for release into the peripheral blood. The release of marrow cells into the blood is only partially understood and is most probably based on a selective type of release of mature cells rather than a random release. It is thought that sub-

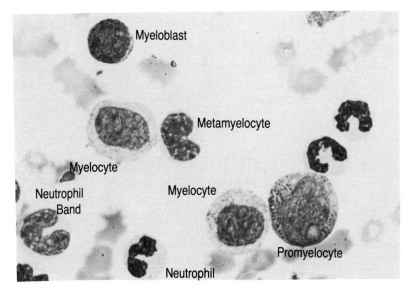

Fig. 93. Myeloblast, promyelocyte, myelocytes (two), metamyelocyte, neutrophilic band, neutrophils. Note the coarsening of the nuclear chromatin as the cell matures.

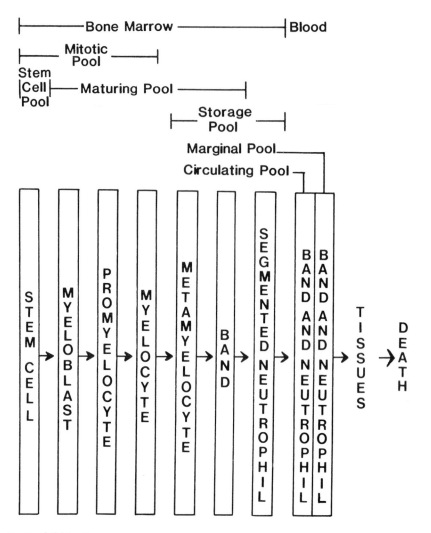

Fig. 94. Neutrophil kinetics.

stances (e.g., a CSF [colony stimulating factor] and a form of granulopoietin) may exist which regulate granulocyte production and control the movement of granulocytes from the bone marrow to the blood. The exact mechanisms and controls are still unknown.

When the mature neutrophils leave the storage pool they enter the peripheral blood, where approximately 50% of the neutrophils circulate freely and make up the *circulating pool.* The remaining 50% adhere to the walls of the blood vessels and constitute the *marginal pool.* (The cells in the marginal pool are not included in the white blood cell count. Therefore, in a blood sample, the number of neutrophils counted in a white blood cell count and differential represents only half the number actually present in the peripheral blood.) The cells are continually changing back and forth between the marginal and circulating pools. A small percentage of bands are also normally released to the peripheral blood along with the mature neutrophils. The segmented neutrophil is generally released to the peripheral blood first, before the band. When the demand for neutrophils in the peripheral blood increases, as soon as the numbers of segmented neutrophils in the storage pool become depleted, the number of bands entering the peripheral blood from the storage pool increases. This is reflected by an increased percentage of bands in the white blood cell differential count. Mathematically, the average time the neutrophil spends in the peripheral blood is considered to be about 10 hours. According to this figure, the neutrophils in the peripheral blood are completely replaced by neutrophils from the bone marrow almost 2.5 times every 24 hours. The neutrophils do not return to the bone marrow once they enter the peripheral blood.

From the marginal pool, the neutrophils randomly enter the tissues and body cavities in which they carry out their major functions. The cells leave the peripheral blood randomly, regardless of the age of the cell or the length of time it has been in the marginal or circulating pool. Normally, the neutrophils enter the tissues at the same rate as other neutrophils leave the storage pool and enter the peripheral blood. Once the neutrophil has entered the tissues, it is utilized to fight infection, or it leaves the body via excretions from the intestinal tract, the urinary tract, the lungs, or the salivary glands. It may also be destroyed by the reticuloendothelial system within 4 or 5 days.

Physiology and Function of the Neutrophil

Neutrophils are metabolically active. They are capable of both aerobic and anaerobic glycolysis. Their major function is to stop or retard the action of foreign material or infectious agents by means of: (1) moving into the area of inflammation or infection, (2) phagocytosis of the foreign material, and (3) killing and digestion of the offending material.

The primary (nonspecific) and secondary (specific) granules of the neutrophil are packaged and released from the Golgi apparatus. In the mature neutrophil, the ratio of specific granules to nonspecific granules is about 2 or 3:1. The primary granules are membrane-bound lysosomes and contain acid phosphatase, peroxidase, esterase, sulfated mucosubstance, β-galactosidase, arylsulfatase, lysozyme, and other basic proteins. The secondary granules contain aminopeptidase, collagenase, muramidase, lactoferrin, lysozyme, and a number of basic proteins. Alkaline phosphatase is no longer thought to be contained in the granules but may reside on the neutrophil plasma membrane.

The neutrophil is capable of both random and directed locomotion (chemotaxis). The cells in the marginal pool move through the unruptured walls of the blood vessels (diapedesis) and travel to the tissues and body cavities. In the presence of infection, inflammation, or a foreign substance, the neutrophils in the area of the foreign matter quickly move, within minutes, by diapedesis to the damaged or infected area. This directed locomotion, chemotaxis, is brought about by chemotactic factors, such as secretions from transformed lymphocytes and macrophages, endotoxins and other products from bacteria, and activated complement. The neutrophils are able to distinguish foreign particles and damaged cells. This is of utmost importance to its function of phagocytosis. Opsonins (specific antibodies, complement, and so on) enhance phagocytosis and increase chemotaxis. They act on the foreign particles by coating them. The surface of the neutrophil membrane contains receptors for complement (C3) and for the Fc portion of IgG. The neutrophil is able to bind the coated matter and phagocytose it.

When the neutrophil phagocytizes the foreign particle, the cell membrane moves inward and encloses the material, forming a phagocytic vacuole (phagosome), the walls of which had been the outer membrane of the neutrophil before phagocytosis (Fig. 95). During phagocytosis, a

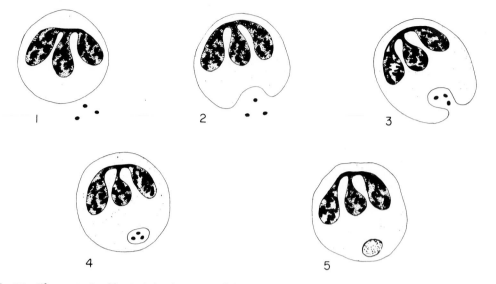

Fig. 95. Phagocytosis of bacteria by the neutrophil.

number of metabolic changes take place: increased glycolysis and lipid synthesis, increased monophosphate shunt activity, a decrease in pH within the phagosome, increased oxygen consumption, and an increased formation of hydrogen peroxide and superoxide (O_2^-).

Once the phagocytic vacuole is formed, the specific neutrophil granules will first fuse with the phagosome membrane, emptying their contents into the phagosome. (This process is known as *degranulation*.) Following this, the nonspecific granules release their contents into the phagosome. Myeloperoxidase from the primary granules in combination with the hydrogen peroxide generated and an intracellular halide is one effective way the neutrophil is able to kill bacteria, viruses, and fungi. When the bacteria has been killed, this phagosome is known as a *secondary lysosome.* The cell may then expel the digested residue *(exocytosis).* The neutrophil is also capable of *pinocytosis* (ingestion of small amounts of liquid). The combination of phagocytosis and pinocytosis is termed *endocytosis.*

In the presence of an inflammatory process, the neutrophils continually move into the infected area, phagocytize, die, and are, in turn, phagocytized by macrophages. The neutrophils are generally the first phagocytic cell to reach infected areas and are followed by the monocyte. These two cell types continue their migration to the area until all of the foreign material has been phagocytized. Under normal conditions, the neutrophil will spend 4 to 5 days in the tissues before senescence (growing old) and destruction.

Neutrophilia

(1) Extreme exercise and also the administration of certain drugs cause a decrease in the proportion of neutrophils in the marginal pool. These cells become part of the circulating pool and are reflected by an increased white blood cell count and an increased percentage of neutrophils in the differential count. (2) In the presence of infection, an increased number of neutrophils are present in the marginal pool. These cells then enter the tissues at a faster rate. The influx of neutrophils from the storage pool increases until the rate of outflow to the tissues is exceeded by the rate of inflow from the storage pool in the bone marrow. (3) In chronic infection, the high rate of influx of neutrophils into the peripheral blood and the corresponding in-

creased outflow may remain unchanged and a steady state of neutrophilia is maintained.

Neutropenia

When the white blood cell count is less than 1,000/μL the patient is prone to recurrent infections. However, when the white count drops to less than 500/μL the patient is very seriously open to infection. (1) Certain drugs cause an increased number of neutrophils to enter the marginal pool, resulting in a lower percentage of neutrophils in the circulating pool. (2) In a severe infection, the outflow of cells to the tissues may exceed the input from the bone marrow storage pool. (3) Decreased production in the bone marrow gives rise to decreased numbers of neutrophils available to the peripheral blood. (4) An increased loss of white blood cells (as might occur with splenomegaly), whereby the spleen sequesters (removes from the blood and holds) and destroys the cells, may also lead to neutropenia.

The Eosinophil

The majority of eosinophils are produced in the bone marrow. They most likely originate from their own committed stem cell and not the same committed stem cell as the neutrophils. The maturation process of the eosinophil, however, closely parallels that of the neutrophil. They are slightly larger than neutrophils and the nuclei of the cells average fewer lobes than found in the mature neutrophil. The eosinophils will average 2.1 lobes in the normal person. The colony stimulating factor (CSF) which stimulates the production of eosinophils from the committed stem cell (CFU-Eo) is produced by the lymphocytes.

The eosinophil is primarily a tissue cell. Once it is released into the peripheral blood from the bone marrow, it will be randomly removed from the blood independently of its age. Its half-life in the blood is about 8 hours. From the blood it moves into the tissues where it localizes in areas exposed to the external environment, most notably in the skin, lungs, and gastrointestinal tract. For each eosinophil in the peripheral blood there are 300 to 500 eosinophils in the tissues where their life span is probably several days. Most likely, once they migrate to the tissues, they do not return to the circulation. The eosinophils are motile and capable of locomotion in a manner similar to the neutrophils.

The eosinophil is metabolically more active than the neutrophil. The mitochondria is larger and the Golgi zones are more developed. Although the eosinophil membranes have receptors for complement and IgG, they are present on fewer of the cells than found in the neutrophils.

The mature eosinophil contains two types of granules. The larger granules are the more numerous and contain a very dense core which primarily consists of what is termed *major basic protein*. Little is known of the function of this protein. Production of these granules stops when the eosinophil becomes mature. The second type of granule present is smaller than the first and may not appear in the cell until after the myelocyte stage. The eosinophilic granules contain peroxidase, β-glucuronidase, acid β-glycerophosphatase, arylsulfatase (contained in small granules), phospholipase, acid phosphatase, ribonuclease, and cathepsin. The peroxidase is a different form than that found in the neutrophil. In addition, the eosinophil granules differ from those in the neutrophil in that they lack lysozyme, phagocytin, and neutrophil bactericidal cationic proteins.

The functions of the eosinophil are not completely understood. They are capable of phagocytizing foreign material and antigen-antibody complexes. However, these are probably not their primary functions. One proposed function describes the eosinophil as an *anti-inflammatory cell* in that they may modulate reactions in which basophils and mast cells are active. Basophils contain eosinophil chemotactic factors. In addition, eosinophils: (1) are thought to prevent basophil and mast cell degranulation, (2) contain histaminase which can inactivate the histamine from mast cells, (3) contain arylsulfatase B which inactivates leukotrienes released by the mast cell, (4) contains phospholipase D to inactivate platelet-activating factor, and (5) are capable of neutralizing the heparin released by mast cells by the action of the major basic protein (present in the large eosinophil granule). The eosinophils also appear to function by providing some defense against helminth parasites by first moving to the site of parasite infection. The cells then attach to the surface of the parasites where they release substances toxic to the parasitic invaders.

Basophils and Mast Cells

It is thought that basophils develop from a cell similar to the myeloblast. The stem cell from which this myeloblast originates has not yet been identified and it may or may not be a separate stem cell from that of the neutrophil and monocyte, or eosinophil. The cell matures in a manner similar to the eosinophil and is produced in the bone marrow. Once released from the bone marrow to the peripheral blood, the basophil remains in the circulation for approximately the same amount of time as the neutrophil before it moves into the tissues. The mast cells are widely distributed throughout the body including the thymus, spleen, and bone marrow, and are of mesenchymal origin. They are normally not present in the peripheral blood.

The granules of the basophil are larger than the azurophilic granules found in the promyelocyte, and may be slighly irregular in shape. They are water soluble and stain a deep purple with Wright stain. During maturation, the nucleus does not segment as completely as the neutrophil and the nuclear chromatin in the mature basophil has a condensed but somewhat smudged appearance. The mast cells are slightly larger than the basophil and contain abundant purple staining (Wright stain) granules which are slightly smaller than the basophil and are less soluble than the basophil granules.

The basophil exhibits chemotaxis and some phagocytic activity. It is also capable of a sluggish motility. The basophil granules contain peroxidase, histamine, and heparin. They synthesize an eosinophil chemotactic factor, a slow reacting substance of anaphylaxis, and platelet activating factor (PAF). The biochemical make up of the mast cell is similar and, in addition, it contains serotonin and some proteolytic enzymes.

Basophils and mast cells appear to function similarly. They appear to participate in immediate hypersensitivity reactions and are also involved in some delayed hypersensitivity reactions. Their membranes readily bind immunoglobulin E and when specific antigens react with the membrane-bound IgE, degranulation occurs and the contents of the basophil/mast cell granules are released to the surrounding area. This, in turn, will lead to the accumulation of eosinophils in the area (due to the eosinophil chemotactic factor released from the cells).

Monocytes

The monocyte is produced in the bone marrow.

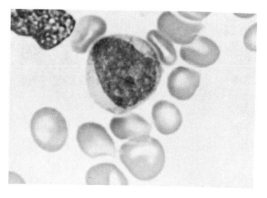

Fig. 96. Promonocyte (immature monocyte).

Promonocyte (immature monocyte) (Fig. 96).

Size: 14 to 18 μm in diameter.

Cytoplasm: Blue-gray.
Contains fine dustlike azurophilic granules.
Ground glass appearance.
Moderate amount.

Nucleus: Oval or indented.
One to five nucleoli.
Fine chromatin pattern.

Monocyte (Fig. 97).

Size: 14 to 20 μm in diameter.

Cytoplasm: Abundant.
Blue-gray.
Many fine azurophilic granules, giving a ground glass appearance.
Vacuoles may sometimes be present.

Nucleus: Round, kidney shaped, or may show slight lobulation. It may be folded over on top of itself, thus showing brainlike convolutions.
No nucleoli are visible.
Chromatin is fine, arranged in skeinlike strands.

PHYSIOLOGY AND BIOLOGY OF THE MONOCYTE

The monocyte arises from the same committed stem cell as the neutrophil.

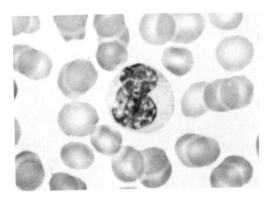

Fig. 97.   Monocyte.

The precursor to the promonocyte is probably the 'myelomonoblast' (also termed 'monoblast' by some) and is normally indistinguishable from the myeloblast. Unlike the other white blood cells in the peripheral blood, the monocyte is considered to be an immature cell. When it leaves the blood, it travels to the tissues, where this cell line spends most of its time maturing and differentiating into various types of macrophages, depending on the local conditions in the various tissues.

The immature monocyte, or promonocyte, is less phagocytic and less motile than the monocyte. Once the promonocyte is formed it will undergo two mitotic divisions within a period of 2 to 2½ days under normal conditions. The mature monocyte in the peripheral blood has a well-developed Golgi apparatus, rough endoplasmic reticulum, numerous mitochondria, and variable amounts of ribosomes and polyribosomes. There are nucleoli present in the nucleus in about 50% of the monocytes, as seen by electron microscopy. The granules in the cytoplasm of the monocyte are packaged by the Golgi apparatus, represent primary lysosomes, and contain acid phosphatase and arylsulfatase activity. The monocyte and macrophage are actively motile cells which are capable of chemotaxis, are able to move through blood vessel walls and migrate to areas of inflammation, and may extend multiple pseudopods. They respond to such substances as MIF (migration inhibition factor), which is produced by the T lymphocytes to immobilize the macrophage, and to chemotactic inhibitors. The monocyte and macrophage are capable of phagocytosis and pinocytosis. When there are areas of inflammation present in the body, the production of monocytes is increased and there are more present in the peripheral blood.

LIFE SPAN OF THE MONOCYTE

The bone marrow contains the developing monocyte precursors and supplies monocytes to the peripheral blood. The proliferation of monocytes in the bone marrow takes about 55 hours. The monocytes undergo no maturation in the bone marrow and leave the marrow randomly, in no specific order. The marginal pool of monocytes in the blood is about 3.5 times the size of the circulating pool. The mature monocyte spends about 12 hours in the peripheral blood before going to the tissues.

DEVELOPMENT OF THE MONOCYTE INTO THE MACROPHAGE

The monocyte moves via diapedesis through the blood vessel walls into the various tissues and transforms into the macrophage, at the same time becoming actively phagocytic. It is also thought that some macrophages are produced by cell division of existing macrophages. As the macrophage develops from the monocyte, the cell increases in size. One or more nucleoli develop and there is an increase in the hydrolytic enzymes. In addition, the Golgi apparatus and the number of mitochondria increase. There is also an increased number of secondary lysosomes as a result of increased phagocytosis. Once the monocyte leaves the circulation it is probably pleuripotential, capable of differentiating into various types of macrophage depending upon the local conditions in the tissues to which it has migrated. They may become the Küpffer cells of the reticuloendothelial system, osteoclasts, macrophages of inflammatory areas, connective tissue macrophages, or pulmonary alveolar macrophages. Overall, the macrophage is more active than the monocyte and has a much richer supply of acid hydrolases. Once the monocyte leaves the blood it may spend several months, or longer, in the tissues where it will eventually die.

THE MACROPHAGE

The macrophage is a large cell, ranging in size from 15 to 80 μm in diameter. It has an eccentric nucleus that may be egg-shaped, indented, or elongated. The chromatin appears spongy, and there are generally one to two nucleoli. The cell has abundant sky blue cytoplasm which contains many coarse azure granules and which is usually vacuolated. There is a large variation in the appearance of the macrophage, depending on the site from which the cell has been derived. Some macrophages may develop epithelioid characteristics and may then fuse to form giant multinucleated cells. Macrophages have been divided into two categories: fixed macrophages and unfixed, or wandering macrophages. When stimulated, some of the fixed macrophages may become actively motile, wandering macrophages. The unfixed, wandering macrophage has also been termed a *histiocyte.* Macrophages are found scattered throughout the body. There are macrophages lining the sinusoids of the spleen and bone marrow, the alveolar macrophages of the lungs, the Küpffer cells of the liver, and freely migrating macrophages of the pleural and peritoneal cavities. These cells are also found at sites of inflammation and in peritoneal, pleural, and synovial fluids. The macrophage lives much longer in the tissues than does the neutrophil. It is capable of cell division and can be stimulated to synthesize a number of enzymes and other substances, depending on the body's needs.

PROPERTIES AND FUNCTIONS OF THE MONOCYTE AND MACROPHAGE

Both the monocyte and macrophage show active chemotaxis and *necrotaxis* (attraction to dead or dying cells). Pinocytosis and micropinocytosis increase as the cell matures toward the macrophage. Phagocytosis of antigens by the monocyte and macrophage requires that certain antigens be coated with an antibody *(opsonization).* The monocytes and macrophages are also capable of *necrophagocytosis* (ingestion of dying cells and cellular debris) that, along with pinocytosis, does not require antibody coating of the material being ingested. The primary functions of the monocyte and macrophage are:

1. *Defense mechanism against intracellular parasites, including certain bacteria, fungi, and protozoa.* They primarily control such microbial infections as mycobacteria, brucella, listeria, and salmonella. When an antibody coated antigen is present, the monocyte or macrophage travels to the site by the use of chemotaxis. It then attaches to the antigen and extends pseudopods around the material, forming a phagosome. Primary lysosomes in the cytoplasm of the monocyte or macrophage then fuse with the phagosome, emptying their acid hydrolases into the area to digest or degrade the antigen and become secondary lysosomes. The material may then be released from the cell *(exocytosis).* It has been suggested that the macrophage contains receptor sites for immunoglobulins on their surface. This then facilitates the recognition and ingestion of the foreign particles. Also, ingestion of particles by these cells is enhanced by certain factors present in the plasma such as antibodies and complement. The macrophage is able to phagocytize more quickly and has a greater capacity for phagocytosis than either the neutrophil or the monocyte. The cell is also capable of anaerobic phagocytosis, functioning in the center of wounds where oxygen is decreased. Unlike the neutrophil, both the monocyte and macrophage are able to synthesize new enzymes and replace lysosomes. Macrophages also are capable of destroying a variety of cells. They may produce substances that destroy some tumor cells or may destroy cells coated with specific antibodies.

2. *Removal of damaged and old cells, plasma proteins and plasma lipids.* They play an important part in the removal of old and damaged red blood cells and also in wound debridement through phagocytosis. The plasma proteins and lipids are removed by the macrophage via pinocytosis. The process by which the macrophage identifies the cells and proteins to be removed is largely unknown. One factor may be the less negative charge of cell membranes due to a decrease in their sialic acid content upon aging.

3. *Participation in iron metabolism.* Some tissue macrophages contain heme oxidase activity which enables them to break down the hemoglobin present in red blood cells. The iron, from the hemoglobin, remains in the macrophage, binding with apoferritin (in the macrophage) to form ferritin. It may subsequently form hemosiderin. The ferritin will later leave the macrophage, bind to transferrin, and be available for use in hemoglobin production.

4. *Processes antigen information for lymphocytes.* Macrophages serve an important role in the immune response. They interact with antigens by membrane attachment, ingestion, and by subsequent modification of the antigen, and will secrete a lymphocyte activating factor, *interleukin-1.* The processed antigen is presented to the lymphocyte on specific cytoplasmic surface sites. The lymphocyte may then undergo blast transformation and antibody production. The macrophage can interact with both B and T lymphocytes and is, therefore, also active in cell mediated immunity.

5. *Production and secretion of various substances.* The macrophages release lysosomal enzymes into the surrounding area which decompose tis-

sue components. These enzymes include acid phosphatase, lipase, nucleases, proteinase, collagenase, elastase, various glycosidases, and plasminogen activator. They are an important source of colony stimulating factor (CSF), which is felt to represent an important ingredient for the control of leukopoiesis. They secrete an erythropoietic factor, substances concerned with the stimulation and differentiation of T and B lymphocytes, substances which suppress lymphocyte function, chemotactic factors, and chemotactic factor inhibitors. The macrophage produces and secretes high levels of pyrogen upon stimulation, which causes fever. They also secrete such miscellaneous substances as thromboplastin, platelet activating factors, transferrin, protease inhibitors (α2-macroglobulin and α1-antitrypsin), and transcobalamin II (vitamin B_{12} transport protein). Complement factors, interferons, lysozymes, hydrogen peroxide, and superoxide are also secreted by the macrophages for use in the body's defense system.

Lymphocytes

Lymphocytes are produced by the lymph nodes, spleen, thymus, and bone marrow.

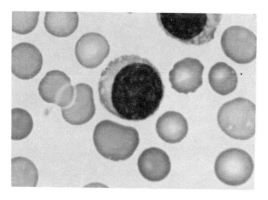

Fig. 98.   Immature lymphocyte (center).

Lymphoblast (nonleukemic lymphoblast) (Fig. 98).

Size: 10 to 18 μm in diameter.

Cytoplasm: No granules present.
            Appears smooth.
            Moderate to dark blue. May stain deep blue at the periphery and a lighter blue near the nucleus.
            More abundant than in the myeloblast.

Nucleus: Chromatin pattern is somewhat coarse.
            Round or oval in shape.
            Generally contains one to two distinct nucleoli.

Prolymphocyte

Size: May be the same size as the lymphoblast or smaller.

Cytoplasm: Moderate to dark blue.
            Usually nongranular.
            More abundant than in the lymphoblast.

Nucleus: Round, oval, or slightly indented.
            Chromatin pattern is more clumped than in the lymphoblast.

MATURE LYMPHOCYTE

The lymphocytes found in the peripheral blood occur in varying sizes. For purposes of description, they are divided into three categories: small, medium, and large, with a size variation of 8 to 16 μm in diameter. In addition to differing in size, the relative amount of cytoplasm varies. Generally, the larger the lymphocyte, the more abundant the cytoplasm.

Small Lymphocyte (Fig. 99).

Size: 8 to 10 μm in diameter.

Cytoplasm: Usually forms a thin rim around the nucleus.
            Moderate to dark blue.

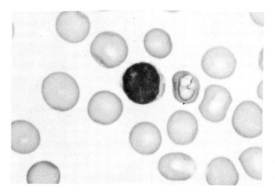

Fig. 99. Small mature lymphocyte.

Nucleus: Chromatin pattern is dense and clumped.
Round or oval in shape and may be slightly indented.
No nucleoli are visible.

Medium Lymphocyte

Size: 10 to 12 μm in diameter.

Cytoplasm: More abundant than in the small lymphocyte.
Pale to moderately blue.
May or may not contain a few nonspecific azurophilic granules.

Nucleus: Round or oval in shape and may be slightly indented.
Chromatin pattern is clumped but not as dense looking as in the small lymphocyte.
No nucleoli are visible.

Large Lymphocyte

Size: 12 to 16 μm in diameter.

Cytoplasm: Abundant.
Very pale blue.
May or may not contain a few nonspecific azurophilic granules.

Nucleus: Round or oval in shape and may be slightly indented.
Chromatin pattern is coarse.
No nucleoli are visible.
May be eccentrically located.

BIOLOGY AND PHYSIOLOGY OF THE LYMPHOCYTE

The lymphocytes are vital to the immune system. They function in the production of circulating antibodies and in the expression of cellular immunity. The mature lymphocyte has little or no endoplasmic reticulum, only a small Golgi apparatus, possesses only a few mitochondria, and the ribosomes are free and in clusters. Depending upon the functional state of the lymphocyte it may have microvilli projections on its outer surface, or, it may have a relatively smooth outside surface. The nucleus of the lymphocyte usually contains a nucleolus, which, because of the denseness of the nucleus, is generally not visible under light microscopy.

Using special staining procedures, the lymphocyte is negative for chloroacetate esterase, alkaline phosphatase, and peroxidase and is positive for acid phosphatase.

The lymphocyte is actively motile and, during locomotion, has the appearance of a hand mirror. When moving, the nucleus is at the leading end of the cell with the cytoplasm trailing behind, appearing as the handle of the mirror.

THE LYMPHOCYTIC SYSTEM

The lymphocytic system in the adult is comprised of the primary lymphopoietic organs, made up of the bone marrow and thymus, and the secondary, or peripheral, lymphatic system, which includes the lymph nodes, spleen, gut-associated lymphoid tissues (lymph nodules of the intestines, which are also termed *Peyer's patches,* and tonsils), and the blood. The lymph tissue is composed of lymphatic vessels that form a dense network in most of the tissues of the body. The smaller vessels unite with each other to form larger vessels until all of the lymphatic vessels come together and form two main trunks: the right lymphatic duct and the thoracic duct. These two main vessels open into the veins of the neck. Lymph nodes are located along these lymphatic vessels. The contents of the vessels pass through the lymph nodes on their way to the thoracic and lymphatic ducts.

The bone marrow is the body's largest lymphopoietic mass. The source of lymphocyte replacement is the stem cell compartment in the bone marrow. Production of lymphocytes in the bone marrow and thymus is independent of antigenic stimulation and events occuring in other areas of the lymphoid system.

These two organs (bone marrow and thymus) provide the peripheral lymph system with a supply of lymphocytes that can become immunocompetent when stimulated by an antigen. The fate of the lymphocytes produced in the bone marrow varies; some of these cells may serve as lymphocyte stem cells, while some lymphocytes may migrate to the peripheral lymphatic system. Most of the marrow lymphocytes, however, probably die randomly in the bone marrow and serve as building blocks for future generations of lymphocytes. In the thymus, most of the lymphocytes are replaced every 3 to 4 days. A few of these lymphocytes will migrate to thymus-dependent areas of the spleen and lymph nodes, whereas the remainder will die in the thymus or migrate out of the thymus and die elsewhere.

LYMPHOCYTE SUBPOPULATIONS

There are two main functional classes of lymphocytes: B lymphocytes and T lymphocytes. These cells are morphologically similar and cannot be distinguished from each other on a Wright-stained smear.

The B lymphocyte is derived from the bone marrow and was so named because it was originally discovered in birds, where it was programmed by an organ called the bursa of Fabricius. (The equivalent organ in the human is thought to be the bone marrow.) The B lymphocyte migrates from the bone marrow to the peripheral lymphatic tissues where it inter-acts with antigens and differentiates into a plasma cell which secretes immunoglobulins for defense against infections (this is termed *humoral immunity*).

T lymphocytes mature in the thymus and then travel to the peripheral tissues where they interact with antigens to form specific effector cells which act in delayed hypersensitivity reactions, suppression of tumors, graft rejection, and against some intracellular organisms. This is termed *cellular immunity*. The T lymphocytes may also assist in regulating both humoral and cellular immune responses.

A third population of lymphocytes appears to exist which lack the characteristics of the mature T and B lymphocytes, and are termed *null* lymphocytes. The *natural killer* (NK) lymphocytes are thought to be in this group of cells.

LIFE SPAN, CIRCULATION AND RECIRCULATION OF LYMPHOCYTES

The majority of lymphocytes are long-lived, with a life span of about 4 years. Some lymphocytes, however, may live as long as 10 years. The remaining lymphocytes, about 15%, are short-lived, lasting 3 to 4 days.

Those lymphocytes present in the peripheral blood are generally in transit from one lymphoid tissue to another or to sites of inflammation. The lymphocytes have two basic patterns of circulation: (1) There is a recirculation of the mature, differentiated lymphocytes continually moving from one area of the lymphatic system to another. (2) Immature lymphocytes will travel from the bone marrow to the thymus and from there to the peripheral or secondary lymphoid organs. These cells then migrate to thymus-dependent areas in the peripheral lymphatic system and most probably become the long-lived T lymphocytes. They make up most of the recirculating pool of lymphocytes, although both the B and T lymphocytes are able to recirculate and will travel back and forth between the blood, bone marrow, and peripheral lymphoid tissue. They will enter the thymus, however, only from the bone marrow. It is thought that T lymphocytes have their own patterns of recirculation in that some T lymphocytes travel only to the lymph nodes, whereas other T lymphocytes only recirculate to the gut area. Antigenic stimulation will convert short-lived, noncirculating lymphocytes into long-lived, recirculating cells, and during an immune response, the rate of blood flow through the lymph nodes may increase as much as fourfold. The major factor that appears to affect the total number of lymphocytes in the body seems to be the amount of exposure to antigen. Because lymphocytes are capable of blast transformation and mitosis, they can serve as their own stem cell compartment in terms of replacement when needed.

T AND B LYMPHOCYTE CELL MARKERS

As the lymphocyte transforms from the immature stem cell, the characteristics of the B and T lymphocyte surface membranes change according to the cell's degree of maturation and differentiation.

B Cell Differentiation. As the intended B cell matures from the stem cell, the pre-B lymphocyte demonstrates: (1) cytoplasmic immunoglobulins (cIg), primarily the μ chains (termed Cμ), (2) TdT antigen (terminal deoxynucleotidyl transferase), and (3) HLA-DR antigens. The immature B lymphocyte will then begin to show surface membrane immunoglobulin (SIg) and other membrane receptors (Fc and C3), but will lose the TdT antigen and Cμ. Mature B cells have a full range of the surface immunoglobulins, sIgM and sIgD, and continue to retain the HLA-DR antigens. The plasma cell is the final stage in this cell type. These are specific cells for the production and secretion of immunoglobulins (cytoplasmic immunoglobulins [CIg]). These cells generally lack the previously described lymphocyte markers.

Development of the T lymphocyte is also characterized by changes in the sur-

face antigens. The immature T cells show the TdT antigen and have heat stable receptors for sheep erythrocytes. As the cells differentiate into the mature peripheral T lymphocytes they lose the TdT antigen and develop heat labile receptors for sheep erythrocytes. During maturation the T cells develop an Fc receptor for IgM (designated Tμ) and IgG (termed Tγ) which correlates with specific functions. Tμ cells function as *helper* cells, while Tγ cells have *suppressor* and *cytotoxic* functions.

The use of monoclonal antibodies against T cell antigens has allowed further identification of T cell populations: the T4 antigen is common to all helper cells, the T8 antigen is a marker of the suppressor/cytotoxic cells, and the T3 antigen is common to all peripheral T lymphocytes. The most immature T lymphocytes contain the T1, T9 (transferrin receptor), and T10 antigens. As the cell matures, the T9 antigen is lost, and the cells acquire the T4, T8, and T11 antigens. The cells will then differentiate and maintain either the T4 or the T8 antigen. Each group will maintain antigens T1, T10, and T11 and take on the T3 antigen. The mature peripheral T lymphocyte loses the T10 antigen and maintains the antigens T1, 3, 11, and T4 or T8. The ratio of T helper to T suppressor cells is normally about 2:1 and is thought to be an important index in some disease states.

T and B lymphocytes may be identified and differentiated from each other by the identification of characteristic antigens and receptors on their membranes. The cell membranes of the B lymphocytes contain immunoglobulin which may be identified by immunofluorescent techniques. On the other hand, T lymphocytes lack immunoglobulins in their membranes, but do contain (on their membranes) a receptor for sheep erythrocytes (sheep erythrocytes will form rosettes with T lymphocytes [three or more sheep red blood cells attach to the membrane of the T lymphocyte]). Other methods of distinguishing T and B cells from each other use differences in their surface membranes, the employment of monoclonal antibodies, and noting their response to the lectins, pokeweed mitogen and phytohemagglutinin. The class I histocompatibility antigens (HLA-A, -B, -C) are contained on both T and B lymphocytes. The class II antigens (HLA-D), however, are present on resting B cells and only on activated T cells. In addition, antigens termed B1, B2, and B4 have been identified on mature B lymphocytes and their precursors. Almost half of the B lymphocytes possess binding sites for the C3b, C3d, and C4 components of complement.

LYMPHOCYTE FUNCTION

The primary function of the lymphocytes is to provide for the recognition and elimination of foreign pathogens, proteins, and altered cells from the body, and to maintain the body's resistance to these offending agents. If the invading or foreign substances are completely phagocytized and disposed of by phagocytes, an immunologic reaction does not take place. If, however, some of these foreign antigens remain, the lymphocytes become activated.

The B lymphocytes function primarily in *humoral immunity* and are responsible for the synthesis of antibodies. T lymphocytes are responsible for *cell-mediated immunity* and function in delayed hypersensitivity reactions, tumor suppression, graft rejection, and in resistance to some intracellular organisms. There is not a clear cut division in the functions of the T and B lymphocytes, however. The T lymphocytes do play a role in both the cellular and humoral immune responses.

During an immune response the T helper lymphocytes become activated. They, in turn, release factors *(lymphokines)* which activate the B lymphocytes. The B lymphocytes will undergo blast transformation and develop clones of plasma cells which secrete the specific antibody necessary, along with a few long-lived memory cells capable of the same antigen-recognition and proliferation as the original parent cell. Other substances released by the T helper lymphocytes activate the antigen-specific T suppressor and cytotoxic lymphocytes. The suppressor cells will secrete suppressor factors which are antigen-specific. The cytotoxic cells are able to lyse 'target' cells. (There are three types of cytotoxic lymphocytes: cytotoxic T lymphocytes, natural killer (NK) lymphocytes, and killer (K) lymphocytes. The NK and K cells appear to belong to the null group of lymphocytes.)

Numerous lymphokines exist which are secreted by both the T and B lymphocytes during an immune response. Some of these are: (1) *Lymphotoxin* enhances and accelerates the action of 'target' cell lysis by the cytotoxic T lymphocytes. (2) *Migration inhibition factor* (MIF) temporarily immobilizes macrophages. (3) *Macrophage chemotactic factor* is chemotactic for monocytes and macrophages. (4) *Macrophage activation factor* changes normal macrophages into killer cells. (5) *Osteoclast activating factor* causes an increase in the number and activity of osteoclasts. (6) *Interferon* has numerous functions in the host's defense against the spread of viral infections, including the enhancement of the actions of cytotoxic T lymphocytes, macrophages, and natural killer lymphocytes. (7) Other substances secreted cause circulating white cells to marginate along the walls of the blood vessels while chemotactic substances then direct their migration to sites of inflammation. (8) *B cell growth factor* stimulates cell division along with *interleukin-1,* while *B cell differentiation factor* stimulates B cell lymphocyte transformation into plasma cells. (9) *Interleukin-2* causes proliferation of the cytotoxic T lymphocytes.

MORPHOLOGY OF LYMPHOCYTES IN DISEASE

Lymphocytes will undergo transformations when they are stimulated. In the laboratory, under certain in-vitro conditions, the lymphocyte can be made to transform into an immature cell that has the appearance of a blast cell. These cells have increased ribosomes, a well-developed Golgi apparatus, and some endoplasmic reticulum development, in addition to actively synthesizing RNA, DNA, immunoglobulins, and complement components. This is similar to the reactions that occur in the body in response to various disease states such as drug reactions and viral infections. These lymphocytes, when found on the Wright-stained blood smear, are collectively termed *atypical lymphocytes.* Various terms have been used to describe these morphologic changes in the lymphocyte in addition to the broad description of atypical lymphocyte: *virocytes, leukocytoid lymphocytes, reticular lymphocytes, reactive lymphocytes,* and *Türk* cells. Two additional terms used frequently are the *plasmacytoid lymphocyte* and *lymphocytoid plasma cell,* which more correctly describes the intermediate forms of the lymphocyte/plasma cell (the B lymphocyte in the process of developing into a plasma cell). When the lymphocyte is stimulated, the morphologic characteristics of the cell are transformed, and various changes take place. The cell first increases in size, and the nucleus becomes less dense and may show one or more nucleoli. Generally, the cytoplasm becomes basophilic and shows a greater increase in amount than the nucleus. As a B lymphocyte transforms into a plasma cell it also increases in size. The cytoplasm becomes basophilic and may show a lighter-staining area near the nucleus. The nuclear chromatin becomes more coarse and clumped and shows increased areas of parachromatin. Other characteristics exhibited by a stimulated lymphocyte are foamy (holes) or vacuolated cytoplasm, an irregularly shaped nucleus, increased numbers of azurophilic granules in the cytoplasm (normally, approximately one third of the lymphocytes contain these granules), radial and/or peripheral basophilia of the cytoplasm, sharper separation of the nuclear chromatin and parachromatin, and more abundant basophilic cytoplasm than is normally present in the cell. These cells have been separated into three groups by Dr. Hal Downey:

Downey type I: The nucleus may be irregularly shaped. The cytoplasm is relatively basophilic and may at times be foamy.

Downey type II: There is an increased amount of cytoplasm that also contains radial or peripheral basophilia. The nuclear chromatin is generally more coarse and clumped.

Downey type III: This group of cells increases in size and shows basophilic cytoplasm. The nucleus usually has visible nucleoli.

Cells of Acute and Subacute Lymphatic Leukemia

The lymphocytic cells present in acute lymphatic leukemia show several morphologic variations from the normal lymphocyte. The leukemic lymphoblast is slightly larger than the lymphocyte of the circulating blood. It has a thin rim of clear, light blue cytoplasm. The chromatin pattern of the nucleus is delicate and fine but somewhat more coarse than that of the myeloblast. There are usually one to two well-defined nucleoli present. The immature lymphocyte or leukemic prolymphocyte is approximately the same size as the leukemic lymphoblast. It has only a small amount of cytoplasm. The nucleus shows more clumping of the chromatin. Nucleoli are usually visible.

Plasma Cells

Plasmablast

Size: 18 to 25 μm in diameter.

Cytoplasm: Basophilic cytoplasm.
Abundant.
Nongranular.

Nucleus: Nuclear chromatin is more clumped than in the reticular lymphocyte.
Eccentric. (The nucleus is off center, located at one side of the cell.)
Round or oval in shape.
Multiple nucleoli that may or may not be visible.

Proplasmacyte

Size: 15 to 25 μm in diameter.

Cytoplasm: Basophilic; usually bluer than in the blast stage.
Nongranular.
Abundant, but slightly less than in the blast stage.
A lighter staining area in the middle of the cell (in the cytoplasm, next to the nucleus) may become visible. This is termed a *hof*.

Plasmacyte (Plasma Cell) (Fig. 100).

Size: 8 to 20 μm in diameter.

Cytoplasm: Moderately abundant, but less than in the previous stage.
Deeply basophilic.
Hof next to nucleus.
Nongranular, usually.

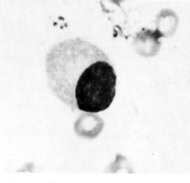

Fig. 100. Plasma cell.

Nucleus: Chromatin is condensed and coarse.
Round or oval in shape.
Eccentric.
No nucleoli are visible.

PLASMA CELLS

The plasma cell represents the end stage of the B lymphocyte. When the mature B lymphocyte is antigenically stimulated, it undergoes transformation first to a blast stage and then develops into a plasma cell. The mature plasma cell contains a Golgi apparatus located in the hof (clear zone or light staining area near the nucleus). The cytoplasm contains a well developed rough endoplasmic reticulum and a few mitochondria. Plasma cells contain no surface immunoglobulin markers.

In certain pathologic states and when manufacturing immunoglobulins, plasma cells may produce striking alterations in their appearance. Some of the changes possible are:
1. Red staining of the cytoplasm *(flame cell)*.
2. Red staining, crystalline, rod shaped bodies present in the cytoplasm.
3. Red staining globules in the cytoplasm *(Russell bodies)*.
4. Globular bodies present in the cytoplasm *(grape, berry,* or *morula cell)*.

The globules present in the cytoplasm are usually perfectly round, and the color may vary from pink, red, blue, or green to colorless. These globules may become so tightly packed as to give a honeycombed appearance. At times, the protein material in the cytoplasm may crystallize, thus giving rise to elongated and pointed structures. Following the secretion of products from the plasma cell, the cytoplasm may have an uneven, tattered appearance to it.

For more details on the plasma cell and immunoglobulins, the reader is referred to the previous section describing B lymphocytes.

MEGAKARYOCYTES

The megakaryoblast develops into the megakaryocyte, which then gives rise to the blood platelet.

Megakaryoblast (Fig. 101).

Size: 20 to 50 μm in diameter.

Cytoplasm: Varying shades of blue. Usually darker than the myeloblast. May have small, blunt pseudopods. Small to moderate amount. Usually a narrow band around the nucleus. As the cell matures, the amount of cytoplasm increases. Usually nongranular.

Nucleus: Round, oval, or may be kidney shaped. Fine chromatin pattern. Multiple nucleoli that generally stain blue.

Promegakaryocyte

Size: 20 to 50 μm in diameter.

Cytoplasm: Usually abundant. Less basophilic than the blast stage. Granules begin to form.

Nucleus: Chromatin becomes more coarse. Multiple nucleoli are visible.

Irregular in shape; may even show slight lobulation.

Megakaryocyte (the largest cell found in the normal bone marrow) (Fig. 102).

Size: 30 to 160 μm in diameter.

Cytoplasm: Abundant. Pinkish blue in color. Very granular. Usually has an irregular peripheral border. The granules begin to aggregate into little bundles that bud off from the cell to become platelets.

Nucleus: Small in comparison to cell size. Multiple nuclei may be visible or the nucleus may show multilobulation. Chromatin is coarser than in the previous stage. No nucleoli are visible.

Platelet (thrombocyte)

Size: 1 to 4 μm in diameter.

Cytoplasm: Light blue to purple. Very granular. Consists of two parts: (1) the *chromomere*, which is granular and located centrally, and (2) the *hyalomere*, which surrounds the chro-

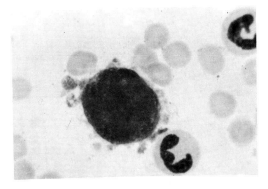

Fig. 101. Megakaryoblast. (Magnification × 1000)

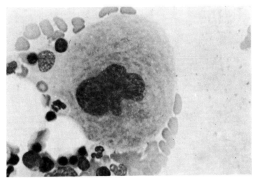

Fig. 102. Megakaryocyte. (Magnification × 500)

momere and is nongranular and clear to light blue.

Nucleus: None present.

MATURATION OF THE MEGAKARYOCYTE

The committed stem cell for the megakaryoblast (CFU-M) most probably arises from the uncommitted hematopoietic stem cell (CFU-C). *Megakaryocyte colony stimulating factor* (MK-CSF) causes the committed stem cells to proliferate, while *thrombopoietin* stimulates differentiation and maturation of the megakaryocytes and also influences their size and thus the number of platelets produced.

The maturation of the megakaryoblast is unique. It is unable to undergo cell division, and, as it matures, the nucleus becomes lobulated and the cytoplasm increases in amount and becomes more granular. Nuclear and cytoplasmic maturation do not occur together or on parallel levels. Initially, the nucleus contains a paired set of chromosomes (termed *diploid*). As the cell begins to mature, DNA synthesis takes place, and the nuclear material duplicates itself, resulting in a two-lobed nucleus in which each nuclear lobe contains a paired set of chromosomes (this process is termed *endomitosis*). The entire nucleus now contains two-paired sets of chromosomes and may be termed 4 N, in which 4 represents the ploidy value of 4 single sets of chromosomes and N stands for nuclear number. The nuclear number generally undergoes further divisions, yielding 4 sets of paired chromosomes (4-lobed nucleus) and is termed 8 N. Further nuclear divisions give rise to 8 sets of paired chromosomes (8-lobed nucleus, or 16 N), then 16 sets of paired chromosomes (16-lobed nucleus, or 32 N), and so on. Another term used to describe the increased numbers of chromosomes over the diploid number is *polyploid.* The majority of mature megakaryocytes in the bone marrow are 16 N (8 nuclear lobes), whereas about 25% are 32 N and a few are

8 N. When the cell has acquired all of its nuclear lobes, the cytoplasm begins to mature, becoming larger in size and more granular. During the entire process of nuclear and cytoplasmic maturation, there is no division of the cytoplasm.

PHYSIOLOGY AND BIOLOGY OF THE MEGAKARYOCYTE

The maturing megakaryocyte contains a Golgi region around the nucleus where specific granules are packed to be distributed throughout the cytoplasm, except at the peripheral borders of the cell, which remain free of granules until platelets begin to form. Polyribosomes and rough endoplasmic reticulum are present at the beginning of cytoplasmic maturation. It takes 4 to 5 days for the megakaryocyte to mature in the bone marrow.

Megakaryocytes, or megakaryocyte fragments, frequently escape from the bone marrow and get into the peripheral blood. They may occasionally be seen on a routine peripheral blood smear, but will more often be found if buffy coat smears are prepared. Megakaryocyte fragments may be seen more frequently in the blood in chronic myelogenous leukemia, various forms of cancer, myelofibrosis, polycythemia vera, Hodgkin's disease, leukocytosis due to infection, and following surgical procedures. The presence of dwarf or micro megakaryocytes indicates an abnormal production, as they are found in myeloproliferative disorders.

PLATELET PRODUCTION

Platelets are produced directly from the megakaryocyte cytoplasm. As the megakaryocyte matures, the granules cluster into small groups, and a network of tubules develops in the cytoplasm, many of which open to the outside of the cell. These tubules fuse to form fissures, which ultimately form the margins and plasma membranes of individual platelets. The megakaryocytes in the bone marrow lie adjacent to the sinus walls. The cytoplasm fragments into individual platelets which are released into the peripheral blood over a period of several hours. The entire megakaryocyte cytoplasm is thus broken away, and the nucleus is left to degenerate and be processed by reticuloendothelial cells. Each megakaryocyte generally produces between 2,000 to 4,000 platelets in this manner. Thus, the platelet is a portion of the megakaryocyte cytoplasm and, as such, contains no nucleus. As a general rule, the more nuclear lobes the megakaryocyte possesses, the larger the cytoplasmic mass, and, therefore, the more platelets that are produced. Increased production of platelets may be accomplished by means of three possible mechanisms: the number of megakaryocytes in the bone marrow may increase, the size of the megakaryocytes may increase, and there may be a decrease in the maturation time of the megakaryocyte. Major platelet production takes place in the bone marrow, where the megakaryocytes make up less than 1% of the nucleated cells of the marrow.

PLATELET LIFE SPAN

Once the platelet is released into the peripheral blood, it has a life span of 9 to 12 days. The young platelets are larger and less dense than older platelets. Also, they are metabolically more active and more effective in hemostasis. At any one time, approximately two thirds of the platelets are in the blood, whereas the remaining one third are in the spleen. The platelets in the spleen are interchangeable with those in the blood. A high percentage of the platelets in the spleen are young platelets. Damaged and nonfunctioning platelets are generally removed from the blood, principally by the spleen. The platelet turnover rate is approximately 35,000 platelets ($\pm 4,300$) per μL each day.

PLATELET STRUCTURE

The circulating platelet is circular to ellipsoidal in shape, 1 to 4 μm in diameter, and has a volume of approximately 6 to 7.5 fL (Fig. 103). It may be divided anatomically into four areas: peripheral zone, sol-gel zone, organelle zone, and the membranous system.

The *peripheral zone* is basically composed of the membranes and is responsible for platelet adhesion (attachment of the platelet to a foreign surface) and aggregation (attachment of the platelets to each other). The platelet membrane originates from the plasma membrane of the megakaryocyte. The peripheral zone may be divided into three areas. The external surface of the platelet has a fuzzy coating, termed the *glycocalyx* (1), and is primarily composed of glycoproteins. It is important in platelet reactions with thrombin, von Willebrand factor, and fibrinogen. The *plasma membrane* (2) lies directly beneath the glycocalyx and is composed of asymmetrically distributed phospholipids. The third portion of this zone is a sub-membranous area where messages from the external membrane are translated into chemical signals causing activation and a physical change in the platelet. A number of platelet membrane receptor sites have been identified for ADP, collagen, serotonin, epinephrine, thrombin, von Willebrand factor, and factors V and Xa.

The *sol-gel zone* lies directly beneath the platelet membrane and is composed of *microfilaments* (3) and *microtubules* (4). They help to maintain platelet shape and are thought to contain the proteins actin and myosin which, upon stimulation of the platelet, will interact to form actomyosin *(thrombosthenin)*, a contractile protein, important in clot retraction.

The *organelle zone* is composed of the mitochondria, alpha granules, dense bodies, and a lysosomal type granule. The *alpha granules* (5) are the most numerous and contain a number of substances including platelet factor 4, β thromboglobulin, platelet derived growth factor (mitogenic factor), thrombospodin, von Willebrand factor, fibrinogen, fibronectin,

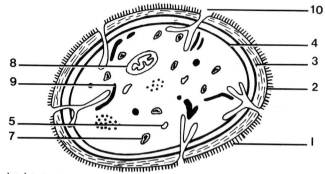

Fig. 103. Normal platelet structure.

and factor V. The *lysosomal type granules* (7) contain ADP, ATP, calcium, serotonin, and pyrophosphate, and play an important role in platelet aggregation. The *mitochondria* (8) are important for ATP synthesis.

The *membranous system* is composed of the *dense tubular system* (9) and the *surface connecting system* (10). The dense tubular system is derived from smooth endoplasmic reticulum and sequesters (holds) calcium for platelet activation processes. It also synthesizes prostaglandin. The surface connecting system acts as a canal for the release of the granule constituents and cytoplasm to the exterior of the platelet. This system is also involved in platelet phagocytosis.

The platelet is composed of about 60% protein, 30% lipid, 8% carbohydrate, various minerals, water, and nucleotides. It contains over ninety different enzymes. Other proteins present include glycoproteins and coagulation factors. Fibrinogen, along with most of the other coagulation factors, has been demonstrated in association with the platelet. In addition, the platelet is able to synthesize amino acids, proteins, fatty acids, and phospholipids, and glycogen is the main carbohydrate present. The platelet has an active energy metabolism, using glucose as its main energy source.

PLATELET FUNCTION

Platelets function primarily in hemostasis (the stoppage of bleeding) and in main-

taining capillary integrity. (This is discussed in greater detail in Chapter 5.)

WHITE BLOOD CELL AND PLATELET MORPHOLOGY

In **toxic granulation** (Plate IVa), dark blue-black cytoplasmic granules are seen in the neutrophil. These are thought to be primary granules and show increased alkaline phosphatase activity. They are found in acute infections, drug poisoning, and burns.

Döhle bodies (Plate IVb) appear as a small, light blue staining area in the cytoplasm of the neutrophil. The blue staining area is rough endoplasmic reticulum containing RNA and may represent localized failure of the cytoplasm to mature. They are found in infections, poisoning, burns, and following chemotherapy.

Hypersegmented neutrophils (Plate IVc) are neutrophils with a six- or more, lobed nucleus. This represents an abnormality in the maturation of the neutrophil and may be acquired (as in megaloblastic erythropoiesis) or inherited *(Undritz anomaly)*. Normally, approximately 50 to 60% of the neutrophils contain three lobes, no more than 20% have four lobes, and there may be an occasional five-lobed neutrophil. Any time there is an increased percentage of four- and/or five-lobed neutrophils present, hypersegmentation should be reported. In cases of pernicious anemia and folic acid deficiency, neutrophils with more than five lobes are commonly found. Hypersegmented neutrophils are also found in chronic infections. The **Barr** (sex chromatin) **body** (Plate IVd) represents the second X chromosome in females and may be seen in 2 to 3% of the neutrophils in females. It is a small, well-defined, round projection of nuclear chromatin that is connected to the nucleus of the neutrophil by a single, fine strand of chromatin. The Barr body can be differentiated from small, nonspecific nodules of chromatin in that these projections are not attached to the nucleus with as fine a strand of chromatin. The number of Barr bodies in a cell is one less than the number of X chromosomes present in a cell. Another term used to describe the Barr body is a *drumstick.* These chromatin bodies are not found in normal males.

Degenerated neutrophil with pyknotic nucleus (Plate IVe) results from condensation of nuclear chromatin to a solid, structureless mass with no pattern. These cells are not counted in a differential cell count.

A **vacuolated neutrophil** (Plate IIIr) results when the degenerating cytoplasm begins to acquire holes or as the result of active phagocytosis (may reflect increased lysosomal activity). This condition may be found in septicemia and severe infection.

Giant neutrophils may be seen occasionally in a normal peripheral blood smear. These cells are much larger than normal neutrophils and are generally hyperlobulated. They may be found normally in a frequency of about 1 in every 20,000 neutrophils but may increase somewhat in frequency in disease states.

Pelger-Huët anomaly (Plate V e, f, g) is indicated by failure of the neutrophil nucleus to segment properly. All of the neutrophils have no more than a bi-lobed nucleus. The nuclear chromatin is coarsely clumped. This benign anomaly may be inherited or acquired, as in certain leukemias. A person heterozygous for this characteristic shows numerous bi-lobed (dumbbell-shaped) nuclei, whereas the homozygous person has round neutrophil nuclei. The neutrophils in this anomaly appear to function normally.

Chédiak-Higashi syndrome (Plate V a, b) is a rare, fatal disorder found in children. It is inherited as an autosomal recessive characteristic. The granulocytes usually contain several large, reddish-purple staining granules in the cytoplasm, whereas they stain bluish purple in the lymphocytes and monocytes. The lymphocytes and monocytes may contain several of these granules or they may contain only a single large granule. These granules represent abnormal lysosomes. Anemia, neutropenia and thrombocytopenia generally develop. Patients with this condition show increased susceptibility to infection.

Alder-Reilly anomaly (Plate IV f) shows heavy azurpohilic granulation of the neutrophils, eosinophils, basophils, and sometimes, the lymphocytes and monocytes. This is an inherited condition and is commonly associated with Hurler's syndrome and Hunter's syndrome.

May-Hegglin anomaly is an inherited anomaly affecting the neutrophils and platelets. Döhle-like inclusion bodies are present in the neutrophils. Bizarre platelets are present, and the platelets may be decreased in number. Some patients are asymptomatic, whereas others may exhibit bleeding tendencies. Platelet function may be abnormal.

Auer rods (Plate Vh) are rod-like bodies that stain a reddish purple. They are found only in the cytoplasm of the blast cells in acute monocytic or acute myelogenous leukemia.

Smudge or **basket cell** (Plate IV j, k) is the disintegrating nucleus of a ruptured white blood cell.

Atypical platelets (Plate III o, p), abnormal in appearance, occur in some diseased states. In such cases, the platelet may have one or more of the following characteristics:

1. Large size.
2. Increased amount of hyalomere.

3. Granules decreased or absent.

4. Zoned appearance.

Platelet satellitosis (platelets encircling the peripheral borders of neutrophils) is seen in a rare patient whose blood is anticoagulated with EDTA. This phenomenon is thought to be due to a serum factor which reacts in the presence of EDTA.

THE RETICULOENDOTHELIAL SYSTEM

The cells comprising the reticuloendothelial system (RES) are the reticulum cells of the lymph nodes and spleen, the Küpffer cells in the sinusoids of the liver, the blood monocytes (since they transform into tissue or fixed macrophages), and the sinusoid cells of the lymph nodes, bone marrow, adrenal gland, and pituitary gland. The reticuloendothelial system is of considerable size and is based on the ability of the cells to engulf particulate matter and damaged or dead cells. The macrophages may quickly kill and digest bacteria or red blood cells or may indefinitely store some particles. In this manner, the RE system functions as a cellular and immunologic defense system. Cells of the RE system also function to clear intravascular fibrin, to conserve and utilize hemoglobin iron, and to neutralize endotoxins.

3

Routine Hematology Procedures

COMPLETE BLOOD COUNT

In most laboratories the complete blood count (CBC) consists of the white blood cell count, the hemoglobin, hematocrit, and red blood cell count. Also included are the red blood cell indices, which give the average red blood cell size and the relative and absolute values for the amount of hemoglobin in the average red blood cell. The last test in the CBC is the differential, in which the different white blood cells present are classified, detailed information about the appearance of the red blood cells is given, and the platelets are reviewed for number and morphologic features. The importance of the CBC cannot be underestimated. In addition to being a screening procedure, it is helpful in the diagnosis of many diseases, it is used to reflect the body's ability to fight disease, it is utilized to monitor the effects of drug and radiation therapy on the blood/bone marrow, and it is employed as an indicator of the patient's progress in certain diseased states such as infection or anemia.

HEMOGLOBIN

The measurement of hemoglobin, along with the hematocrit (and reticulocyte count), is used to follow the treatment of anemias.

The normal values for hemoglobin in the peripheral blood vary with the age and sex of the individual. (Altitude also plays a role in that the normal hemoglobin concentration for persons at high altitudes is higher than for those individuals living at sea level.) At birth, the hemoglobin concentration is normally in the range of 17 to 23 g/dL. This value decreases to about 9 to 14 g/dL at 2 months. By 10 years of age, the normal hemoglobin is between 12 and 14 g/dL. Normal adult values range from 13 to 15 g/dL for women and from 14 to 17 g/dL for men. There is a slight decrease in the hemoglobin level after 50 years of age.

Cyanmethemoglobin Method

REAGENTS AND EQUIPMENT

1. Cyanmethemoglobin (hemiglobin-cyanide (HiCN) reagent. Contains potassium cyanide and potassium ferricyanide. This reagent also contains either dihydrogen potassium phosphate (KH_2PO_4) or sodium bicarbonate ($NaHCO_3$) which aids in red cell lysis and also decreases turbidity due to lipoproteins. Store reagent in a brown bottle at room temperature where it is stable for several months. This reagent may be obtained commercially.
2. Test tubes, 13 × 100 mm.
3. Pipets, 0.02 mL, or, Sahli pipets.
4. Spectrophotometer.

79

SPECIMEN

Whole blood, using EDTA as the anticoagulant. Capillary blood may also be used.

PRINCIPLE

Whole blood is added to cyanmethemoglobin (HiCN) reagent (containing potassium cyanide and potassium ferricyanide). The ferricyanide converts the hemoglobin iron from the ferrous state (Fe^{++}) to the ferric state (Fe^{+++}) to form methemoglobin (Hi) which then combines with potassium cyanide to form the stable pigment, cyanmethemoglobin (HiCN). (Hi = hemiglobin = hemoglobin in which the iron has been oxidized to the ferric state. HiCN = hemiglobin cyanide = Hi which has been banded to the cyanide ions.) The color intensity of this mixture is measured in a spectrophotometer at a wavelength of 540 nm. The optical density of the solution is proportional to the concentration of hemoglobin. All forms of hemoglobin are measured with this method except sulfhemoglobin.

PROCEDURE

1. For each patient to be tested, place exactly 5.0 mL of HiCN reagent into an appropriately labeled test tube. Place 5.0 mL of the reagent into a test tube to be used as the blank.
2. Add 0.02 mL of well-mixed whole blood (or capillary blood) to the appropriately labeled tube. Rinse the pipet 3 to 5 times with the HiCN reagent until all blood is removed from the pipet.
3. Mix the preceding solutions well and allow to stand at room temperature for at least 3 to 15 minutes (see #1 under Discussion) to allow adequate time for the formation of HiCN.
4. Transfer the mixture to a cuvette and read in a spectrophotometer at a wavelength of 540 nm using the HiCN reagent in the blank tube to set the optical density (O.D.) at 0.0. Record the readings for the patient samples from the O.D. scale and refer to the precalibrated chart for the actual value of the hemoglobin in g/dL.

DISCUSSION

1. If the HiCN reagent contains KH_2PO_4, the final mixture should stand for 3 minutes before reading. If $NaHCO_3$ is used in the reagent, allow at least 15 minutes for complete red cell lysis and HiCN formation before reading on the spectrophotometer.
2. Before the unknown sample is read, the solution must be crystal clear. If any turbidity is present, a falsely elevated result is obtained. Clouding may be due to:
   a. An exceptionally high white blood cell count. (In such cases, centrifuge the mixture and use the supernatant as the test sample.)
   b. Hemoglobin S and hemoglobin C. (Dilute the mixture 1:1 with distilled water, read on the spectrophotometer, and multiply the result by 2.)
   c. Lipemic blood. (Add 0.01 mL of the patient's plasma to 5.0 mL of HiCN reagent and use this mixture for the patient blank.)
3. Over-anticoagulation of the blood does not affect the hemoglobin results.
4. The HiCN reagent should have an O.D. reading of 0.0 when measured on a spectrophotometer at a wavelength of 540 nm, against a water blank.

Preparation of a Standard Hemoglobin Curve

Using the stock solution of HiCN standard, set up at least 4 dilutions according to the directions received with the reagent, or as shown in Table 2.

Using graph paper, plot hemoglobin in g/dL on the abscissa (horizontal axis)

TABLE 2.   DILUTIONS FOR A HEMOGLOBIN CURVE

TUBE	HiCN REAGENT	STOCK STANDARD	CONCENTRATION OF HEMOGLOBIN
1	0.0 mL	5.0 mL	100% of assay value of hgb standard
2	1.0 mL	4.0 mL	80% of assay value of hgb standard
3	2.0 mL	3.0 mL	60% of assay value of hgb standard
4	3.0 mL	2.0 mL	40% of assay value of hgb standard

against O.D. on the ordinate (vertical axis)—this is a straight line curve. (If % transmittance is read, use semilogarithmic graph paper and plot as for O.D. This will also be a straight line curve.) A chart should then be made to facilitate reading the test results.

Abnormal Hemoglobin Pigments

If hemoglobin is converted to an abnormal hemoglobin pigment, it is no longer capable of oxygen transport and, if this impairment is severe enough, a condition of hypoxia or cyanosis occurs. The three abnormal hemoglobin pigments of most significance are discussed briefly below.

1. *Carboxyhemoglobin* is formed by the combination of hemoglobin with carbon monoxide. The hemoglobin molecule has a much greater affinity for carbon monoxide than for oxygen and, therefore, readily combines with carbon monoxide, even when it is present in low concentrations. The formation of carboxyhemoglobin is reversible. It is found in the blood of tobacco smokers in concentrations of 1 to 10%.
2. *Methemoglobin* is a type of hemoglobin in which the ferrous ion has been oxidized to the ferric state and is, therefore, incapable of combining with or transporting the oxygen molecule which is replaced by a hydroxyl radical. Methemoglobin formation is reversible and is normally present in the blood in concentrations of 1 to 2%.
3. *Sulfhemoglobin* is not normally found in the blood. When it is present, its formation is irreversible, and

it remains for the life of the carrier red blood cell. Its exact nature is unknown, but it is thought to be formed by the action of certain drugs and chemicals such as sulfonamides and aromatic amines. It is incapable of transporting oxygen.

HEMATOCRIT

When anticoagulated whole blood is centrifuged, the space occupied by the packed red blood cells is termed the *hematocrit* reading and is expressed as the % of red blood cells in a volume of whole blood. It is also, less commonly, known as the *PCV* (packed [red] cell volume). The values for the hematocrit closely parallel the values for the hemoglobin and red blood cell count.

When whole blood is centrifuged, the heavier particles fall to the bottom of the tube and the lighter particles (white blood cells and platelets) precipitate out on top of them as shown in Figure 104. When reading the hematocrit, it is important to take the reading at the top of the red blood cell layer. This is most significant in cases in which there is an extremely elevated white blood cell or platelet count. The

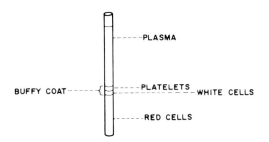

Fig. 104.   Cell layers in centrifuged whole blood.

white blood cell and platelet layers comprise the *buffy coat*.

As with the hemoglobin and the red blood cell count, the normal values for the hematocrit vary with the age and sex of the individual. Altitude also plays a role in that the normal hematocrit for residents at high altitudes is higher than that of individuals living at sea level, due to decreased concentration of oxygen in the air. At birth, the normal range for the hematocrit is 50 to 62%. This range decreases to 37 to 45% by 1 year of age. The normal hematocrit value gradually increases to the adult levels of 36 to 48% for women and 39 to 55% for men. There is a slight decrease in the hematocrit level after 50 years of age. The hematocrit is decreased in anemia and increased in the various forms of polycythemia. It is also used to calculate the MCV and the MCHC (RBC indices).

Microhematocrit Method

REAGENTS AND EQUIPMENT

1. Microhematocrit tube, approximately 75 mm long with an inner bore of approximately 1.2 mm (Fig. 105). Commercially obtained microhematocrit tubes are generally color coded and show a blue ring (at the end of the tube) if the tube contains no anticoagulant, and a red ring if it contains anticoagulant (heparin). If anticoagulated whole blood is used, the blue-tipped microhematocrit tube should be used. If capillary

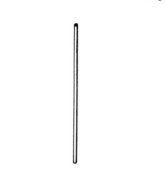

Fig. 105. Capillary hematocrit tube.

blood is employed, the red-tipped microhematocrit tube should be used.
2. Clay-like sealing compound, to seal one end of the microhematocrit tube.
3. Microhematocrit centrifuge capable of producing an RCF of 10,000 to 15,000 g. The centrifuge should be able to reach maximum speed within 30 seconds of starting.
4. Microhematocrit tube reader.

SPECIMEN

Whole blood using disodium ethylenediaminetetraacetic acid (Na_2EDTA) as the anticoagulant. (The tripotassium salt of EDTA [K_3EDTA] is thought to possibly cause a small amount of shrinkage of the red blood cells.) Capillary blood should be collected in the red tipped microhematocrit tubes (containing heparin).

PRINCIPLE

Whole blood is centrifuged for maximum red blood cell packing. The space occupied by the red blood cells is measured and expressed as a percentage of the whole blood volume.

PROCEDURE

1. Allow the capillary or well-mixed anticoagulated whole blood to enter two microhematocrit tubes until they are approximately two-third's filled with blood. (Air bubbles denote poor technique but do not affect the results of the test.)
2. Seal one end of the microhematocrit tube with the clay material by placing the dry end of the tube into the clay in a vertical position (the microhematocrit tube forms a 90° angle with the tray of clay). The plug should be 4 to 6 mm long. Make certain blood is not forced out the top of the microhematocrit tube during this process.
3. Place the two microhematocrit tubes in the radial grooves of the centrifuge

head exactly opposite each other, with the sealed end away from the center of the centrifuge.

4. Centrifuge for 5 minutes.

5. Remove the hematocrit tubes as soon as the centrifuge has stopped spinning. Obtain the results for both microhematocrits, using the microhematocrit tube reading device. Results should agree within ±2% of the hematocrit result. If they do not, repeat the preceding procedure.

DISCUSSION

1. Incomplete sealing of the microhematocrit tubes generally give falsely low results since, as the tubes spin, there is a greater loss of red blood cells than of plasma.

2. Inadequate centrifugation of the microhematocrit tubes or allowing the tubes to stand longer than 10 minutes after centrifugation, yields falsely elevated values. The time and speed of centrifugation are extremely important to obtain maximum red blood cell packing. To determine the maximum packing time of the microhematocrit centrifuge, perform the microhematocrit procedure on two different blood samples, centrifuging them for 2 minutes. Read and record results. Prepare two more microhematocrits from the same blood samples and centrifuge for 2½ minutes. Read and record results. Repeat this procedure, increasing the centrifugation time by ½ minute each time until the hematocrit reading remains the same for two consecutive time periods. One of the two samples should have a hematocrit of >50%. Two sets of consistent readings should be obtained with 3 to 5 minutes of centrifugation.

3. If blood is overanticoagulated, the hematocrit reading will be falsely low due to shrinkage of the red blood cells.

4. When the microhematocrit is spun for the correct time period and at the proper speed, a small amount of plasma still remains in the red blood cell portion. This is termed *trapped plasma.* When comparing spun microhematocrit results with hematocrit results obtained from an electronic cell counter, the spun hematocrit results are generally 1.3 to 3% higher due to this trapped plasma (unless the cell counter has been calibrated against spun microhematocrits uncorrected for trapped plasma). An increased amount of trapped plasma is found in macrocytic anemias, spherocytosis, thalassemia, hypochromic anemias, and sickle cell anemia (the amount of trapped plasma increases as the % of affected sickle shaped red blood cells increases).

5. For accurate results, anticoagulated blood samples should be centrifuged within 6 hours of collection when the blood is stored at room temperature.

6. It is recommended that heat sealing of the microhematocrit tubes not be used since it is difficult to obtain a flat sealing of the tube and the heat may cause damage to the red blood cells.

7. A macrohematocrit method for determining the packed red blood cell volume has been used in the past, but this method is of little use today since it is more time consuming, requires large amounts of blood, and contains a higher degree of plasma trapping. In this method, a Wintrobe tube, calibrated from 0 to 100, is filled with blood and centrifuged at 2000 to 2300 g for 30 minutes. The ratio of the volume of the red blood cells to the total volume of blood is then determined and reported as the hematocrit reading.

BLOOD CELL COUNTS

Units of Reporting

The International Committee for Standardization in Hematology has recommended that all units of volume be measured in liters (L). In terms of cell counts this means that these tests are expressed as the number of cells or formed elements (e.g., platelets, white blood cells, red blood cells) per liter of blood. The previous, traditional unit of reporting was cubic millimeters (cu mm, or, mm³). Since the difference between 1 cu mm and 1 microliter (μL) (1 cu mm = 1.00003 μL) is felt to be insignificant, 1 μL is considered equivalent to 1 cu mm. Therefore:

$$1 \text{ cu mm} = 1 \text{ μL} = 10^{-6} \text{ liters}$$
$$1 \times 10^6 \text{ μL} = 1 \text{ liter}$$

A white blood count of $6{,}500 \times 10^6$/liter =

6.5×10^9/L
6.5×10^3/μL (or, 6,500/μL)
6.5×10^3/cu mm (or, 6,500/cu mm)

THE UNOPETTE SYSTEM

The Unopette System affords the technologist a method for collecting and testing micro blood specimens for hematology. The Unopette may also be used for diluting and/or staining the specimen once it is in the laboratory, preparatory to testing. This system is a method for standardizing the pipetting and diluting of specimens.

The standard Unopette (Fig. 106) is made up of the following parts:

1. The *reservoir* contains a premeasured volume of diluting fluid and is sealed by a thin covering of plastic (*diaphragm*) located in the neck of the reservoir.
2. The *pipet* is self-filling and is available in various sizes (3 μL, 3.3 μL, 10 μL, 20 μL, 25 μL, and 44.7 μL), depending on the procedure to be performed. Each pipet is color coded according to its size. The end opposite the pipet tip is termed the *overflow chamber.*
3. The *pipet shield* protects the pipet and is also utilized to puncture the reservoir diaphragm just prior to use.

PROCEDURE

1. Immediately before use, remove the pipet from the pipet shield. Using the pointed end of the pipet shield, pierce the reservoir diaphragm firmly, inserting the shield as far as possible to obtain an opening large enough for the pipet.
2. Holding the pipet almost horizontal (about a 15° angle above the horizontal), touch the tip of the pipet to the blood sample. The pipet will automatically fill by capillary action. When the sample reaches the neck of the pipet, no more blood will enter. (If the pipet is tilted too low, or below the horizontal, it will overfill.) Carefully wipe excess blood from the outside of the pipet without removing any blood from inside the pipet tip. Place index finger firmly over the top of the overflow chamber.
3. Squeeze the reservoir slightly (do not lose any liquid) with other hand. With the pipet in a vertical position (finger covering the overflow chamber), carefully place the pipet into the reservoir and seat it firmly in the neck of the reservoir.
4. Release the pressure on the reservoir and index finger from the overflow chamber. The sample will be drawn from the pipet into the diluting fluid. Squeeze and release the reservoir several times in order to remove all blood from the pipet. (This must be done carefully to prevent the diluted sample from escaping through the top of the overflow chamber.)
5. Place index finger over the overflow chamber and invert the reservoir several times in order to completely mix the dilution.
6. Immediately prior to performing the test, carefully mix the dilution by in-

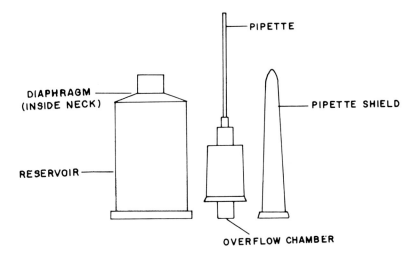

Fig. 106. Unopette.

verting the reservoir several times. In between mixing, rinse the pipet several times (by carefully squeezing the reservoir) in case some of the sample entered the pipet upon standing.

7. Any one of several methods may be used to remove the diluted sample from the reservoir, dependent upon the test being performed.

   a. For cell counting, as soon as the sample is well mixed, squeeze the reservoir, forcing the diluted sample up into (but not out of) the overflow chamber. Place index finger over the pipet (top of overflow chamber) and remove from the reservoir. The sample will drain from the pipet upon removal or partial removal of the index finger from the top of the overflow chamber.

   b. The reservoir may be converted into a dropper assembly by removing the pipet and replacing it in the reservoir in a reverse position, with the overflow chamber seated firmly in the neck of the reservoir. In this method, the diluted sample may then be completely expelled from the reservoir by squeezing, or this method

may be used in performing cell counts, in which case, the first three or four drops would be expelled from the reservoir and then the counting chamber filled by gentle squeezing of the reservoir.

   c. If the entire diluted sample is to be removed from the reservoir, the pipet may be removed and the reservoir inverted and squeezed to expel the entire contents through the neck of the reservoir.

8. To store a diluted sample, the pipet shield may be installed on the top of the overflow chamber (of the pipet), or the pipet may be removed from the reservoir, and the tip of the pipet shield inserted firmly into the reservoir opening.

DISCUSSION

1. Specific Unopettes are available for the following manual procedures: red blood cell count, white blood cell count, platelet count, hemoglobin, reticulocyte count, eosinophil count, and the red blood cell fragility test. Unopettes are also available for automated counting: red blood cell count and white blood cell count (Coulter Counter Models A, B, F, Fn,

and ZBI, and the Fisher Autocytometer), platelet count (Coulter Counter Models F, Fn, ZBI, and Thrombocounter, and the Technicon Autocounter System), and microdilutions on the Coulter Counter Model S and Coulter Counter Model S Plus. A collection system is also available for the blood lead and the sodium and potassium determination (by flame photometer).

WHITE BLOOD CELL COUNT

The white blood cell count (WBC) denotes the number of white blood cells in 1 liter (L) of whole blood. In a normal, healthy individual, the WBC falls in the range of 4,500 to 11,000 × 10^6/L (or 4.5 to 11.0 × 10^9/L). This count varies with age. The WBC of a newborn baby is 10.0 to 30.0 × 10^9/L at birth. It decreases to about 12.0 × 10^9/L after about the first week and drops to normal levels by about 21 years of age.

The WBC is a useful measurement to the physician. It is utilized to indicate infection and may also be employed to follow the progress of certain diseases. The WBC may be elevated in bacterial infections, appendicitis, leukemia, pregnancy, hemolytic disease of the newborn, uremia, ulcers, and normally at birth. The WBC may drop below normal values in viral diseases (such as measles), brucellosis, typhoid fever, infectious hepatitis, rheumatoid arthritis, cirrhosis of the liver, and lupus erythematosus. Radiation or drug therapy tends to lower the WBC. In these cases, patients have white counts done while receiving therapy to ensure that the WBC does not become too low. A white count above 11.0 × 10^9/L is termed *leukocytosis;* a white count below normal is known as *leukopenia.* The white count in children usually shows a greater variation during disease. For example, during infection, a child's WBC reaches much higher elevations than does an adult's white count in response to a corresponding infection. An

individual's normal WBC is subject to variations, being slightly higher in the afternoon than in the morning. There is also an increase in the WBC following strenuous exercise, emotional stress, and anxiety.

Two methods are currently used to determine the WBC. The older method is the manual, or microscopic, method. Over the past 20 to 30 years, there has been a changeover to the electronic method of counting white blood cells. The manual WBC is discussed in this section. Please refer to Chapter 7, Automation, for electronic methods of counting blood cells.

Manual White Blood Cell Count

The following procedure for the manual WBC is presented in detail. The techniques outlined are the same as those employed in the manual red blood cell count, platelet count, and direct eosinophil count. Therefore, these detailed methods are presented only once. Familiarize yourself with this procedure before progressing to the other manual counts outlined later in this chapter. It takes many attempts before these techniques are mastered, but do not be discouraged.

REAGENTS AND EQUIPMENT

1. White count pipet and aspirator (Fig. 107). A Stop-it mouthpiece (Fig. 108) (obtainable from Medical Device Division, Gelman Sciences, Inc., Ann Arbor, Michigan) may be used in place of the regular mouthpiece. This safety device contains a Gelman microporous membrane that will prevent the passage of aqueous liquids through it. Air passes through the membrane so that it does not interfere with pipetting. (Vapors from strong acids, bases, or solvents may penetrate the filter and make it ineffective.) Alternatively, the WBC Unopette (1:20 dilution) may be used.

2. White count diluting fluid. Any one

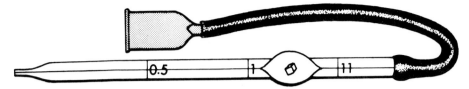

Fig. 107. White count pipet with aspirator.

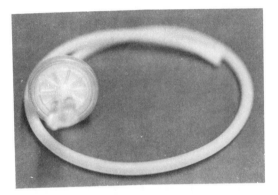

Fig. 108. Stop-it mouthpiece and aspirator.

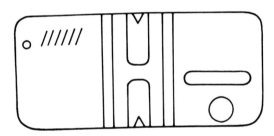

Fig. 109. Neubauer hemocytometer.

of the following diluting fluids may be used:

a. Acetic acid, 2% v/v, in distilled water.

b. Hydrochloric acid, 1% v/v, in distilled water.

c. Turk's diluting fluid.

Glacial acetic acid	3 mL
Aqueous gentian violet, 1% w/v	1 mL
Distilled water	100 mL

Note: If the WBC Unopette is used, diluting fluid is unnecessary since it is contained in the Unopette.

3. Microscope.

4. Clean gauze or Kimwipes.

5. Hemocytometer (counting chamber) (Fig. 109) with coverglass.

   a. The hemocytometer with Neubauer ruling consists of two raised platforms.

   b. There is a raised ridge on both sides of the two platforms on which a cover glass is placed.

   c. The space between the top of the platform and the cover glass over it is 0.1 mm (Fig. 110).

   d. Each of the platforms contains a ruled area composed of nine large squares of equal size (Fig. 111). The entire ruled area of the platform (nine large squares) is 3 mm wide and 3 mm long, each large square measuring 1 mm by 1 mm.

   e. The volume of the entire ruled area on one platform is 0.9 μL. The volume of one large square is 0.1 μL.

   f. The four large corner squares, each of which is subdivided into sixteen smaller squares, are labeled 'W' and are the 4 squares used for counting white blood cells.

All hemocytometers used in the clinical laboratory must meet the specifications of the National Bureau of Standards (NBS) and are identified by those initials.

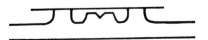

Fig. 110. Neubauer hemocytometer (side view).

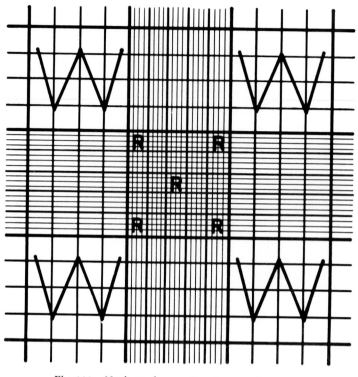

Fig. 111. Neubauer hemocytometer, counting area.

SPECIMEN

Whole blood, using EDTA as the anticoagulant. Capillary blood may also be used.

PRINCIPLE

Whole blood is mixed with a weak acid solution to dilute the blood and hemolyze the red blood cells.

PROCEDURE

1. Dilution of blood (using a white count pipet).
   a. Mix the specimen of blood for approximately 1 minute. Using the aspirator and white cell pipet, draw the blood up to the 0.5 mark in the pipet. It is permissible for the blood to go slightly beyond the 0.5 mark. (If the blood is drawn up too far beyond this mark, however, the dilution is inaccurate, because a small amount of blood continues to adhere to the inside of the stem when the excess blood is withdrawn from the pipet.)
   b. Remove the blood from the outside of the pipet with a clean gauze or Kimwipe. Be careful that the material does not withdraw any blood from the stem of the pipet. Place a nonabsorbent material to the end of the pipet, bringing the blood down to exactly the 0.5 mark. (If an absorbent material is used to remove the excess blood from the stem, the material tends to absorb the liquid portion of the blood and, therefore, the blood will have a higher concentration of cells.)
   c. Holding the pipet almost vertically, place the tip of the pipet into the white count diluting fluid. Draw the diluting fluid into

the pipet slowly, while gently rotating the pipet with your hand to ensure a proper amount of mixing. Aspirate the diluting fluid until the mixture reaches the 11 mark. (If the level of blood falls below the 0.5 mark at any time during this step, repeat the entire procedure, beginning with a clean pipet. Use fresh diluting fluid if any blood has dropped into the bottle, contaminating the fluid. If the pipet has not been held in a vertical position while aspirating the diluting fluid, air bubbles may form in the bulb. If this occurs, the dilution is inaccurate, and the procedure must be repeated, using a clean pipet. It is permissible for the level of the mixture to go slightly above or below the 11 mark.)

d. Place the pipet in a horizontal position and firmly hold the index finger of either hand over the opening in the tip of the pipet. Detach the aspirator from the other end of the pipet.

e. The dilution of blood is now complete. The white cell pipet is divided into units or volumes: 0.5, 1.0, and 11 (refer to the diagram of the white cell pipet, if necessary). The stem contains 1.0 unit and the bulb holds 10 units. The blood is drawn up into the pipet first. As the diluting fluid is aspirated, all of the blood is drawn up into the bulb. Therefore, if the blood is drawn up to the 0.5 mark and diluted to the 11 mark, there is 0.5 volumes of blood and 9.5 volumes of diluting fluid in the bulb of the pipet, for a total of 10 volumes. The stem contains the last 1.0 volume of diluting fluid and contains no blood. The dilution of blood is, therefore, 0.5 in 10, or a 1:20 dilution.

f. Repeat the preceding procedure on the same blood sample so that there are two white count dilutions on the same specimen of blood.

2. Dilution of blood (using the WBC Unopette). Make duplicate dilutions of well mixed whole blood using two WBC Unopettes. Follow the procedure outlined in the Unopette section.

3. Clean the counting chamber and cover glass with a clean, lint free cloth. The use of 95% (v/v) ethanol also facilitates the cleaning process. Carefully replace the cover glass on top of the ruled area of the counting chamber.

4. Mix the diluted white blood cell counts for approximately 3 minutes to ensure hemolysis of the red blood cells and adequate mixing. This may be done with a mechanical shaker. If there is no shaker available to mix the dilution in the WBC pipet, place your thumb over the tip of the pipet and your middle finger over the other end of the pipet. Moving your hand only, mix the pipet in the direction shown in Figure 112. If the WBC Unopette is used, follow the instructions outlined in that section for mixing the Unopette dilution.

5. Filling the counting chamber.

a. Using the WBC pipet, hold the pipet in a vertical position with the right index finger covering the top of the pipet. Discard the first four drops of the mixture onto a piece of gauze. (If the WBC Unopette is used, refer to that section for this step of the procedure.)

b. Remove any excess liquid from the outside of the pipet with a piece of gauze.

c. Using the right index finger to control the rate of flow, place the tip of the pipet on the edge of the ruled area of the counting cham-

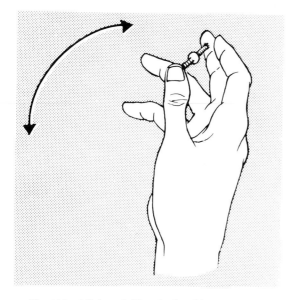

Fig. 112. Mixing of diluted white blood cell count.

ber. Allow the mixture to seep under the cover glass gradually and exactly fill this area. (If the pipet is removed just before the area looks filled, the area will fill without becoming flooded.) Care should be taken not to move the cover glass. (Steps 5a, b, and c must be done quickly so that the white blood cells in the mixture do not begin to settle out. Figure 113 illustrates the proper and improper filling of the counting chamber. If the counting chamber is filled improperly, reclean the counting chamber and cover

glass. If there is enough diluted blood remaining in the white cell pipet, remix, expel three drops of the mixture, and refill the counting chamber. Otherwise, repeat the entire procedure beginning at step 1.)

  d. Fill the opposite side of the counting chamber with the second white count dilution.

  e. When the counting chamber is filled, care should be taken that it is not jarred or the cover glass moved. The filled counting chamber should be allowed to stand for approximately 1 minute prior to performing the count to give the white blood cells time to settle.

6. Count the white blood cells.

  a. Carefully, keeping the counting chamber horizontal at all times, place the hemocytometer on the stage of the microscope.

  b. Using low power only (10× objective), make certain that the microscope light is adjusted properly. In proper focus, the white blood cells should look like small dark or black dots.

  c. Scan the four large corner squares marked 'W' on the counting chamber (Fig. 111). For accurate white counts, there should be an even distribution of cells in all four large squares, with no more than a ten-cell variation between the four squares.

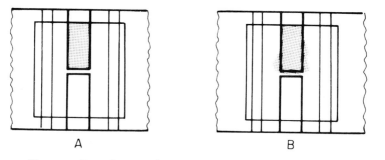

A   B

Fig. 113. Properly (A) and improperly (B) filled counting chamber.

d. Beginning with the upper left square, count all white blood cells in the four large corner squares and add the results together to obtain the total number of cells counted. In counting the cells that touch the outside lines of the large square, count only those that touch the left and upper outside lines (in counting chambers with double lines), disregarding those that touch the right and lower outside margin. If the chamber has triple lines, count those cells that touch the middle of the three outside lines on two sides and disregard those touching the corresponding lines on the other two sides. (That is, count the cells touching either the right margin or the left margin and the cells on the upper margin or lower margin. Whichever you choose is immaterial, but it is important to be consistent and count the cells touching the same two lines every time.)

e. Count the cells on the opposite side of the counting chamber and record the number of cells counted in these four large squares. This total should be close to the first count. (If not, repeat the entire procedure starting with step 1. The number of cells in each of the eight squares should not differ from each other by more than fifteen cells.)

7. Calculation of the WBC.

a. For each of the two white counts performed, calculate the number of white blood cells/µL, as shown below:

Number of white blood cells counted $\times$ Correction for volume $\times$ Correction for dilution

Number of white blood cells counted. Add up the total number of white blood cells counted in the four large squares of the counting chamber. For example:

Square 1	25 white cells	25
Square 2	34 white cells	34
Square 3	32 white cells	32
Square 4	31 white cells	31

Number of cells counted = 122

Correction for volume. Obtain the WBC as the number of white blood cells in 1 µL of blood. Therefore, if the cells are counted in four large squares, the total volume counted is 4 (1.0 $\times$ 1.0 $\times$ 0.1) µL, or 0.4 µL. To obtain a volume of 1.0 µL, 0.4 is multiplied by 2.5 (1.0 ÷ 0.4). The correction factor for volume is then 2.5.

Correction for dilution. Since the blood was initially diluted 1:20, the correction factor for dilution is 20.

b. Therefore:
WBC/µL = 122 $\times$ 2.5 $\times$ 20 = 6,100 WBC/µL.

c. WBC/L = 6,100 $\times$ 10^6 = 6.1 $\times$ 10^9/L.

d. Calculate the WBC for the second white count and average the two results for the final report.

DISCUSSION

1. In certain conditions, such as leukemia, the WBC may be extremely high. If the white count is above 30.0 $\times$ 10^9/L, it is advisable to employ a larger dilution of blood. Using a red cell pipet (see the section entitled Red Blood Cell Count), the blood is drawn up to the 1.0 mark and diluted to the 101 mark with the white count diluting fluid, thus obtaining a 1:100 dilution. (Alternatively, the platelet Unopette may be used.) If the white count is markedly elevated, as in some leukemias, in which it may be

as high as 100 to 300 $\times$ 10^9/L, a 1:200 dilution is used. This is accomplished by drawing the blood up to the 0.5 mark in the red cell pipet and diluting to the 101 mark with white count diluting fluid. The procedure for the WBC then proceeds as previously described. The correction factor for the dilution, however, changes accordingly.

2. Whenever the WBC drops below 3.0 $\times$ 10^9/L, a smaller dilution of the blood should be used to achieve a more accurate count. In this situation, the blood is drawn up to the 1.0 mark in a white cell pipet and diluted to the 11 mark with the white count diluting fluid for a dilution of 1:10. The white count then proceeds as previously outlined, with a correction factor of 10 for the dilution.

3. It is important that the diluting fluid remain free from contamination. Often, small amounts of blood collect in the diluting fluid, causing inaccuracies and difficulties in distinguishing and counting the white blood cells.

4. It is imperative that the counting chamber and cover glass be free from dirt and lint. Again, contamination may cause inaccuracies and difficulties in counting white blood cells. (The counting chamber and cover glass should be cleaned off immediately after completion of the count.)

5. Pipets must be free of dirt and dried blood. Never leave undiluted blood in a pipet. It quickly hardens and plugs up the pipet. Draw water or diluting fluid into the pipet and place it in a container of 0.1% aqueous Clorox solution.

6. There is an approximate 15% error for the manual WBC procedure.

7. The diluting fluids used for the white cell counts destroy or hemolyze all non-nucleated red blood cells. In certain disease states, nucleated red blood cells (NRBC) are present in the peripheral blood. These cells, because they contain a nucleus, cannot be distinguished from the white blood cells. Therefore, any time there are five or more nucleated red blood cells per 100 white blood cells in a differential, the white blood cell count should be corrected as follows:

$$\text{Corrected WBC} = \frac{\text{Uncorrected WBC}}{100 + \text{\# of NRBC/100 WBC}} \times 100$$

The white count is then reported as the 'corrected' WBC.

8. Once the hemocytometer is filled, the counting of cells must proceed without delay. If too much time elapses, the fluid in the chamber begins to evaporate, causing inaccuracies in the white count.

RED BLOOD CELL COUNT

The red blood cell count (RBC) is the number of red blood cells in 1 liter (L) of whole blood.

The normal RBC is 3.6 to 5.6 $\times$ 10^{12}/L for females and 4.2 to 5.8 $\times$ 10^{12}/L for males. The newborn shows an RBC of 5.0 to 6.5 $\times$ 10^{12}/L at birth, which gradually decreases to 4.3 $\pm$ 0.8 $\times$ 10^{12}/L at 1 year of age. During childhood and adolescence, the normal values for the RBC are slightly below the normal adult values. There is also a slight decrease in the RBC after 50 years of age. In addition to the effects of age on the red cell count, strenuous physical activity tends to increase the red cell count. There may also be daily fluctuations with the red count being highest in the morning and at its lowest in the evening. An increased red cell count is found in polycythemia vera and secondary polycythemia due to other causes, such as dehydration. The red count is below normal in anemia and secondarily in numerous other disorders.

As in the WBC, there are two methods used for counting red blood cells: the manual method and the procedure employing an electronic cell counter. The manual method for the RBC is similar to that for the WBC. It is suggested that the student master the WBC procedure before attempting to perform the RBC. For this reason, and to avoid duplication of material, the RBC is not presented in as detailed a manner as the WBC. When in doubt, refer to the section entitled White Blood Cell Count.

REAGENTS AND EQUIPMENT

1. Red count pipet and aspirator (Fig. 114), with or without the Stop-it mouthpiece (Fig. 108). Alternatively, the RBC Unopette may be used.
2. Red count diluting fluid. Any one of the following diluting fluids may be used:
   a. Hayem's solution

Sodium sulfate	2.50 g
Sodium chloride	0.50 g
Mercuric chloride	0.25 g
Distilled water	100 mL

   Certain conditions, such as hyperglobulinemia, cause precipitation of protein, rouleaux, and clumping of the red blood cells when Hayem's solution is used.
   b. Gower's solution

Sodium sulfate	12.5 g
Glacial acetic acid	33.3 mL
Distilled water	200 mL

   Gower's solution is superior to Hayem's solution in that it prevents rouleaux and clumping of the red blood cells.
   c. Sodium chloride, 0.85% w/v

Sodium chloride	0.85 g
Distilled water	100 mL

   If the RBC Unopette is employed,

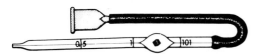

Fig. 114. Red count pipet with aspirator.

none of the above diluting fluids is needed.
3. Microscope.
4. Clean gauze or Kimwipes.
5. Hemocytometer and cover glass. Referring to Figure 111 and the explanation of the hemocytometer in the section entitled White Blood Cell Count, note the large middle square containing twenty-five smaller squares of equal size.
   a. The five small squares labeled 'R' are the areas to be counted for the RBC.
   b. The large center square has a volume of 0.1 μL. Therefore, the volume of each of the twenty-five smaller squares is 0.004 μL, or a total volume for the five small squares of 0.02 μL.

SPECIMEN

Whole blood, using EDTA or heparin as the anticoagulant. Capillary blood may also be used.

PRINCIPLE

To facilitate counting and prevent lysis of the red blood cells, whole blood is diluted with an isotonic diluting fluid.

PROCEDURE

1. Draw the blood up to exactly the 0.5 mark in the red count pipet and dilute to the 101 mark with red count diluting fluid, thus making a 1:200 dilution of blood. Repeat, making a second dilution on the same specimen. Alternatively, use two RBC Unopettes for diluting the blood.
2. Clean the counting chamber.
3. Mix both pipets (or Unopettes) for 3 minutes.
4. Fill the counting chamber, using both pipets (or Unopettes) (1 red count dilution filling each side of the hemocytometer). Expel the first four drops of each mixture (if the red count pipet is used) onto a piece of

gauze. Once the counting chamber is filled, allow approximately 3 minutes for the red blood cells to settle before proceeding to step 5.

5. Count the red blood cells as described in the following steps.

   a. Carefully place the filled counting chamber on the microscope stage.

   b. Using low power (10× objective), place the large center square in the middle of the field of vision. Carefully examine the entire large square for even distribution of red blood cells.

   c. Carefully change to the high dry objective (40×).

   d. Move the counting chamber so that the small upper left corner square is completely in the field of vision. This square is further subdivided into sixteen even smaller squares. This facilitates cell counting.

   e. Count all the cells in this square, remembering to count the cells on two of the outer margins but excluding those lying on the other two outside edges.

   f. Some of the red blood cells may be lying on their sides and, therefore, do not appear as round as the majority of cells in the area. These cells are to be included in the count.

   g. If there are any white blood cells in the area being counted, do not include these cells in your count. (The white blood cell is usually much larger than the red blood cell and does not have as smooth an appearance.)

   h. Count the red blood cells on the opposite side of the counting chamber in the corresponding center square.

6. Calculate the red blood cell count for each of the red counts performed and average the two results for the final report.

RBC/L =
$$\frac{\text{\# Cells in}}{\text{five squares}} \times \frac{\text{Correction}}{\text{for volume}} \times \frac{\text{Correction}}{\text{for dilution}} \times 10^6$$

For example:

# Cells in five small squares = 400
Dilution = 1:200
Volume counted = five small squares
Conversion to liter = × 10^6

$$\text{RBC/L} = 400 \times \frac{1.0}{.02} \times 200 \times 10^6$$
$$= 4.0 \times 10^{12}$$

DISCUSSION

1. In certain conditions, such as polycythemia, the red blood cell count may be extremely high, which makes it difficult to obtain an accurate count. In this instance, make a larger dilution of blood by drawing the blood to the 0.3 mark in the red cell pipet and dilute to the 101 mark. The dilution factor is then 333.

2. For a patient who has severe anemia and in whom the RBC is low, draw the blood up to the 1.0 mark and dilute to the 101 mark. The dilution factor is then 100.

3. Ensure that the diluting fluid is free from blood and other contamination.

4. Make certain that the pipets, hemocytometer, and cover glass are free from dirt, lint, and dried blood.

5. An RBC takes longer to perform than a WBC because of the larger number of cells. Therefore, proceed as quickly as possible once the cells have settled. Drying of the dilution in the counting chamber causes inaccuracies in the final cell count.

6. If the red blood cells show agglutination with Hayem's diluting fluid, this should be noted. It may be helpful in diagnosing the patient's condition. Proceed with the RBC by diluting the blood with 0.85% sodium chloride or Gower's solution.

7. The range of error for a manual RBC usually falls within 10 to 20%.

PREPARATION AND STAINING PROCEDURES FOR THE BLOOD SMEAR

There are three different types of blood smear used in the laboratory: (1) the *cover glass smear,* (2) the *wedge smear,* and (3) the *spun smear.* The cover glass smear is thought by many to contain a more even distribution of white cells than the wedge smear. However, it is more time consuming, the technique is somewhat more difficult to master, cover glasses are too small for most automated stainers, and they are difficult to label. The spun smear is used primarily in conjunction with automated differential counters, although it may be used in laboratories in which differentials are performed manually by the technologists.

There are two additional methods used for preparing blood smears under certain circumstances. It is sometimes desirable to prepare a *buffy coat smear* when the patient's white blood cell count is less than 500 or 1000/μL in order to perform a 100-cell differential. This procedure concentrates the nucleated cells present in the blood. *Thick blood smears* are commonly used when specifically looking for blood parasites such as malaria.

Once the blood smear is made, it is stained with Wright stain or Wright-Giemsa stain, so that a differential white blood cell count and morphology study may be performed. Smears using blood anticoagulated with EDTA should be made within 2 hours of blood collection.

Cover Glass Method for Making Blood Smears

1. Obtain two clean cover glasses, 22 mm square and 0.13 to 0.17 mm thick (number 1 or 1.5).
2. Hold one cover glass by its two adjacent corners with the thumb and index finger of one hand.

3. Place a small drop of blood on this cover glass.
4. With the other hand, hold a second cover glass in the same manner as the first.
5. Gently place the second cover glass over the cover glass containing the drop of blood (with the drop of blood in between the two cover glasses), so that the two cover glasses, one on top of the other, form a sixteen-sided figure (Fig. 115). As soon as the two cover glasses come together, the blood begins to spread.
6. Just before the spreading of the blood is complete, separate the two cover glasses by a rapid, even, horizontal, lateral pull. Care should be taken to avoid squeezing the cover glasses together.
7. Allow the smears to air dry completely.
8. The cover glass smears are now ready for Wright staining.

DISCUSSION

1. The cover glasses must be scrupulously clean.
2. When obtaining blood from a finger tip puncture (or heel), the skin must not touch the cover glass.
3. As soon as the drop of blood is placed on the cover glass, the two cover glasses should be brought together without delay. If the drop of blood

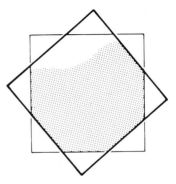

Fig. 115. Cover glass method of making a blood smear.

sits for longer than 3 to 5 seconds, clumping of the platelets and white blood cells, and rouleaux formation of the red blood cells occur.

4. Do not put too large a drop of blood on the cover glass. This results in smears too thick for accurate study.

5. A modified cover glass smear may be prepared on a glass slide by substituting a slide for one of the cover glasses. In this technique, place a drop of blood on the center of a glass slide. While holding a cover glass by opposite corners with the thumb and index finger, place it over the drop of blood on the glass slide. Just before the spreading of blood is complete, remove the cover glass from the slide by a rapid, even, lateral pull. The resultant blood smear on the slide is similar to a coverslip smear.

Manual Method for Making Wedge Blood Smears

1. Obtain two clean glass slides, one spreader slide, and, if using anticoagulated blood, a plain microhematocrit tube. (The spreader slide is merely a glass slide with specially ground ends to ensure even spreading of the blood.)

2. If anticoagulated blood is used, partially fill a microhematocrit tube with well-mixed blood. Carefully place a small drop of blood in the middle of the slide, approximately 1 cm from one end.

3. When using blood from the finger or heel, place a drop of blood on the slide as described in step 2 above, being careful not to touch the skin of the finger (or heel) with the slide.

4. Place the slide on a flat table top with the drop of blood on the right. (For left handed people, it may be easier to reverse all techniques to the opposite hand.)

5. With the thumb and index finger of the left hand, hold the two edges of

the slide. With the right hand, hold the spreader slide with the thumb on the edge of one side and the other four fingers on the edge of the other side (Fig. 116). Place the end of the spreader slide slightly in front of the drop of blood on the other slide. There should be an approximate 25° angle between the two slides (Fig. 117).

6. Draw the spreader slide back toward the drop of blood. As soon as the spreader slide comes in contact with the drop of blood, the blood will begin to spread to the edge of the spreader slide. If this does not occur, wiggle the spreader slide a little until it does so. (Be careful that blood does not get in front of the spreader slide.)

7. Keeping the spreader slide at a 25° angle and the edge of the spreader slide firmly against the horizontal slide, push the spreader slide rapidly over the entire length of the slide. This step should be performed at the moment when the blood has spread to within about $\frac{1}{8}$ inch of the edges of the slide.

8. When the blood smears have air dried, they are ready to be Wright stained.

DISCUSSION

1. The glass slides must be scrupulously clean.

2. As soon as the drop of blood is placed on the glass slide, the smear should be made without delay. Any delay whatsoever results in an abnormal distribution of the white blood cells, with many of the larger white cells accumulating at the thin edge of the smear. Rouleaux of the red blood cells and platelet clumping may also occur.

3. Common causes of a poor blood smear:
   a. Drop of blood too large or too small.

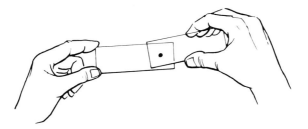

Fig. 116. Method of holding slides for preparation of blood smear.

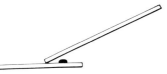

Fig. 117. Proper 25° angle for spreader slide.

  b. Spreader slide pushed across the slide in a jerky manner.
  c. Failure to keep the entire edge of the spreader slide against the slide while making the smear.
  d. Failure to keep the spreader slide at a 25° angle with the slide. (Increasing the angle results in a thicker smear, whereas a smaller angle gives a thin smear.)
  e. Failure to push the spreader slide completely across the slide.
4. The Miniprep automatic blood smearing instrument affords the technologist a semiautomated method for preparing consistently good quality wedge smears. This instrument is described in Chapter 7.

Automated Spun Smear

The spun smear is prepared on an instrument called a spinner. A clean glass slide is seated on a platen, and three to four drops of blood are placed in the middle of the slide. When the top of the instrument is closed, the platen spins at high speed for a period of time, during which excess blood is thrown from the slide into a catch basin, and the resultant slide is completely covered with a thin monolayer of cells. The more sophisticated spinners contain an optical system. During spinning, a beam of light passes up through the glass slide onto a sensor. When the cells have separated the proper amount, the sensor detects this and the platen automatically stops spinning. In this way, spreading of the blood is consistent from one smear to the next, regardless of the patient's hematocrit. (The Hemaspinner is more fully described in Chapter 7.)

Preparation of Buffy Coat Smears

1. Using a capillary pipet, fill a Wintrobe sedimentation tube with well-mixed whole blood.
2. Centrifuge the filled Wintrobe tube for 15 minutes at 1500 g.
3. Examine the centrifuged specimen, locating the buffy coat. Remove and discard all of the plasma except for a small amount near the buffy coat.
4. Using the capillary pipet, remove the small amount of remaining plasma, the entire buffy coat and a small amount of red blood cells.
5. Place the specimen on a glass slide and mix as well as possible. (Do not spread the specimen out too much on the slide.)
6. Transfer a small amount of the blood to each of two slides and immediately prepare wedge or cover glass smears.

DISCUSSION

1. The amount of plasma mixed with the buffy coat and red cells should be approximately equal to the vol-

ume of the cellular portion of the mixture.

2. Alternatively, microhematocrit tubes may be used to centrifuge the specimen. After centrifugation, cut the hematocrit tube slightly above the buffy coat layer. Cut the sealed end of the hematocrit tube from the bottom of the tube. Allow the small plasma layer, buffy coat layer, and a few red blood cells to drain from the microhematocrit tube directly onto a glass slide. Mix this blood well and prepare wedge or cover glass smears.

3. The distribution of the different types of nucleated cells on a buffy coat smear may be affected, due to the fact that the nucleated cells will tend to sediment in layers according to cell type, during the centrifugation process. In cases of leukopenia, however, the differentials from well made buffy coat smears are thought to correlate relatively well with the standard blood smear.

Preparation of Thick Blood Films

1. Place one large drop of well-mixed blood in the center of a glass slide.
2. Using the corner of a second slide, carefully spread the drop of blood over an area the size of a dime. (To determine the correct thickness of the blood film, place the slide on a piece of newspaper. Spread the drop of blood until the newspaper print is just visible through the blood.)
3. Allow the blood film to completely air dry before staining. This will take at least 2 to 4 hours at room temperature, or preferably overnight. If the smear is not completely dry, the blood will be washed from the slide during the staining process since this type of smear is not fixed prior to staining.

Staining Procedure for Blood Smears

For best results, blood smears should be stained within 1 to 2 hours after they are prepared. The stain used for routine examination of blood and bone marrow smears is Wright stain or Wright-Giemsa stain.

PRINCIPLE

Wright stain is a polychromatic stain: the dyes present in the stain produce multiple colors when applied to cells. Wright stain is a mixture of methylene blue, azure B (obtained from oxidation of the methylene blue), and eosin Y dissolved in methanol. The quantities of the dyes used in preparing the Wright stain powder must be carefully controlled to yield a neutral compound dye and optimum staining results. During the staining process, when the buffer solution is added to the stain, ionization occurs, during which time the process of staining the cells takes place. The eosin ions are negatively charged and stain the basic components of the cells an orange to pink color. The acid structures of the cell are stained varying shades of blue to purple by the positively charged, basic, ions. The neutral components of the cells are probably stained by all components of the dye. Because of the complexity of preparing the dyes, Wright stain powder may vary slightly from one lot to another.

REAGENTS AND EQUIPMENT

1. Wright-Giemsa stain.

Wright stain powder	9.0 g
Giemsa stain powder	1.0 g
Glycerin	90 mL
Methanol (absolute,	2,910 mL
anhydrous, acetone free)	

(Mallinckrodt methanol is recommended for use in the Wright stain.) Mix the above reagents in a large tightly stoppered brown bottle. The stain should be allowed to age for approximately 30 days prior to use. During this time, the stain should be shaken once a day. Incubation at 37°C speeds the aging process. The stain should be freshly filtered at the beginning of each day.

2. Phosphate buffer (pH 6.4).

Anhydrous monobasic potassium phosphate (KH_2PO_4)   6.63 g

Anhydrous dibasic sodium   2.56 g phosphate (Na_2HPO_4)

Distilled water   1 liter

The pH of the buffer solution should be within a pH range of 6.4 to 6.7, depending on the staining times and the Wright stain or Wright-Giemsa stain used. If a more alkaline pH (than 6.4) is desired, it is prepared by decreasing the amount of monobasic potassium phosphate and increasing the amount of dibasic sodium phosphate. A pH of 6.7 is obtained by dissolving and diluting 5.13 g of monobasic potassium phosphate and 4.12 g of dibasic sodium phosphate to 1 liter with distilled water. In place of the phosphate buffer, distilled water may be used. However, it is not advisable because the pH of water varies from day to day.

3. Methanol, Mallinckrodt (absolute, anhydrous, acetone free).

4. Staining rack.

PROCEDURE

1. Place the air dried blood smears on a level staining rack, with the smear side up.

2. Fix the smears by flooding the slides with methanol. Drain the excess methanol off the slides. (An alternative method is to dip the smears into a coplin jar containing methanol and then place the slides on the staining rack. However, the utmost care must be taken to change the methanol in the coplin jar several times a day and to keep the jar covered when not in use because methanol readily takes up water. If anhydrous copper sulfate is placed in the coplin jar, the uptake of water by the methanol is minimized.)

3. Flood the slides with Wright-Giemsa stain and time for 4 minutes.

4. Without removing the stain, add an equal volume of phosphate buffer to the slide. Mix the two solutions on the slide by gently blowing back and forth over the solutions. A metallic green sheen should now form on top of this mixture. Time for 7 minutes.

5. Rinse the slide off thoroughly with a stream of tap water or distilled water.

6. Wipe the back of the slides with a piece of gauze to remove any stain.

7. Stand the slides up on end to air dry. Never blot the smears dry.

8. A well-stained smear shows pink to orange red blood cells, pinkish gray reticulocytes, dark purple nuclei in the lymphocytes and neutrophils, a lighter purple nucleus in the monocyte, bright orange granules in the eosinophil, dark blue black granules in the basophil, and violet to purple platelet granules. The cytoplasm of the monocyte is a gray blue with fine reddish granules. The neutrophil has a light pink cytoplasm with lilac granules, and the lymphocyte shows varying shades of blue cytoplasm.

DISCUSSION

1. Generally, when bone marrow smears are stained, the staining times must be increased.

2. The staining times for both peripheral blood and bone marrow smears vary from one laboratory to another, and may also change when a new lot of Wright stain is used.

3. During staining, the phosphate buffer controls the pH of the stain. If the pH is too acid, those cells or cell parts taking up an acid dye stain well, whereas those cell parts which stain at a more alkaline pH appear pale. For example, eosinophils and red blood cells take up an acid dye, whereas nuclei and platelets prefer a more basic pH. Therefore, to stain all

cells and cell parts well, the pH of the phosphate buffer is critical.

4. The staining rack must be exactly level to guard against uneven staining of the smear.
5. Insufficient washing of the smears when removing the stain and buffer mixture causes precipitate on the smear.
6. Leaving water on the smear after rinsing or prolonged rinsing causes the stain to fade.
7. If it is desirable to restain a slide, the original Wright stain may be removed with methanol. Flood the smear with methanol and rinse with tap water as many times as necessary to remove the stain and then restain the slide according to the previously described procedure. This is not recommended, however. For best results, make a new smear.
8. For cover glass smears, after the stained smears have dried, mount the cover glass, blood side down, on a slide using a mounting medium.

DIFFERENTIAL CELL COUNT

The differential white blood cell count is performed to determine the relative number of each type of white blood cell present in the blood. At the same time, a study of red blood cell, white blood cell, and platelet morphology is performed. A rough estimate of the platelet and white counts is also made. More information can be obtained from a detailed examination of the stained blood smear than from any other single laboratory test. The differential and smear review should be performed after the blood counts have been completed. In this way, examination of the smear may be used to double check the white blood cell count, and a rough estimate of the hemoglobin, hematocrit, and red blood cell count may be made.

In disease states, a particular white blood cell type may show an absolute increase in number in the blood. Common diseases showing an increased number of a specific cell type are listed below.

1. *Neutrophilia* (absolute increase in the number of neutrophils):
   a. Appendicitis
   b. Myelogenous leukemia
   c. Bacterial infections
2. *Eosinophilia* (absolute increase in the number of eosinophils):
   a. Allergies ad allergenic reactions
   b. Scarlet fever
   c. Parasitic infections
   d. Eosinophilic leukemia
3. *Lymphocytosis* (absolute increase in the number of lymphocytes):
   a. Viral infections
   b. Whooping cough
   c. Infectious mononucleosis
   d. Lymphocytic leukemia
4. *Monocytosis* (absolute increase in the number of monocytes):
   a. Brucellosis
   b. Tuberculosis
   c. Monocytic leukemia
   d. Subacute bacterial endocarditis
   e. Typhoid
   f. Rickettsial infections
   g. Collagen disease
   h. Hodgkin's disease
   i. Gaucher's disease

Procedure for Examination of the Stained Blood Smear

1. Place the slide (smear side up) on the microscope stage. (It is a good idea to place the thick end of the smear on the same side of the microscope stage each time a differential is performed when the wedge smear is used.)
2. Examine the blood smear using the low power (10×) objective.
   a. Check that there is even distribution of the white blood cells on the smear.
   b. Estimate the white blood cell count (by noting the number of white cells/field and the number of white cells in relation to the

number of red blood cells). It should agree with the test result obtained. If it does not, the white count should be repeated.

c. Examine the thin peripheral edge of the smear (if the wedge type smear is being used). If there is an increased number of white cells in this area, the differential cell count may be inaccurate. Most of the cells at the edge of the smear are usually the larger white blood cells, namely, neutrophils and monocytes. This, therefore, shows poor distribution of white blood cell types in the smear. If there are clumps of platelets in this area, the smear will then show a decrease in platelets. In such situations, the blood smear should be discarded and another made.

d. In scanning the blood smear, it is important to note anything unusual or irregular, such as large, abnormal looking cells or rouleaux formation of the red blood cells.

e. Choose that portion of the blood smear where there is only a slight overlapping of the red blood cells. Place a drop of oil on the slide and carefully change to the oil immersion objective (100×).

3. Perform the differential cell count and, at the same time, examine the morphology of the white blood cells.

a. Begin in the thin area of the slide where the red blood cells are slightly overlapping. Gradually move the slide as shown in Figure 118. Count each white blood cell seen and record on a differential cell counter until 100 white blood cells have been counted. If any nucleated red blood cells (NRBC) are seen during the differential count, enumerate them on a separate counter. These cells are not to be included in the 100-cell differential count, but are reported as the # of NRBC/100 WBC. (If any megakaryocytic cells or fragments, smudge cells, or epithelial cells are seen, these cells should also be enumerated in the same manner as the NRBC, and reported as the #/100 WBC.

4. Examine the red blood cell morphology in a thin area of the slide where only a few of the red blood cells slightly overlap. Note any variations from normal and classify these irregularities as slight, moderate, or marked (or 1+, 2+, 3+).

5. Examine the platelets on the smear for morphology and number present. Using the same fields on various parts of the smear, as in step 4 above for the red blood cell morphology, determine the approximate number of platelets per field. A normal (wedge) blood smear (normal red blood cell count and normal platelet count) should show approximately 8 to 20 platelets per field in this area. One method for reporting platelet estimates is to determine the average number of platelets per field (using 5 to 10 different fields) and multiply this result by 20,000 (for a wedge smear) to obtain an approximation of the platelet count. For example:

Platelet Est. of	Report Platelet Est. as:
0–49,000/µL	Marked decrease
50,000–99,000/µL	Moderate decrease
100,000–149,000/µL	Slight decrease
150,000–199,000/µL	Low normal
200,000–400,000/µL	Normal
401,000–599,000/µL	Slight increase
600,000–800,000/µL	Moderate increase
Above 800,000/µL	Marked increase

A patient with a red blood cell count of $5.0 \times 10^{12}/L$ and a platelet count of $300 \times 10^9/L$ has 30 platelets for every 500 red blood cells. This must be kept in mind when performing a platelet estimate and adjustments

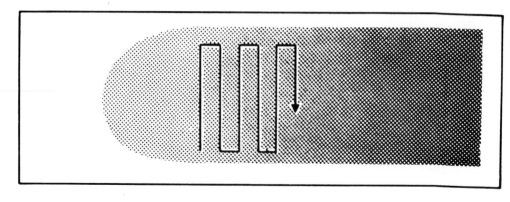

Fig. 118. Pathway for the differential cell count.

made when the patient's red count is greater or less than 5.0×10^{12}/L. For example, if a patient's red count is 2.5×10^{12}/L and the platelet count is 300×10^9/L, there are 30 platelets for every 250 red blood cells, or 60 platelets for every 500 red blood cells. It is, therefore, helpful to know the patient's red blood cell count (hemoglobin or hematocrit) when performing a platelet estimate.

DISCUSSION

1. The differential white count gives the relative number of each type of white blood cell. At times, however, it is helpful to know the actual number of each white blood cell type/L of blood. This is referred to as the *absolute count* and is calculated as follows:

$$\begin{array}{l} \text{Absolute \#} \\ \text{of cells/L} \end{array} = \begin{array}{l} \text{\% of cell type in} \\ \text{differential} \times \text{WBC/L} \end{array}$$

2. When performing a differential, the following outline may be followed.
   a. White blood cells.
      1) Check for even distribution and estimate the number present (also, look for any gross abnormalities present on the smear).
      2) Perform the differential count.
      3) Examine for morphologic abnormalities.
   b. Red blood cells.
      1) Examine for:
         a) Size and shape.
         b) Relative hemoglobin content.
         c) Polychromatophilia.
         d) Inclusions.
         e) Rouleaux formation or agglutination.
   c. Platelets.
      1) Estimate number present.
      2) Examine for morphologic abnormalities.

3. When studying a stained smear, do not progress too far into the thick area of the slide. The morphologic characteristics of the cells are difficult to distinguish in this area. Also, do not use the very thin portion of the smear where the red blood cells appear completely filled with hemoglobin and show no area of central pallor. The cells in this area are generally distorted and do not show a true morphologic picture.

4. When the white count is below 1.0×10^9/L, it may be difficult to find many white blood cells on the stained smear. In this situation, a differential may be performed by counting 50 white blood cells. A notation on the report must then be made that

only 50 white blood cells were counted. (Alternatively, a buffy coat smear may be prepared.)

5. On a differential showing an abnormal distribution of cell types (as listed below):
   a. Over 10% eosinophils,
   b. Over 2% basophils,
   c. Over 11% monocytes, or
   d. More lymphocytes than neutrophils (except in children) 200 white blood cells should be counted. The results are then averaged (divided by 2) and a notation made on the report that 200 white blood cells were counted.

6. Before reporting platelets as being decreased, scan the slide on low power, especially the feathered edge, for platelet clumps. Also recheck the tube of blood for a clot.

7. When the differential count is complete, the results may show the presence of immature granulocytic cells. This is termed a *shift to the left* and may be found in such disorders as leukemias and bacterial infections. A *shift to the right* refers to an increased number of hypersegmented neutrophils.

8. Do not hesitate to ask questions concerning the morphology or identification of cells. The differential is the most difficult laboratory test to learn. In fact, learning about cells and their morphologic features is a process that should continue for as long as you perform differentials.

9. There is a relatively large range of variability in the results of the 100-cell differential count. As the number of total cells counted increases, the amount of variability will decrease. The 95% confidence limit (±2 S.D.) improves somewhat more remarkably when counting 200 white cells rather than the routine 100 cell count. Although the accuracy of the count improves with a 500 or 1000

cell count, the change is not as great as seen between 100 and 200 cell counts. (See below.)

Actual # of cell type	±2 S.D. when counting			
	100	200	500	1000
2	0–8	0–6	0–4	1–4
25	16–35	19–32	21–30	22–28
45	35–56	38–53	40–50	41–49
60	54–68	56–66	57–63	58–63
80	71–90	73–87	76–85	77–83

(From: Nelson, D.A., and Morris, M.W.: Basic methodology, In: *Clinical Diagnosis and Management*, Henry, J.B., ed., Philadelphia, W.B. Saunders Co., 1984, p. 611.)

RED BLOOD CELL INDICES

The red blood cell indices are used to define the size and hemoglobin content of the red blood cell. They consist of the mean corpuscular volume (MCV), mean corpuscular hemoglobin (MCH), and mean corpuscular hemoglobin concentration (MCHC). The red blood cell indices are used as an aid in differentiating anemias. When these indices are combined with an examination of the red blood cells on the stained smear, a clear picture of red blood cell morphology may be obtained.

The derivation of the formulas for the calculation of red blood cell indices is given on the following pages. It is not important that the student memorize how to derive these formulas, but should be aware of what the equations mean.

The size of the individual red blood cell is small, and the amount of hemoglobin in a single cell is rather minute.

Mean Corpuscular Volume (MCV)

The MCV indicates the average volume of the red blood cells in femtoliters (fL).

$$MCV = \frac{\text{Volume of red blood cells in femtoliters (fL) of blood}}{RBC/L}$$

If: Hematocrit = 45% (or, .45 L)
     RBC = $5.0 \times 10^{12}/L$
     1 µL = 10^9 fL
     1 L = 10^{15} fL

Then:

$$MCV = \frac{.45 \times 10^{15} \text{ fL/L}}{5.0 \times 10^{12}/\text{L}}$$
$$= .09 \times 10^3 \text{ fL}$$
$$= 90 \text{ fL}$$

Therefore, the formula:

$$MCV = \frac{\text{Hct} \times 10^3 \text{ fL}}{\text{RBC/L}}$$

Normal range for the MCV: 80 to 100 fL

DISCUSSION

The MCV indicates whether the red blood cells appear normocytic, microcytic, or macrocytic. If the MCV is less than 80 fL, the red blood cells are *microcytic*. If the MCV is greater than 100 fL, the red blood cells are considered *macrocytic*. If the MCV is within the normal range, the red blood cells are *normocytic*.

Mean Corpuscular Hemoglobin Concentration (MCHC)

The MCHC is an expression of the average concentration of hemoglobin in the red blood cells. It gives the ratio of the weight of hemoglobin to the volume of the red blood cell.

$$MCHC = \frac{\text{Hgb in g/dL}}{\text{Hct (vol. of RBC in g/dL)}}$$
$$\times 100 \text{ (to convert to \%)}$$

If: Hgb = 15.0 g/dL
      Hct = 45%

Then:

$$MCHC = \frac{15.0 \text{ g/dL}}{45 \text{ g/dL}} \times 100\%$$
$$= .333 \times 100\%$$
$$= 33.3\%$$

Therefore, the formula:

$$MCHC = \frac{\text{Hgb} \times 100\%}{\text{Hct}}$$

Normal range for the MCHC = 31 to 36%

DISCUSSION

The MCHC indicates whether the red blood cells are normochromic, hypochromic, or hyperchromic. An MCHC below 31% indicates *hypochromia,* an MCHC above 36% indicates *hyperchromia,* and red blood cells with a normal MCHC are termed *normochromic.* Please note that an MCHC above 38% should not occur. Such a result is usually due to incorrect calculation of the MCHC, or, the patient's red blood cells may be agglutinated (cold agglutinin), thereby causing a falsely low red blood cell count (the hematocrit may also be falsely low if measured by an electronic cell counter which calculates the hematocrit from the MCV and RBC). Alternatively, the MCHC will not usually go below 27 to 29% when hypochromia is present. If the MCHC does fall below this value, it may be due to a lipemic plasma causing an invalidly high hemoglobin.

Mean Corpuscular Hemoglobin (MCH)

The MCH indicates the averge weight of hemoglobin in the red blood cell.

$$MCH = \frac{\text{Weight of hgb in 1 L of blood}}{\text{\# of red cells in 1 L of blood}}$$

If: 1 g = 10^{12} pg
      1 L = 10 dL

Then:

$$MCH = \frac{\text{Hgb} \times 10 \times 10^{12} \text{ pg/L}}{\text{RBC/L}}$$

If: Hgb = 15.0 g/dL
      RBC = 5.0 × 10^{12}/L

Then:

$$MCH: = \frac{15 \times 10^{13} \text{ pg/L}}{5.0 \times 10^{12}/\text{L}}$$
$$= \frac{15 \times 10 \text{ pg/L}}{5.0/\text{L}}$$
$$= 30 \text{ pg}$$

Therefore, the formula:

$$MCH = \frac{\text{Hgb (g/L)}}{\text{RBC (/L)}} \text{ pg}$$

Normal range for the MCH: = 27 to 31 pg

DISCUSSION

The MCH indicates the average amount of hemoglobin in the red blood cell and should always correlate with the MCV and MCHC. An MCH lower than 27 pg is found in microcytic anemia and also with normocytic, hypochromic red blood cells. An elevated MCH occurs in macrocytic anemias and in some cases of spherocytosis in which hyperchromia may be present.

Examples of Red Blood Cell Indices with Corresponding Red Blood Cell Morphology

1. Hgb = 14.0 g/dl   Hct = 41%
        RBC = 4.5 × 10^{12}/L

                        The red blood cells are

   MCV = 91.1 fL   normocytic
   MCH = 31.1 pg   and
   MCHC = 34.1%   normochromic.

2. Hgb = 9.8 g/dL   Hct = 30%
        RBC = 4.5 × 10^{12}/L

                        The red blood cells are

   MCV = 66.7 fL   microcytic
   MCH = 21.8 pg   and
   MCHC = 32.7%   normochromic.

3. Hgb = 9.0 g/dL   Hct = 30%
        RBC = 4.5 × 10^{12}/L

                        The red blood cells are

   MCV = 66.7 fL   microcytic
   MCH = 20.0 pg   and
   MCHC = 30.0%   hypochromic.

4. Hgb = 15.0 g/dL   Hct = 45%
        RBC = 4.0 × 10^{12}/L

                        The red blood cells are

   MCV = 112.5 fL   macrocytic
   MCH = 37.5 pg   and
   MCHC = 33.3%   normochromic.

5. Hgb = 11.8 g/dL   Hct = 41%
        RBC = 4.5 × 10^{12}/L

                        The red blood cells are

   MCV = 91.1 fL   normocytic
   MCH = 26.2 pg   and
   MCHC = 28.8%   hypochromic.

ERYTHROCYTE SEDIMENTATION RATE

When anticoagulated whole blood is allowed to stand for a period of time, the red blood cells settle out from the plasma. The distance the red blood cells fall after a specific time period (1 hour) is known as the *erythrocyte sedimentation rate* (ESR).

The ESR is affected by three factors: erythrocytes, plasma, and mechanical and technical factors.

ERYTHROCYTES

A factor of chief importance in determining the distance the red blood cells fall is the size or mass of the falling particle. The larger the particle, the faster its rate of fall. In normal blood, the red blood cells remain more or less separated from each other. They are negatively charged and, therefore, repel each other. In certain diseases, however, plasma proteins, namely fibrinogen and globulin, may be altered, causing rouleaux formation (Fig. 119). This leads to a larger mass and an increased sedimentation velocity. Agglutination of the red blood cells due to changes in the erythrocyte surface also leads to an increased red blood cell mass and a more rapid sedimentation rate. Macrocytes tend to settle more rapidly than microcytes. Red blood cells which show an alteration in shape, such as sickle cells and spherocytes, are unable to agglutinate or form rouleaux and the sedimentation distance is decreased (normal). Anisocytosis and poikilocytosis reduce the ability of the red cell to form large aggregates and thereby tend to falsely lower an ESR. In severe anemia, the ESR is markedly elevated. The concentration of the erythrocytes in the blood is decreased and they, therefore, settle out more easily and rapidly. (A chart has been devised by Wintrobe and Landsberg [for use with the Wintrobe ESR method] to correct for anemia. This graph utilizes the patient's hematocrit and theoretically yields the ESR value which results when the patient is not anemic. This value is then termed the *corrected ESR.* There are, however, serious objections to

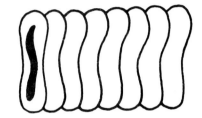

Fig. 119. Rouleaux formation of the red blood cells.

this procedure, and it is not commonly used today.) In polycythemia, in which the red blood cell count is high, the ESR is generally normal.

PLASMA COMPOSITION

The plasma composition is the single most important factor determining the ESR. Rouleaux and aggregation of the red blood cells are affected mainly by the levels of fibrinogen, alpha-1 globulin, and alpha-2 globulin, increasing as these three plasma protein levels are increased in the blood. The viscosity of the plasma is generally increased in the presence of an increased protein concentration and this will also cause an increase in the ESR. Increased concentrations of albumin, however, will tend to lower the ESR even in the presence of abnormal proteins.

MECHANICAL AND TECHNICAL FACTORS

It is important that the ESR tube be exactly perpendicular. A tilt of 3° can cause errors up to 30%. Also, the rack holding the tubes should not be subject to any movement or vibration. Minor, everyday variations in room temperature do not significantly affect the ESR. With large changes in temperature, however, the sedimentation rate increases as the temperature increases. The length and inner diameter of the ESR tube also affect the final test results. ESR tubes with a narrower than standard bore will generally yield lower sedimentation rates.

SIGNIFICANCE OF THE ERYTHROCYTE SEDIMENTATION RATE

Adults over 60 years of age frequently have a slightly higher ESR value due primarily to decreased concentrations of plasma albumin. The ESR mainly reflects changes in the plasma proteins which accompany most of the acute and chronic infections, tumors, and degenerative diseases. It may be used to follow the progress of certain diseases such as tuberculosis and rheumatism. The ESR represents a nonspecific response to tissue damage and inflammation and denotes the presence of disease, but not its severity. An elevated ESR may be found in pregnancy (after the third month), acute and chronic infections, rheumatic fever, rheumatoid arthritis, myocardial infarction, nephrosis, acute hepatitis, menstruation, tuberculosis, macroglobulinemia, cryoglobulinemia, hypothyroidism, and hyperthyroidism, to name a few.

Modified Westergren Method

REFERENCES

Gambino, R.S., DiRe, J.J., Monteleone, M., and Budd, D.C.: The Westergren sedimentation rate, using K$_3$EDTA, Techn. Bull. Regist. Med. Techn., *35*, 1, 1965.

National Committee for Clinical Laboratory Standards: *Reference Procedure for the Human Erythrocyte Sedimentation Rate (E.S.R.) Test,* Code #H2-T2, National Committee for Clinical Laboratory Standards, Villanova, Pa., 1983.

REAGENTS AND EQUIPMENT

1. Applicator sticks.
2. Sodium chloride, 0.85% (w/v).
3. Pipets, 2.0 and 0.5 mL.
4. Test tubes, 13 × 100 mm.
5. Westergren pipet, calibrated in millimeters (Fig. 120). The National Committee for Clinical Laboratory Standards has set specific dimensions for the pipets to be used:
   Length = 300.5 mm (±0.5 mm)
   External diameter =
   5.5 mm (±0.5 mm)
   Internal bore = 2.7 mm (±0.1 mm)
   Bore uniformity = ±0.05 mm
   Graduated scale on pipet =
   200 mm (±0.35 mm)
6. Westergren pipet rack. All racks should contain a leveling bulb in order to ensure that the position of the tubes is vertical (±1°).

SPECIMEN

Whole blood, 3 mL, using EDTA as the anticoagulant.

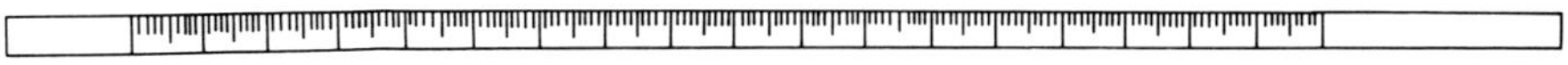

Fig. 120. Westergren pipet.

PRINCIPLE

Well-mixed, whole blood is diluted with 0.85% sodium chloride, placed in a Westergren pipet, and allowed to stand for exactly 1 hour in a vertical position. The number of millimeters the red blood cells fall during this timed period constitutes the ESR. The normal values for the modified Westergren ESR are 0 to 15 mm/hour for women, 0 to 10 mm/hour for men, and 0 to 10 mm/hour for children.

PROCEDURE

1. Mix the whole blood for at least 2 minutes on a rotator. (The blood should be at room temperature.) Check the tube for clots using two applicator sticks.
2. Place 0.5 mL of 0.85% sodium chloride in a plain 13 × 100 mm test tube.
3. Add 2.0 ml of well mixed whole blood to the test tube.
4. Mix the tube for 2 minutes.
5. Make certain the Westergren ESR rack is exactly level.
6. Fill the Westergren pipet to exactly the 0 mark, making certain there are no air bubbles in the blood.
7. Place the pipet in the rack. Be certain the pipet fits snugly and evenly into the grooves provided.
8. Allow the pipet to stand for exactly 60 minutes.
9. At the end of 60 minutes, record the number of millimeters the red blood cells have fallen. This result is the erythrocyte sedimentation rate in millimeters/hour.

Wintrobe and Landsberg Method

REAGENTS AND EQUIPMENT

1. Wintrobe tube, calibrated in millimeters (Fig. 121).
2. Wintrobe pipet rack.
3. Disposable capillary pipet.

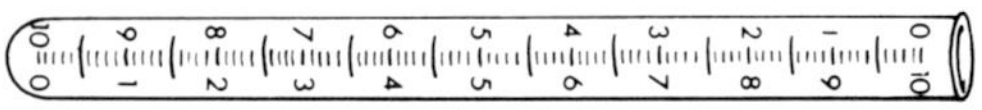

Fig. 121. Wintrobe sedimentation tube.

SPECIMEN

Whole blood, 1 ml, using EDTA as the anticoagulant.

PRINCIPLE

Well-mixed, whole blood is placed in a Wintrobe tube and allowed to stand for 1 hour. The number of millimeters the red blood cells fall during this time constitutes the ESR. In the Wintrobe and Landsberg method, normal values for women are 0 to 20 mm/hour and 0 to 9 mm/hour for men.

PROCEDURE

1. Mix the whole blood for at least 2 minutes on a rotator. (Make certain the blood is at room temperature.)
2. With a capillary pipet, fill the Wintrobe tube to the 0 mark.
3. Place the tube in an exactly vertical position in the rack. Time for 60 minutes.
4. At the end of 60 minutes, record the level of the erythrocyte column. This result is the erythrocyte sedimentation rate in millimeters/hour.

DISCUSSION

1. The sedimentation of red blood cells takes place in three stages: (1) In the first stage rouleaux formation occurs and the sedimentation rate is slight, (2) sedimentation then occurs at a fairly rapid rate, and (3) during the last stage, the sedimentation rate is slow because of the accumulation of red blood cells in the bottom of the tube.
2. Although care may be taken in filling the sedimentation tube to the 0 mark,

occasionally the upper level of the blood may only reach the 1- or 2-mm mark. In such a case, care should be taken in reading the final result. Subtract these 1 or 2 mm from the final result. For example, if the sedimentation tube is filled to the 2-mm mark and the red blood cells fall to the 18-mm mark, the ESR is reported as 16 mm/hour. If the level of blood falls below the 5-mm mark, the test should be repeated to ensure that valid results are obtained.

3. All sedimentation racks should be equipped with leveling screws and a spirit level.

4. Sources of error:

   a. If the concentration of the anticoagulant is greater than recommended, the ESR will be falsely low.

   b. If the ESR stands for more than 60 minutes, the results will be falsely elevated. If the test is timed for less than 60 minutes, invalidly low values are obtained.

   c. A marked increase (or decrease) in room temperature leads to increased (or decreased) ESR results.

   d. Tilting of the ESR tube increases the sedimentation rate.

   e. Bubbles in the blood cause invalid results.

   f. Fibrin clots present in the blood invalidate the test results.

5. The ESR should be set up within 2 hours of blood collection. If EDTA is used as the anticoagulant, the test must be set up within 6 hours if the blood has been refrigerated. It has been reported that blood refrigerated up to 24 hours and diluted with sodium chloride immediately before testing will give valid results by the Westergren technique.

6. The Wintrobe technique is thought to be more sensitive when the ESR is low and when the patient is in the acute phase of disease. The Westergren procedure more reliably reflects the over all clinical state of the patient. The Westergren method has been chosen as the standard method by the International Committee for Standardization in Hematology.

7. A second type of Westergren ESR tube contains a cotton plug located at the top of the 0-mm mark (Fig. 122). The cotton plug prevents blood from being drawn up into the tube beyond the 0-mark. In this method, an inexpensive rubber bulb is used to draw the diluted blood up into the ESR tube. The excess blood drawn up is absorbed into the cotton plug. When the pipetting bulb is removed from the tube, the blood remains in the ESR tube, prevented from leaking out of the tube by the cotton plug at the top of the column of blood. The cotton plug does not appear to have any effect on the ESR results. This pipet, manufactured by Chase Instruments, Poultney, Vermont, is the same size recommended by the National Committee for Clinical Laboratory Standards. It affords the technologist a quick method for setting up the ESR without the necessity of using more cumbersome pipet fillers. Also, because of the cotton plug, the chances of the blood leaking out of the ESR tube while standing, are minimal.

8. The internal bore and the length of the graduated scale on the Westergren pipet are critical measurements. Any tube of a different size in these two dimensions will generally give results different from those obtained using the standard size pipet. If a smaller bore and/or length tube is used (for pediatric samples) a new set of normal values needs to be determined. It must also be kept in mind that even with the new set of nor-

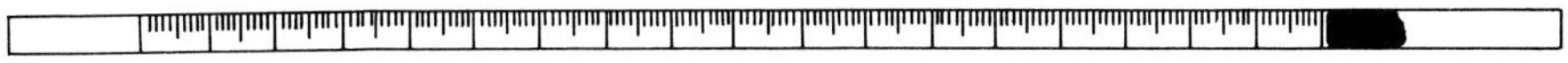

Fig. 122. Westergren pipet with cotton plug.

mals, the results may still not be comparable with the reference technique.

9. Blood for the Westergren ESR may be collected in 0.109 M sodium citrate. If this anticoagulant is used, obtain the blood specimen and immediately mix exactly 4 volumes of whole blood with 1 volume of sodium citrate. Mix the blood well. When performing the ESR, the blood should not be diluted with 0.85% sodium chloride solution as previously described since the blood has already been diluted with the sodium citrate anticoagulant.

10. A reference procedure for the ESR has been devised which uses a standardized hematocrit. The whole blood specimen (anticoagulated with EDTA) is adjusted to a hematocrit of 35% (by adding or removing the patient's own plasma). The Westergren ESR is then set up (do not further dilute the specimen with sodium chloride). This procedure, however, is too cumbersome for routine use.

RETICULOCYTE COUNT

The red blood cell goes through six stages of development: pronormoblast, basophilic normoblast, polychromatophilic normoblast, orthochromic normoblast, reticulocyte, and mature red blood cell. The first four stages are normally confined to the bone marrow. The reticulocyte, however, is found in both the bone marrow and peripheral blood. In the bone marrow, it spends approximately 2 to 3 days maturing and is then released into the blood, where it matures for another day before becoming a mature red blood cell.

The reticulocyte count is an important diagnostic tool. It is a relatively accurate reflection of the amount of effective red blood cell production taking place in the bone marrow. Since the life span of a red blood cell is 120 days, ± 20 days, the bone marrow replaces approximately 1% of the adult red blood cells every day. The normal value for a reticulocyte count is therefore, 0.5 to 1.5%. The reticulocyte count is expressed as the number of reticulocytes present per 100 red blood cells (in percent). A decreased reticulocyte count is found in aplastic anemia and in conditions in which the bone marrow is not producing red blood cells. Increased reticulocyte counts are found in hemolytic anemias, individuals with iron deficiency anemia receiving iron therapy, thalassemia, sideroblastic anemia, and in acute and chronic blood loss.

CORRECTED RETICULOCYTE COUNT

A reticulocyte count should reflect the total production of red blood cells, regardless of the concentration of red cells in the blood (red blood cell count). As an example, compare the following two patients. Patient #1 has a hematocrit of 42% and a reticulocyte count of 1.0%. Patient #2 has a hematocrit of 21% and a reticulocyte count of 2.0%. Patient #2, theoretically, has ½ as many red blood cells as patient #1 but has the same number of reticulocytes as patient #1 because the reticulocytes are diluted by only ½ the number of red blood cells, as in patient #1. To compensate for this, a corrected reticulocyte count is calculated based on a normal hematocrit of 45%. The formula for this correction is:

$$\text{Corrected reticulocyte count (percent)} = \frac{\text{Patient's hematocrit}}{\text{Normal hematocrit}} \times \text{Reticulocyte count (percent)}$$

In addition to correcting a reticulocyte count for an abnormally low hematocrit, consideration may also be given to the presence of marrow reticulocytes present in the peripheral blood. In this circumstance, the reticulocyte production index is calculated. As previously stated, the reticulocytes spend approximately 2 to 3 days in the bone marrow before being released into the blood where they spend 1 day in the peripheral circulation to mature. In certain situations, these marrow reticulocytes are released directly into the blood prior to maturation in the bone marrow. This is detected by nucleated red blood cells and/or polychromatophilic macrocytes *(shift cells)* present in the circulating blood. To correct for this reticulocyte maturation delay, the reticulocyte production index is calculated by dividing the corrected reticulocyte count by the number of days the reticulocyte most probably takes to mature in the blood. These times will vary, but are thought to be approximately 1 day in patients with a normal hematocrit, 1.5 days with a hematocrit of 35%, 2 days when the patient's hematocrit is in the range of 25%, and 3 days when the hematocrit level is at 15%. In patients with a normal hematocrit and showing no nucleated red cells or shift cells, the corrected reticulocyte count is divided by 1 (normal reticulocyte maturation time), and the reticulocyte production index is equal to the corrected reticulocyte count. If a patient has a hematocrit of 25% and has shift cells or nucleated red blood cells present in the peripheral blood, the corrected reticulocyte count may be divided by 2 in order to obtain the reticulocyte production index.

REFERENCE

National Committee for Clinical Laboratory Standards, *Method for Reticulocyte Counting. Proposed standard.* Document #H16-P. NCCLS, Villanova, Pa., 1985.

REAGENTS AND EQUIPMENT

1. New methylene blue stain solution
   New methylene blue   1.0 g
   (certified by the U.S. Biological
   Stain Commission)
   Sodium chloride   0.89 g
   Distilled water   100 mL
   Mix, filter, and store at room temperature.
2. Glass slides.
3. Microhematocrit tubes.
4. Microscope.

SPECIMEN

Whole blood (1 mL), using EDTA or heparin as the anticoagulant. Capillary blood may also be used.

PRINCIPLE

After the orthochromic normoblast loses its nucleus, a small amount of RNA remains in the red blood cell, and the cell is known as a reticulocyte. To detect the presence of RNA, the red blood cells must be stained while they are still living. This process is called *supravital staining.* Whole blood is incubated with new methylene blue. Smears of this mixture are then prepared and examined. The number of reticulocytes in 1000 red blood cells is determined. This number is divided by 10 to obtain the reticulocyte count in percent.

PROCEDURE

1. Place three drops of filtered reticulocyte stain in a small test tube.
2. Add three drops of well-mixed whole blood to the tube containing the stain.
3. Mix the tube and allow to stand at room temperature, or incubate at 37°C, for 15 minutes. This allows the reticulocytes adequate time to take up the stain.
4. At the end of 15 minutes, mix the contents of the tube well.
5. Using a microhematocrit tube, place a drop of the mixture on each of three slides and make smears.
6. Allow the smears to air dry.
7. Place the first slide on the microscope stage and, using the low power objective (10×), find an area in the thin portion of the smear in which

the red blood cells are evenly distributed and are not touching each other. Carefully change to the oil immersion objective (100×) and further locate an area in which there are approximately 100 to 200 red blood cells per oil immersion field.

8. As soon as the proper area is selected, the reticulocytes may be counted. The red blood cells will be a light to medium green in color. The RNA present in the reticulocytes stains a deep blue. The reticulum may be abundant or sparse, depending on the cell's stage of development. The youngest reticulocyte shows a larger amount of RNA (Fig. 123A), whereas the more mature reticulocyte shows only a small amount of RNA (Fig. 123C). Count all of the red blood cells in the first field on 1 cell counter. At the same time, enumerate the reticulocytes (Fig. 124) in the same field with a second cell counter. Move the slide as described in the section entitled Differential Cell Count, until all reticulocytes in 1000 red blood cells have been counted.

9. A second technologist should repeat the reticulocyte count in the same manner as described in step 8 on the second reticulocyte smear. The two results should agree within ±20% of each other. If they do not, repeat the reticulocyte count on the third smear.

10. Average the two results and calculate the reticulocyte count as shown below.

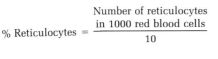

$$\% \text{ Reticulocytes} = \frac{\text{Number of reticulocytes in 1000 red blood cells}}{10}$$

11. Calculate the corrected reticulocyte count and the reticulocyte production index if applicable and/or desired.

DISCUSSION

1. The blood-to-stain ratio does not have to be exactly equal. For best results, a larger proportion of blood should be added to the stain when the patient's hematocrit is low. Add a smaller amount of blood to the stain when the patient has an unusually high hematocrit.

2. The time allowed for staining of the reticulocyte is not critical. It should, however, not be less than 10 minutes.

3. It is extremely important that the blood and stain be mixed well prior to making smears. The reticulocytes have a lower specific gravity than mature red blood cells and, therefore, settle on top of the red blood cells in the mixture.

4. Red blood cells containing areas of high refractility may be noted on the smear. These cells should not be confused with reticulocytes. This condition is probably due to moisture in the air and poor drying of the smear.

5. The presence of a high blood sugar (glucose) or the use of heparin as the anticoagulant may cause the reticulocytes to have a pale stain.

6. The range of error in the reticulocyte count varies, depending on the number of reticulocytes counted. Using the previously outlined procedure, there is an error of approximately ±25% in the reticulocyte counts within the normal range. This de-

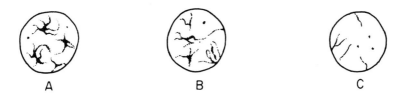

A   B   C

Fig. 123.   Stages of maturation in the reticulocyte count.

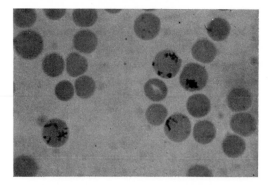

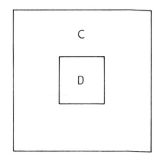

Fig. 126. Miller disk (newer model).

Fig. 124. Reticulocytes. (Supravital staining of the red blood cells with new methylene blue.) (Magnification × 1000.)

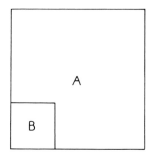

Fig. 125. Miller disk (older model).

creases to ±10% in a reticulocyte count of 5% and decreases even further as the uncorrected reticulocyte count increases.

7. There are several methods of counting reticulocytes once the smears have been made:

(1) A Miller disk may be placed inside the microscope eyepiece. This disk consists of two squares, as shown in Figures 125 and 126. The area of the smaller square (B) or (D) is one ninth that of square A or C. When employing this method to count reticulocytes, the red blood cells in square B or D are counted in successive fields on the slide until a total of twenty fields have been counted. At the same time, the reticulocytes in the large square A or C are enumerated. The reticulocyte count is

then calculated by dividing the total number of reticulocytes counted by 9 times the number of red blood cells counted in square B or D. The count may be performed in duplicate, using a second smear, and the results averaged to obtain the test value.

(2) Place a small 'window' in the eyepiece of the microscope. This makes the field smaller and the counting of cells easier. (Cut out a round piece of paper the same diameter as the eyepiece and cut a square hole in the center. Unscrew the top lens of the eyepiece, insert the paper, and replace the top lens.)

(3) For reticulocyte counts less than 10%, count at least 100 reticulocytes (except in extremely low counts where this would not be practical). Instead of counting the number of red blood cells in every field, count the red blood cells in every eight to ten fields and also keep track of the number of fields examined. Calculate the reticulocyte count as follows:

$$\frac{\text{\# of RBCs}}{\text{examined}} = \frac{\dfrac{\text{\# of RBCs}}{\text{counted}}}{\substack{\text{\# of fields} \\ \text{in which RBCs} \\ \text{were counted}}} \times \frac{\text{\# of fields}}{\text{examined}}$$

$$\text{\% Reticulocytes} = \frac{\dfrac{\text{\# of retics}}{\text{counted}}}{\substack{\text{\# of RBC's} \\ \text{examined}}} \times 100$$

(4) Use of 15× eyepieces (instead of 10×) makes the field smaller and, at the same time, enables the technologist to see the reticulocytes much more clearly.

8. There are several red blood cell inclusions that are stained by the new methylene blue stain, in addition to the RNA of the reticulocytes. Howell-Jolly bodies appear as one, sometimes two, round, deep purple staining structures. Heinz bodies stain a light blue green and are usually present at the peripheral edge of the red blood cell (Fig. 127). Pappenheimer bodies are most often confused with reticulocytes and are the most difficult to distinguish from reticulocytes. These purple staining deposits generally appear as several granules in a small cluster and will usually be a darker shade of blue than the reticulocyte. If Pappenheimer bodies are suspected, a Wright-stained smear may be examined to verify their presence. Hemoglobin H bodies will appear as round greenish blue inclusions.

9. The normal range for an absolute reticulocyte count is approximately 50×10^9/L and may be calculated by multiplying the % reticulocyte count by the red blood cell count.

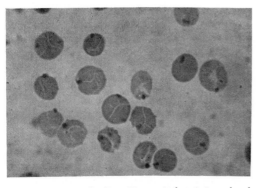

Fig. 127. Heinz bodies. (Supravital staining of red blood cells with new methylene blue. Compare with reticulocytes stained similarly.) (Magnification ×1000.)

10. It is advisable not to counterstain the reticulocyte smears with Wright stain since any precipitated stain may cause confusion in the identification of reticulocytes.

PLATELET COUNT

Platelet counts are of great importance in helping to diagnose bleeding disorders. As stated previously, platelets function primarily in hemostasis (the stoppage of bleeding) and in maintaining capillary integrity (injuries to capillary walls are plugged by platelets to inhibit bleeding and to maintain the sealing function of the capillary walls).

The normal range for the platelet count is 150,000 to 400,000/μL (150 to 400 × 10^9/L). An increased platelet count, *thrombocytosis,* is found in polycythemia vera, idiopathic thrombocythemia, chronic myelogenous leukemia, and following a splenectomy. A decreased platelet count, *thrombocytopenia,* occurs in thrombocytopenia purpura, aplastic anemia, acute leukemia, Gaucher's disease, pernicious anemia, and sometimes following chemotherapy and radiation therapy. A prolonged bleeding time and poor clot retraction are found when there is marked thrombocytopenia.

Platelets are difficult to count. They are small, disintegrate easily, and are hard to distinguish from dirt. They readily adhere to each other (aggregation) and also become easily attached to any foreign body (adhesiveness). The use of EDTA as an anticoagulant helps to decrease the clumping of platelets. In EDTA, platelet volume increases during the first hour in the tube, and they will generally then maintain a constant size between 1 and 3 hours. After this period of time, the platelet will again begin increasing in size. Although fingertip (or heel) blood may be used, the results are generally less satisfactory and significantly lower than platelet counts performed on venous blood. (A significant number of the platelets are probably lost at the puncture site.) When obtaining capillary blood, it is important that the platelet count be obtained first.

There are two general methods for the direct counting of platelets. The phase microscope is employed in one method (outlined below) and an electronic cell counter is the second procedure for counting platelets (the most accurate and reproducible).

REFERENCE

Brecker, G., and Cronkite, E.P.: Morphology and enumeration of human blood platelets, J. Appl. Physiol., 3:365, 1950.

REAGENTS AND EQUIPMENT

1. Ammonium oxalate, 1% (w/v), in distilled water. Store in refrigerator and filter before use.
2. Red count pipets. Alternatively, platelet count Unopettes (containing ammonium oxalate) may be used in this procedure.
3. Phase (flat-bottomed) hemocytometer. (The hemocytometer used on a light microscope has a concave area on the underside, beneath the platform counting areas.) A thin disposable coverslip (#1 or #1½) should be used rather than the thick standard hemocytometer cover glass.
4. Glass slides.
5. Wright's stain and buffer.
6. Phase microscope.
7. Petri dish.
8. Filter paper.
9. Pipet rotator.

SPECIMEN

Whole blood, using EDTA as the anticoagulant, is recommended. Blood from the fingertip (or heel) may be used if it is not feasible to obtain venous blood.

PRINCIPLE

Whole blood is diluted with 1% ammonium oxalate, which hemolyzes the red blood cells. The platelets are then counted, using the phase hemocytometer and phase microscopy. Results are double-checked by examination of the platelets on a Wright stained smear.

PROCEDURE

1. Gently mix blood for approximately 2 minutes.
2. Prepare a blood smear and Wright stain.
3. Using two red cell pipets (or two platelet Unopettes), draw blood to exactly the 1.0 mark and dilute to the 101 mark with 1% ammonium oxalate (1:100 dilution).
4. Place the pipets on a pipet rotator for 10 to 15 minutes. This ensures proper mixing and complete hemolysis of the red blood cells.
5. Clean the hemocytometer thoroughly and make certain it is completely free of all dirt and lint. The use of 95% (v/v) ethyl alcohol and a lint free cloth is recommended for this process.
6. Prepare a moist chamber as follows: obtain a Petri dish and a piece of filter paper of approximately the same diameter as the Petri dish. (Either the top or the bottom of the dish may be used.) Thoroughly moisten the filter paper and place in the top of the Petri dish so that it adheres to the dish.
7. When the pipets are adequately mixed, fill the counting chamber. Discard the first four drops from the red cell pipet and fill one side of the hemocytometer. Repeat, using the second pipet and fill the opposite side of the hemocytometer.
8. Place the moist chamber over the hemocytometer and allow the preparation to stand for 20 to 30 minutes. This allows time for the platelets to settle and prevents evaporation of the fluid in the counting chamber.
9. Place the hemocytometer on the phase microscope stage.
   a. Focus the large middle square of the hemocytometer under low

power (10 ×). The background appears black, with the white blood cells, platelets, debris, and markings of the hemocytometer giving an illuminated appearance.

b. Carefully change to the 43 × phase objective. The platelets appear as round or oval bodies with a light purplish sheen. When focusing up and down with the fine adjuster, the platelets may be seen to have 1 or more fine processes. Dirt and debris are distinguishable because of their high refractility.

c. The platelets in 10 of the 25 small squares in the large central square are counted. The suggested squares to use are those labeled with a P (Fig. 128).

d. Enumerate the platelets in the same area on both sides of the counting chamber. The total number of platelets counted on each side should agree with each other by ±10 when the platelet count is in the normal range.

e. Add the two counts together and divide by 2 to determine the average number of platelets counted.

10. Calculate the number of platelets/L as shown below:

Plts/µL =

$$\frac{\text{Av \# plts}}{\text{counted}} \times \frac{\text{Correction}}{\text{for dilution}} \times \frac{\text{Correction}}{\text{for volume}}$$

Plts/L = plts/µL × 10^6

11. A second technologist should scan a Wright-stained smear and make a platelet estimate. If the platelet count does not reasonably agree with the platelet estimate, the count should be repeated. (If the platelets do not show even distribution on the smear, a second smear and platelet estimate may be made before repeating the count.)

DISCUSSION

1. If clumps of platelets are noted in the platelet count, the procedure should be repeated. This may be due to inadequate mixing or poor technique in obtaining the blood sample.

2. There should always be an even distribution of platelets in the counting chamber.

3. It is imperative that the hemocytometer and pipets be scrupulously clean and the diluting fluid freshly filtered.

4. If fewer than 80 platelets are counted in the 10 small squares, all of the platelets in the large center square (25 small squares) on both sides of the hemocytometer should be counted. Then, if fewer than 50 platelets are counted per side, the platelet count may be repeated, diluting the original blood sample 1:20 using a white count pipet.

5. If the platelet count is extremely high, a dilution of 1:200 may be made, using the red count pipet.

6. With experience, it is possible to perform platelet counts by phase microscopy with an error of ±10%.

7. Once the blood has been diluted with 1% ammonium oxalate, the dilution is stable for at least 8 hours.

8. As soon as the platelet count has been removed from the mixer, it

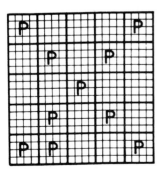

Fig. 128. Suggested squares to use for the platelet count.

should not stand for more than 8 to 10 seconds without being remixed.

9. The blood should be diluted and smears made within 5 hours of blood collection, or within 24 hours if the blood has been refrigerated.

10. The use of 15× eyepieces on the phase microscope greatly facilitates the counting of platelets.

11. If a phase microscope is not available, a routine bright light microscope may be used. The light in the microscopic field should not be too bright which may be accomplished by moving the condensor down. The platelets will appear as small, highly refractile bodies.

12. The Rees-Ecker platelet procedure utilizes a brilliant cresyl blue staining solution: sodium citrate, 3.8 g; brilliant cresyl blue, 0.1 g; formaldehyde (37%), 0.2 mL; distilled water, 100 mL. This diluting fluid must be filtered before use. Follow the procedure as described above for diluting the blood and performing the count. This diluting fluid will not hemolyze the red blood cells. On the bright light microscope, platelets appear as small, round, oval, or elongated particles that are highly refractile and stain a light bluish color. The utmost care must be taken not to confuse the platelets with dirt or debris. Using this diluting fluid, the platelet count must be completed within 30 minutes of diluting in order to ensure against platelet disintegration. The range of error for this method is estimated to be approximately 16 to 25%.

EOSINOPHIL COUNT

Although the relative number of eosinophils in the blood may be determined by the differential white count, it is sometimes necessary to more accurately determine the total number of eosinophils/L of blood. A direct method for counting eosinophils has been devised that is similar to the method used for the red and white blood cell counts.

The normal values for the eosinophil count are approximately 50 to 350 × 10^6/ L. A low eosinophil count (eosinopenia) is found in hyperadrenalism (Cushing's disease), shock, and following the administration of adrenocorticotropic hormone (ACTH). Increased numbers of eosinophils (eosinophilia) occur in allergic reactions, parasitic infestations, brucellosis, and certain leukemias. In addition, there may be a considerable variation in the eosinophil count over a 24-hour period, with the lowest count generally present at midmorning and the highest count present during the night (midnight and later).

There are two general methods for counting eosinophils: the indirect method (white blood cell count multiplied by the % of eosinophils in the differential) and the direct method. The ideal procedure is to perform the eosinophil count by the direct method and double-check these results using the indirect method. This procedure is outlined below.

REFERENCE

Randolph, T.G.: Differentiation and enumeration of eosinophils in the counting chamber with a glycol stain: A valuable technique in appraising ACTH dosage. J. Lab. Clin. Med., *34*:1696, 1949.

REAGENTS AND EQUIPMENT

1. Any one of the following diluting fluids may be employed.
   a. Phyloxine diluting fluid

Propylene glycol	50 mL
Distilled water	40 mL
Aqueous solution of phyloxine, 1%, w/v	10 mL
Aqueous solution of sodium carbonate, 10%, w/v	1 mL

   Mix, filter, and store at room temperature.
   Stable for 1 month.
   b. Pilot's solution is prepared in the same manner as phyloxine dilut-

Color Plates

Plate I

Normoblasts and megaloblasts contrasted (photomicrographs, ×1000; Wright stain).

   A, B, C, D, E, Normoblasts: A, pronormoblasts; B, basophilic normoblast; C, early; D, late, polychromatophilic normoblasts; E, orthochromic normoblast with stippling.
   F–O. Various stages of megaloblasts (pernicious anemia): F, promegaloblast (left) and basophilic megaloblast (right); G, H, I, J, K, mainly polychromatophilic megaloblasts; L, M, N, O, mainly orthochromic megaloblasts, O being from the blood. All other cells are from the bone marrow. (From Wintrobe, M.M., et al.: Clinical Hematology, 8th ed. Philadelphia, Lea & Febiger, 1981.)

PLATE I

(Legend on opposite page)

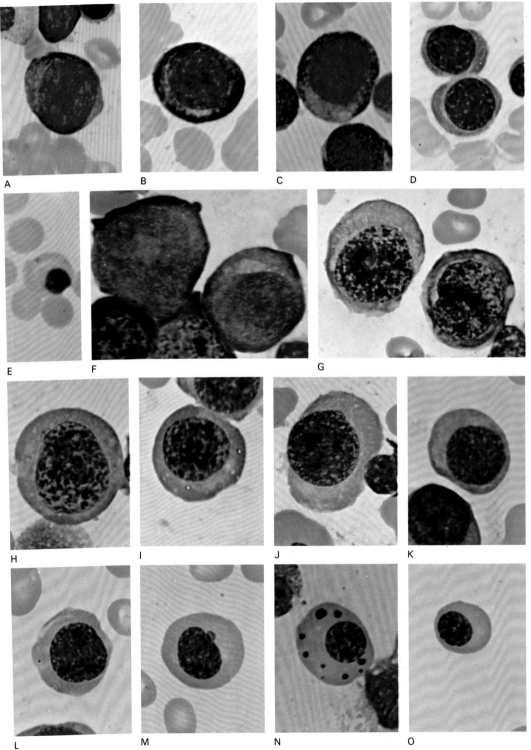

Plate II

Normal leukocytes from bone marrow and blood (photomicrographs, ×1000 [approx.]; Wright stain).

A, myeloblast; B, myeloblasts, with myelocyte and late metamyelocyte; C, two promyelocytes; D, promyelocyte; E, late promyelocyte or myelocyte; F, myelocyte; G, myelocyte; H, late myelocyte or early metamyelocyte; I, metamyelocyte; J, band neutrophil; K, band neutrophil; L, polymorphonuclear neutrophil; M, polymorphonuclear neutrophil; N, polymorphonuclear neutrophil; O, eosinophil; P, basophil, Q, monocyte; R, monocyte. (From Wintrobe, M.M., et al.: Clinical Hematology, 8th ed. Philadelphia, Lea & Febiger, 1981.)

PLATE II

(Legend on opposite page)

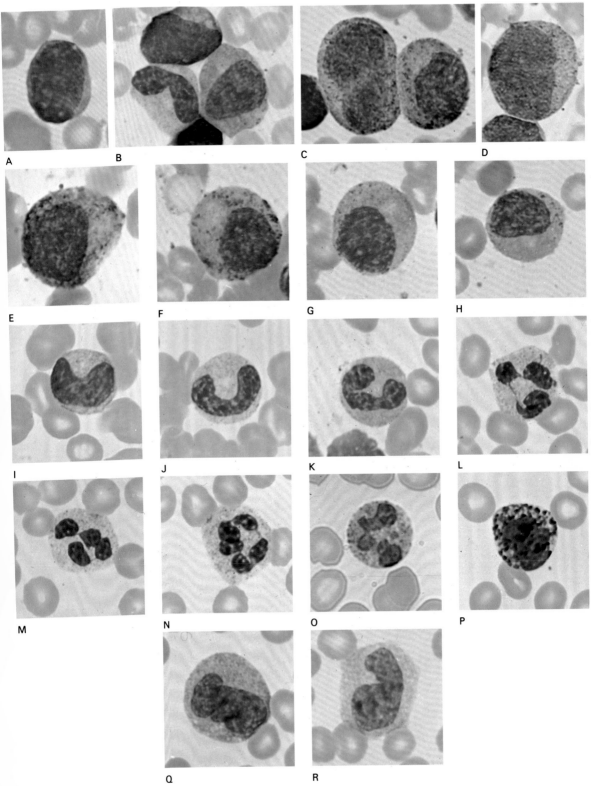

Plate III

Immature and mature white blood cells, red blood cells, megakaryocytes and platelets. (Wright stain. Magnification ×1000.)

A, leukemic lymphoblast; B, prolymphocyte (larger cell) and normal lymphocyte; C, small lymphocyte; D, medium-sized lymphocyte; E, large lymphocyte; F, blast (acute monocytic leukemia); G, promonocyte; H, monocyte; I, macrophage; J, myeloblast; K, rubriblast (bone marrow); L, promegaloblast (bone marrow); M, megakaryoblast (bone marrow); N, megakaryocyte (bone marrow) (×450); O, giant platelet; P, abnormal platelet; Q, vacuolated monocyte; R, vacuolated neutrophil.

PLATE III
(Legend on opposite page)

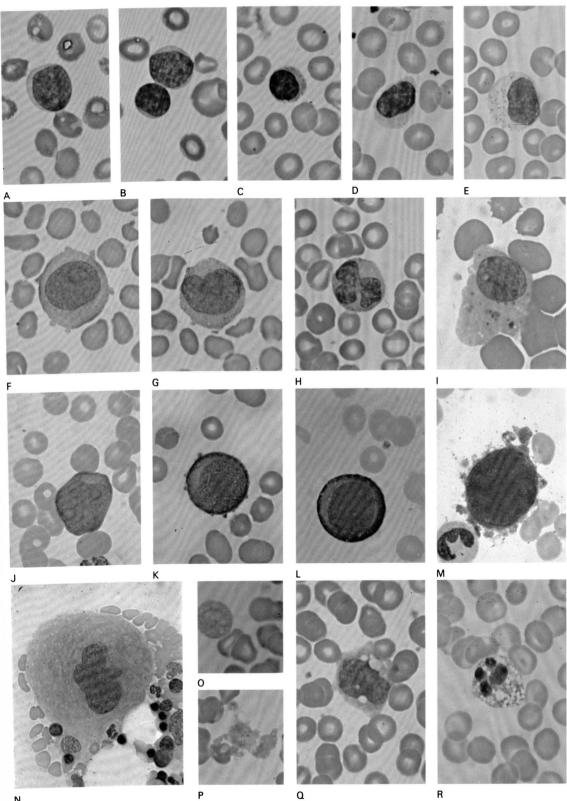

A   B   C   D   E

F   G   H   I

J   K   L   M

N   O   P   Q   R

Plate IV

Heinz bodies, reticulocytes, white blood cell morphology, and abnormal white blood cells. (Wright stain, except where indicated. Magnification ×1000.)

A, neutrophilic band showing toxic granulation; B, neutrophil containing Döhle body; C, hypersegmented neutrophil; D, neutrophil showing a Barr body; E, neutrophil with a pyknotic nucleus; F, neutrophil and lymphocyte from a patient with Alder Reilly anomaly; G, reticulocytes (new methylene blue N stain); H, Heinz bodies (new methylene blue N stain); I, mitotic figure; J, basket cell; K, smudge cell; L, plasma cell; M, lymphoma cell; N, micromegakaryoblast; O, Reed-Sternberg cell; P, lipid histiocyte from a patient with Gaucher's disease; Q, lipid histiocyte from a patient with Niemann-Pick disease.

PLATE IV

(Legend on opposite page)

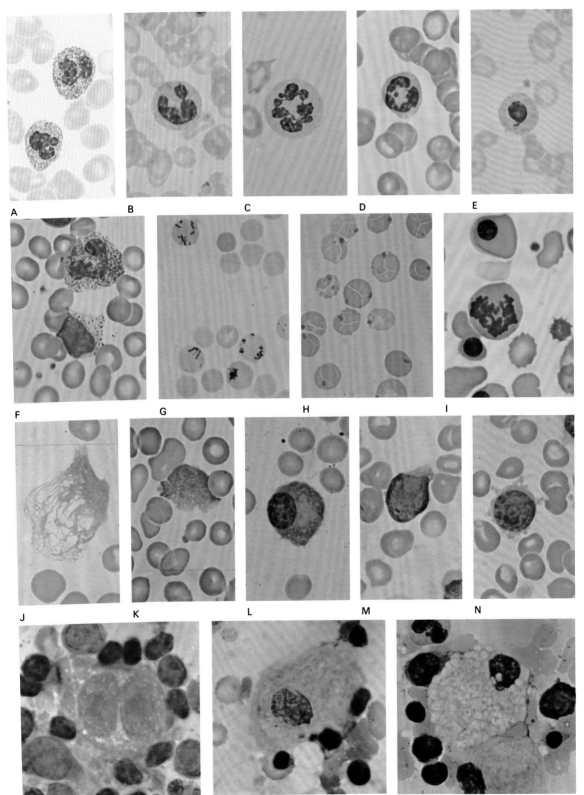

Plate V

Red blood cell and white blood cell morphology and malaria. (Wright stain. Magnification ×403.)

A, neutrophil from a patient with Chédiak-Higashi anomaly; B, lymphocyte from a patient with Chédiak-Higashi anomaly; C, D, L.E. cell; E–G, neutrophils from a patient with Pelger-Huët anomaly; H, myeloblast containing an Auer rod; I, plasma cells containing crystals; J, red blood cells showing polychromatophilia; K–N, various stages of malaria parasites; O, platelet on top of a red blood cell (compare with malaria parasites in photographs L, M, N).

PLATE V

(Legend on opposite page)

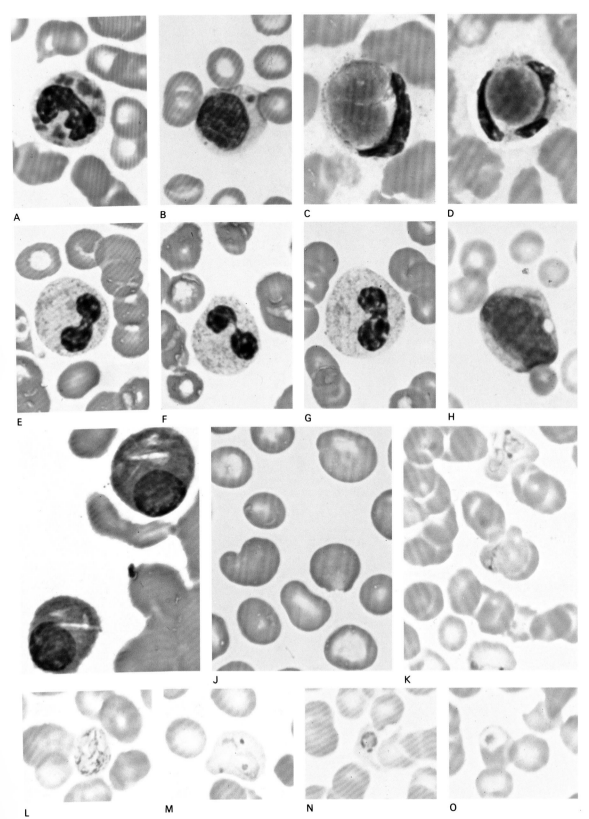

A

B

C

D

E

F

G

H

J

K

L

M

N

O

Plate VI

Atypical lymphocytes and hairy cell leukemia. (Wright stain. Magnification ×403.)

A–L, atypical lymphocytes; M, hairy cell and normal lymphocyte; N, hairy cell; O, hairy cell and normal lymphocyte.

PLATE VI

(Legend on opposite page)

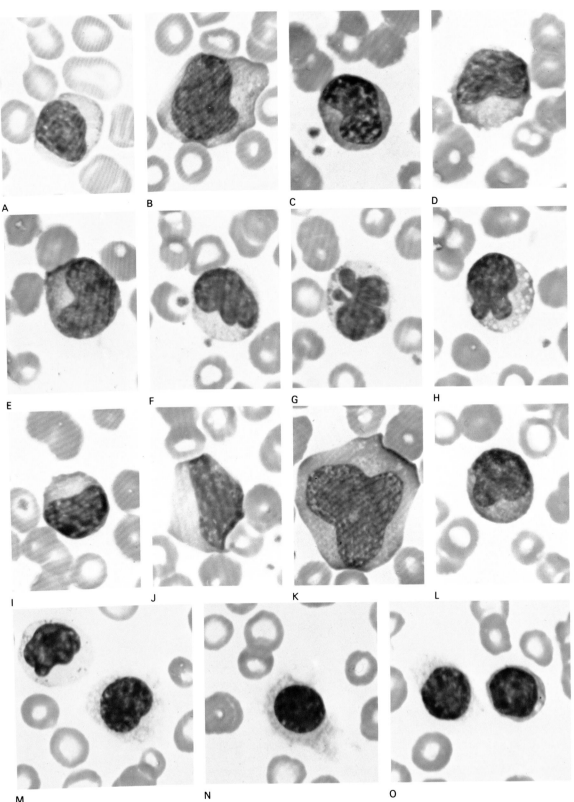

Plate VII

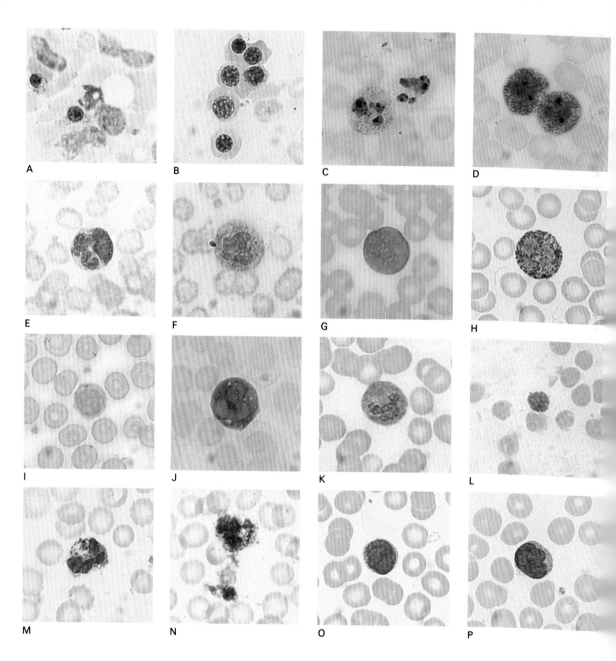

Special stains, NBT, and Sézary cells. (Stained as indicated. Magnification ×403.)

A–B, iron (Prussian blue) stain (showing sideroblasts); C, leukocyte alkaline phosphatase stain (one neutrophil shows 0 activity, the second neutrophil shows 2+ activity); D, leukocyte alkaline phosphatase stain (both neutrophils show 4+ activity); E, peroxidase stain (neutrophil shows strongly positive staining); F, peroxidase stain (neutrophil shows very weak staining); G, periodic acid-Schiff stain (neutrophil); H, sudan black B stain (neutrophil); I, acid phosphatase (note red staining granule in the cytoplasm of the lymphocyte); J, nonspecific esterase stain (monocyte); K, chloroacetate esterase stain (neutrophil); L, red blood cell containing hemoglobin H bodies (brilliant cresyl blue stain) (note the reticulocyte in the same field); M–N, NBT positive neutrophils (Wright stain) (note black staining particles); O–P, Sézary cells (Wright stain).

Plate VIII

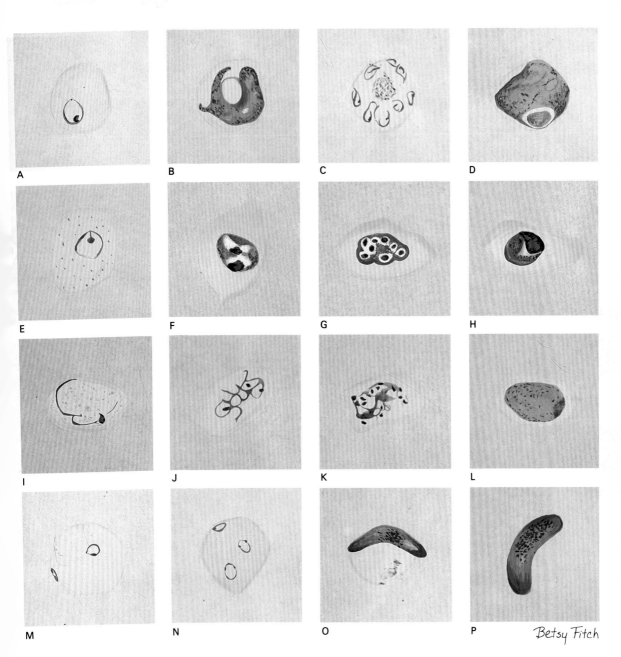

A–D, Plasmodium malariae: A, ring form (trophozoite); B, trophozoite; C, schizont; D, macrogametocyte.

E–H, Plasmodium ovale: E, ring form (trophozoite); F, G, schizonts; H, gametocyte.

I–L, Plasmodium vivax: I, trophozoite; J, trophozoite (ameboid); K, schizont; L, macrogametocyte.

M–P, Plasmodium falciparum: M, double ring (trophozoite); N, multiple rings (trophozoite); O, macrogametocyte; P, microgametocyte.

ing fluid (above) except that 100 units of heparin is added to the final mixture.

c. Randolph's stain
   Solution 1
   Methylene blue,   50 mL
       0.1% (w/v), in
       propylene glycol
   Distilled water   50 mL
   Solution 2
   Phyloxine, 0.1%   50 mL
       (w/v), in methylene blue
   Distilled water   50 mL
   Store solutions 1 and 2 at room temperature. Prior to use, mix equal volumes of both solutions together. This mixture is stable for 4 hours.

2. White count pipets. The eosinophil Unopette containing phloxine B as the diluting fluid may also be used.

3. Counting chamber. There are three different types of counting chambers available for use in the eosinophil count.

   a. Hemocytometer with Neubauer ruling. This is the counting chamber previously described for the red and white blood cell counts. However, it is not recommended for the eosinophil count because of its relatively small volume.

   b. Fuchs-Rosenthal hemocytometer (Fig. 129). The Fuchs-Rosenthal counting chamber consists of two platforms, or counting areas. The chamber is 0.2 mm deep. Each ruled counting area consists of 1 large square, 4 mm × 4 mm × 0.2 mm, or 3.2 μL in volume. The large square is divided into 16 smaller squares, each of which is 1 mm long and 1 mm wide. Each of these squares is further subdivided into 16 smaller squares.

   c. Speirs-Levy hemocytometer (Fig. 130). The Speirs-Levy counting chamber consists of 4 platforms, or counting areas. The chamber is

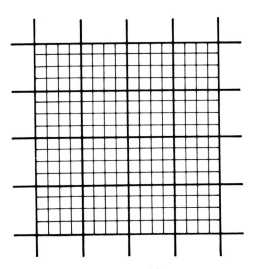

Fig. 129. Fuchs-Rosenthal hemocytometer.

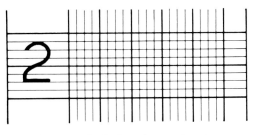

Fig. 130. Speirs-Levy hemocytometer.

0.2 mm deep. Each counting area consists of 10 squares, 1 mm long and 1 mm wide, arranged in 2 horizontal rows of 5 squares. Each of these 10 squares is further subdivided into 16 smaller squares. The volume of 1 counting area is 2 mm × 5 mm × 0.2 mm, or 2.0 μL.

4. Microscope.
5. Moist chamber.
6. Glass slides.
7. Wright's stain and buffer.

SPECIMEN

Collect 1 mL of whole blood using EDTA or heparin as the anticoagulant. Capillary blood may also be used.

PRINCIPLE

Whole blood is diluted with the staining solution. The phyloxine present in the diluting fluid serves to stain the eosinophils red; the sodium carbonate and water help to lyse the white blood cells (except the eosinophils); and the red blood cells are lysed by the propylene glycol. Heparin, if present in the diluting fluid, prevents clumping of the white blood cells. The sodium carbonate also enhances the staining of the eosinophil granules.

PROCEDURE

1. Using a white count pipet, draw the blood up to the 1.0 mark. Wipe off the outside of the pipet carefully. Draw the eosinophil diluting fluid up to the 11 mark to make a 1:10 dilution. If the eosinophil Unopette is used, draw the blood up in a 25 μL pipet and dilute in the Unopette (1:32 dilution).
2. Repeat step 1, making a second dilution on the same specimen.
3. Mix both pipets (or Unopettes) for approximately 2 minutes.
4. Expel the first four drops of the mixture from the first pipet and fill one side of the counting chamber. Repeat, using the second pipet, and fill the opposite side of the hemocytometer. (If the Speirs-Levy counting chamber is used, fill both counting areas on one side with the first pipet and the two opposite counting areas with the second pipet.)
5. Place a moist chamber (a Petri dish with a piece of wet filter paper in the top) over the filled counting chamber.
6. Allow 15 minutes for the cells to settle. Lysis of the red blood cells and staining of the eosinophils also take place during this time.
7. Using the low power objective (10 ×), count the eosinophils, which are stained red. Count the following areas, depending on which hemocytometer is used:
   a. Hemocytometer with Neubauer ruling: count the entire ruled area

on both sides of the counting chamber. This gives a total volume counted of 1.8 μL.
   b. Fuchs-Rosenthal hemocytometer: count the entire ruled area on both sides of the counting chamber. This gives a total volume counted of 6.4 μL.
   c. Speirs-Levy hemocytometer: count the entire ruled area on two platforms, one on each side of the counting chamber. This gives a total volume counted of 4 μL.
8. Calculate the number of eosinophils/L as shown below:

$$\text{Eosinophils/L} = \frac{\text{Eosinophils}}{\text{counted}} \times \frac{\text{Correction}}{\text{for dilution}}$$

$$\times \frac{\text{Correction}}{\text{for volume of}} \times 10^6$$
$$\text{chamber used}$$

9. As a means of double-checking the preceding results, the indirect method for the eosinophil count should now be performed.
   a. Perform a white blood cell count on the specimen of blood. Make 2 blood smears and Wright stain.
   b. Perform a differential white count on the blood smear.
   c. Calculate the indirect eosinophil count as follows:

   Eosinophils/L
   $$= \frac{\text{Percent}}{\text{Eosinophils}} \times \text{WBC/L}$$
   $$\text{in differential}$$

   d. The results obtained should correlate with the eosinophil count by the direct method. If there is too large a variation, repeat the preceding procedures for the direct and indirect eosinophil counts.

DISCUSSION

1. A single eosinophil count may be ordered on a patient, or, the eosinophil counts may be ordered in conjunction with the Thorn test for adrenal

cortical function. This test, however, is now rarely performed.

2. The indirect method for counting eosinophils is not as accurate as the direct method. Therefore, a close correlation between the results of the two methods is not always possible.
3. Once the eosinophil count is diluted, it should be counted within 30 minutes. The eosinophils will easily disintegrate in the diluting fluid if left diluted for too long a period of time. If the Unopette is used, the count should be completed within 1 hour of being diluted.
4. The approximate error in the eosinophil count is ±30% when the hemocytometer with Neubauer ruling is used. Errors of approximately ±20% are found when the Speirs-Levy or Fuchs-Rosenthal counting chambers are employed.

SICKLE CELL TESTS

Sickle shaped red blood cells are found under certain conditions in the peripheral blood of people who have sickle cell anemia, and rarely, in patients with sickle cell trait. This sickling phenomenon may also be demonstrated in the laboratory by depriving the red blood cells of oxygen. The anemia and the trait are inherited and are usually confined to the black race. They are discussed in more detail in the Disease section of this book.

Sickle cell anemia and sickle cell trait are caused by an abnormal hemoglobin, hemoglobin S. In the presence of hemoglobin S, the red blood cells take on a sickle like shape when the oxygen supply to the red blood cell is decreased. The degree of sickling depends on the concentration of hemoglobin S in the red blood cell. When the concentration of hemoglobin S is 80 to 100% (as in sickle cell anemia), sickling of the red blood cell occurs readily at only slightly reduced oxygen concentrations. When the concentration of hemoglobin S is only 20 to 40% (as in the

sickle cell trait), oxygen concentrations must be much lower before sickling occurs.

Sodium Metabisulfite Method

REFERENCE

Daland, G.A., and Castle, W.B.: A simple and rapid method for demonstrating sickling of the red blood cells: The use of reducing agents. J. Lab. Clin. Med., *33*:1082, 1948.

REAGENTS AND EQUIPMENT

1. Sodium metabisulfite, 2% (w/v)
   Sodium metabisulfite   0.2 g
   Distilled water   10 mL
   Stable for 8 hours at room temperature.
2. Syringe (5 mL) filled with petroleum jelly.
3. 19-gauge needle.
4. Glass slide.
5. Cover glass.
6. Microscope.

SPECIMEN

Whole blood, using EDTA or heparin as the anticoagulant. Capillary blood may also be used.

PRINCIPLE

Whole blood is mixed with sodium metabisulfite, a strong reducing agent which deoxygenates the hemoglobin. Under these conditions, hemoglobin S present in the red blood cell causes the formation of sickle shaped red cells.

PROCEDURE

1. Place one drop of the blood to be tested on a glass slide.
2. Add one to two drops of 2% sodium metabisulfite to the drop of blood (two drops if the hemoglobin is normal, a single drop if the hematocrit is decreased).
3. Mix well with an applicator stick.
4. Place a cover glass on top of the sample and press down lightly on it to remove any air bubbles and to form

a thin layer of the mixture. Wipe off the excess sample.

5. Using the syringe and 19-gauge needle, carefully rim the cover glass with the petroleum jelly, completely sealing the mixture under the coverslip.

6. Examine the preparation for the presence of sickle cells after 30 minutes, using the high dry objective (40×). (Take care that when the objective is changed to high dry, it does not come in contact with the petroleum jelly.) In some instances, the red blood cells may take on a 'holly-leaf' form, as shown in Figure 131. This shape is often found in the sickle cell trait, and, when present, the test is reported as positive.

7. If there is no sickling present at the end of 30 minutes, allow the preparation to stand at room temperature for 24 hours and reexamine at that time.

8. When sickle cells or the 'holly-leaf' form of the red blood cells are present, the results are reported as positive. Normal looking red blood cells or slightly crenated red blood cells are reported as negative.

DISCUSSION

1. The sickle cells or the 'holly-leaf' form of the cell must come to a point or points to be considered positive. Elongated cells with a rounded end must not be confused with sickle cells.

2. Sickling of the red blood cells is maximal at 37°C and decreases as the temperature decreases. Sickling also occurs more readily at a decreased pH.

3. With this method, it is difficult to distinguish sickle cell trait from sickle cell anemia. (In sickle cell anemia, the sickling reaction occurs more rapidly than in sickle cell trait. This, however, must not be relied upon to differentiate between the two conditions.) If the sickle cell preparation is positive, it is advisable to perform a hemoglobin electrophoresis to determine the presence of the trait or the anemia.

4. Either sodium metabisulfite or sodium bisulfite may be used in this procedure.

5. It is advantageous to run a positive control each time this test is performed in case the reagent has deteriorated.

6. In infants with a sickling hemoglobin, this test may be negative until they reach approximately 2 months of age.

Solubility Test

REFERENCES

Nalbandian, R.M., Nichols, B.M., Camp, F.R., Jr., Lusher, J.M., Conte, N.F., Henry, R.L., and Wolf, P.L.: Dithionite tube test—a rapid, inexpensive technique for the detection of hemoglobin. Clin. Chem., *17*:1028, 1971.

National Committee for Clinical Laboratory Standards, *Solubility test for confirming the presence of sickling hemoglobins,* Document #H10-A, NCCLS, Villanova, Pa., 1986.

REAGENTS AND EQUIPMENT

1. Stock solution
   Dibasic potassium phosphate, 216 g

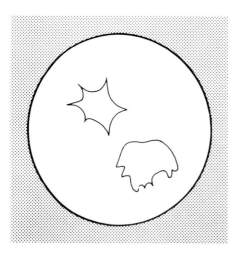

Fig. 131. Holly-leaf shaped red blood cells.

anhydrous (K_2HPO_4)

Monobasic potassium 169 g
  phosphate, crystals (KH_2PO_4)
Saponin 10 g
Sodium hydrosulfite 5 g
  (dithionite) ($NA_2S_2O_4$)

Place approximately 500 mL of distilled water into a 1-liter volumetric flask. Add the dibasic potassium phosphate and mix until dissolved. Add the remaining reagents, one at a time, dissolving each one in the mixture before adding the next reagent. This solution is stable for approximately 1 month stored at 4°C.

2. Working solution
   Stock solution 10 mL
   Sodium hydrosulfite 50 mg
     (dithionite)
   Prepare fresh, on the day of testing. Pre-prepared reagent is available commercially from most laboratory supply companies.
3. Test tubes, 12 × 75 mm.
4. Lined reader scale. This may be prepared by obtaining a piece of white cardboard and drawing relatively fine black parallel lines on it.
5. Pipets, 2.0 mL and 10 μL.

SPECIMEN

Whole blood, using EDTA, heparin, or sodium citrate as the anticoagulant.

PRINCIPLE

When red blood cells are added to the working solution, the red cells immediately lyse due to the saponin present. Hemoglobin S (and non-S sickling hemoglobins), in the reduced state, in a concentrated buffer solution, forms liquid crystals and gives a turbid appearance to the mixture.

PROCEDURE

1. Centrifuge a small portion (1 mL) of whole blood at 1200 g for 5 minutes. Remove the plasma and buffy coat layers.

2. Make certain the stock solution is at room temperature. Prepare the working solution and add 2 mL of the working solution to a 12 × 75 mm test tube for each patient and control (positive and negative) to be tested.
3. Add 10 μL of the centrifuged red blood cells to each appropriately labeled tube. Mix.
4. Allow tubes to stand at room temperature for 5 to 6 minutes.
5. Place the tube approximately 1 inch in front of the lined reader scale. If there is no sickling hemoglobin present, the solution will be clear and the lines on the reader scale will be visible through the solution. If a sickling hemoglobin is present, the solution will be turbid and the scale will not be visible through the solution (Fig. 132).
6. If the lines on the reader scale are visible through the test solution, report the results as negative. Failure to see these lines because of turbidity should be reported as a positive test.

DISCUSSION

1. Whole blood may be used for this

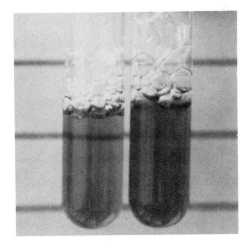

Fig. 132. Sodium dithionite tube test. (Negative results are indicated by the clear solution, where the black lines on the reader scale are visible through the test solution. Positive results are shown as a turbid solution, where the reader scale is not visible through the test solution.)

procedure, in which case, 20 μL of whole blood is added to 2.0 mL of working solution. However, when whole blood is used, the results are more liable to false negatives or false positives: hemoglobins of less than 7 g/dL will cause false negative results, while certain abnormal plasma proteins, hyperproteinemia, or extremely high hemoglobins may cause false positive test results.

2. If the solubility test is positive, a hemoglobin electrophoresis should be performed on the specimen. Conversely, hemoglobin electrophoresis results showing the presence of hemoglobin S should be verified by a positive solubility test.

3. The purity of the saponin reagent is important. Fisher saponin has been found to be effective in this procedure. Also, care should be taken in handling the anhydrous dibasic potassium phosphate. This reagent absorbs moisture upon excessive exposure to the air.

4. The size of the test tube is important. Use of 10 × 75 mm test tubes may result in false negative results.

5. Fresh blood specimens are not necessary for this test. Reliable results have been obtained on specimens up to 20 days old.

6. The solubility test is more sensitive to sickling hemoglobins than the sodium metabisulfite method, however, false negative results may be obtained on infants 1 or 2 months old.

7. A positive solubility test may be found in hemoglobin Bart's and Hemoglobin C$_{HARLEM}$.

8. Deterioration of reagents is an important factor in causing false negative and false positive results. It is, therefore, important to use positive and negative controls each time this procedure is performed.

4

Special Hematology Procedures

EXAMINATION OF THE BONE MARROW

Examination of the bone marrow is a widely used method of diagnosing many hematologic disorders. It is a valuable procedure in conditions where diagnostic cells are present in the bone marrow but absent in the peripheral blood. Such conditions are found in Gaucher's disease, multiple myeloma, Niemann-Pick disease, some megaloblastic anemias, and when tumor cells are metastasizing (spreading) from other organs of the body. When pancytopenia exists, a bone marrow examination is helpful to rule out the diagnosis of leukemia and, where possible, to determine the cause of the pancytopenia. In addition to determining the presence of specific cells, the bone marrow procedure offers the opportunity for assessing the iron stores and cellularity of the marrow. Alterations in the normal distribution of cells may be noted, and the marrow cells may also be studied with special staining techniques.

Samples of bone marrow may be obtained from the sternum, the iliac crest, the spinous process of the lumbar vertebrae, and from the tibia in children under 2 years of age. The usual site of puncture in adults is the sternum, in the midline of the bone between the second and third ribs. The anterior or posterior iliac crest is also a common site for bone marrow biopsy. This area is advantageous in that there are no vital organs near the site of puncture and the patient is unable to see what is happening, which is helpful if the person is apprehensive.

Bone Marrow Biopsy

The bone marrow biopsy is carried out using sterile techniques. If necessary, the skin at the puncture site may be shaved. A wide area around the site is washed and cleaned with a suitable antiseptic solution, the same as for any minor surgical procedure. The area surrounding the puncture site is draped with sterile towels and a local anesthetic is injected into the skin and periosteum of the bone. After 1 or 2 minutes, a small ⅛ inch stab wound is made in the skin at the puncture site to avoid pushing the skin into the bone marrow. The area is now ready for the biopsy. A special needle is employed, of which there are several varieties available. These needles generally consist of a heavy duty, short, outer needle and a stylet which fits inside the needle. The outer needle has an adjustable guard to prevent it from entering too deeply into the bone. With the stylet in place, the needle is inserted until it impinges on the outer surface of the bone. The guard is screwed down until it comes in contact with the skin. It is then screwed back a set distance, between 3 and 5 mm. The needle is inserted through the bone until the guard comes in contact with the skin and in this way the needle only advances the preset distance into the bone. The stylet is removed from inside the needle and a small syringe is attached. Firm, sharp pressure is applied to the plunger of the syringe to withdraw marrow. When this is done, the patient usually feels some pain. As soon as a few drops of marrow have entered the syringe, it is removed and passed to a technologist for the preparation of smears. If more marrow is desired, a second syringe may be attached to the needle and approximately 0.5 ml of marrow withdrawn. The syringe is removed, and the blood placed in a tube containing the proper amount of EDTA or heparin. The needle is removed from the bone, and a sterile dressing is applied.

Preparation of the Bone Marrow for Study

The exact procedures to be followed in preparing the bone marrow will vary according to the possible diagnosis of the patient. The most frequently used techniques are outlined below.

1. Using the first syringe containing only a few drops of marrow:
   a. Place the marrow on a slide in the form of a large drop.
   b. Using a spreader slide, immediately make 5 to 8 thin smears. (Dip one end of the spreader slide into the pool of marrow. Transfer the marrow on the end of the slide to a clean glass slide and spread as for a routine blood smear.) It may also be desirable at this time to prepare several coverslip preparations. (The small clumps present in the specimen are marrow particles.)
   c. To prepare *particle* smears, place several of the marrow particles, from the slide, onto three or four clean slides or coverslips using the broken end of an applicator stick. Gently crush these marrow particles by covering with a glass slide or coverslip and exerting a small amount of pressure. Pull the slides or coverslips apart with a smooth motion. This will spread the crushed particle.
   d. When the pool of marrow remaining on the original slide has clotted, transfer this to a small bottle of suitable fixative for the cytology department, where stained sections of the clot will be made.
2. Place the marrow obtained from the second syringe into a tube containing EDTA or heparin to prevent clotting, and return this specimen to the laboratory.
3. Using the fingerstick procedure, prepare several routine peripheral blood smears from the patient.
4. After adequate mixing of the anticoagulated bone marrow, place in a Wintrobe tube and centrifuge at 1500 × g for 10 minutes. Four layers should then be seen (fat, plasma, nucleated cells, and red blood cells), and their relative volumes should be noted. Normally, there is 1 to 3% fat and 5 to 8% nucleated cells. Marrow which has been diluted with peripheral blood contains a smaller proportion of fat and nucleated cells. As the percent of nucleated cells increases and the amount of fat present decreases, the marrow is termed *hypercellular.* If the fat layer increases and the percent of nucleated cells decreases, the marrow is *hypocellular.* The volumes of the plasma and red cell layers will vary depending upon how much sinusoidal blood is present. Remove the plasma and fat layers from the Wintrobe tube. Using a clean, disposable dropper, withdraw the nucleated cell layer, dilute with an equal volume of the plasma on a watch glass, and make several smears of this material. These are called *concentrate,* or *buffy coat,* smears.
5. The following smears are generally Wright stained:

a. Thin direct smears (2).

b. Concentrate smear (1).

c. Particle smear (1).

d. Peripheral blood smear (1).

(When Wright-staining bone marrow smears, it is advisable to double the staining times, especially when there is increased marrow cellularity.)

6. It is often advisable to routinely stain a concentrate smear with the Prussian blue stain for iron. Other stains in widespread use for bone marrow smears are the peroxidase, Sudan black B, and the periodic acid-Schiff, among others. The stains requested depend on the possible diagnosis of the patient.

7. The sections of clot prepared by the cytology department are generally stained with the hematoxylin and eosin stain in addition to special stains as indicated.

Examination of Marrow Slides

The bone marrow slides are studied and reported by the attending pathologist, with or without the aid of a technologist experienced in this area of hematology. A general outline of this procedure follows:

1. Examine the marrow section to determine the relative cellularity of the marrow. At this time, with experience, it is possible to detect certain abnormal cells if they are present. A differentiation between myeloid and erythroid cells is also possible.

2. A systematic examination of the direct marrow slide is made. The Wright stained smear is examined first, using low power (10 ×). In scanning, megakaryocytes, abnormal cells of large size, and groups of abnormal cells may be detected. Using the oil immersion objective (100 ×), a differential cell count is made, based on a count of 200 to 500 nucleated cells. This will determine abnormalities present in the distribution of cells, including alteration in

the myeloid:erythroid ratio. At the same time, the cells are also examined for morphologic abnormalities. (If the direct smear is very hypocellular, the concentrate smear may be examined.) Normal ranges for a differential count on bone marrow is shown in Table 3.

3. The Prussian blue stained concentrate smear is examined, and an estimate is made of the sideroblasts and particulate iron present.

4. Any marrow smears which had special stains are examined, evaluated, and reported.

IRON (PRUSSIAN-BLUE) STAIN

Siderocytes are red blood cells that have one or more iron containing granules. When these granules are found in nucleated red blood cells, the cell is called a *sideroblast*. (See Plate VII A, B.) These iron containing granules stain positively with the Prussian-blue stain but do not stain with Wright's stain. In contrast, *Pappenheimer bodies* (iron deposits in the mitochondria) stain positively with both the Prussian-blue and the Wright stains. *Basophilic stippling* (clusters of ribosomes) does not stain with Prussian-blue.

It is thought that siderotic granules represent iron that has not yet been incorporated into hemoglobin. Normally, these granules are found in 20 to 60% of the nucleated red blood cells in the bone marrow. These granules are also found in some marrow reticulocytes but are not normally present in the mature red blood cell of the peripheral blood. In certain diseases in which the synthesis of hemoglobin is disturbed, an increased number of siderocyte granules are found. Also, the granules are generally larger in size. In sideroblastic anemias, the granules may be arranged in a ring around the nucleus of the nucleated red blood cell *(ringed sideroblast)*. The iron stores of the body and the serum iron level are related to the percent of sideroblasts in the bone marrow. In iron defi-

TABLE 3. NORMAL RANGES FOR THE BONE MARROW IN ADULTS

CELL	PERCENT
Myeloblast	0.3–4.0
Promyelocyte	1.0–5.0
Myelocytes	
Neutrophil	5.0–19.0
Eosinophil	0.5–3.0
Basophil	0.0–0.5
Metamyelocytes	13.0–32.0
Neutrophils	7.0–25.0
Eosinophils	0.5–4.0
Basophils	0.0–0.7
Lymphocytes	3.0–20.0
Monocytes	0.5–3.0
Megakaryocytes	0.1–3.0
Plasma cells	0.1–3.0
Reticulum cells	0.1–2.0
Pronormoblast	1.0–5.0
Basophilic normoblast	
Polychromatophilic normoblast	7.0–32.0
Orthochromic normoblast	
Mitotic cells	0.0–2.0
Myeloid:erythroid ratio	2:1–5:1

ciency anemia, in which the iron stores are markedly decreased, the number of marrow sideroblasts is also reduced. Siderocytes are usually present in the peripheral blood following splenectomy since the spleen, as one of its functions, removes the red blood cell from the circulation until heme synthesis is complete. The spleen may also remove these granules from the red blood cell.

REFERENCE

Lillie, R.D., and Fullmer, H.M.: *Histopathologic Technic and Practical Histochemistry*, New York, McGraw-Hill Book Co., 1976.

REAGENTS AND EQUIPMENT

1. Methyl alcohol, Mallinckrodt (absolute anhydrous, acetone free).
2. Prussian-blue reagent.

Potassium ferrocyanide	2.0 g
Distilled water	36 mL
Hydrochloric acid, concentrated	4 mL

   Use immediately after preparation.
3. Buffered neutral red, 1% w/v in acetate buffer, 0.1 N, pH 5.0.
4. Coplin jars, 2.
5. Coverslips.
6. Permount mounting medium.

SPECIMEN

Air dried blood or bone marrow slides.

PRINCIPLE

Prussian-blue reagent stains nonheme iron a vivid blue or green color. Nuclei and red cells are stained red or pink by the neutral red.

PROCEDURE

1. Fix blood or bone marrow smears by flooding the slide with methanol for 30 seconds. Allow to air dry.
2. Place the smears in a coplin jar containing Prussian-blue reagent for 30 minutes.
3. Rinse the smears in distilled water.
4. Place the smears in a coplin jar containing neutral red and counterstain for 10 minutes.
5. Wash smears under running tap water.
6. Allow to air dry and coverslip with Permount mounting medium.

DISCUSSION

1. A positive control smear should be run each time this test is performed.
2. Wright-stained smears several years

old may be effectively stained with Prussian-blue reagent.

LEUKOCYTE ALKALINE PHOSPHATASE STAIN

Alkaline phosphatase activity is present in varying degrees in the neutrophilic granulocytes and, sometimes, to a very small degree in certain B lymphocytes. (See Plate VII, C, D.) The amount of alkaline phosphatase present will vary in different diseases. Increased values for this test are found during pregnancy (the last trimester), in infections accompanied by neutrophilia, polycythemia vera, people receiving corticosteroids, aplastic anemia, multiple myeloma, myelosclerosis, and obstructive jaundice. In Hodgkin's disease the results of this stain closely parallels the progression of the disease, being elevated in untreated cases. In one type of lymphocytic lymphoma some lymphocytes will show alkaline phosphatase activity. Decreased scores for this test will be found in chronic myelogenous leukemia, paroxysmal nocturnal hemoglobinuria, sickle cell anemia, hereditary hypophosphatasemia, marked eosinophilia, sideroblastic anemia, and rarely, in normal people. Normal alkaline phosphatase activity will be found in untreated hemolytic anemia, lymphosarcoma, viral hepatitis, and secondary polycythemia.

REFERENCES

Ackerman, G.A.: Substituted naphthol AS phosphate derivatives for the localization of leukocyte alkaline phosphatase activity, Lab. Invest., *11,* 563, 1962.

Sigma Diagnostics: Alkaline Phosphatase, pkg. insert, St. Louis, Sigma Chemical Co., 1984.

REAGENTS AND EQUIPMENT

1. Acetone.
2. The following reagents are available from Sigma Chemical Co., St. Louis, Mo.:
   a. Citrate concentrated solution. Store at room temperature. Do not use if contamination is evident.
      (1) Citrate working solution. Dilute 2 mL of citrate concentrated solution to 100 mL with distilled water. Store in refrigerator.
      (2) Citrate buffered acetone, 60% w/v, (fixative). Prepare just prior to use. Add 20 mL of the citrate working solution (must be at room temperature) to 30 mL of acetone, while constantly stirring the mixture. Discard after using.
   b. Naphthol AS-MX phosphate alkaline solution, 0.25%, pH 8.6. Store in refrigerator.
   c. Fast blue RR salt (capsules). Store at 0°C.
   d. Mayer's hematoxylin solution, 1 g/L. Store at room temperature.
3. Coplin jars, 3.

SPECIMEN

Capillary blood is recommended: collect five or six well-made fingerstick blood smears from the patient, from a positive control (pregnant woman in the last trimester), and from a normal control. Alternatively, blood may be collected using heparin as the anticoagulant.

PRINCIPLE

The blood smears are fixed, and when placed in the incubating solution, the alkaline phosphatase present in the white blood cells liberates naphthol, which couples with fast blue RR to form an insoluble blue compound. The smears are then counterstained. The degree of reactivity is determined by scoring each neutrophil according to the amount of precipitated dye present.

PROCEDURE

1. Immediately after collection, place the air dried blood smears in a coplin jar containing citrate buffered acetone (fixative) for 30 seconds.

2. Carefully rinse the smears in running tap water for 10 to 20 seconds.
3. Allow smears to air dry for at least 15 minutes. (If staining is to be delayed for more than 2 hours, store smears in the dark at room temperature.)
4. Prepare the staining solution immediately before use:
   a. Dissolve the contents of 1 capsule of fast blue RR in 48 mL of distilled water.
   b. Add 2 mL of naphthol AS-MX phosphate alkaline solution and mix.
   c. Place stain in a coplin jar. Discard stain after use.
5. Place smears in the staining solution for 30 minutes at room temperature.
6. Wash smears in running tap water.
7. Counterstain with Mayer's hematoxylin for 10 minutes. Allow smears to air dry.
8. Examine the smears microscopically, using the oil immersion objective $(100 \times)$. Count 100 consecutive neutrophils and grade each one from 0 to 4 on the basis of the appearance of the precipitated dye in the cytoplasm.
   0 = No staining.
   1 = Faint and diffuse blue cytoplasm.
   2 = Pale, with a moderate amount of blue staining.
   3 = Strong blue staining of the cytoplasm.
   4 = Deep blue or brilliant staining of the entire cytoplasm.
9. The total of the rating for 100 neutrophils is the score reported. The normal range for this test will generally fall in the vicinity of 30 to 185, but should be determined by each laboratory.

DISCUSSION

1. Smears should be stained within 8 hours of blood collection. If this is not possible, the smears may be prepared, fixed, and stored at room temperature for a short period of time. Delay in staining will cause gradual loss of alkaline phosphatase activity.
2. The entire staining procedure should be carried out with the slides protected from direct light as much as possible.
3. Various mounting media have been found to adversely affect the dye in the stain. It is therefore preferable not to coverslip the smears.

PEROXIDASE STAIN

The peroxidase stain is generally used to identify granulocytes and monocytes. (See Plate VII E, F.) Myeloperoxidase is present in neutrophils, eosinophils and monocytes, but is not found in lymphocytes. This stain is often used in the classification of acute leukemias where the blasts present in myeloblastic and myelomonocytic leukemias will show peroxidase activity.

REFERENCES

Graham, R.C., Lundholm, U., and Karnovsky, M.J.: Cytochemical demonstration of peroxidase activity with 3-amino-9-ethylcarbazole, J. Histochem. Cytochem., 13, 150, 1965.

Kaplow, L.S.: Substitute for benzidine in myeloperoxidase stains, Am. J. Clin. Path., 63, 451, 1975.

REAGENTS AND EQUIPMENT

1. Phosphate buffered formalin acetone fixative, pH 6.6 to 6.8.
2. Acetic acid, 0.02 M.
   Glacial acetic acid   1.16 mL
   Dilute to 1 liter with distilled water.
3. Sodium acetate, 0.02 M.
   Sodium acetate   2.72 g
   $(CH_3COONa \cdot 3H_2O)$
   Dilute to 1 liter with distilled water.
4. Acetate buffer, 0.02 M, pH 5.0 to 5.2.
   Acetic acid, 0.02 M   176 mL
   Sodium acetate, 0.02 M   800 mL
   Store in the refrigerator.
5. Hydrogen peroxide, 0.3%.

Hydrogen peroxide, 30%   0.1 mL
Distilled water   9.9 mL
Prepare immediately before use.

6. Stain, pH 5.5.
   3-Amino-9-ethylcarbazole   10 mg
   (obtainable from Sigma Chemical
   Co., St. Louis, Mo.)
   Dimethyl sulfoxide   6.0 mL
   Acetate buffer, 0.02 M,   50 mL
   pH 5.0 to 5.2
   Hydrogen peroxide,   0.4 mL
   0.3% v/v
   Filter before use. Allow stain to age
   at room temperature for 30 minutes
   prior to use.
7. Mayer's hematoxylin.
8. PVP mounting medium.
9. Coplin jars, 3.
10. Coverslips.

SPECIMEN

Fresh blood smears made from capillary blood are recommended, or, use fresh whole blood anticoagulated with EDTA.

PROCEDURE

1. Prepare thin blood or bone marrow smears and allow to air dry.
2. Place the smears in a coplin jar containing phosphate buffered formalin acetone for 30 seconds at room temperature.
3. Wash the smears under gently running tap water.
4. Place the smears in a coplin jar containing the stain mixture for 12 minutes.
5. Wash the smears under gently running tap water.
6. Counterstain the smears in a coplin jar containing Mayer's hematoxylin for 5 minutes.
7. Wash the smears under gently running tap water.
8. Allow the smears to air dry and immediately mount and coverslip in PVP mounting medium to prevent the stain from fading.
9. Examine the smears microscopically,

using the oil immersion objective (100×). The presence of peroxidases is indicated by reddish-brown deposits present in the cytoplasm of the granulocytes and monocytes. The cytoplasm of the neutrophils is packed with these red-brown granules. The monocytes show a small to moderate number of the granules. The eosinophil exhibits darkly stained granules, whereas the basophil and lymphocyte remain unstained. The early myeloblast may give a negative reaction.

PERIODIC ACID-SCHIFF (PAS) REACTION

The periodic acid-Schiff stain indicates the presence of mucoproteins, glycoproteins, and high molecular weight carbohydrates. In blood cells it is primarily glycogen which stains positively. Normally, almost all blood cells, except erythroblasts, show positive staining. The intensity of the stain and the pattern of staining will vary with the cell type. (See Plate VII G.) Granulocytes normally show a diffuse staining pattern, while lymphocyte staining has a granular pattern. Granulocytes show a positive reaction in all stages of development, the mature neutrophils reacting the most strongly. Myelocytes and myeloblasts contain fewer positively stained granules. Eosinophil granules do not take up the stain, but the background cytoplasm stains positively. Lymphocytes contain a few fine or coarse, positively stained granules. Monocyte granules exhibit a small amount of positive staining, and nucleated red blood cells generally show no positively stained granules. In disease states, the PAS staining reaction will differ from the normal and this is of some diagnostic value. In chronic lymphocytic leukemia, lymphosarcoma, and Hodgkin's disease, the lymphocytes contain an increased number of positively stained granules. In erythroleukemia (Di Guglielmo's disease) and thalassemia, the nucleated red blood cells often show a positive reaction. Some positive staining of the nucleated red blood cells has also been found in iron deficiency anemia, some hemolytic anemias, pernicious anemia, aplastic anemia, and polycythemia.

REFERENCES

McManus, J.F.A.: Histological demonstration of mucin after periodic acid, Nature, *158,* 202, 1946.

Dacie, J.V., and Lewis, S.M.: *Practical Hematology,* 6th ed., New York, Churchill Livingstone Inc., 1984.

REAGENTS AND EQUIPMENT

1. Methanol.
2. Periodic acid solution, 1% w/v. Store in refrigerator in a brown bottle. Stable for 3 to 4 months.
3. Schiff's reagent.

    Basic fuchsin   1.0 g
    Boiling distilled water   400 mL
    Allow the preceding solution to cool to 50°C and filter. Add 1.0 g of thionyl chloride ($SOCl_2$). Allow the mixture to stand in the dark for 12 hours. Add 2.0 g of activated charcoal to the mixture, shake for 1 minute, filter, and store in the dark at 0 to 4°C. (This reagent may be obtained commercially from Rowley Biochemical Institute, Rowley, Ma., 01969.)
4. Mayer's hematoxylin.
5. Coplin jars.
6. Permount mounting medium.

SPECIMEN

Air dried blood or bone marrow smears.

PROCEDURE

1. Fix and place smears in a coplin jar containing methanol.
2. Wash smears in running tap water for 15 minutes.
3. Place smears in a coplin jar containing 1% periodic acid for 10 minutes.
4. Drain smears and place in a coplin jar containing Schiff's reagent for 30 minutes.
5. Rinse smears in tap water and then wash in distilled water for 5 minutes.
6. Counterstain smears in a coplin jar containing Mayer's hematoxylin for 5 minutes.
7. Rinse smears with tap water and allow to air dry.
8. Coverslip smears using Permount mounting medium.
9. Examine the smears microscopically, using the oil immersion objective (100×). The glycogen present in the cells will stain positively, taking on a reddish purple color.

DISCUSSION

1. Blood or bone marrow smears that have been Wright stained may be successfully stained according to the preceding procedure.
2. Smears several years old, whether Wright-stained or not, may also be stained by the PAS stain.
3. To make certain the Schiff's reagent is still effective it may be tested by adding a few drops of the reagent to 10 mL of formaldehyde (37%). The mixture should change to a light purple color. If it does not, this indicates that the Schiff's reagent is no longer good and it should be discarded.

SUDAN BLACK B STAIN

Sudan black B stains various lipids, among which are sterols, phospholipids, and neutral fats. As a stain, it is most often employed to distinguish the different types of acute leukemia. Lymphocytic granules do not stain. The myelogenous cells show coarse staining granules with faint staining in the myeloblast. (See Plate VII H.) The monocytic cells show positive staining of the finely scattered granules. This stain is similar to the peroxidase stain in the types of cells which stain positively. It is also similar in sensitivity to the peroxidase stain, but is more sensitive than the chloroacetate esterase in the staining of myeloblasts. It may be noted that vacuolated immature cells found in Burkitt's lymphoma may show positive staining of the lipid present in the vacuoles.

REFERENCE

Sheehan, H.L., and Storey, G.W.: An improved method of staining leukocyte granules with Sudan black B, J. Path. Bact., *59*, 336, 1947.

REAGENTS AND EQUIPMENT

1. Stock buffer solution.

Crystalline phenol	16 g
Ethanol	30 mL

   Add the preceding two reagents to 100 mL of distilled water containing 0.3 g of disodium phosphate ($Na_2HPO_4 \cdot 12H_2O$).

2. Stock Sudan solution.

Sudan black B	0.3 g
Ethanol	100 mL

   Prepare this solution several days prior to use. Allow it to sit at room temperature and shake frequently to ensure that all of the dye is dissolved.

3. Sudan black B staining solution.

Stock buffer solution	20 mL
Stock Sudan solution	30 mL

   Stable for 2 to 3 months.

4. Formaldehyde, 37%.
5. Buffered neutral red, 1% w/v in acetate buffer, 0.1 N, pH 5.0.
6. Ethyl alcohol, 70% v/v.
7. Coplin jars, 2.
8. PVP mounting medium.

SPECIMEN

Air dried blood or bone marrow smears.

PROCEDURE

1. Place torn up filter paper in the bottom of a coplin jar and moisten with 37% formaldehyde.
2. Place the air dried smears in the coplin jar and cover. Allow the smears to fix in the vapor for 10 minutes. Wash gently in tap water, allowing excess water to drain from the smear (avoid washing smear off slide).
3. Place the smears in a coplin jar containing Sudan black B staining solution for 30 minutes. (The time is variable, between 10 and 60 minutes depending on the age of the staining solution.)
4. Rinse each slide with 70% ethyl alcohol just long enough to remove the excess stain.
5. Wash the smears gently in running tap water for 2 minutes.
6. Place the smears in a coplin jar containing 1% neutral red and counterstain for 10 minutes.
7. Wash the slides very gently in tap water, air dry, and coverslip with PVP mounting medium.
8. Examine the smears microscopically, using the oil immersion objective (100×). The neutrophils are packed with fine granules taking up the black stain. The eosinophils have a similar appearance, whereas the monocytes have a moderate number of black-staining granules distributed evenly throughout the cell. The lymphocyte granules remain unstained.

DISCUSSION

1. Bone marrow or blood smears need not be fresh to obtain good results with the Sudan black B stain.
2. As the Sudan black B stain ages, it may be necessary to increase the staining time.
3. The granules are not readily decolorized by the 70% ethyl alcohol.

ACID PHOSPHATASE STAIN (WITH TARTRATE RESISTANCE)

Acid phosphatase is present in myelogenous cells, lymphocytes, plasma cells, monocytes, and platelets. In this test, the acid phosphatase in the cytoplasm of the cells stain a red color. (See Plate VII I.) L(+) tartaric acid inhibits acid phosphatase activity, and when added to the incubation mixture, the preceding cells exhibit no acid phosphatase activity (stain negatively). The acid phosphatase present in the 'hairy' cells of hairy cell leukemia (leukemic reticuloendotheliosis), however, is resistant to L(+) tartaric acid and stains strongly positive even when this chemical has been added to the incubation mixture. The atypical lymphocyte of infectious mononucleosis and, rarely, the lymphocytes in chronic lymphocytic leukemia and lymphosarcoma may show less than complete resistance to L(+) tartaric acid. (They may stain very faintly positive.)

REFERENCE

Katayama, I., and Yang, J.P.S.: Reassessment of a cytochemical test for differential diagnosis of leukemic reticuloendotheliosis, Am. J. Clin. Path., *68*, 268, 1977.

REAGENTS AND EQUIPMENT

1. Phosphate buffered formalin acetone fixative, pH 6.6 to 6.8.
2. Sodium nitrite, 4% w/v. Prepare immediately before use.
3. Pararosanilin solution, 4% w/v in 20% (v/v) hydrochloric acid.
4. Saturated sodium hydroxide.
5. Solution A.
   Sodium nitrite, 4%   2.4 mL
   Pararosanilin solution,   2.4 mL
      4%, in 20% HCl
   Mix immediately before use in a 250 mL beaker.
6. Solution B.
   Naphthol AS-BI   40 mg
      phosphoric acid
      (obtainable from Sigma Chemical Co., St. Louis, Mo.)
   N,N-dimethyl formamide   4.0 mL
   Acetate buffer,   71.2 mL
      0.1 N, pH 5.0
   Prepare immediately before use.
7. Incubation mixture I.
   Add solution B to solution A. Mix and place 40 mL in a separate beaker. Adjust the pH of mixture I to pH 5.1 with saturated sodium hydroxide. Filter into a coplin jar in the 37°C water bath and use immediately.

8. Incubation mixture II.
   L(+) tartaric acid   0.3 g
   Incubation mixture I   40 mL
   Mix and adjust pH to 5.1 with saturated sodium hydroxide. Filter into a coplin jar and use immediately.
9. Methyl green, 1% w/v, in acetate buffer, 0.1 N, pH 5.0.
10. PVP mounting medium.
11. 37°C water bath.
12. Coplin jars, 7.
13. Coverslips.

SPECIMEN

Air dried blood or bone marrow smears.

PROCEDURE

1. Prepare thin blood or bone marrow smears and allow to air dry. At least two smears should be prepared on each patient and normal control. Label one smear from each patient and normal control, I, and the second smear, II.
2. Place the slides in a coplin jar containing cold phosphate buffered formalin acetone for 30 seconds.
3. Wash smears in three changes of distilled water.
4. Place the appropriately labeled slide for each patient and normal control into a coplin jar containing incubation mixture I and into a coplin jar containing incubation mixture II. Incubate the smears at 37°C for 60 minutes.
5. Wash smears in two changes of distilled water.
6. Place smears into a coplin jar containing 1% methyl green for 2 minutes.
7. Wash smears quickly in running tap water.
8. Allow the smears to air dry, mount, and coverslip in PVP mounting medium.
9. Examine the smears microscopically using oil immersion objective (100×). Those smears from incuba-

tion mixture I should show acid phosphate activity in the cytoplasm of the white blood cells and the platelets (varying degrees of reddish staining). The smears from incubation mixture II should show no acid phosphatase activity or only a minute amount of red staining. The 'hairy' cells of hairy cell leukemia exhibit positive red staining from both incubation mixtures I and II.

NONSPECIFIC ESTERASE STAIN (WITH FLUORIDE INHIBITION)

White blood cells contain esterases, a group of lysosomal enzymes. The esterase stains (nonspecific and specific [chloroacetate]) are primarily utilized to differentiate granulocytic and monocytic leukemias. The nonspecific esterase stain, using α-naphthyl acetate as substrate, is more specific for monocytic cells and shows positive staining in the monocytes, macrophages, megakaryocytes, and platelets. (See Plate VII J.) In the presence of fluoride, however, the staining reaction is inhibited and these cells show no staining for nonspecific esterase activity. The lymphoblasts of acute lymphocytic leukemia may show a few weakly positive coarse granules which are not inhibited by fluoride. The nonspecific esterase stain is negative in acute myelogenous leukemia. Acute monocytic leukemia generally shows 80 to 100% of the cells with a positive stain, while in myelomonocytic leukemia, the monocytes will not stain as positively and the granulocytes may show some positive staining which is not inhibited by fluoride. The erythroblasts present in erythroleukemia and DiGuglielmo's syndrome may stain positively for nonspecific esterase.

REFERENCE

Yam, L.T., Li, C.Y., and Crosby, W.H.: Cytochemical identification of monocytes and granulocytes, Am. J. Clin. Path., *55*, 283, 1971.

REAGENTS AND EQUIPMENT

1. Cold phosphate buffered formalin acetone, fixative, pH 6.6 to 6.8.
2. Pararosanilin, 4% w/v in 20% (v/v) hydrochloric acid.
3. Sodium nitrite, 4% w/v. Make fresh, just prior to use.
4. Phosphate buffer, M/15, pH 6.3.
   Dibasic sodium phosphate   1.183 g
       (Na_2HPO_4)
   Monobasic potassium   3.399 g
       phosphate (KH_2PO_4)
   Dilute to 500 mL with distilled water. Store in the refrigerator. Reagent must be at room temperature when used.
5. Sodium hydroxide, 1 N.
6. Sodium fluoride, 0.1 M.
   Sodium fluoride   0.42 g
   Dilute to 100 mL with distilled water. Store at room temperature.
7. α-Naphthyl acetate in ethylene glycol monomethyl ether. Prepare just prior to use.
   α-Naphthyl acetate   0.2 g
   Ethylene glycol   10.0 mL
       monomethyl ether
8. Incubation mixture (A) without fluoride. Prepare just prior to use.
   Pararosanilin   3.0 mL
       (4% w/v in 20% HCl)
   Sodium nitrite, 4% w/v   3.0 mL
   Mix in a 200-mL beaker. Allow to sit for 1 minute and add:
   Phosphate buffer M/15,   89.0 mL
       pH 6.3
   α-Naphthyl acetate   5.0 mL
       in ethylene glycol
       monomethyl ether
   Mix. Remove 50 mL of this solution and place in a 100-mL beaker. This will be used to prepare the incubation mixture (B) with fluoride. Adjust the pH of incubation mixture A to approximately 6.1 (5.8 to 6.5), using 1 N sodium hydroxide. Filter directly into a coplin jar and use immediately.
9. Incubation mixture (B) with fluoride.

Add 0.5 mL of 0.1 M sodium fluoride to 50 mL of incubation mixture (A) (which was set aside). Adjust the pH to 6.1 (5.8 to 6.5) using 1 N sodium hydroxide. Filter directly into a coplin jar and use immediately.

10. Buffered methyl green, 1% w/v in acetate buffer, 0.1 N, pH 5.0.
11. Permount mounting medium.
12. Coplin jars.
13. Coverslips.

SPECIMEN

Air-dried blood or bone marrow smears.

PROCEDURE

1. Prepare thin blood or bone-marrow smears and allow to air dry. At least two smears should be prepared for each patient and normal control. Label one smear from each patient and normal control, A, and the second smear from each, B.
2. Fix the above smears in a coplin jar containing cold phosphate buffered formalin acetone for 30 to 60 seconds.
3. Wash smears in three changes of distilled water.
4. Allow smears to air dry for 10 to 30 minutes while making up the incubation mixtures.
5. Place the appropriately labeled slide for each patient and normal control into a coplin jar containing incubation mixture A and into a second coplin jar containing incubation mixture B. Incubate the smears at room temperature for 60 minutes.
6. Wash smears in three changes of distilled water.
7. Counterstain, by placing the smears in a coplin jar containing 1% methyl green for 1 to 2 minutes.
8. Wash smears in running tap water.
9. Allow the smears to air dry and coverslip with Permount.
10. Examine the smears microscopically using the oil immersion objective (100×). Nonspecific esterase activity is indicated by the presence of dark red-staining granules in the cytoplasm of the cell. Those smears from incubation mixture A (without fluoride) will show strong esterase activity in the cytoplasm of the monocytes, macrophages, megakaryocytes, and platelets. There may also be positive staining in some T-lymphocytes and plasma cells. Immature granulocytes and normal erythroblasts will show very weak to no nonspecific esterase activity. With fluoride, nonspecific esterase staining is inhibited in the monocytes, macrophages, megakaryocytes, and platelets.

CHLOROACETATE ESTERASE STAIN

The chloroacetate stain is specific for esterases found in the granulocytic cells and is frequently performed in combination with the nonspecific esterase stain to differentiate monocytic from granulocytic cells. (See Plate VII K.)

REFERENCE

Yam, L.T., Li, C.Y., and Crosby, W.H.: Cytochemical identification of monocytes and granulocytes, Am. J. Clin. Path., 55, 283, 1971.

REAGENTS AND EQUIPMENT

1. Cold phosphate buffered formalin acetone fixative pH 6.6 to 6.8.
2. Buffered methyl green, 1% w/v in acetate buffer, 0.1 N, pH 5.0.
3. Phosphate buffer, M/15, pH 7.4.
   Dibasic sodium phosphate   3.786 g
   (Na_2HPO_4)
   Monobasic potassium   0.907 g
   phosphate (KH_2PO_4)
   Dilute to 500 mL with distilled water.
   Adjust the pH to 7.4.
4. Naphthol AS-D chloroacetate (0.2% w/v in N,N-dimethlyformamide).
   Naphthol AS-D chloroacetate 10 mg
   N,N-dimethylformamide   5.0 mL
   Prepare immediately before use.

5. Incubation mixture.

Phosphate buffer (M/15, pH 7.4)	47.5 mL
Naphthol AS-D chloro- acetate (0.2% w/v in N,N- dimethylformamide)	2.5 mL
Fast blue BB	30 mg

Mix and filter directly into a coplin jar. Prepare immediately before use.
6. Permount mounting medium.
7. Coplin jars.
8. Coverslips.

SPECIMEN

Air-dried blood or bone marrow smears.

PROCEDURE

1. Prepare thin blood or bone marrow smears on the patient and the normal control and allow to air-dry.
2. Fix the smears in a coplin jar containing cold, phosphate buffered formalin acetone for 30 to 60 seconds.
3. Wash smears in three changes of distilled water.
4. Allow smears to air dry for 10 to 30 minutes while preparing the incubation mixture.
5. Place smears in a coplin jar containing the incubation mixture for 20 minutes.
6. Wash smears in three changes of distilled water.
7. Counterstain by placing the smears in a coplin jar containing 1% methyl green for 1 to 2 minutes.
8. Wash smears in running tap water.
9. Allow smears to air-dry and coverslip using Permount.
10. Examine the smears microscopically using the high immersion objective (100 ×). Chloroacetate esterase activity will show up as blue-staining granules in the granulocytic cells. Basophils show little to no chloroacetate esterase activity. Granulocytes, including promyelocytes, will show very strong activity, as do many, but not all, myeloblasts. Monocytes show little to no activity. Lymphocytes, eosinophils, plasma cells, megakaryocytes, and erythroblasts show no chloroacetate esterase activity.

DISCUSSION

1. Unfixed smears up to 2 weeks old that were stored at room temperature may be successfully stained by this procedure. There appears to be no loss of enzyme activity during this time.
2. The nonspecific esterase stain and the chloroacetate esterase stain may be combined and performed on the same patient and control slides. To do the combined nonspecific esterase stain and chloroacetate esterase stain, perform steps 1 through 6 as outlined for the nonspecific esterase stain. Continue the procedure by performing steps 5 through 9 as described above for the chloroacetate esterase stain. The staining results for the combined stain are similar to the individual stain results. Nonspecific esterase activity is indicated by dark red granules in the monocytes, histiocytes, and megakaryocytes. Blue staining granules in the cytoplasm of the granulocytes indicates chloroacetate esterase activity.

NITROBLUE TETRAZOLIUM (NBT) NEUTROPHIL REDUCTION TEST

The nitroblue tetrazolium reduction test is helpful in diagnosing chronic granulomatous disease. In this disorder, markedly decreased values for the NBT reduction test are obtained. The test may also be used to monitor patients who have a high susceptibility to bacterial infections, to differentiate bacterial infections from nonbacterial infections, and to determine a patient's response to antibiotic therapy. This procedure may also be used in diagnosing other disease states by incubating the blood with substances capable of stimulating the phagocytic system.

REFERENCES

Sigma Chemical Co.: Nitroblue tetrazolium (NBT) reduction, histochemical demonstration in neutrophils, pkg. insert, St. Louis, Mo., Sigma Chemical Co., 1985.

Park, B.H., Fikrig, S.M., and Smithwick, E.M.: Infection and nitroblue tetrazolium reduction by neutrophils, Lancet, 2, 532, 1968.

REAGENTS AND EQUIPMENT

1. The following reagents and equipment are available from Sigma Chemical Co.:
   a. Siliconized collection vial containing 20 units of heparin (#840–20).
   b. Nitroblue tetrazolium, 1 mg, (#840–10). Store in the dark at 2 to 6°C. Reconstitute with 1.0 mL of distilled water. Mix vigorously. Once reconstituted the reagent is stable for 1 day stored in the refrigerator.
2. Plastic syringe, 5 mL.
3. Test tubes, plastic, 12 × 75 mm, with caps.
4. Pipets, 1.0 and 0.1 mL.
5. Water bath, 37°C.
6. Glass microscope slides.
7. Wright stain and buffer.

SPECIMEN

Heparinized whole blood, 1.0 mL. Using a plastic syringe, carefully obtain 1.5 to 2 ml of whole blood making certain the specimen is not contaminated with tissue juice. Remove the needle from the syringe and slowly add 1.0 ml of blood to the heparinized tube (containing 20 units of heparin). Cap the tube and gently mix by tilting the tube for about 30 seconds. Do not allow the blood to come in contact with the tube cap. Collect blood for a normal control at the same time the patient's blood is obtained.

PRINCIPLE

Increased enzyme activity normally present in neutrophils during a bacterial infection is capable of reducing nitroblue tetrazolium to formazan, which forms a black precipitate. In fatal granulomatous disease, the neutrophils do not have a normal ability to kill certain organisms and are also unable to reduce nitroblue tetrazolium. In this procedure, blood is mixed with nitroblue tetrazolium, allowed to incubate, and smears made and counterstained with Wright stain. The smears are examined microscopically for neutrophils containing formazan. In healthy adults 10% or less of the neutrophils contain formazan. (Some normal samples may show up to 17% neutrophils containing formazan.) In the presence of a bacterial infection, up to 70% of the neutrophils normally reduce the nitroblue tetrazolium.

PROCEDURE

1. Pipet 0.1 mL of NBT reagent into an appropriately labeled plastic test tube, 12 × 75 mm, for each specimen and control to be tested.
2. Add 0.1 mL of well-mixed whole blood to the above tube. Mix thoroughly by gently tilting the tube using a rolling motion. Cap tube.
3. Incubate each tube for 10 minutes at 37°C. At the end of this period, remove the tubes from the incubator and allow to stand at room temperature for an additional 10 minutes.
4. Mix the tubes very gently. Transfer a small drop of each mixture onto labelled microscopic slides and prepare a moderately thick blood smear on each specimen. (A thick smear is prepared in order to cause less mechanical damage to the neutrophils.) Allow smears to air dry.
5. Wright stain the above blood smears according to your laboratory's procedure. Allow smears to air dry.
6. Using the oil immersion objective (100×), count 100 neutrophils, enumerating those neutrophils that contain the reduced nitroblue tetrazolium. The formazan appears as

large black deposits in the neutrophil. Report results as the percent of neutrophils containing reduced nitroblue tetrazolium (% of NBT positive neutrophils). (See Plate VII M, N.)

DISCUSSION

1. Control blood from a normal person should be tested along with the patient's blood.
2. The absolute number of NBT positive neutrophils may be determined by performing a white count and 100 cell differential on the test blood. Calculate the absolute number of neutrophils present by multiplying the percent of neutrophils by the white count. Multiply the absolute number of neutrophils by the percent of NBT positive neutrophils to obtain the absolute number of NBT positive neutrophils.
3. In chronic granulomatous disease, there is negligible to 0 reduction of the nitroblue tetrazolium.
4. An increased concentration of heparin may give false positive results.
5. As an aid in detecting metabolic defects of neutrophil function, this procedure may be performed using a stimulating agent (a nonviable bacterial extract is available from Sigma Chemical Co. for this purpose [Stimulant—#840-15]). In this test, the procedure as described above is performed in exactly the same manner by mixing 1.0 mL of NBT solution with 0.05 mL of whole blood and 0.05 mL of stimulant. Normal results with this modification are quite variable but will usually be increased by an additional 10 to 50% NBT positive cells. This modification may be performed simultaneously with the unstimulated procedure.
6. The whole blood specimens for this test should be treated gently through-

out the procedure to avoid break-up of the neutrophils.
7. Each laboratory should determine its own normal range for this procedure.

LUPUS ERYTHEMATOSUS PREPARATION (L.E. PREP)

Antinuclear antibodies occur in the serum of patients with a number of disorders including systemic lupus erythematosus. This antinuclear antibody is also termed the LE factor and is a component of the γ globulin fraction of the serum protein. Four different methods are available for detection of the LE factor: (1) immunofluorescence procedure, (2) radioimmunoassay procedure, (3) a serologic procedure using coated latex particles, and (4) demonstration of LE cells (as described below) where the LE factor in the serum causes the lysis of neutrophil nuclei, with subsequent phagocytosis of this nuclear material by other neutrophils.

REFERENCES

Dacie, J.V., and Lewis, S.M.: *Practical Haematology*, New York, Churchill Livingstone, Inc., 1984.

Magath, T.B., and Winkle, V.: Technic for demonstrating "L.E." (lupus erythematosus) cells in blood, Am. J. Clin. Path., *22*, 586, 1952.

Zinkham, W.H., and Conley, C.L.: Some factors influencing the formation of L.E. cells. A method for enhancing L.E. cell production. Bullet. Johns Hopkins Hosp., *98*, 102, 1956.

L.E. Cell Technique Using Heparinized Blood

REAGENTS AND EQUIPMENT

1. Glass beads, 4 mm in diameter.
2. Test tube rotator.
3. Wintrobe ESR tubes, 3 to 4.
4. Glass slides.
5. Wright stain.
6. Disposable dropper pipets with a long narrow tip for filling the Wintrobe tubes.
7. Incubator or water bath, 37°C.

SPECIMEN

Five mL of whole blood using heparin as the anticoagulant. Make certain there is no excess heparin present in the tube (for the amount of patient blood added). (Heparin concentration must be the minimum amount to prevent clotting.)

PRINCIPLE

In order for the LE factor (present in a patient's plasma) to lyse the neutrophil nuclei, the neutrophils must first be damaged to allow for liberation of the nuclei from the cells. Glass beads are therefore added to whole blood which is then mixed for a period of time in order to damage some of the neutrophils. The blood is then incubated for a period of time to allow for lysis of the neutrophil nuclei. The whole blood is centrifuged and buffy coat smears prepared, stained and examined for phagocytized nuclear material (L.E. cells).

PROCEDURE

1. Place 5 to 10 glass beads in the tube of blood.
2. Place blood on a mechanical rotator and mix for 30 minutes.
3. Incubate tube of blood at 37°C for 15 to 30 minutes.
4. Fill three to four Wintrobe tubes with well-mixed blood.
5. Centrifuge tubes at 200 × g for 10 minutes.
6. Discard the plasma from each of the tubes. Remove the buffy coat from each tube and prepare three to four smears. Wright stain.

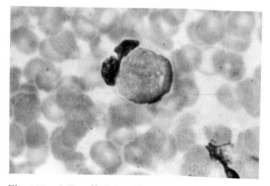

Fig. 134. L.E. cell. (Magnification × 1000.)

7. Examine each smear for the presence of L. E. cells (Figs. 133 and 134). Report results as positive or negative. The slides should be examined for at least 10 minutes. The smear should be studied using the low oil objective (50×), or on low power (10×) when enough experience has been gained. All suspicious cells should be examined under the high oil immersion objective (100×). The characteristic L.E. cell appears as a neutrophil containing a large spherical body in its cytoplasm. Ordinarily, the nucleus of the neutrophil is pushed to one side of the cell and may appear to wrap itself around the ingested material. The inclusion shows no nuclear structure and stains as a pale purple homogeneous mass. It has a velvety appearance. In rare instances, the ingesting cell may be a monocyte or eosinophil. The L.E. phenomenon also includes *rosettes,* which consist of free lysed nuclear material surrounded by neutrophils. These are readily seen using the low power objective (10×). The *tart cell,* which may be confused with the L.E. cell, is usually a monocyte which has ingested another cell or the nucleus of another cell. In this case, the ingested material generally resembles a lymphocyte nucleus or phagocytized material with a definite nuclear pattern.

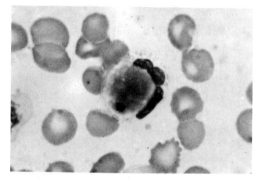

Fig. 133. L.E. cell. (Magnification × 1000.)

Another form of ingested material found in the tart cell is an intensely stained body termed a *pyknotic nucleus.* The significance of these cells is not known. Their presence in an L.E. preparation does not signify a positive test for systemic lupus erythematosus.

L.E. Cell Technique Using Clotted Blood

REAGENTS AND EQUIPMENT
1. Wire sieve and pestle.
2. Petri dish.
3. Wintrobe ESR tubes, three to four.
4. Glass slides.
5. Wright stain.
6. Disposable dropper pipets with a long narrow tip for filling the Wintrobe tubes.
7. Incubator or water bath, 37°C.

SPECIMEN
Clotted whole blood, 10 ml.

PRINCIPLE
Clotted blood is allowed to sit at room temperature for 2 hours. The clot is then macerated by forcing it through a sieve. The trauma produced when the blood is forced through the strainer causes extrusion of nuclei from the polymorphonuclear cells. The LE factor present in the blood lyses the nuclear material, which is then phagocytized by other neutrophils. This forms the L.E. cell.

PROCEDURE
1. Place 10 ml of whole blood in a plain test tube and allow the blood to clot.
2. Incubate the tube of clotted blood at room temperature for 2 hours.
3. Place the sieve over a petri dish.
4. Transfer the clot and serum to the sieve and mash the clot through the sieve, using the pestle.
5. Transfer the blood from the petri dish to three or four Wintrobe tubes.
6. Incubate the filled Wintrobe tubes at 37°C for 2 hours.
7. Centrifuge the Wintrobe tubes at 200 × g for 10 minutes.
8. Remove the serum from each of the tubes, using a disposable dropper. Remove the buffy coat from each tube and prepare three to four blood smears. Wright stain.
9. Examine smears as described in step 7 above for the procedure using heparinized blood.

DISCUSSION
1. The presence of one L.E. cell is not a substantial basis for reporting a positive result. Several typical L.E. cells should be seen before a positive report is made.
2. If a patient has severe leukopenia, a false-negative result may be obtained due to the decrease in neutrophils present. Therefore, because the LE factor is present in the serum, 5 mL of patient's serum may be added to 5 mL of washed red and white blood cells (type O blood) obtained from a normal individual. The test should then be carried out as previously described.
3. Occasionally, false-positive results are obtained in patients with drug reactions, hepatitis, and rheumatoid arthritis.
4. This test is positive only in about 75% of the patients with systemic lupus erythematosus. False-negative results may also be obtained on patients with the disease who are receiving adrenocorticosteroid therapy.

OSMOTIC FRAGILITY TEST

The osmotic fragility test using fresh red blood cells is a measure of the ability of the red cells to take up fluid without lysing. This test is employed to help diagnose different types of anemias in which the physical properties of the red blood cell are altered. The main factor affecting the osmotic fragility test is the shape of the red blood cell, which, in turn, is dependent on the volume, surface area, and functional state of the red blood cell membrane. An increased osmotic fragility is found in hemolytic anemias, hereditary spherocytosis, and whenever spherocytes are found. Decreased osmotic fragility occurs following splenectomy, in liver disease, sickle cell anemia, iron-deficiency anemia, thalassemia, polycythemia vera, and in conditions in which target cells are present. Reticulocytes also show a decreased osmotic fragility.

REFERENCES

Dacie, J.V., and Lewis, S.M.: *Practical Hematology*, 6th ed., New York, Churchill Livingstone, Inc., 1984.

Parpart, A.K., Lorenz, P.B., Parpart, E.R., Gregg, J.R., and Chase, A.M.: The osmotic resistance (fragility) of human red cells, J. Clin. Invest., *26*, 636, 1947.

REAGENTS AND EQUIPMENT

1. Buffered sodium chloride stock solution (osmotically equivalent to 10% of sodium chloride).

   Sodium chloride   90 g
   (Dry for 24 hours in a desiccator with calcium chloride prior to weighing out.)

   Dibasic sodium   13.76 g
     phosphate (Na_2HPO_4)
   Monobasic sodium   2.43 g
     phosphate ($NaH_2PO_4 \cdot 2\ H_2O$)

   Dilute to 1 liter with distilled water. This solution is stable for several months at room temperature if it is kept well stoppered.

2. Buffered sodium chloride working solution.

   Buffered sodium chloride   20 mL
     stock solution
   Distilled water   180 mL

3. Distilled water.
4. Erlenmeyer flask (250 mL) and glass beads (3 to 4 mm in diameter), if defibrinated whole blood is used.
5. Pipets, 10, 5, and 0.05 mL.
6. Test tubes 13 × 100 mm.
7. Parafilm.
8. Centrifuge.
9. Spectrophotometer.

SPECIMEN

Heparinized venous blood, or, 15 to 20 mL of defibrinated whole blood. A normal control blood should be collected in the same manner and at the same time the patient's blood is drawn. The test should be set up within 2 hours of collection, or within 6 hours of collection if the blood is refrigerated.

PRINCIPLE

If red blood cells are placed in an isotonic solution, 0.85% sodium chloride, fluid will neither enter nor leave the red blood cell. If red blood cells are placed in a hypotonic solution (0.25% sodium chloride), however, fluid enters the red blood cell, the cell swells up, and eventually hemolyzes or ruptures. A spherocyte, which is almost round, swells up in a hypotonic solution and ruptures much more quickly than a normal red blood cell or more quickly than cells that have a large surface area per volume, such as target cells or sickle cells. The fragility of the red blood cell is said to be increased when the rate of hemolysis is increased. When the rate of hemolysis is decreased, the fragility of the red blood cells is considered to be decreased. In the osmotic fragility test, whole blood is added to varying concentrations of buffered sodium chloride solution and allowed to incubate at room temperature. The amount of hemolysis is then determined by reading the supernatants on a spectrophotometer. A normal control blood is run at the same time the patient's blood is being tested.

PROCEDURE

1. Prepare dilutions of buffered sodium chloride and place in the appropriately labeled test tube (Table 4).
2. Mix the preceding dilutions well, using Parafilm to cover each test tube while mixing.

TABLE 4. DILUTIONS AND NORMAL RANGES FOR THE OSMOTIC FRAGILITY TEST

TEST TUBE #	1% BUFFERED SODIUM CHLORIDE (mL)	DISTILLED WATER (mL)	FINAL CONCEN. BUFF. SODIUM CHLORIDE (%)	% HEMOLYSIS
1	10.0	0.0	1.00	0
2	8.5	1.5	0.85	0
3	7.5	2.5	0.75	0
4	6.5	3.5	0.65	0
5	6.0	4.0	0.60	0
6	5.5	4.5	0.55	0
7	5.0	5.0	0.50	0–5
8	4.5	5.5	0.45	0–45
9	4.0	6.0	0.40	50–90
10	3.5	6.5	0.35	90–99
11	3.0	7.0	0.30	97–100
12	2.0	8.0	0.20	100
13	1.0	9.0	0.10	100
14	0.0	10.0	0.00	100

3. Transfer 5 mL of each dilution to a second set of test tubes, labeled #1 through #14. This set of dilutions will be used for the normal control blood.

4. If defibrinated blood is to be used, proceed as follows:
   a. Place 15 to 20 mL of whole blood into an Erlenmeyer flask containing 15 glass beads.
   b. Gently rotate the flask until the hum or noise of the beads on the glass can no longer be heard (about 10 minutes).
   c. Repeat steps 4a and 4b for the normal control blood.

5. Add 0.05 mL of the patient's heparinized or defibrinated blood to each of the 14 test tubes. Repeat, adding the normal control blood to the set of 14 control test tubes.

6. Mix each test tube immediately by gentle inversion.

7. Allow the test tubes to stand at room temperature for 30 minutes.

8. Remix the test tubes gently and centrifuge at 1200 to 1500 g for 5 minutes.

9. Carefully transfer the supernatants to cuvettes and read on a spectrophotometer at a wavelength of 540 nm. Set the optical density at 0, using the supernatant in test tube #1, which represents the blank, or 0% hemolysis. Test tube #14 represents 100% hemolysis.

10. Calculate the percent hemolysis for each supernatant as follows:

$$\text{Percent hemolysis} = \frac{\text{O.D. of supernatant}}{\text{O.D. supernatant tube \#14}} \times 100$$

11. The results of the test may then be graphed, with the percent hemolysis plotted on the ordinate (vertical axis) and the sodium chloride concentration on the abscissa (horizontal axis) as shown in Figure 135 (shows normal range).

12. Normal results are shown in Table 4.

DISCUSSION

1. Instead of determining the amount of hemolysis on the sperctrophotometer, the test may be read visually. In this method, the first test tube (the highest concentration of sodium chloride) showing a trace of hemolysis in the supernatant determines the beginning of hemolysis. The first test tube, having the highest concentration of sodium chloride in which hemolysis is complete, determines complete hemolysis. Hemolysis should be complete in 0.3% sodium chloride. Beginning hemolysis

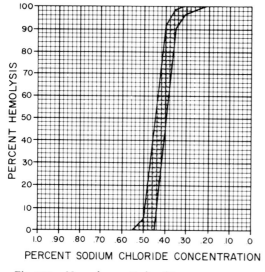

Fig. 135. Normal osmotic fragility curve.

should not occur in a concentration over 0.45% sodium chloride.

2. The pH of the blood-saline mixture is important and should be 7.4.

3. There are many possible sources of technical error in this procedure. It is, therefore, important to report the control results and interpret the patient's test in light of the normal control values.

4. If anticoagulated blood is used for this test, use only heparin as the anticoagulant, in order to avoid adding more salts to the blood.

5. Becton-Dickinson manufactures a Unopette test kit for determination of the red cell osmotic fragility test. This reagent set is made up of 10 buffered saline concentrations (0.85%, 0.65%, 0.60%, 0.55%, 0.50%, 0.45%, 0.40%, 0.35%, 0.30%, and 0.0%) contained in Unopette reservoirs. Each Unopette contains 1.98 mL of a buffered saline reagent with preservative (to inhibit bacterial growth). For testing, 20 μL of well-mixed whole blood (heparinized or defibrinated) is added to each Unopette dilution, mixed, incubated at room temperature for 20 minutes, re-

mixed, transferred to 12 × 75 mm test tubes, centrifuged at 2000 RPM for 5 minutes, and the supernatants read on a spectrophotometer at a wavelength of 540 nm. The normal ranges for this method are similar to those for the procedure outlined above.

OSMOTIC FRAGILITY TEST WITH INCUBATION

The osmotic fragility of red cells after 24 hours of incubation at 37°C is also a measure of their ability to take up fluid without lysing. There are, however, other factors which affect this ability. Normally, after incubation, the red blood cells have increased osmotic fragility due to an accumulation of sodium in the red cells which is greater than the loss of potassium. This is determined by the membrane properties of the red cell and the metabolic activity of the cell. The metabolism of the red cell during incubation is stressed due to a lack of glucose. Those red cells with an abnormal membrane (hereditary spherocytosis, elliptocytosis) show an abnormal increase in osmotic fragility. Red cells having a glycolytic deficiency (pyruvate kinase deficiency) will show variable results: if the deficiency is severe, the osmotic fragility may increase greatly, or the fragility may decrease due to a greater loss of potassium in proportion to the increases in sodium in the red cell. Thalassemias major and minor generally show markedly reduced fragility due to a large loss of potassium. Iron deficiency anemia usually shows a less marked decrease in osmotic fragility. Therefore, abnormal results in the incubated osmotic fragility indicate an abnormality but are not always diagnostic of a specific disorder.

REFERENCE

Dacie, J.V., and Lewis, S.M.: *Practical Hematology,*
6th ed., New York, Churchill Livingstone, Inc.,
1984.

REAGENTS AND EQUIPMENT

1. Water bath 37°C.
2. Buffered sodium chloride stock solution. (See Osmotic Fragility Test, Reagents and Equipment.)
3. Buffered sodium chloride working solution. (See Osmotic Fragility Test, Reagents and Equipment.)
4. Sterile Erlenmeyer flask (250 mL), sterile glass beads (3 to 4 mm in diameter), and 10 mL sterile screw cap vials (2/specimen), if defibrinated whole blood is used.
5. Distilled water.
6. Pipets, 10, 5, and 0.05 mL.
7. Test tubes, 13 × 100 mm.
8. Parafilm.
9. Centrifuge.
10. Spectrophotometer.

SPECIMEN

Heparinized venous blood, or, 15 to 20 mL of defibrinated whole blood. A normal control blood should be collected in the same manner and at the same time the patient's blood is drawn.

PROCEDURE

1. Place unopened heparinized tube of patient and normal control blood in the 37°C water bath and incubate for 24 hours.
2. If defibrinated blood is to be used, proceed as follows:
   a. Place 15 to 20 mL of whole blood into a sterile Erlenmeyer flask containing 15 glass beads.
   b. Gently rotate the flask until the hum or noise of the beads on the glass can no longer be heard (about 10 minutes).
   c. Place 5 mL of the patient's defibrinated blood into each of two sterile screw-cap vials. Repeat, using the control blood.
   d. Incubate the above specimens of blood at 37°C for 24 hours.
3. At the end of the 24 hours of incubation, number two sets of test tubes #1 through 17.
4. Prepare the dilutions (see Table 5) of buffered sodium chloride and place in the appropriately labeled test tubes.
5. Mix the preceding dilutions well, using Parafilm to cover each test tube while mixing.
6. Transfer 5 mL of each dilution to the second set of labeled test tubes. This is to be used for the normal control blood.
7. Gently mix the incubated blood samples. (Pool the contents of the two patient test tubes together and combine the contents of the two control test tubes, if defibrinated blood was used. Do not pool the samples if one appears to be contaminated.) The blood should not be grossly hemolyzed.
8. Add 0.05 mL of the patient's incubated blood to each of the 17 test tubes. Repeat, adding the normal incubated control blood to the set of 17 control test tubes.
9. Mix each test tube immediately by gentle inversion.
10. Allow the test tubes to stand at room temperature for 30 minutes.
11. Remix the test tubes gently and centrifuge at 1200 to 1500 g for 5 minutes.
12. Carefully transfer the supernatants to cuvettes and read on a spectrophotometer at a wavelength of 540. Set 0 optical density using the supernatant in test tube #1, which represents the blank, or 0% hemolysis. Test tube #17 represent 100% hemolysis.
13. Calculate the percent hemolysis for each supernatant:

$$\text{Percent hemolysis} = \frac{\text{O.D. of supernatant}}{\text{O.D. supernatant tube \#17}} \times 100$$

14. The results of the test should be graphed with the percent hemolysis

TABLE 5.   DILUTIONS AND NORMAL RANGES FOR THE INCUBATED OSMOTIC FRAGILITY TEST

TEST TUBE #	1% BUFFERED SODIUM CHLORIDE (mL)	DISTILLED WATER (mL)	FINAL CONCEN. BUFF. SODIUM CHLORIDE (%)	% HEMOLYSIS
1	10.0	0.0	1.00	0
2	9.0	1.0	0.90	0
3	8.5	1.5	0.85	0
4	8.0	2.0	0.80	0
5	7.5	2.5	0.75	0
6	7.0	3.0	0.70	0–5
7	6.5	3.5	0.65	0–10
8	6.0	4.0	0.60	0–40
9	5.5	4.5	0.55	15–70
10	5.0	5.0	0.50	40–85
11	4.5	5.5	0.45	55–95
12	4.0	6.0	0.40	65–100
13	3.5	6.5	0.35	75–100
14	3.0	7.0	0.30	85–100
15	2.5	7.5	0.25	90–100
16	2.0	8.0	0.20	95–100
17	1.0	9.0	0.10	100

plotted on the ordinate (vertical axis) and the sodium chloride concentration on the abscissa (horizontal axis) as shown in Figure 136 (shows normal range).

15. Normal results are shown in Table 5.

DISCUSSION

1. It is important to maintain the sterility of the blood during incubation at 37°C. Bacterial contamination may produce hemolysis and inaccurate test results. The test may be performed in duplicate if desired.

2. The Becton-Dickinson Unopette test kit for the red cell osmotic fragility test may also be used in this procedure, in the same manner as outlined for the non-incubated osmotic fragility test.

AUTOHEMOLYSIS TEST

The primary purpose of the autohemolysis test is in the diagnosis of hereditary spherocytosis. In the past, it was useful in differentiating several types of congenital nonspherocytic hemolytic anemias, namely type I (Dacie) congenital nonspherocytic hemolytic anemia (paroxysmal nocturnal hemoglobinuria, glucose-6-phosphate dehydrogenase deficiency), and type II (Dacie) congenital nonspherocytic hemolytic anemia (pyruvate kinase deficiency). The development of less complicated and more specific enzyme assays have made the test unnecessary for this purpose.

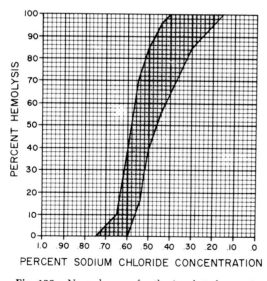

Fig. 136.   Normal curve for the incubated osmotic fragility test.

REFERENCE

Dacie, J.V., and Lewis, S.M.: *Practical Hematology*, New York, Churchill Livingstone, Inc., 1984.

REAGENTS AND EQUIPMENT

1. Water bath, 37°C.
2. Glass beads, 3 to 4 mm in diameter.
3. Cyanmethemoglobin (HiCN) reagent.
4. Glucose solution, 10%.

Glucose	10.0 g
Sodium chloride, 0.85% (w/v)	100 mL

   This solution must be sterile. Autoclave or sterilize by Seitz filtration.
5. Sterile 0.85% sodium chloride (w/v).
6. Sterile screw-cap test tubes.
7. Sterile Erlenmeyer flask, 125 mL.
8. Sterile pipets, 2.0 and 0.1 mL.

SPECIMEN

Whole defibrinated blood (15 to 20 mL) from the patient and a normal control.

PRINCIPLE

Sterile, defibrinated blood is incubated for 48 hours at 37°C. A second sample of defibrinated blood is incubated with a specific amount of glucose. The percent hemolysis in each specimen is determined spectrophotometrically. Normally, and in certain disorders, such as herditary spherocytosis, glucose inhibits or reduces the amount of autohemolysis. In other pathologic states, the presence of added glucose does not effectively decrease the autohemolysis.

PROCEDURE

1. The entire test procedure must be run under sterile conditions.
2. Defibrinate the patient and control bloods according to the following procedure:
   a. Place 15 to 20 mL of whole blood in a 125 mL sterile Erlenmeyer flask containing 15 glass beads.
   b. Gently rotate the flask until the hum or noise of the beads on the glass can no longer be heard (about 10 minutes).
3. Label 8 sterile screw cap tubes, #1 through #8.
4. Place 2 mL of the patient's defibrinated blood into test tubes #1, 2, 3, and 4. Place the remainder of the patient's defibrinated blood in an empty sterile screw cap tube and centrifuge at 1500 × g for 10 minutes. Remove the serum and place in a sterile screw cap tube in the refrigerator.
5. Repeat step 4 above for the normal control blood. (Label test tubes #5, 6, 7, and 8.)
6. Add 0.1 mL of 0.85% sodium chloride to tubes #1, 2, 5, and 6. Gently mix the tubes.
7. Add 0.1 ml of 10% glucose solution to test tubes #3, 4, 7, and 8. Mix the tubes gently.
8. Incubate the 8 test tubes at 37°C for 24 hours.
9. At the end of 24 hours, gently mix the test tubes by carefully inverting them 5 to 10 times. Incubate the tubes for an additional 24 hours.
10. At the end of 48 hours, inspect each test tube for contamination (a greenish discoloration or bad odor).
11. If there is no contamination, pool test tubes #1 and 2 together, #3 and 4 together, #5 and 6 together, #7 and 8 together.
12. Perform a duplicate hematocrit on each of the four specimens. Average the duplicate readings and record the results.
13. Pipet 0.02 mL of well-mixed blood from each test tube to four separate tubes containing 5.0 ml of cyanmethemoglobin reagent (1:251 dilution).
14. Centrifuge the four tubes of pooled blood at 1500 × g for 10 minutes.
15. Remove the supernatant serums from each tube and pipet 0.5 mL of each serum into appropriately labeled test tubes containing 5.0 mL of cyanmethemoglobin reagent (1:11 dilution).
16. Pipet 0.5 mL of the nonincubated (refrigerated) patient's serum into an appropriately labeled test tube con-

taining 5.0 mL of cyanmethemoglobin reagent. Repeat, pipetting 0.5 mL of the nonincubated (refrigerated) control serum into a second test tube containing 5.0 mL of cyanmethemoglobin reagent.

17. Record the optical density of the following solutions diluted with cyanmethemoglobin reagent, using a spectrophotometer set at a wavelength of 550 nm and using the cyanmethemoglobin reagent as the solution blank (0 O.D.):

a. Patient's incubated whole blood.
b. Patient's incubated serum without glucose.
c. Patient's incubated serum with glucose.
d. Patient's nonincubated serum.
e. Control's incubated whole blood.
f. Control's incubated serum without glucose.
g. Control's incubated serum with glucose.
h. Control's nonincubated serum.

18. Calculate the percent hemolysis for the control and patient bloods incubated with, and without, glucose according to the following formula:

$$\% \text{ Hemolysis} = (D_2 - D_3) \times \frac{\text{Dilution factor}}{\text{of serum}}$$

$$\times \frac{100 - \text{hematocrit}}{D_1 \times \text{Dilution factor of blood}}$$

D_1 = The optical density of diluted whole blood.

D_2 = The optical density of the diluted serum after incubation.

D_3 = The optical density of the diluted nonincubated serum.

Dilution factor of serum = 11.

Dilution factor of whole blood = 251.

19. Interpretation of test results. Normally, there is less than 2.0% hemolysis in the blood specimen with no added glucose, and less than 0.9% hemolysis in the specimen with added glucose. In hereditary spherocytosis, autohemolysis in the absence of added glucose is generally greatly increased. With the addition of glucose, however, autohemolysis is usually reduced.

DISCUSSION

1. There may be considerable methemoglobin formation in the preceding procedure. Therefore, the cyanmethemoglobin method must be employed for measuring the amount of hemoglobin in the serum.

2. Hemolysis may be increased by bacterial contamination.

ASCORBATE-CYANIDE SCREENING TEST

The ascorbate-cyanide test is a nonspecific screening procedure which detects deficiencies in the pentose phosphate pathway. Positive results will be found, most commonly, in glucose-6-phosphate dehydrogenase deficiency, but the procedure also detects deficiencies in glutathione, glutathione peroxidase, and glutathione reductase.

Jacob and Jandl Method

REFERENCES

Jacob, H.S., and Jandl, J.H.: A simple visual screening test for glucose-6-phosphate dehydrogenase deficiency employing ascorbate and cyanide, N. Engl. J. Med., 274, 1162, 1966.

Deacon-Smith, R.: The ascorbate cyanide test and the detection of females heterozygous for glucose-6-phosphate dehydrogenase deficiency, Med. Lab. Sciences, 39, 139, 1982.

REAGENTS AND EQUIPMENT

1. Ascorbate and glucose tubes for testing.

Place:

Sodium ascorbate	10.0 mg
Glucose	5.0 mg

into each of several 13 × 100 mm test tubes. (One tube is used for each test and control.) These tubes may be stoppered and stored at −20°C indefinitely.

2. Iso-osmotic phosphate buffer, pH 7.4.

Solution 1

Monobasic sodium phosphate ($NaH_2PO_4 \cdot 2H_2O$)   23.4 g

Dilute to 1 liter with distilled water.

Solution 2

Dibasic sodium phosphate (Na_2HPO_4)   21.3 g

Dilute to 1 liter with distilled water.

For iso-osmotic phosphate buffer, pH 7.4, mix together:

Solution 1   18 mL
Solution 2   82 mL

3. Sodium cyanide.

Sodium cyanide   500 mg
Distilled water   50 mL
Iso-osmotic phosphate buffer 20 mL

Adjust the above mixture to a pH of 7.0 using 3 N hydrochloric acid. Dilute to 100 ml with distilled water. This solution is stable at room temperature indefinitely.

4. Pipets, 2.0 and 0.1 mL.
5. Water bath, 37°C.

SPECIMEN

Collect 3 ml of whole blood, using heparin or EDTA as the anticoagulant. A normal control blood should be collected at the same time the patient's blood is obtained. (EDTA is the anticoagulant of choice.)

PRINCIPLE

In the red blood cell, catalase normally inhibits, or decomposes, hydrogen peroxide. Sodium cyanide, however, added to the blood inhibits catalase and allows hydrogen peroxide to be generated. If the enzymes in the pentose phosphate pathway are not able to utilize the added glucose, the red blood cells are oxidized by the hydrogen peroxide and converted to methemoglobin (brown color).

PROCEDURE

1. Aerate both patient and control bloods to a bright red color by gently swirling the blood under air.

2. Add 2 mL of well-mixed whole blood to a test tube containing sodium ascorbate and glucose. Repeat, for each specimen and control to be tested.

3. Mix each tube well.

4. Add 0.1 mL of sodium cyanide solution to each of the preceding test tubes.

5. Gently mix the tubes and place, unstoppered, in a 37°C water bath for 2 to 4 hours.

6. During the incubation, gently shake each mixture at the end of 2, 3, and 4 hours and inspect the color of the solutions each time.

7. The normal control mixture should be a red color. If the patient's mixture is red, the test result is normal. If, however, the patient's solution has turned a brown color, the test is positive, and there is probably an enzyme deficiency in the pentose phosphate pathway, most often a glucose-6-phosphate dehydrogenase deficiency. (Generally, the color change is not very great when positive results are obtained. A certain amount of experience is required to correctly detect the end point. As soon as the tube of blood is shaken, note the color of the film of blood as it moves down the side of the test tube.) If EDTA is used as the anticoagulant and the result is positive, the color change to brown is most evident within 1½ to 2 hours of incubation. With the use of heparin, however, this color change will take 3 to 4 hours.

DISCUSSION

1. If the blood specimen has a hematocrit below 20%, the volume of blood added to the ascorbate tube should be adjusted so that the amount of red blood cells added is equivalent to a hematocrit of 30 to 40%. For exam-

ple, if the hematocrit is 20%, add 3 to 4 ml of whole blood to the ascorbate tube. As an alternative method, an appropriate amount of plasma may be removed from the whole blood until a hematocrit reading of 30 to 40% is attained.

2. To increase the sensitivity of this test, the red blood cells may be stained and examined for inclusions at the conclusion of the test. Add 2 drops of the test mixture to 8 drops of 0.5% methyl violet (w/v, in 0.85% [w/v sodium chloride]) (filter before use) and incubate at room temperature for 10 minutes. Prepare several blood smears, allow to air dry, and examine the red blood cells for inclusions. Normal blood will show less than 5% of the red cells containing inclusion bodies. A specimen from a patient heterozygous for glucose-6-phosphate dehydrogenase deficiency will show an increased number of red cells containing inclusion bodies in a variable number of the red blood cells. Homozygotes will show virtually all red blood cells with inclusions.

3. Due to normally decreased concentrations of gluthathione peroxidase in newborns, this age group may also show positive results when tested by this procedure.

GLUCOSE-6-PHOSPHATE DEHYDROGENASE TEST

When red blood cells are exposed to an oxidant drug, the activity of the hexose monophosphate shunt increases. If one of the enzymes in this pathway is decreased or absent, reduced glutathione cannot be produced and oxidation of the hemoglobin takes place.

REFERENCES

Beutler, E.: A series of new screening procedures for pyruvate kinase deficiency, glucose-6-phosphate dehydrogenase deficiency, and gluthathione reductase deficiency, Blood, *28,* 553, 1966.

Sigma Diagnostics: Glucose-6-Phosphate Dehydrogenase (G-6-PDH) Deficiency, pkg. insert, St. Louis, Sigma Chemical Co., 1984.

REAGENTS AND EQUIPMENT

1. The following reagents are obtainable from Sigma Chemical Co., St. Louis:
   a. Phosphate buffer, 0.075 M, pH 7.4. Store in refrigerator. Discard if solution becomes cloudy.
   b. G-6-PDH screening test substrate, containing glucose-6-phosphate, nicotinamide-adenine dinucleotide phosphate (NADP), and a hemolytic reagent. Reconstitute with 2.0 mL of phosphate buffer, 0.075 M, pH 7.4. Allow to stand for 2 minutes. Mix carefully by inversion. Use as quickly as possible. (When reconstituted, this reagent is stable for approximately 2 weeks when it is stored at 0°C.)
2. Sodium chloride, 0.85% w/v.
3. Test tubes, 12 × 75 mm.
4. Microhematocrit tubes (without anticoagulant).
5. Pipets, 2 mL, 0.2 mL, and 10 µL.
6. Filter paper, 32 cm, No. 1.
7. Long-wave, ultraviolet lamp. (This is available from various laboratory suppliers for about $125.)
8. Water bath, 37°C.
9. Timer.

SPECIMEN

Whole blood, 1 mL, using EDTA, heparin, or ACD (acid citrate dextrose) as the anticoagulant. Obtain a normal control specimen.

PRINCIPLE

When red blood cells containing glucose-6-phosphate dehydrogenase (G-6-PDH) are mixed with the test reagent (containing glucose-6-phosphate and NADP), the following reaction occurs:

Glucose-6-phosphate

$$+ \text{ NADP} \xrightarrow{\text{G-6-PDH}} \text{NADPH}$$
$$+ \text{ 6-phosphogluconate}$$

The resultant NADPH fluoresces under long wave ultraviolet light. NADP does not fluoresce.

PROCEDURE

1. Reconstitute one vial of the G-6-PDH substrate as described previously.
2. Label one 12 × 75 mm test for each patient and control to be tested. Label one tube as a blank.
3. Pipet 0.2 mL of G-6-PDH substrate into each of the preceding test tubes.
4. Fold a piece of 32 cm filter paper in half as shown in Figure 137.
5. Pipet 10 μL of whole well-mixed blood from the first specimen and add to the appropriately labeled test tube containing the G-6-PDH substrate. Rinse the pipet several times. Mix the contents of the test tube and, using a microhematocrit tube, quickly place a drop of the mixture on the filter paper (diameter of the drop should be about ½ inch) under the 0 column (0 time) across from the appropriate name. Place the test tube in a 37°C water bath and set a clock for 5 minutes.
6. Repeat step 5 for each specimen and control. (Add 10 μL of 0.85% sodium chloride to the blank.)
7. At the end of the first 5-minute incubation period, place 1 small drop of each mixture in the appropriate line in the 5 minute column on the filter paper. Reset the clock for a second 5-minute incubation period. At the completion of the incubation period, place a small drop of each mixture in the appropriate place on the filter paper.
8. Allow 10 to 15 minutes for the sample applications to dry. In a dark room, place the filter paper under a long-wave ultraviolet light and observe for fluorescence. Record the results, using + for the presence of fluorescence, and − for lack of fluorescence, and ± for weak fluorescence (outer rim fluoresces, whereas the center of the spot does not).
9. Interpretation of results. There should be little to no fluorescence at 0 time. (The reaction occurs very quickly causing possible fluorescence at 0 time.) Normal G-6-PDH activity is indicated by maximum fluorescence at 10 minutes. Little or no fluorescence is seen in the 10-minute column on patients with a gross G-6-PDH deficiency. The normal control should show strong fluorescence at 10 minutes, whereas the blank should show no fluorescence. Patients with a mild deficiency (about 50%) generally show about half the fluorescence that is seen with the normal control.

DISCUSSION

1. Whole blood samples can be stored for several days at 4°C without loss of G-6-PDH activity.
2. This test may be performed at room temperature. However, the amount of fluorescence will be less than if the specimens were incubated at 37°C.
3. The 32-cm filter paper should be folded in half (not torn in half). The drops placed on the filter paper generally seep through one layer of the filter paper and, unless they are pro-

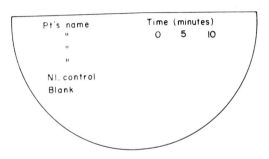

Fig. 137. Folded filter paper for G-6-PD procedure.

tected, may pick up contamination from the counter top (from a previous drop).

4. Hemoglobin has a quenching effect on fluorescence.

5. Once the drop of mixture has been placed on the filter paper, the reaction will continue until the drop completely dries.

6. No fluorescence or decreased fluorescence will be present as long as the drop is moist.

7. The fluorescent spots on the filter paper are stable for several hours but will begin to fade within 24 hours.

8. In this procedure, the rate of formation of fluorescence generally parallels the concentration of G-6-PDH in the blood sample. For example, a blood sample with G-6-PDH concentration that is 50% of normal will take twice as long to form fluorescence as a normal blood sample.

9. Quantitative assays should be performed when abnormal results are obtained by this procedure.

10. This test procedure may be used to differentiate normal and grossly deficient levels of G-6-PDH.

11. If the G-6-PDH substrate solution has deteriorated, it may show fluorescence under long-wave ultraviolet light, or a normal patient specimen may show a dull fluorescence.

12. When excessive numbers of reticulocytes, white cells, or platelets are present, test results may be erroneous.

PYRUVATE KINASE TEST

Pyruvate kinase is an enzyme in the Embden-Meyerhof pathway. A deficiency in this enzyme causes congenital nonspherocytic hemolytic anemia and is probably the most common cause of this type of anemia. Crenated red blood cells and irregularly contracted red blood cells may also be found in this deficiency.

REFERENCES

Beutler, E.: A series of new screening procedures for pyruvate kinase deficiency, glucose-6-phosphate dehydrogenase deficiency, and glutathione reductase deficiency, Blood, *28*, 553, 1966.

Sigma Diagnostics: Pyruvate Kinase Deficiency, Qualitative, Visual Fluorescence Determination in Red Cells, pkg. insert, St. Louis, Sigma Chemical Co., 1984.

REAGENTS AND EQUIPMENT

1. Pyruvate kinase deficiency screening test reagent. Reconstitute with 2.0 mL of distilled water. Allow to stand for 2 minutes. Mix gently. Reconstituted reagent may be stored at 0°C for approximately 5 days. (Available from Sigma Chemical Co., St. Louis.)
2. Test tubes, 12 × 75 mm.
3. Microhematocrit tubes.
4. Pipets, 2.0 mL, 0.2 mL, 0.1 mL, and 20 μL.
5. Sodium chloride, 0.85% w/v.
6. Filter paper, 32 cm, No. 1.
7. Long-wave, ultraviolet lamp.
8. Water bath, 37°C.
9. Timer.

PRINCIPLE

The pyruvate kinase reagent contains phosphoenolpyruvate, adenosine diphosphate (ADP), and reduced nicotinamide-adenine dinucleotide (NADH). When red blood cells containing pyruvate kinase and lactate dehydrogenase (LDH) are added to the test reagent, the following reactions occur:

$$\text{Phosphoenolpyruvate} + \text{ADP} \xrightarrow{\text{Pyruvate kinase}} \text{ATP} + \text{Pyruvate}$$

$$\text{Pyruvate} + \text{NADH} \xrightarrow{\text{LDH}} \text{Lactate} + \text{NAD}$$

Under long-wave, ultraviolet light, NADH fluoresces, whereas NAD does not fluoresce. Normally, all fluorescence should disappear within 30 minutes after the patient's red blood cells have been mixed with the pyruvate kinase test reagent.

SPECIMEN

Whole blood, 1 mL, using EDTA, heparin, or ACD as the anticoagulant. For a fingerstick specimen, obtain about 1 mL of whole blood, using heparinized microcollection tubes. Obtain a specimen for a normal control at the same time.

PROCEDURE

1. Place approximately 1 mL of patient's whole blood into an appropriately labeled tube. Repeat, using a normal control blood. Centrifuge at 1200 to 1500 g for 5 minutes. Remove the supernatant plasma and buffy coat.

2. Place 0.4 mL of 0.85% sodium chloride into 12 × 75 mm test tubes appropriately labeled for each of the preceding specimens.

3. Carefully remove 0.1 mL of packed red blood cells from the bottom of the tube. (Do not contaminate the red cells with any remaining buffy coat cells.) Wipe off the outside of the pipet and transfer the cells to the appropriately labeled tube containing 0.4 mL of sodium chloride. Rinse the pipet several times with the mixture.

4. Reconstitute the pyruvate kinase reaction mixture.

5. Pipet 0.2 mL of pyruvate kinase reaction mixture into appropriately labeled 12 × 75 mm test tubes (one tube for the normal control, one tube for the blank, and one tube for each patient).

6. Fold a piece of 32 cm filter paper in half and label with the patients' names, control and blank as shown in Figure 137 for the glucose-6-phosphate dehydrogenase test procedure. Insert reading times of 0, 10, 20, and 30 minutes.

7. Pipet 20 μL of well-mixed diluted red blood cell suspension into the appropriately labeled test tube containing 0.2 mL of reaction mixture. Mix the test tube and, using a microhe-matocrit tube, quickly place a drop of the mixture on the filter paper under the 0 column (0 time). Place the test tube in a 37°C water bath. Set the clock for 30 minutes.

8. Repeat step 7 for each specimen and control, working as quickly as possible. (Use only one clock.) Add 20 μL of 0.85% sodium chloride to the blank in place of the red blood cell suspension.

9. When 10 minutes have elapsed on the clock, place one drop of each mixture in the 10-minute column. (Each drop should be about ½ inch in diameter.) Repeat at 20 and 30 minutes.

10. Allow 10 to 15 minutes for the sample applications to dry. In a dark room, place the filter paper under a long wave ultraviolet light and observe for fluorescence. Record the results, using + for the presence of fluorescence, − for lack of fluorescence, and ± for weak fluorescence (outer rim fluoresces, whereas the center of the spot does not).

11. Interpretation of results. There should be strong fluorescence at 0 time. With normal pyruvate kinase activity, all NADH should have been oxidized to NAD and there should be no fluorescence at 30 minutes. Any fluorescence present at 30 minutes or after indicates decreased pyruvate kinase activity. The normal control blood should show no fluorescence at 30 minutes, whereas the blank mixture shows fluorescence throughout the 30 minutes. Normally, fluorescence disappears within 10 to 20 minutes.

DISCUSSION

1. Pyruvate kinase is present in the plasma and in the white blood cells. Since this procedure is used to test the pyruvate kinase activity of the red blood cells, it is important that

no plasma or white blood cells contaminate the red blood cell suspension. The red cells may be washed 1 time using 0.85% sodium chloride if desired.

2. The 32 cm filter paper should be folded in half (not torn in half). The drops placed on the filter paper generally seep through one layer of the filter paper and, unless they are protected, may pick up contamination from the counter top (from a previous drop).
3. Once the drop of mixture has been placed on the filter paper, the reaction will continue until the drop completely dries.
4. Hemoglobin has a quenching effect on fluorescence.
5. No fluorescence, or decreased fluorescence, will be present as long as the drop is moist.
6. The fluorescent spots on the filter paper are stable for several hours but will begin to fade within 24 hours.
7. Pyruvate kinase activity in the red blood cells is stable for 2 to 3 weeks when the blood is stored at refrigerator temperature.
8. Quantitative assays should be performed when abnormal results are obtained by this procedure.
9. This test procedure may be utilized to differentiate normal and grossly deficient levels of pyruvate kinase.

GLUTATHIONE REDUCTASE TEST

Glutathione reductase is a red blood cell enzyme. It functions in the hexose monophosphate shunt to catalyze the reaction of the transfer of electrons from NADPH to glutathione in forming reduced glutathione.

A severe hemolytic anemia, frequently drug-induced, is caused by a deficiency in glutathione reductase.

REFERENCES

Beutler, E.: A series of new screening procedures for pyruvate kinase deficiency, glucose-6-phosphate dehydrogenase deficiency, and gluthathione reductase deficiency, Blood, *28,* 553, 1966.
Sigma Chemical Co.: Glutathione Reductase Deficiency in Blood, pkg. insert, St. Louis, Sigma Chemical Co., 1982.

REAGENTS AND EQUIPMENT

1. Glutathione reductase deficiency screening test reagent. Reconstitute with 2.0 mL of distilled water. Allow to stand for 2 minutes. Mix gently. Reconstituted reaction mixture can be stored at 0°C for 5 days without losing activity. (Available from Sigma Chemical Co., St. Louis, Mo.)
2. Test tubes, 12 × 75 mm.
3. Microhematocrit tubes.
4. Pipets, 2.0 mL, 0.2 mL, and 20 μL.
5. Filter paper, 32 cm., No. 1.
6. Long-wave, ultraviolet lamp.
7. Sodium chloride, 0.85% w/v.
8. Water bath, 37°C.
9. Timer.

SPECIMEN

Whole blood using EDTA, heparin, or ACD as the anticoagulant. For fingerstick specimens, obtain 6 or 7 heparinized microhematocrit tubes (about three-fourths full). As soon as each tube is collected, allow the blood to flow back and forth several times to ensure complete anticoagulation of the blood. Obtain a normal control specimen at the same time.

PRINCIPLE

The glutathione reductase reagent contains oxidized glutathione (GSSG) and reduced nicotinamide-adenine dinucleotide phosphate (NADPH). When red blood cells containing glutathione reductase (GSSG-R) are added to the reaction mixture, the following reactions occur:

$$GSSG + NADPH \xrightarrow{\text{GSSG-R}} \text{Reduced glutathione} + NADP$$

Under long-wave ultraviolet light, NADPH shows fluorescence, whereas NADP does not. Generally, in normal patients, fluorescence begins to disappear within 20 minutes after the patient's red blood cells have been mixed with the glutathione reductase test reagent. In blood samples from patients with decreased activity of glutathione reductase, fluorescence may continue for 1 hour or longer.

PROCEDURE

1. Reconstitute the glutathione reductase test reagent.
2. Pipet 0.2 mL of glutathione reductase reagent into the appropriately labeled 12 × 75 mm test tubes (one tube for the normal control, one tube for the blank, and one tube for each patient).
3. Fold a piece of 32 cm filter paper in half and label with the patient's name, control and blank, as shown in Figure 137 for the glucose-6-phosphate dehydrogenase test procedure. Insert reading times of 0, 20, 40, and 60 minutes.
4. Pipet 20 μL of whole, well-mixed blood from the first specimen into the appropriately labeled test tube containing 0.2 mL of reaction mixture. Rinse the pipet several times. Mix the test tube and, using a microhematocrit tube, quickly place a drop of the mixture on the filter paper under the 0 column (0 time). Place the tube in the 37°C water bath. Set the timer for 60 minutes.
5. Repeat step 4 for each specimen, working as quickly as possible. (Use only 1 clock.) (Add 20 μL of 0.85% sodium chloride to the blank in place of the whole blood.)
6. When 20 minutes have elapsed on the clock, place 1 small drop of the mixtures in the 20 minute column. Repeat at 40 and 60 minutes.
7. Allow 10 to 15 minutes for the sample applications to dry. In a dark room, place the filter paper under a long-wave, ultraviolet light and observe for fluorescence. Record the results, using + for the presence of fluorescence, − for lack of fluorescence, and ± for weak fluorescence (outer rim fluoresces, whereas the center of the spot does not).
8. Interpretation of results. There should be strong fluorescence at 0 time. With normal glutathione reductase activity, all NADPH is generally oxidized to NADP and there is little to no fluorescence at 20 minutes. Fluorescence at 60 minutes is abnormal. The normal control blood should show almost no fluorescence at 20 minutes, whereas the blank mixture does show fluorescence in all samples.

DISCUSSION

1. Blood samples may be stored at refrigerator temperature for 3 weeks without a loss of glutathione reductase activity.
2. The 32-cm filter paper should be folded in half (not torn in half). The drops placed on the filter paper generally seep through one layer of the filter paper and, unless they are protected, may pick up contamination from the counter top (from a previous drop).
3. Hemoglobin has a quenching effect on fluorescence.
4. Once the drop of mixture has been placed on the filter paper, the reaction continues until the drop completely dries.
5. No fluorescence or decreased fluorescence is present as long as the drop is moist.
6. Quantitative assays should be performed when abnormal results are obtained by this procedure.
7. This test procedure may be used to differentiate normal and grossly deficient levels of glutathione reductase.

8. The fluorescent spots on the filter paper are stable for several hours but will begin to fade within 24 hours.

SUGAR WATER SCREENING TEST

The sugar water test is a simple screening procedure for paroxysmal nocturnal hemoglobinuria (PNH), an acquired disorder in which the patient's red blood cells are abnormally sensitive to destruction by normal constituents in plasma. Usually this disorder is characterized by red cell hemolysis during sleep (nocturnal hemoglobinuria).

If the sugar water test is positive, the sucrose hemolysis procedure should be performed before a diagnosis of PNH is made.

REFERENCE

Hartmann, R.C., Jenkins, D.E., Jr., and Arnold, A.B.: Diagnostic specificity of sucrose hemolysis test for paroxysmal nocturnal hemoglobinuria, Blood, *35*, 462, 1970.

REAGENTS AND EQUIPMENT

1. Sugar water solution, pH 7.4 ± 0.1.
   Sucrose (commercial   9.5 g
     granulated sugar)
   Distilled water   100 mL
   Prepare fresh.
2. Cyanmethemoglobin reagent.
3. Test tubes, 12 × 75 mm and 13 × 100 mm.
4. Pipets, 10, 2, 1, and 0.2 mL.
5. Spectrophotometer.

SPECIMEN

Citrated whole blood: 1 part 0.109 M sodium citrate to 9 parts whole bood. Obtain a blood specimen for the normal control at the same time the patient's blood is collected.

PRINCIPLE

Whole blood is mixed with a sugar water solution and incubated at room temperature. PNH red blood cells are abnormally susceptible to lysis by complement and under the conditions of this test will show hemolysis. The presence of hemolysis in this test, therefore, indicates a positive result for paroxysmal nocturnal hemoglobinuria.

PROCEDURE

1. Pipet 1.8 mL of sugar water solution into each of two 12 × 75 mm test tubes, labeled patient and control.
2. Add 0.2 mL of well-mixed control and patient's whole blood to the respective test tubes.
3. Invert each test tube gently to mix.
4. Incubate both tubes at room temperature for 30 minutes.
5. While the tubes are incubating, label 13 × 100 mm test tubes, 'Total' and 'Test' for each patient and control. Label one tube as the blank. Pipet 9.5 mL of cyanmethemoglobin reagent into each tube.
6. At the end of the 30-minutes incubation, remix each tube very gently. Remove 0.5 mL of the mixture from each tube and add to the appropriately labeled 'Total' tube containing cyanmethemoglonin reagent. Mix well by inversion. Allow to sit at room temperature for 10 minutes.
7. Centrifuge the remaining blood-sugar water mixtures at 1200 to 1500 g for 5 minutes.
8. Add 0.5 mL of each supernatant to the appropriately labelled 'Test' tube containing cyanmethemoglobin reagent. Add 0.5 mL of the sugar water reagent to the tube labeled 'Blank.' Mix all tubes well by inversion and allow to sit at room temperature for 10 minutes.
9. Transfer all above mixtures to a cuvet and read in a spectrophotometer at a wavelength of 540 nm, setting the blank at 0.0 optical density. Record the O.D. readings for each sample.
10. Calculate the percent of hemolysis for each specimen as shown below.

$$\text{Percent Hemolysis} = \frac{\text{O.D. Test}}{\text{O.D. Total}} \times 100$$

11. Interpretation of results. Hemolysis of 5%, or less is considered negative and within normal limits. Hemolysis of 6 to 10% is thought to be borderline. Positive results will show greater than 10% hemolysis, and should be followed up by the confirmatory sucrose hemolysis test and/or the acid-serum test.

DISCUSSION

1. Prior to performing the test it is suggested that a small portion of the patient and control bloods be centrifuged to make certain there is no initial hemolysis present in the plasma.
2. In the presence of anemia, hemolysis may be slightly increased in PNH negative specimens.
3. The use of defibrinated blood may cause false positive results due to hemolysis of the traumatized red blood cells.
4. The test should be performed within 2 hours of obtaining the specimen.

SUCROSE HEMOLYSIS TEST

The sucrose hemolysis test is used as a confirmatory test for paroxysmal nocturnal hemoglobinuria when the sugar water test is positive.

REFERENCE

Hartmann, R.C., Jenkins, D.E., Jr., and Arnold, A.B.: Diagnostic specificity of sucrose hemolysis test for paroxysmal nocturnal hemoglobinuria, Blood, *35,* 462, 1970.

REAGENTS AND EQUIPMENT

1. Sodium phosphate,   7.8 g
   50 mmol/L ($NaH_2PO_4 \cdot 2H_2O$)
   Dissolve and dilute to 1 liter with distilled water.
2. Sodium phosphate,   7.1 g
   50 mmol/L (Na_2HPO_4)
   Dissolve and dilute to 1 liter with distilled water.
3. Sucrose solution (isotonic).
   Sucrose (reagent grade)   92.4 g

NaH_2PO_4 (50 mmol/L)   91 mL
Na_2HPO_4 (50 mmol/L)   9 mL
Mix and adjust pH to 6.1, if necessary, using dilute NaOH or HCl. Dilute to 1 liter with distilled water. Reagent is stable at refrigerator temperature for 2 weeks.
4. Cyanmethemoglobin reagent.
5. Test tubes, 12 × 75 mm and 13 × 100 mm.
6. ABO compatible serum, or, serum from type AB blood, from a normal donor. Specimen must be fresh.
7. Sodium chloride, 0.85% w/v.
8. Pipets, 10, 2, 1, 0.2, and 0.1 mL.
9. Spectrophotometer.

SPECIMEN

Citrated whole blood: 1 part 0.109 M sodium citrate to 9 parts whole blood. Obtain a blood specimen (preferably the same blood type) for the normal control at the same time the patient's blood is collected.

PRINCIPLE

Washed red blood cells are incubated in an isotonic sucrose solution containing normal ABO compatible serum. At the end of the incubation period, the mixture is examined for hemolysis. Red blood cells will absorb complement components from serum at low ionic concentrations. PNH red blood cells are much more sensitive than normal red blood cells and under these conditions will hemolyze.

PROCEDURE

1. Place 1 mL of patient and control bloods in respective 12 × 75 mm test tubes. Wash red cells by adding 0.85% sodium chloride to each tube. Centrifuge specimens at 1200 to 1500 g for 5 minutes. Carefully remove all of supernatant. Wash the red blood cells a second time in the same manner.
2. Prepare a 50% solution of red cells for both patient and control: add 3 drops of washed red blood cells to 3

drops of 0.85% sodium chloride. Mix.

3. Into appropriately labeled 12 × 75 mm test tubes (one tube for each patient and control, and one tube for the blank), pipet 1.7 mL of sucrose solution. Add 0.1 mL of ABO compatible serum (or serum from a type AB donor) to each tube.

4. Add 0.2 mL of the 50% suspension of red cells to each appropriately labeled tube. Gently mix each tube by inversion.

5. Incubate all tubes at room temperature for 30 minutes.

6. While the tubes are incubating, label 13 × 100 mm test tubes, 'Total' and 'Test' for each patient and control, and 1 tube for the blank. Pipet 9.5 mL of cyanmethemoglobin reagent into each tube.

7. At the end of the 30-minutes incubation, remix each blood-sucrose tube very gently. Remove 0.5 mL of the mixture from each tube and add to the appropriately labeled 'Total' tube containing cyanmethemoglobin reagent. Transfer 0.5 mL from the tube labeled blank to the cyanmethemoglobin tube labeled blank. Mix well by inversion. Allow to sit for 10 minutes.

8. Centrifuge the remaining blood-sucrose mixtures at 1200 to 1500 g for 5 minutes.

9. Add 0.5 mL of each supernatant to the appropriately labeled 'Test' tube containing cyanmethemoglobin reagent. Mix all tubes well by inversion and allow to sit for 10 minutes.

10. Transfer all above mixtures to a cuvet and read in a spectrophotometer at a wavelength of 540 nm, setting the blank at 0.0 optical density. Record the O.D. readings for each sample.

11. Calculate the percent hemolysis for each specimen as shown below.

$$\text{Percent Hemolysis} = \frac{\text{O.D. Test}}{\text{O.D. Total}} \times 100$$

12. Interpretation of results. Hemolysis of 5%, or less is considered negative and within normal limits. Hemolysis of 6 to 10% is thought to be borderline. Positive results should show greater than 10% hemolysis.

ACID-SERUM TEST

Paroxysmal nocturnal hemoglobinuria (PNH) may also be reliably diagnosed by means of the acid-serum test.

Ham Method

REFERENCES

Ham, T.H.: Studies on destruction of red blood cells, Arch. Intern. Med., *64*, 1271, 1939.
Dacie, J.V., and Lewis, S.M.: *Practical Haematology*, New York, Churchill Livingstone, Inc., 1984.
Sirchia, G., Soldano, F., and Mercuriali, F.: The action of two sulfhydryl compounds on normal human red cells. Relationship to red cells of paroxysmal nocturnal hemoglobinuria, Blood, *25*, 502, 1965.

REAGENTS AND EQUIPMENT

1. Glass beads, 3 to 4 mm in diameter.
2. Sodium chloride, 0.85% (w/v).
3. Test tubes, 12 × 75 mm.
4. Hydrochloric acid, 0.2 N.
5. Water bath, 37°C.
6. Water bath, 56°C.
7. Erlenmeyer flasks, 125 mL.
8. Ammonium hydroxide, 0.04% (v/v), or cyanmethemoglobin (HiCN) reagent.
9. Graduated centrifuge tubes, 15 mL.

SPECIMEN

Whole blood, 10 ml, to be defibrinated. Collect blood to use as a normal control and, preferably, process in the same manner as the patient's blood. (The normal control [serum and cells] may be obtained from blood allowed to clot at room temperature. Patient blood, however, must not be allowed to clot in the normal manner, since PNH red cells would most likely lyse while the blood was sitting at room temperature or 37°C.) (The control blood must be of the same ABO blood group, or, one compatible with the patient's blood group.)

PRINCIPLE

The red blood cells of patients with paroxysmal nocturnal hemoglobinuria are unusually susceptible to lysis by complement. In this procedure the patient's red blood cells are mixed with normal serum and also with the patient's own serum and incubated at 37°C. Selected serum samples are inactivated to destroy the complement, and a weak acid is added to several tubes to adjust the pH of the mixture for maximum hemolytic activity. After incubation, all tubes are inspected for hemolysis. Normally, there should be no lysis of the red blood cells in any of the tubes of the test. In PNH, the patient's red blood cells will hemolyze in the presence of noninactivated, acidified, normal serum and in the patient's own noninactivated, acidified serum.

PROCEDURE

1. Defibrinate the patient and control blood in the following manner.
   a. Place 10 ml of whole blood in an Erlenmeyer flask containing 10 glass beads.
   b. Gently rotate the flask until the hum or noise of the beads on the glass can no longer be heard (about 10 minutes).
2. Decant the blood into a graduated centrifuge tube and centrifuge at 1500 × g for 5 minutes.
3. Remove the serum. Save the red cells for step 6 below.
4. Repeat steps 1, 2, and 3 for each specimen and control to be tested.
5. Number eight 12 × 75 mm test tubes for each patient to be tested. Pipet 0.5 mL of normal control serum into tubes #1 through #6. Add 0.5 mL of patient's serum into tubes #7 and #8. Place tubes #3 and #6 in a 56°C

water bath for 30 minutes (to inactivate the serum and destroy the complement).

6. While the serum is incubating, fill each graduated centrifuge tube containing the red blood cells (step 3 above) with 0.85% sodium chloride. Mix and centrifuge at 1500 × g for 5 minutes. Remove the supernatant and wash the red cells two more times. After the last wash, note the volume of the packed red blood cells.
7. Add an equal volume of 0.85% sodium chloride to the packed red blood cells. Mix. This gives a 50% suspension of red cells.
8. Add 0.05 mL of the patient's red blood cells to tubes #1, 2, 3, 7 and 8. Add 0.05 mL of normal control red blood cells to tubes #4, 5, and 6. (See Table 6.) Mix all tubes gently.
9. Add 0.05 mL of 0.2 N hydrochloric acid to tubes #2, 3, 5, 6, and 7. Mix tubes gently.
10. Place all tubes in the 37°C water bath for 1 hour.
11. At the end of 1 hour, centrifuge the 8 tubes (per patient) at 800 × g for 2 minutes, and examine the supernatants for hemolysis.
12. The percent hemolysis present in each tube may be quantitated as follows.
    a. For each patient, add 0.05 mL of the original cell suspension (in step 7) to 0.55 mL of 0.85% sodium chloride. This mixture represents 100% hemolysis for those tubes to which 0.05 mL of hydrochloric acid was added. Label tube appropriately. To represent 100% hemolysis for the other tubes which contain no hydrochloric acid (and, therefore, a lesser volume), add 0.05 mL of the red blood cell suspension to 0.5 mL of 0.85% sodium chloride. Label tube.
    b. Add 5 mL of 0.04% ammonium

TABLE 6.   ACID SERUM TEST RESULTS INDICATING PAROXYSMAL NOCTURNAL HEMOGLOBINURIA

TUBE	0.05 mL RBC	0.5 mL SERUM	0.5 mL INACTIVATED SERUM	mL OF 0.2 N HCl	HEMOLYSIS
1	P	N			Trace
2	P	N		0.05	+
3	P		N	0.05	0
4	N	N			0
5	N	N		0.05	0
6	N		N	0.05	0
7	P	P		0.05	+
8	P	P			Trace

hydroxide (or cyanmethemoglobin reagent) to 12 test tubes and label #1 through #12.

c. Add 0.3 mL of the supernatants to the respectively numbered test tubes containing ammonium hydroxide (or cyanmethemoglobin reagent).

d. To tube #9, add 0.3 mL of the cell suspension representing 100% hemolysis (for the acidified mixtures). Add 0.3 mL of the red cell suspension representing no addition of acid, to tube #10.

e. To tube #11 add 0.3 mL of normal preincubated serum. This represents 0% hemolysis for those tubes using normal serum. Tube #12 represents 0% hemolysis for the tubes containing the patient's serum and contains 0.3 mL of the preincubated patient's serum.

f. Read the above solutions in a spectrophotometer at a wavelength of 540 nm, using tube #11 or #12 (whichever is appropriate) to set the instrument at 0 optical density.

g. Calculate the percent hemolysis as shown below (use the appropriate tube to represent 100% hemolysis):

$$\text{Percent Hemolysis} = \frac{\text{O.D. of test}}{\text{O.D. of tube representing 100\% hemolysis}} \times 100$$

h. A positive test usually shows 10 to 50% hemolysis. Ranges from 5 to 80% hemolysis, however, may be considered positive.

13. Interpretation of test results.

a. Normal—no hemolysis in any tubes.

b. Paroxysmal nocturnal hemoglobinuria—hemolysis present in tubes #2 and #7. There may also be a trace of hemolysis present in tubes #1 and #8. There should be no hemolysis in tubes #3 or #6 since the complement in the serum has been destroyed. Tubes #4 and #5 contain normal red cells so there should be no hemolysis in these tubes. Rarely, there may be decreased or no hemolysis in tube #7 (patient's serum) possibly due to complement depletion.

c. In the rare disorder, dyserythropoietic anemia type II (also termed HEMPAS, or *h*ereditary *e*rythroblast *m*ultinuclearity with a *p*ositive *a*cid *s*erum test), tube #2 will show hemolysis. However, in these patients their red cells will not be lysed by their own serum and, therefore, tube #7 will show no lysis.

DISCUSSION

1. Hemolysis in test tubes #2, 3, and 7 may indicate the presence of markedly spherocytic red blood cells.

This can be differentiated from paroxysmal nocturnal hemoglobinuria because lysis of the spherocytes is unaffected by heating the serum at 56°C.

2. Inactivating the serum in test tubes #3 and #6 at 56°C destroys the hemolytic system. Therefore, lysis present in these tubes rules out the possibility of a positive test for PNH.

3. When the patient has received blood transfusions, less lysis occurs because of the presence of normal red blood cells from the transfusion.

4. A positive control should be run with this test and may be prepared by treating normal red blood cells with 2-aminoethylisothiouronium bromide (AET). Normal blood is collected in ACD anticoagulant and the red cells washed two times with 0.85% sodium chloride (w/v). An 8% (w/v) aqueous solution of AET is prepared and the pH of the solution adjusted to 8.0 with 5 N sodium hydroxide. Four volumes of 8% AET (pH 8.0) is added to one volume of packed washed red blood cells, placed in a flat bottomed beaker, mixed well, and incubated at 37°C for 19 minutes. At the end of this period, the red cells are washed repeatedly with relatively large amounts of 0.85% sodium chloride until the supernatant is clear. (Each time the cells are washed the red cells should be mixed well to ensure resuspension before centrifuging. After the first wash the red blood cells will be clumped together and the mixing and resuspension are very important.) At the end of the last wash, remove as much of the supernatant as possible. The red cells are then ready for use as a positive PNH control.

HEMOGLOBIN ELECTROPHORESIS BY CELLULOSE ACETATE

The hemoglobin molecule is made up of globin and heme. There are numerous types of hemoglobins, based on the structure of the globin chains. These polypeptide chains differ in the number, type, and sequence of amino acids, depending on the type of hemoglobin involved. The normal adult hemoglobin is hemoglobin A, in addition to which small amounts of hemoglobins A_2 (up to 3.5%) and F (less than 2%) are also present. Two of the most commonly seen hemoglobin variants (abnormal hemoglobins) are hemoglobins C and S. Other, less common mutants seen are hemoglobins E, G, D, and Lepore. Numerous other abnormal hemoglobins exist, but are rare in occurrence. Hemoglobin electrophoresis is a procedure used to detect the types of hemoglobin present in a patient's red blood cells.

There are several electrophoretic methods in use for differentiating the various types of hemoglobin. To date, the most widely used technique employs the use of cellulose acetate. Other media used are starch gel and agar gel.

The technical details of this procedure vary between different laboratories and according to the apparatus used. The following procedure is easy to perform and uses primarily reagents and equipment from Helena Laboratories, Beaumont, Texas 77704.

REFERENCES

Helena Laboratories: Hemoglobin Electrophoresis Procedure, Beaumont, Texas, Helena Laboratories, 1985.

Schmidt, R.M., and Brosius, E.M.: *Basic Laboratory Methods of Hemoglobinopathy Detection,* HEW Pub. No. (CDC) 74-8266, U.S. Department of Health, Education, and Welfare, Public Health Service, Atlanta, Center for Disease Control, 1974.

REAGENTS AND EQUIPMENT

(Item #1 through 9 below are obtainable from Helena Laboratories.)

1. Supre-Heme buffer (tris-EDTA-boric acid buffer, pH 8.2 to 8.6). Dissolve 1 package of buffer in 980 mL distilled water. Stable for 1 month at 4°C.
2. Hemolysate reagent.

3. Ponceau S stain.
4. Disposable wicks.
5. Titan III-H cellulose acetate strips with mylar backing.
6. Super Z sample applicator (Fig. 138).
7. Sample plate (holds hemolysate samples to be tested) (Fig. 138).
8. Aligning base (holds cellulose acetate strip for inoculation). (Fig. 138).
9. Electrophoresis chamber (Fig. 139).
10. Large filter paper (for blotting cellulose acetate strips).
11. Test tubes, 10 × 75 mm.
12. Pipet, 5 μL.
13. Disposable pipet droppers.
14. Squeeze bottle of distilled water for rinsing applicator and sample plate.
15. Small shallow pans, 5, for buffer, stain, and acetic acid rinse.
16. Hemostats, 2 pair.
17. Acetic acid, 5% (v/v).
18. DC-regulated power supply (Fig. 140).
19. Microhematocrit tubes, plain.
20. Glass slides, 1 × 3 inch.
21. Sodium chloride, 0.85% (v/v).
22. Known control samples. These may be liquid or frozen red cell hemolysates and may be prepared from blood with known abnormal hemoglobins, or purchased from any one of several commerical laboratory distributors.

SPECIMEN

Whole blood using EDTA or heparin as the anticoagulant. Capillary blood may also be used. When using whole blood, at least 0.5 mL of blood should be obtained. When utilizing capillary blood, 3 to 4 microhematocrit tubes ¾ filled should be collected. Whole blood samples may be stored in the refrigerator for up to 1 week, or, once the hemolysate has been prepared, it may be frozen for several months.

PRINCIPLE

The hemoglobin molecule contains globin chains which are composed of amino acids. The sequence of these amino acids influences the properties of the globin chain and, therefore, the hemoglobin molecule. Basically, the globin chain consists of a carboxyl group (COOH), an amino group (NH$_3$), and an R group (chain of amino acids) attached to a carbon atom. The following equation, as shown, has no net charge (is neutral).

$$\begin{array}{c} NH_3{}^+ \\ | \\ H-C-COO^- \\ | \\ R \end{array}$$

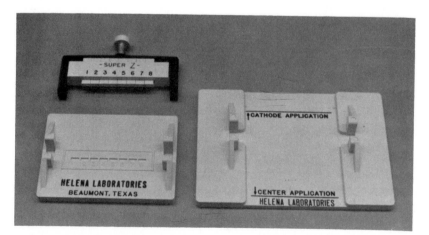

Fig. 138.   Equipment used in hemoglobin electrophoresis by cellulose acetate. Sample applicator (top left), sample plate (left), and aligning base (right).

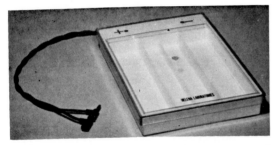

Fig. 139. Electrophoresis chamber. (Courtesy of Helena Laboratories, Beaumont, Texas.)

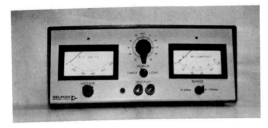

Fig. 140. Power supply. (Courtesy of Gelman Instrument Co., Ann Arbor, Michigan.)

As indicated, the carboxyl and amino groups are able to carry a charge. The protein will have a positive or negative charge, depending upon the pH of the solution it is in. For example, in an alkaline solution, where there is an excess of negative charges, the amino group is neutralized and the globin shows a net negative charge (as shown in the following diagram).

$$\underset{R}{\overset{NH_3{}^+}{H-C-COO^-}} \xrightarrow[\substack{Solution \\ (OH^-)}]{Alkaline} \underset{R}{\overset{NH_2}{H-C-COO^-}} + H_2O$$

In an acid solution, in which there is an excess of hydrogen ions, the negative charges are neutralized and the protein has a net positive charge.

$$\underset{R}{\overset{NH_3{}^+}{H-C-COO^-}} \xrightarrow[\substack{Solution\ (H^+)}]{Acid} \underset{R}{\overset{NH_3{}^+}{H-C-COOH}}$$

Electrophoresis is the movement of charged molecules or particles in an elec-

tric field. In hemoglobin electrophoresis, the hemoglobin is placed in an alkaline buffer solution (pH of 8.2 to 8.6). The net negative charge of the various hemoglobins depends on the amino acids (the R group) making up the hemoglobin molecule.

The first step in hemoglobin electrophoresis is the preparation of a hemolysate to destroy the red blood cell membranes and free the hemoglobin. A small quantity of hemolysate is then placed on a cellulose acetate membrane and positioned in an electrophoresis tray with the inoculated hemolysate near the cathode (−). One end of the cellulose acetate strip is immersed in the buffer (pH 8.2 to 8.6) on the cathode side and the other end is placed in the buffer on the anode (+) side. An electric current of specific voltage and milliamps is allowed to run for a specified period of time. During this period, the hemoglobin molecules migrate toward the anode because of their net negative charge. The difference in the net charge of the hemoglobin molecule determines its mobility in an electric field and manifests itself by the speed with which it migrates to the positive pole. The cellulose acetate membrane is then placed in a stain which colors the proteins (hemoglobins) red. By noting the distance each hemoglobin has migrated and comparing this distance with the migration distance of known controls, the types of hemoglobins are identified.

PROCEDURE

1. Preparation of hemolysate.
   a. *Washed packed red cell procedure.* Place ½ to 1 mL of well-mixed whole blood into an appropriately labeled 10 × 75 mm test tube. Wash red cells 1 to 3 times with sodium chloride (0.85%, v/v): fill tube with sodium chloride and centrifuge at 1200 to 1500 g for 5 minutes; remove supernatant; repeat cell washing two more times. Place 1 drop of

washed, packed red blood cells into an appropriately labeled 10 × 75 mm test tube. Add 6 drops of hemolysate reagent. Mix and allow to sit for 5 minutes for complete hemolysis of the red cells. If the hemolysate is at all cloudy, place the hemolysate in the freezer for about 10 minutes. Upon thawing the hemolysate should be crystal clear.

b. *Whole blood procedure.* Place 1 drop of whole blood into a 10 × 75 mm test tube. Add 3 drops of hemolysate reagent. Mix and allow to stand for 5 minutes. If the hemolysate is not crystal clear, freeze and thaw specimen as described in step a above.

c. *From microhematocrit tubes.* Centrifuge two microhematocrit tubes. Using a file, cut the packed red cell layer into three or four sections, discarding the plasma and buffy coat portions and the sealed end. Place the open sections containing the red cells, into a 10 × 75 mm test tube. Repeat this procedure for the second microhematocrit tube, placing the red cells in the same tube with the sections from the first hematocrit. Add 6 drops of hemolysate reagent to the tube. Mix vigorously by drawing across the top of a test tube rack numerous times. Allow to sit for 10 minutes for hemolysis to occur.

d. *From capillary blood collected on filter paper* (available from Rochester Paper Co., Rochester, Mi., as ROPACO #1023, 0.038 inch). The specimen is collected by placing a large drop of blood (minimum of 12 mm diameter) onto the filter paper. The specimen may then be stored in the refrigerator. To prepare hemolysate, cut out a circular sample of the blood 1 cm in diameter. Place in a test tube and add 2 drops of hemolysate reagent. Mix and allow to elute for 30 minutes. Remove filter paper. The hemolysate may now be tested or may be frozen for future testing.

2. Fill a pan with approximately 40 mL of buffer solution.

3. Using a clean, dry hemostat, slowly and uniformly immerse a cellulose acetate strip into the buffer solution. This should take 10 to 15 seconds. If the membrane is immersed too quickly, white areas appear on the cellulose acetate and it must be discarded. Allow the entire strip to soak in the buffer for a minimum of 5 minutes prior to use. (Make certain your hands are clean and free of any oil or grease if you touch the cellulose acetate strip prior to the last step of this procedure [staining].)

4. Pour 100 mL of buffer into each of the outer compartments of the electrophoresis chamber. Moisten two disposable paper wicks in the buffer and drape one over each of the two middle support bridges, ensuring that one side is immersed in the buffer and that there are no air bubbles under the wicks.

5. Place 5 μL of hemolysate in the sample well plate (one sample/well). Place the known control hemolysate in well number 1 and/or 2. Cover the sample well plate with glass slide if the hemolysates will not be inoculated within 5 minutes.

6. Remove the cellulose acetate strip from the buffer, and carefully blot the strip between two pieces of filter paper in order to remove the excess surface buffer. Proceed quickly to the next step.

7. With the mylar (plastic) backing facing up, label the strip in one corner.

8. Place a drop of buffer on the middle of the aligning base (prevents slip-

page of the strip). Quickly turn the strip over (cellulose acetate side up) and place it in the aligning base with the bottom edge lined up with the line marked 'cathode application.'

9. Depress the applicator tips into the sample wells 3 or 4 times. Quickly transfer the applicator to the aligning base. Press the button down and hold it on the strip for 3 to 5 seconds.

10. Quickly place the strip, cellulose acetate side down and with the long side of the strip on the horizontal, in the chamber with the application site nearest the cathode (−) side. Place 1 or 2 glass slides on top of the strip to act as a weight. Carefully place the cover on top of the chamber.

11. Attach the electrode terminal pins to the power supply. Turn the power supply on and electrophorese for 25 minutes at a setting of 350 volts.

12. At the end of 25 minutes, turn the power supply off, carefully remove the strips from the chamber, and blot the side edges to remove the excess buffer.

13. Place the strips in a pan containing Ponceau S stain for 5 minutes.

14. Remove the strip from the stain and place it in a 5% acetic acid solution to rinse the excess stain off. Agitate the membrane gently.

15. Repeat step 14, 2 or 3 more times, in clean 5% acetic acid until all of the excess stain is removed. The strip should return to its white color, with only the hemoglobin taking up the stain.

16. After the last acetic acid wash, remove the excess moisture by blotting on filter paper. Allow 5 to 10 minutes for air-drying.

17. Identify the hemoglobin types present in the patient samples by comparing the migration distances with the known controls. See Figure 141 for the mobilities of various hemoglobins.

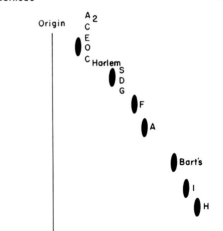

Fig. 141. Electrophoretic mobility of various hemoglobins at pH 8.2 to 8.4

DISCUSSION

1. It is easy and economical for a laboratory to prepare its own hemoglobin electrophoresis controls. Using known blood samples, prepare any number of hemolysates as outlined in step 1 of the previous procedure. Stopper the test tubes tightly and place in the freezer. Each time hemoglobin electrophoresis is performed, remove one test tube of each known hemoglobin control from the freezer, and thaw. Discard the remaining hemolysate after use. In the frozen state, these hemolysates will remain effective controls for several months.

2. If the Ponceaus S stain is kept tightly covered, it may be used for approximately 1 month. Also, the staining time in this procedure is not critical.

3. The buffer solution used for soaking the cellulose acetate strips may be used for soaking up to 12 strips or for 5 working days, if it is kept covered when not in use.

4. Fresh chamber buffer should be used daily.

5. On patients showing hemoglobin S, perform the sodium dithionite sickle cell test. (The results should be posi-

tive.) If the sickle cell test is negative and the patient shows hemoglobin S electrophoretically, the hemoglobin is most probably hemoglobin D. Agar gel electrophoresis may then be performed for further identification.

6. Three cellulose acetate strips may be run in the electrophoresis chamber at one time.

7. Generally, when eight samples are inoculated on a strip, distortion may occur in the first and eighth samples. For consistently good results, use only the second through seventh slots in the sample well plate.

8. If semiquantitative results are desired, the membrane may be placed in a densitometer and scanned. Prior to quantitation, however, the cellulose acetate strip must be cleared in order to develop a transparent background. For accurate quantitation of hemoglobin F and hemoglobin A_2, the alkali denaturation test and a quantitative test specifically for hemoglobin A_2, must be performed.

9. When interpreting the hemoglobin electrophoresis results, the unknown hemoglobins may only be identified by comparing their mobility (distance traveled) with the mobility of known hemoglobins run on the same membrane.

10. There may be a small amount of hemoglobin that distributes itself along the pathway of the migrating hemoglobin. This is called *trailing.* A small amount of this trailing is not unusual. Excessive amounts may be due to: (1) denaturation of the hemoglobin because of excessive heat, or samples that are too old, (2) too large a sample of hemolysate used, or, (3) a dirty membrane.

CITRATE AGAR GEL ELECTROPHORESIS

There are numerous abnormal hemoglobins which are structurally different from each other but have the same electrophoretic mobility on cellulose acetate. Because of this, the citrate agar gel electrophoresis procedure is used as a confirmatory test for some abnormal hemoglobins detected in the cellulose acetate electrophoresis procedure. The citrate agar gel procedure is also the method of choice when testing newborns or infants under 3 months of age for an abnormal hemoglobin. This procedure is much more sensitive to small amounts of a hemoglobin than the cellulose acetate procedure, is helpful in detecting hemoglobin S in the infant or in cord blood, and is, therefore, a helpful procedure for screening cord bloods.

The reader should be familiar with the cellulose acetate hemoglobin electrophoresis procedure before continuing with this test.

REFERENCES

Helena Laboratories: Titan IV citrate hemoglobin electrophoresis procedure, pkg. insert, Beaumont Tex., Helena Laboratories, 1983.
National Committee for Clinical Laboratory Standards: *Proposed Guidelines for Citrate Agar Electrophoresis for Confirming Identification of Mutant Hemoglobins,* NCCLS, Villanova, Pa., 1981.

REAGENTS AND EQUIPMENT

1. The following reagents and supplies are obtainable from Helena Laboratories.

   a. Citrate buffer (contains sodium citrate and citric acid), 0.05 M, pH 6.0 to 6.3. Dilute 1 package of citrate buffer to 1 liter with distilled water. Stable for 1 month stored at 2 to 8°C. Discard if the dry powder is discolored or if the solution is cloudy.

   b. Citrate agar plates (Titan® IV) (contains a preservative and 1.5% [w/v] agarose in citrate buffer).

   c. Zip Zone® sponge wicks.

   d. o-Tolidine, 0.2% (or 0.2% O-Diansidine).

   e. Electrophoresis chamber.

f. Zip Zone® sample applicator (with the spring removed).

g. Zip Zone® sample well plate (Items e, f, and g are the same as those used for the cellulose acetate hemoglobin electrophoresis procedure.)

h. Titan® IV aligning base.

i. Microdispenser (for measuring 5 μl amounts).

j. Hemolysate reagent.

k. AFSC hemoglobin control.

2. DC-regulated power supply.
3. Pipets, 1, 5, and 10 mL.
4. Test tubes, 10 × 75 mm.
5. Polypropylene centrifuge tubes, 15 mL.
6. Acetic acid, 5% (v/v).
7. Sodium nitroferricyanide, 1% (w/v).
8. Hydrogen peroxide, 30%.
9. Parafilm.
10. Glass slides, 1 × 3 inch.

SPECIMEN

Whole blood using EDTA as the anticoagulant. If capillary blood is being used, collect 4 to 6 hematocrit tubes three-fourths filled with blood. Whole blood may be refrigerated for up to 1 week before testing.

PRINCIPLE

A red blood cell hemolysate is prepared in order to destroy the red blood cell membrane and free the hemoglobin. The patient's hemolysate, along with known controls, is placed on a slide containing a thin layer of agar gel. This slide is placed, agar side down, across the support bridges of the electrophoresis tray. An electric current of specific voltage and milliamps is allowed to run for a specific period of time. At the end of electrophoresing, the agar gel slide is placed in a stain that colors the hemoglobins. By noting the distance each hemoglobin has migrated and comparing this distance with the migration distance of known controls, the different types of hemoglobins present can be identified. Using agar gel, there are four major zones of hemoglobin migration: at this acid pH, hemoglobin F has a positive charge and migrates to the cathode (−) side, the negatively charged molecules of hemoglobins C and S move toward the anode (+), and hemoglobin A remains near the site of inoculation. A large majority of the abnormal hemoglobins migrate with hemoglobin A (except C and S). The media through which the hemoglobins travel and the difference in the net charge of the hemoglobin in an acid pH determine the mobility of each type of hemoglobin. The results of this procedure must be correlated with the results of the cellulose acetate hemoglobin electrophoresis.

PROCEDURE

1. Remove the necessary number of Titan® citrate agar plates from the refrigerator and allow to warm up to room temperature. (Up to 16 samples, including controls, may be run on each citrate agar plate.)

2. Prepare the patient sample hemolysates by adding 1 drop of patient whole blood to 19 drops of hemolysate reagent. Mix vigorously and make certain the resultant dilution is crystal clear. Prepare the control hemolysate by adding 1 drop of Helena hemolysate to 1 drop of the Helena AFSC control. Mix well. (If the patient sample has a hemoglobin value of less than 8 g/dL, prepare the hemolysate by washing approximately 1 mL of whole blood one time with 0.85% sodium chloride. Remove the supernatant and mix 1 drop of the packed cells with 20 drops of hemolysate reagent.)

3. Fill the electrophoresis tray with cold citrate buffer, pH 6.0 to 6.3. Place approximately 100 mL of buffer into each of the outer compartments of the electrophoresis chamber. Thoroughly wet two of the sponges in the citrate buffer and

place one in each of the outer chambers, against the inner chamber wall, such that the top surface protrudes approximately 2 mm above the wall.

4. Record, in a workbook, each patient's name and each control to be run, numbering each sample from 1 through 8 to correspond to the sample well plate and thus to their order on the agar gel plate. (Samples run in the first and last positions on the agar gel plate may not electrophorese as well as the centrally located samples. For this reason, it may be preferable to use only sections 2 through 7.)

5. Using the microdispenser, or a 5-µL pipet, add 5 µL of each hemolysate to the appropriate well of the sample plate. Cover the sample well plate with a glass slide if the hemolysates are not to be inoculated within 2 minutes. Position the sample applicator directly over the sample well plate.

6. Prime the sample applicator by lowering the tips into the sample wells several times. Apply this first loading to a piece of filter paper or blotter. This action primes the applicator to ensure more uniform inoculation of the agar gel.

7. Remove the citrate agar plate from the plastic bag, peel off the tape around the cover, and remove the cover from the plate. Label the plate by writing an identifying number on the top right corner. Also, label the right end of the plate with a '+' for anode and the other end of the plate '−' for cathode. Immediately, place the agar gel plate in the Titan IV aligning base with both ends flush with the back and front edges of the base.

8. Load the applicator by depressing the tips into the wells of the sample plate several times. Place the applicator in the set of grooves closest to the + end of the plate and slowly and carefully lower the applicator tips down onto the top surface of the agar. Allow the applicator tips to remain on the agar surface for 1 minute so that the hemolysates will absorb onto the agar. Be extremely careful that the applicator tips do not at any time break the surface of the agar. (A second set of samples may be inoculated and run on this plate by placing the sample applicator in the second set of grooves and inoculating the plate as described.)

9. Very quickly, place the agar plate, gel side down, in the electrophoresis chamber so that the gel layer makes a good contact with the top surface of the sponges. The (first) application should be nearest the anode.

10. Carefully place the cover on the electrophoresis chamber. Attach the electrode terminal pins to the power supply. Turn the power supply on and adjust the voltage so that there are 40 milliamps per agar gel plate. The voltage will be approximately 50 volts. Electrophorese for 45 minutes.

11. Approximately 10 minutes before electrophoresing is complete, prepare the stain. Mix together:

5% Acetic acid	10.0 mL
O-Tolidine (or O-Diansidine), 0.2%	5.0 mL
1% Sodium nitroferri-cyanide	1.0 mL
Distilled water	0.9 mL
Hydrogen peroxide	0.1 mL

12. At the end of the electrophoresing period, remove the agar gel plates from the electrophoresis chamber. Place each plate, agar side up, on a level surface (near a sink is advisable). Using a disposable dropper pipet, carefully flood each plate with a thin layer of stain. Allow to stain until all hemoglobin components are stained (generally takes 2 to 5 minutes using fresh stain).

13. When staining is complete, carefully

rinse the plates under running tap water. Place each plate, agar side down, on blotter or filter paper until the moisture is absorbed (10 to 15 minutes).

14. When the majority of the moisture has been removed, allow the slides to air dry and read. The top may be replaced on the agar gel plate once all moisture has been removed, and the plate may then be stored for future reference, if desired.

15. Identify the hemoglobin types present in the patient samples by comparing the migration distances with the known controls. See Figure 142 for the mobilities of various hemoglobins. The interpretation of agar gel results must be correlated with the hemoglobin types found on cellulose acetate hemoglobin electrophoresis.

DISCUSSION

1. For best results, the hemoglobin concentration of the patient hemolysates should be slightly less than 1 g/dL. Cord blood sample hemolysates should have a concentration of approximately 4 g/dL.

2. Preparation of agar gel plates. Pre-coat one side of a 2 × 3-inch slide by pouring a thin layer of Bacto-agar (0.1% [w/v] in distilled water) over the entire surface of the slide. Allow excess to drain off slide and air dry at 37°C for several hours or overnight at room temperature. Prepare a 1% Bacto-agar (w/v) solution in 0.05 M citrate buffer. Evenly distribute 3 to 4 mL of the melted agar solution over the pre-coated side of the 2 × 3-inch slide. Allow agar to cool and set. If the slides will not be used immediately, wrap in plastic and store in the refrigerator. It is critical that agar does not become dried out before or during testing.

3. The same hemolysate used for the cellulose acetate procedure may also be used for agar gel electrophoresis by adding 1 drop of the original hemolysate (cellulose acetate) to 4 drops of Helena hemolysate reagent.

4. On agar gel the mobility of the hemoglobins will tend to vary more than on cellulose acetate and is more dependent on the concentration of hemoglobin, size of inoculation, and composition of the buffer.

HEMOGLOBIN A_2

Very small amounts of hemoglobin A_2 (up to about 3.5%) are normally found in the adult. Elevated levels of hemoglobin A_2 generally indicate β-thalassemia trait, although some patients with homozygous β thalassemia may show an increased hemoglobin A_2. Decreased amounts of hemoglobin A_2 may be found in iron deficiency anemia, hemoglobin H disease, hereditary persistence of fetal hemoglobin, sideroblastic anemia, and in carriers of α thalassemia.

The anion exchange microchromatography procedure outlined below is an accurate method for hemoglobin A_2 quantitation, and requires no special instrumentation or training.

REFERENCE

Helena Laboratories: *Beta-Thal Hemoglobin A_2 Quik Column*™ *Procedure*, Beaumont, Tex., Helena Laboratories, 1984.

REAGENTS AND EQUIPMENT

1. Beta-Thal HbA$_2$ Quik Column™ test

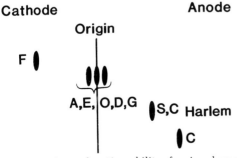

Fig. 142. Electrophoretic mobility of various hemoglobins on agar gel at pH 6.0 to 6.3.

kit (available from Helena Laboratories) contains the following:

a. Beta Thal HbA$_2$ Quik Columns™ (see Fig. 143) containing, primarily, DE52 (diethylaminaethylcellulose) resin in a glycine buffer. Small amounts of potassium cyanide and sodium azide are also present. Store at 2° to 6°C.

b. HbA$_2$ developer (contains glycine and potassium cyanide). Refrigerate when not in use.

c. Hemolysate reagent-C containing Triton X-100. May be stored in refrigerator, or, at room temperature.

2. Additional materials needed (also obtainable from Helena Laboratories):

a. Rack for holding the columns during testing.

b. Total Fraction tubes.

c. HbA$_2$ Collection tubes.

d. Normal and abnormal hgb A$_2$ controls.

3. Pipets, 0.05, 0.2, and 1.0 mL.
4. Disposable pasteur pipets.
5. Parafilm.
6. Distilled water.
7. Test tubes, 10 × 75 mm and 13 × 100 mm.
8. Stopwatch.
9. Spectrophotometer.

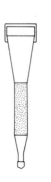

Fig. 143. HbA$_2$ Quik Column™.

SPECIMEN

Whole blood (minimum of 0.1 mL) anticoagulated with EDTA. Fresh blood is desirable, but hemolysates stored up to 14 days at 2° to 6°C may be used.

PRINCIPLE

A hemolysate is prepared from the patient's red blood cells (freeing the hemoglobin from the red cells). A specific amount of hemolysate is then added to the top of the resin column. The DE52 is a preparation of cellulose attached to positively charged molecules, thus giving the cellulose a positive charge. Due to the buffer and the pH level, when the hemolysate is added to the column, the hemoglobins contain a net negative charge and therefore bind to the cellulose resin. When the HbA$_2$ developer is added to the column and allowed to drain through the resin, due to the pH (or ionic strength) of the developer, the hemoglobin A$_2$ (originally bound to the resin) is released from the resin and is eluted by the developer as it passes through the column. Most other hemoglobins remain bound to the resin in the column. The eluted hemoglobin A$_2$ is then measured spectrophotometrically and compared with the amount of total hemoglobin in the specimen to calculate the percent of hemoglobin A$_2$ present.

PROCEDURE

1. Remove all reagents and equipment from the refrigerator and allow to warm to room temperature.
2. Prepare the patient hemolysate.
   a. Pipet 0.05 mL of well-mixed whole blood into a 10 × 75 mm test tube for each patient to be tested.
   b. Add 0.25 mL of Hemolysate Reagent-C to each tube. Vigorously mix each tube by drawing across the top of a test tube rack several times.
   c. Allow each mixture to sit for 5 to

10 minutes to allow for complete hemolysis of the red cells.

3. Label one Quik Column™ tube, one Total Fraction (TF) tube, and one HbA_2 Collection (A_2) tube for each patient and control to be tested. Place the column tubes and the A_2 tubes in the top and bottom portions of the rack respectively. Place the labeled TF tubes in a separate rack.

4. When the hemolysates are ready for testing, prepare a Quik Column™ tube for use:

   a. Carefully invert the column tube two times in order to remove any resin that may be adhering to the cap or side of the tube.

   b. Remove the top screw cap and, using a pasteur pipet, carefully resuspend the resin by aspirating and expelling the resin several times. Perform this procedure carefully so as not to disturb the filter at the bottom of the resin column. Proceed to the next step quickly before the resin begins to settle. Start a stopwatch.

   c. Carefully loosen and remove the small plastic cap at the bottom of the tube and place the tube in the rack, above a 13 × 100 mm empty test tube. The buffer should drain through the resin, out of the tube, and into the 13 × 100 mm test tube as the resin settles. Proceed to the next step quickly.

   d. Carefully watch the resin repack. You will be able to see three different concentrations of the resin-buffer mixture; the top portion will quickly become clear, the middle portion will be cloudy, and, as the resin begins packing a definite line of demarcation will form between the packed resin and the second or cloudy portion. As soon as the cloudy portion disappears and there are only two layers seen (packed resin on bottom and clear liquid portion on top) (approximately 2 minutes 15 seconds will have elapsed on the stopwatch), carefully aspirate and remove all of the clear buffer portion on top, using a pasteur pipet. Discard. Halt the stopwatch.

   e. The above steps must be accomplished without delay in order that the resin does not become too tightly packed.

5. Immediately after the excess buffer is removed from the top of the resin column in the above step, the sample must be applied to the resin column:

   a. Carefully, apply 0.1 mL of the sample hemolysate to the top of the resin column, ensuring that the resin is not disturbed. The sample must not run down the inside of the tube, the pipet tip must not touch the top of the resin, and no bubbles should form in the sample. Start the stopwatch as soon as the sample has been added to the column.

   b. Add 0.1 mL of the patient's hemolysate to the appropriately labeled TF tube. Fill the tube to the 15 mL line with distilled water and mix.

6. Allow the sample to completely absorb into the resin. When 1 to 2 minutes have elapsed on the stopwatch, the top of the resin should have a dull mat-like finish to it indicating complete absorption of the hemolysate.

7. Wipe the bottom of the Quik Column tube and place the tube directly above the appropriately labeled A_2 tube. Add 2.5 mL of the HbA_2 Developer to the top of the Quik Column without disturbing the resin or hemolysate. Halt the stopwatch. Less than 5 minutes should have elapsed since step 5 was completed.

8. Allow 15 to 20 minutes for the Developer to drain through the column. If this step takes any longer than this,

there is most likely a problem with the resin column and the test should be repeated using a new Quik Column™ tube.

9. Repeat steps 4 through 8 above for each patient and control.

10. When all of the Developer has passed through the resin columns, fill the A_2 tubes to the 3-mL mark with distilled water. Mix.

11. Set the spectrophotometer at a wavelength of 415 nm and set 0.00 absorbance using distilled water. Record the absorbance readings for all total hemoglobins (TF tubes) and all hemoglobin A_2 samples.

12. Calculate the concentration of hemoglobin A_2 for each specimen and control:

$$\text{Hgb } A_2 = \frac{\text{Absorb. of } A_2}{\text{Absorb. of Total hgb} \times 5} \times 100$$

DISCUSSION

1. A number of abnormal hemoglobins (S, C, E, O, D, and S-G hybrid), if present, will be eluted along with the hemoglobin A_2 in this procedure. This will be evident in cases where the results of the test procedure show a greater than 7 or 8% hemoglobin A_2 result. In these cases the Sickle-Thal Quik Column™ kit (available from Helena Laboratories) may be used. This procedure is similar to the one described above. The column of resin is slightly different in this test kit. This column allows elution of hemoglobin A_2 in the presence of hemoglobins A, F, S, and numerous other abnormal hemoglobins. In addition, an HbS Developer reagent is included in this kit and allows for quantitation of hemoglobin S, if present. This test kit may also be used routinely for quantitating hemoglobin A_2, rather than having to keep two different kits on hand.

2. The final test dilutions are stable for 4 hours.

3. It is advisable for each laboratory to determine its own normal range for this test procedure.

4. The preparation of the Quik Columns™ in step 4 above are critical. Also, any bubbles present in the resin will cause erroneous results.

5. If the Developer does not flow through the column correctly, the test should be repeated using a new column.

6. Any disturbance of the resin during testing will cause invalid results. The top of the resin should not be allowed to dry out at any time during the procedure.

7. If developer is added to the column too quickly, results will be invalidly low.

8. If a patient heterozygous for β-thalassemia also has iron deficiency, the hemoglobin A_2 may be within the normal range.

ALKALI DENATURATION TEST

The alkali denaturation test measures the amount of fetal hemoglobin present in the red blood cells. A result of less than 2% for this method is normal. Values between 0.8 and 2.0% are borderline, and results above 2.0% are considered abnormal. Approximately 65 to 90% of the total hemoglobin at birth is hemoglobin F. By the age of 4 months there is approximately 10% hemoglobin F present, and by 6 to 12 months of age the level of hemoglobin F is less than 2%. Increased amounts of fetal hemoglobin are also present in hereditary persistence of fetal hemoglobin, sickle cell anemia, acquired aplastic anemia, and in other hemoglobinopathies.

REFERENCES

Betke, K., Marti, H.R., and Schlict, I.: Estimation of small percentages of fetal hemoglobin, Nature, *184*, 1877, 1959.

Singer, K., Chernoff, A.I., and Singer, L.: Studies on abnormal hemoglobin. 1. Their demonstration in sickle cell anemia and other hematologic disorders by means of alkali denaturation, Blood, 6, 413, 1951.

REAGENTS AND EQUIPMENT

1. Cyanmethemoglobin (HiCN) reagent.
2. Saturated ammonium sulfate.
   Ammonium sulfate   160 g
   Add 200 mL of distilled water.
   Mix the above solution until all possible ammonium sulfate goes into solution. Mix frequently over the next several hours and allow to stand overnight. Remix solution and add more ammonium sulfate, if necessary, until no more reagent will go into solution. A small amount of reagent must always be present, undissolved, in the bottom of the reagent bottle. When using this reagent, handle bottle carefully so that the undissolved reagent in the bottom of the bottle is not unnecessarily disturbed.
3. Sodium hydroxide, 1.25 N.
4. Sodium chloride, 0.85%, w/v.
5. Carbon tetrachloride (CCl_4).
6. Whatman #42 filter paper.
7. Graduated centrifuge tube, polypropylene, 15 mL.
8. Normal and abnormal hemolysate controls.
9. Test tubes, 13 × 100 mm.
10. Water bath, 20°C.

SPECIMEN

Whole blood anticoagulated with EDTA: 2 to 3 mL. The hemolysate for this procedure must be prepared from fresh blood, the same day the specimen is collected.

PRINCIPLE

A red blood cell hemolysate is prepared to lyse the red blood cells completely. This test utilizes the characteristic of fetal hemoglobin to resist denaturation in an alkaline solution. The hemolysate is added to the cyanmethemoglobin reagent and then exposed to an alkaline reagent, sodium hydroxide, for a specified period. During this time, normal hemoglobin is denatured or destroyed, but the fetal hemoglobin remains intact. Ammonium sulfate is added to halt the denaturation process and to precipitate the denatured hemoglobin. The solution is filtered, measured spectrophotometrically, and compared with the spectrophotometric readings of the original cyanmethemoglobin solution to determine the percent hemoglobin F present.

PROCEDURE

1. Preparation of hemolysate.
   a. Place 2 to 3 mL of the patient's whole blood into a graduated, polypropylene centrifuge tube. Prepare a normal and abnormal control blood in the same manner.
   b. Fill both tubes with 0.85% sodium chloride to wash the red blood cells. Centrifuge at 1200 to 1500 g for 5 minutes. Remove the supernatant.
   c. Wash the red blood cells two more times by repeating step b above.
   d. Remove 1 mL of washed red blood cells from each tube and place in a clean, labeled, polypropylene centrifuge tube. Add 1 mL of distilled water to each tube. Mix. Add 0.5 mL of CCl_4 to each tube. Stopper tubes.
   e. Vortex, or vigorously shake, each tube for 5 minutes.
   f. Centrifuge the tubes at 1500 g for 25 to 30 minutes. Carefully remove tubes from the centrifuge.
   g. Remove the upper hemolysate layer from each tube, being careful not to disturb the lower stroma and CCl_4 layers.
   h. Determine the hemoglobin content of the hemolysate. It should be between 9 and 11 g/dL. Adjust, if necessary, using distilled water.
2. Pipet 0.5 mL of the patient's he-

molysate and the normal and abnormal control hemolysates into respective tubes containing 9.5 mL of cyanmethemoglobin reagent. Label tubes 'Total Hgb.' This gives a hemoglobin concentration of approximately 0.5 g/dL.

3. Mix and transfer 2.8 mL of each of the preceding cyanmethemoglobin solutions into each of two labeled test tubes. (Each test is performed in duplicate.) Label tubes 'Alkali Res Hgb.' Place the test tubes in a 20°C water bath for 5 to 10 minutes to reach the proper temperature.

4. Add 0.2 mL of 1.2 N sodium hydroxide to the first test tube and rapidly mix. Allow to incubate for exactly 2 minutes.

5. At exactly 2 minutes, add 2 mL of saturated ammonium sulfate to the tube, directly into the solution, and quickly mix the tube to stop the reaction. Allow the tube to stand at room temperature for 5 to 10 minutes.

6. Repeat steps 4 and 5 above for each patient and control sample in step 3.

7. Filter each of the preceding solutions through Whatman #42 filter paper. If the filtrate is not absolutely clear, refilter the solution using the same filter paper.

8. Prepare the total hemoglobin specimen for the patients and controls: add 0.4 mL of each of the 'Total Hgb' solutions (step 2) to 6.75 mL of distilled water. Prepare this dilution in duplicate.

9. Transfer the filtrates and total hemoglobin solutions to cuvettes and read in a spectrophotometer at a wavelength of 540 nm, using cyanmethemoglobin reagent to set the instrument at 0 optical density. Record the absorbance of all specimens. The optical density readings should fall within a range of 0.05 to 0.50 for maximum sensitivity. If the filtrate is too concentrated, dilute it, using distilled water.

10. Calculate the results as follows:

$$\frac{\text{Percent Alk.}}{\text{Res. Hgb.}} = \frac{\text{O.D. Alk. Res. Hgb.}}{\text{O.D. Total Hgb.} \times 10} \times 100$$

The optical density of the total hemoglobin is multiplied by 10 because this solution is 10 times more dilute than the alkali-resistant solution.

DISCUSSION

1. The following aspects of the procedure are critical and must be carried out as indicated.
   a. Concentration of 1.2 N sodium hydroxide.
   b. Incubation time and temperature of the hemolysate with sodium hydroxide.
   c. The hemoglobin concentration of the hemolysate must be within 9 and 11 g/dL.
   d. The filtrate must be crystal clear.

2. The hemolysate must be prepared on the same day the blood specimen is obtained from the patient. The hemolysate may then be placed in the freezer at −20°C until testing occurs.

3. In circumstances where the hemolysate has a hemoglobin concentration of less than 9 g/dL, the 'Total Hgb' dilution (as prepared in step 2 above) may be altered to compensate for this. The following calculations may be used:

$$\frac{A}{10.0} = \frac{0.5}{C} \qquad \text{then: } B = 10 - C$$

   where: A = hgb in g/dL of the heolysate

   B = am't of cyanmethemoglobin reagent to be used in step 2 above

   C = amount of hemolysate to add to the cyanmethemoglobin reagent (step 2)

4. This method is generally very accu-

rate for concentrations up to 10 to 15% hemoglobin F. At concentrations higher than this the results are usually falsely low.

5. A radial immunodiffusion procedure for quantitation of hemoglobin F is manufactured by Helena Laboratories, Beaumont, Texas. This method has the advantage of taking little technologist time to perform, uses 0.2 mL of whole blood, and is easy to read. After inoculation with an easily prepared hemolysate, the plates are incubated at room temperature for 24 hours.

6. Patients with sickle cell anemia may have levels of hemoglobin F as low as normal, to as high as 20%. In hereditary persistence of fetal hemoglobin the hemoglobin F concentration is generally above 15%. Patients with β-thalassemia trait will usually show levels of 2 to 5% hemoglobin F, while patients homozygous for β-thalassemia will have hemoglobin F levels of 15 to 100%.

7. The concentration of the sodium hydroxide and ammonium sulfate are critical for accurate results.

ACID ELUTION TEST

The acid elution test is employed to determine the distribution of hemoglobin F in the red blood cell: to determine whether hemoglobin F is present in the same amount in all red blood cells, or whether it is present in varying amounts in only some of the red blood cells. It is useful in differentiating hereditary persistence of fetal hemoglobin and in determining the presence of fetal red cells in the maternal circulation during pregnancy. Approximately 80% of the total hemoglobin at birth is hemoglobin F. By the age of 4 months, there is approximately 10% hemoglobin F present, and at the end of infancy only trace amounts remain. Normal adult blood will generally contain less than 2% hemoglobin F. Increased amounts

of hemoglobin F in the red cell are found in hereditary persistence of fetal hemoglobin, sickle cell anemia, thalassemia, various other hemoglobinopathies, aplastic anemia, some leukemias, polycythemia vera, Down's syndrome, in a number of other hematological disorders, and in some complications of pregnancy.

REFERENCES

Division of Host Factors, Center for Infectious Diseases, CDC: *Laboratory Methods for Detecting Hemoglobinopathies,* Atlanta, Centers for Disease Control, 1984.

Shepard, M.K., Weatherall, D.J., and Conley, C.L.: Semiquantitative estimation of the distribution of fetal hemoglobin in red cell populations, Bull. Johns Hopkins Hosp., *110*, 293, 1962.

REAGENTS AND EQUIPMENT

1. Ethyl alcohol, 80% (v/v). Stable in the refrigerator for 1 month (or 100 slides), unless the solution becomes cloudy.

2. Citric acid-phosphate buffer, pH 3.1 to 3.3.

   Dibasic sodium phosphate, 0.2 M

      Dibasic sodium phosphate   14.2 g (Na_2HPO_4)

      Dilute to 500 mL with distilled water.

      Stable for 6 months when stored in the refrigerator.

   Citric acid, 0.1 M

      Citric acid   10.5 g ($C_6H_8O_7 \cdot H_2O$)

      Dilute to 500 mL with distilled water.

      Stable for 6 months when stored in the refrigerator.

   Prior to use, prepare the citric acid-phosphate buffer:

      Dibasic sodium   13.3 mL phosphate, 0.2 M

      Citric acid, 0.1 M   36.7 mL

   Check the pH of this mixture on a pH meter. The pH must be within 3.1 and 3.3. This reagent is available from Sigma Diagnostics™, #285-1.

3. Erythrosin B (eosin B) stain, 0.1%

(w/v), aqueous solution. Eosin yellowish, 1.25% (w/v), may be used as an alternative (0.5 g of eosin yellowish in 120 mL of absolute alcohol and 280 mL of distilled water). Add 2 to 3 drops of glacial acetic acid. Eosin B reagent is available from Sigma Diagnostics™, #285-3.

4. Ehrlich's acid hematoxylin.

Hematoxylin, crystalline	4.0 g
Ethyl alcohol, 80% (v/v)	200 mL
10% aqueous solution of sodium iodate	8 mL
Distilled water	200 mL

Heat the above solution until it boils, cool until lukewarm, and add the following:

Glycerine	200 mL
Aluminum sulfate	6.0 g
Glacial acetic acid	200 mL

Mix, and store at room temperature. This stain is also available from Sigma Diagnostics™, #285-2.

5. Coplin jars.
6. Waterbath, 37°C.

SPECIMEN

Obtain 4 blood smears from the fingertip (toe or heel), or make blood smears from venous blood collected in EDTA anticoagulant. Obtain a similar blood specimen for a normal and abnormal control at the same time the patient's blood is collected.

PRINCIPLE

Blood smears are fixed with ethyl alcohol and then incubated in a citric acid-buffer solution. In an acid medium (pH 3.1 to 3.3), hemoglobin F is more resistant to elution from the red blood cell, while other hemoglobins are removed from the red cells. The slides are stained with hematoxylin (stains the white cell nuclei) and erythrosin B (stains the red cells). The smears are then reviewed microscopically to determine the presence of hemoglobin F in the red cells.

PROCEDURE

1. Prewarm citric acid-phosphate buffer. Place 50 mL of the buffer solution into a coplin jar and cover. Incubate at 37°C for 30 minutes.
2. Preparation of blood smears.
   a. Patient—Make four thin (a monolayer of cells) blood smears.
   b. Normal control—Make two thin blood smears from a normal adult.
   c. Positive control—Mix two drops of cord blood with two drops of normal, ABO compatible, whole blood. Make two thin blood smears. (As an alternative, use cord blood, alone, as the positive control.)
3. Allow the blood smears to air-dry for at least 10 minutes.
4. Place the 80% ethyl alcohol in a coplin jar and fix blood smears (patient and controls) in the alcohol for 5 minutes.
5. Rinse the smears carefully in distilled water and allow to air-dry.
6. Place the dry smears in the prewarmed citric acid-phosphate buffer solution for 5 minutes. Carefully agitate the coplin jar 3 times after 1 and 3 minutes of incubation.
7. After 5 minutes, remove the slides from the citric acid-phosphate buffer solution and rinse with distilled water. Air-dry.
8. Stain the dry smears in acid hematoxylin for 3 minutes. Rinse with distilled water and remove as much of the water as possible from the smears by gentle tapping on an absorbent material.
9. Counterstain the smears with erythrosin B for 4 minutes. Rinse with distilled water and allow to air-dry and coverslip (if desired).
10. Examine the slides microscopically, using the oil immersion objective (100 ×), for the presence of red blood cells containing hemoglobin F. Red cells containing large amounts of hemoglobin F will stain a deep pink.

The intensity of the pink staining is directly proportional to the amount of hemoglobin F present in the red cell. Cells containing normal amounts (less than 2%) of hemoglobin F will stain as very pale ghost cells.

11. In order to determine the percent of the red blood cells containing hemoglobin F, perform the following procedure:

   a. Count the number of red blood cells in 3 to 5 microscopic fields and determine the average # of red cells/field.

   b. Examine 20 to 25 microscopic fields, counting the number of red cells containing hemoglobin F. Divide the total number of red cells with hemoglobin F, by the number of fields counted. This is the number of red cells containing hemoglobin F/field.

   c. Divide the number of red cells containing hemoglobin F by the average number of red blood cells/field (step a above). Multiply this result by 100 to obtain the percent of red blood cells containing hemoglobin F.

DISCUSSION

1. Reticulocytes may resist elution and would, therefore, give the appearance of cells containing hemoglobin F.

2. In hereditary persistence of fetal hemoglobin, the amount of hemoglobin F in each cell is constant and, therefore, all of the red blood cells are consistently stained.

3. In diseases such as sickle cell anemia, thalassemia, acquired aplastic anemia, and several other hemoglobinopathies, the amount of hemoglobin F present in the red blood cells varies. This shows up as an inconsistent staining of the red cells.

4. For best results, blood should be less than 6 hours old, and the smears should be fixed within 2 hours of preparation.

5. The pH of the citric acid-phosphate buffer is critical. A pH below 3.1 may cause elution of hemoglobin F from the red cells, while a pH above 3.3 may retard the elution of non-F hemoglobin from the red blood cells.

6. A temperature above 25°C during fixation in the ethyl alcohol will inhibit elution of normal hemoglobin.

7. Ethyl alcohol concentrations above 80% may cause the elution of hemoglobin F, while concentrations below 80% may cause morphologic alterations.

8. Positive control smears may be prepared in advance. Add cord blood to EDTA (1 drop of 2% EDTA/1 mL of whole blood). Prepare blood smears and fix in 80% ethyl alcohol. Place fixed smears in tightly sealed cardboard slide boxes and store at −20°C. These smears should be good for 1 year, prepared and stored in this manner.

HEINZ BODY PREPARATION

Heinz bodies represent precipitated hemoglobin and appear as single or multiple, round, oval, or serrated bodies in the red blood cells. (See Plate IVh.) They will be found in the presence of unstable hemoglobins such as hemoglobin Zurich. In this condition, however, the spleen will generally remove the Heinz bodies from the red cell. They are, therefore, more readily found in splenectomized patients (with an unstable hemoglobin). Heinz bodies are also present in a number of hemolytic disorders and are formed when the glycolytic enzymes in the red blood cell are unable to prevent the oxidation of hemoglobin. As a result, the hemoglobin is eventually denatured and precipitated to form Heinz bodies. In some hemolytic anemias (G-6-PD deficiency and glutathione deficiency) Heinz bodies will form secondary to the action of certain oxidant drugs (e.g., primaquine, sulfanilamide, phenacetin, Furadantin, acetanilid, and probenecid). Because the normal aging of a red blood cell is accompanied by a decrease in the red blood cell enzyme systems, some Heinz bodies will normally be seen with crystal violet stain.

The test for Heinz bodies may be performed with or without acetylphenylhydrazine, which tests for sensitivity to oxidant drugs. The test for Heinz bodies may first be performed without the addition of acetylphenylhydrazine, in order to detect an unstable hemoglobin or a hemolytic anemia secondary to the presence of oxidizing drugs. If the test results are negative, the addition of acetylphenylhydrazine will detect red cells susceptible to the formation of Heinz bodies due to defective reducing systems.

REFERENCE

Beutler, E., Dern, R.J., and Alving, A.S.: The hemolytic effect of primaquine. VI. An in vitro test for sensitivity of erythrocytes to primaquine, J. Lab. & Clin. Med., *45*, 40, 1955.

SPECIMEN

Freshly drawn whole blood specimen, using heparin or EDTA as the anticoagulant. A normal control blood should be obtained at the same time the patient sample is drawn.

Stain for Heinz Bodies

REAGENTS AND EQUIPMENT

1. Test tubes, 10 × 75 mm.
2. Sodium chloride, 0.73%, w/v.
3. Crystal violet, 1%, w/v, in 0.73% sodium chloride.
   Crystal violet   2.0 g
   (Color index 681. Obtainable from National Aniline Division, Allied Chemical Corp., Morristown, N. J.)
   Dilute to 100 mL with 0.73% sodium chloride. Shake mixture for 5 minutes and filter. Dilute the filtered stain with an equal volume of 0.73%

sodium chloride. This stain is stable at room temperature for approximately 5 months.
4. Coverslips.
5. Glass slides.

PRINCIPLE

Whole blood is mixed with crystal violet stain. Slides are prepared and examined for the presence of Heinz bodies.

PROCEDURE

1. Place 5 drops (1 volume) of well-mixed whole blood into a labeled 10 × 75 mm test tube for each sample to be tested.
2. Add 10 drops (2 volumes) of 1% crystal violet stain to each tube.
3. Mix well and incubate at room temperature for 15 minutes.
4. At the end of 15 minutes, and again after 24 hours, remix the blood and stain solution. Place a small drop on each of two slides and cover with a cover glass. Allow approximately 10 minutes for the cells to settle. If desired, more permanent wedge smears may be prepared for examination, in place of the wet preparation.
5. Examine the red blood cells microscopically, using the oil immersion objective (100×). The Heinz bodies appear as purple, irregularly shaped bodies of varying sizes, from 1 to 4 μm in diameter. There may be more than one Heinz body present in a red blood cell, and they generally lie close to the cell membrane.

DISCUSSION

1. The presence of Heinz bodies in a freshly drawn sample of blood may indicate:
   a. An oxidizing drug or chemical has been ingested in such a quantity to overwhelm the normal red cell reducing system causing denaturation of the hemoglobin.
   b. A drug, such as primaquine, has

been ingested by an individual with a red blood cell glycolytic enzyme deficiency, so that hemoglobin is not protected from oxidative denaturation.

c. The patient has thalassemia or an unstable hemoglobin.

Heinz Body Preparation with Acetylphenylhydrazine

REAGENTS AND EQUIPMENT

1. Phosphate buffer, pH 7.6.
   Potassium phosphate   9.1 g
   monobasic (KH_2PO_4)
   Dilute to 1 liter with distilled water.
   Sodium phosphate dibasic,   9.5 g
   anhydrous (Na_2HPO_4), or,
   Sodium phosphate dibasic 11.9 g
   ($Na_2HPO_4 \cdot H_2O$)
   Dilute to 1 liter with distilled water. For the working buffer, pH 7.6, mix 13 mL of monobasic potassium phosphate solution with 87 mL of dibasic sodium phosphate solution. Add 0.2 g of glucose. Store in the refrigerator. Stable for several months.
2. Acetylphenylhydrazine solution.
   Acetylphenylhydrazine   0.1 g
   Dilute to 100 mL with the working phosphate buffer, pH 7.6. This reagent should be used within 1 hour of preparation.
3. Crystal violet solution, 1%, w/v, in 0.73% sodium chloride. See Stain for Heinz Bodies procedure, for method of preparation.
4. Test tubes, 10 × 75 mm.
5. Glass slides.
6. Coverslips.
7. Pipet, 0.1 mL.
8. Water bath, 37°C.

PRINCIPLE

Whole blood is mixed and incubated with acetylphenylhydrazine. A normal control blood is prepared in the same manner as the patient specimen. Heinz bodies will be formed when the red cells are exposed to the reducing substance (acetyl-phenylhydrazine). The blood specimens are then stained with crystal violet. Patients whose red cells have defective reducing systems will show greater than 32% of their red cells with 5 or more Heinz bodies. Normal individuals will have less than 32% of the red cells showing 5 or more Heinz bodies.

PROCEDURE

1. Perform test on a normal control blood at the same time the patient sample is tested.
2. Place 2 mL of acetlyphenylhydrazine solution into a labeled 10 × 75 mm test tube for each sample to be tested.
3. Add 0.1 mL of well-mixed whole blood to the above tube. Gently shake mixture 2 to 3 times to mix. Using a 0.1 mL pipet whiffle the mixture (force air through the mixture), 3 times, using the 0.1 mL pipet.
4. Place tubes in the 37°C water bath for 2 hours.
5. After 2-hours incubation, whiffle mixture by bubbling air through it 4 to 5 times, using the 0.1 mL pipet.
6. At the end of the 4-hours incubation, gently shake the mixture and place 5 drops into a 10 × 75 mm test tube. Add 10 drops of 1% crystal violet stain. Allow to incubate (stain) at room temperature for 10 to 15 minutes.
7. Gently shake the mixture and place a small drop on each of two slides. Coverslip and allow cells to settle for about 10 minutes. As an alternative procedure, wedge smears may be prepared for examination.
8. Using the oil immersion objective, count 200 red blood cells, enumerating those cells containing five or more Heinz bodies. Divide the number of red cells containing five or more Heinz bodies by two in order to determine the percent (test result).

DISCUSSION

1. The following conditions are felt to

be critical to the accurate performance of this test.

a. The phosphate buffer should be at pH 7.6. At an increased pH there will be faster development of Heinz body formation, while a decreased pH slows down Heinz body formation.

b. The amount and speed of Heinz body formation will increase with increased concentrations of acetylphenylhydrazine. A decrease in the ratio of reagent to red blood cells will decrease Heinz body formation. Therefore, in the presence of anemia, the concentration of red blood cells should be adjusted to near normal values (by removing plasma) in order to obtain valid results.

c. The amount of oxygenation (determined by the amount of whiffling) greatly influences the results of the test. The more oxygenation, the greater the development of Heinz bodies. Because of this, capillary blood should not be used when performing the test and using the normal range as outlined above.

d. The acetylphenylhydrazine solution is relatively unstable and should be used as soon as possible after preparation.

2. In this procedure, Heinz body formation is increased in G-6-PD deficiency, 6-phosphogluconate dehydrogenase deficiency, glutathione reductase deficiency, glutathione synthetase deficiency, glutathione peroxidase deficiency, and triosephosphate isomerase deficiency.

HEMOGLOBIN H PREPARATION

Patients suspected of having thalassemia trait, who have an MCV below 80 fL, are not iron deficient, have a normal hemoglobin electrophoresis, and have normal levels of hemoglobins F and A_2, may have α thalassemia. In this disorder, there is an excess of β chains (due to a deficiency in the production of α chains). The excess β chains will form β_4 tetramers (hemoglobin H). Due to the small amount of hemoglobin H formed, it will generally not be seen on cellulose acetate hemoglobin electrophoresis. However, in the presence of an oxidant, such as brilliant cresyl blue, this abnormal hemoglobin will precipitate within the red cell and form many small inclusions. (See Plate VII L.) Unstable hemoglobins may also be detected and stained with this method. In addition, inclusion bodies may be found in the red cells of some patients with enzyme deficiencies (e.g., G-6-PD deficiency) and after exposure to oxidant drugs. Normal hemoglobin will not denature or precipitate in this procedure and will therefore be negative for inclusion bodies.

REFERENCES

Jones, J.A., Broszeit, H.K., LeCrone, C.N., and Detter, J.C.: An improved method for detection of red cell hemoglobin H inclusions, Am. J. Med. Tech., 47, 94, 1981.

Raven, J.L., and Tooze, J.A.: α-thalassaemia in Britain, Br. Med. J., 4, 486, 1973.

REAGENTS AND EQUIPMENT

1. Microhematocrit tubes, non-heparinized.
2. Microhematocrit centrifuge.
3. Clay, to seal the end of the microhematocrit tube.
4. Water bath, 37°C.
5. Small file to cut microhematocrit tubes.
6. Glass slides, 25 × 75 mm.
7. Test tubes, 55 × 12 mm.
8. Microscope.
9. Citrate saline solution.
   Sodium citrate   0.4 g
     $(Na_3C_6H_5O_7 \cdot 2H_2O)$
   Dissolve and dilute to 100 mL with 0.9% (w/v) sodium chloride.
10. Brilliant cresyl blue, 1%, w/v, in citrate saline solution. Filter before use.

Store at room temperature. Stain is good for 1 month.

SPECIMEN

Whole blood, using EDTA (or ACD) as the anticoagulant. Excess amounts of anticoagulant may interfere with the staining process. Fresh blood samples, less than 8 hours old are preferable.

PRINCIPLE

It is thought that red cells containing hemoglobin H are removed more quickly from the circulation by the reticuloendothelial system. Therefore, the red cells containing hemoglobin H, which are present in the blood, are relatively young cells, and, when centrifuged, will lie near the top of the red cell layer. In this procedure, the blood is centrifuged in several microhematocrit tubes. The top layers of red blood cells are removed and incubated with brilliant cresyl blue stain. During incubation, hemoglobin H (an unstable hemoglobin) present in the red cell will denature and precipitate within the cell. The hemoglobin H bodies and any other denatured hemoglobin will be stained by the brilliant cresyl blue. Smears are made, air-dried, and examined for the presence of hemoglobin H bodies.

PROCEDURE

1. Fill four microhematocrit tubes with well-mixed whole blood. Seal tubes. Centrifuge in the microhematocrit centrifuge for 5 minutes.
2. Using a file, score each hematocrit tube approximately 3 mm above, and 5 mm, below the plasma-red cell interface.
3. Place each of the 4 hematocrit sections into a 55 × 12 mm test tube. Add 1 drop of 1% brilliant cresyl blue stain. Mix tube vigorously by drawing back and forth over the top of a test tube rack.
4. Incubate blood and stain mixture at 37°C for 1 hour.

5. Fill a microhematocrit tube with the blood-stain mixture. Centrifuge for 5 minutes.
6. With the file, score and break the hematocrit tube midway between the clay seal and the interface of the plasma-stain and red cell layers. Discard the lower red cell portion. While holding the index finger over the top of the hematocrit tube, allow all of the red cells and a small amount of stain to be expelled from the hematocrit tube onto a glass slide. Mix well and make two wedge smears.
7. The smears may be coverslipped with Permount if desired.
8. Examine approximately 50,000 red cells (200 oil immersion fields containing 200 to 300 red cells per field). Hemoglobin H bodies are multiple, evenly distributed, bodies in the red cell. They stain a bluish-green in color (in contrast to the blue-purple of a reticulocyte). The red cell may also be described as resembling the even pattern of a golf ball.
9. Report results as positive or negative for hemoglobin H bodies.

DISCUSSION

1. In hemoglobin H disease, 10 to 100% of the red cells may contain these inclusion bodies. However, in α thalassemia trait only a few red cells (1 to 2 per 10,000 red blood cells up to 1% of the red cells) will be seen with H bodies.
2. In order to detect other unstable hemoglobins by this technique, the blood-stain mixture should be incubated for longer periods of time (from 4 to 24 hours) since these unstable hemoglobins require a longer incubation for denaturation and precipitation.
3. Heinz bodies may stain with this procedure and may be differentiated from the H bodies by the fact that they are larger, fewer in number, and

most often appear along the membrane of the red cell.

4. Diagnosis of an unstable hemoglobin should also be confirmed by other tests, such as the heat precipitation, isopropanol precipitation, etc.

HEAT PRECIPITATION TEST

Some unstable hemoglobins are not able to be detected by hemoglobin electrophoresis and may only be found using hemoglobin stability tests. The heat precipitation test is one method used to demonstrate unstable hemoglobins. Normally, less than 5% of the hemoglobin precipitates out when the test is performed by the following procedure.

REFERENCES

Dacie, J.V., and Lewis, S.M.: *Practical Hematology*, New York, Churchill Livingstone, Inc., 1984.
Schneiderman, L.J., Junga, I.G., and Fawley, D.E.: Effect of phosphate and non-phosphate buffers on thermolability of unstable haemoglobins, Nature, *225,* 1041, 1970.

REAGENTS AND EQUIPMENT

1. Tris buffer, 0.1 M, pH 7.4.
2. Cyanmethemoglobin (HiCN) reagent.
3. Sodium chloride, 0.85% (w/v).
4. Centrifuge tubes, 15 mL.
5. Waterbath, 50°C.
6. Spectrophotometer.
7. Disposable pipet droppers.
8. Test tubes, 10 × 55 mm, with caps.
9. Test tubes, 13 × 100 mm.

SPECIMEN

Whole blood, using EDTA or heparin as the anticoagulant. A normal control blood must be collected at the same time the patient's blood is obtained.

PRINCIPLE

Washed red blood cells are hemolyzed with water and then mixed with a tris buffer. This mixture is incubated at 50°C for 2 hours. A duplicate mixture is refrigerated. Most unstable hemoglobins will precipitate out more rapidly than normal hemoglobins at this elevated temperature (50°C). The hemoglobin content of the supernatants are then determined and the percentage of unstable hemoglobin precipitated during incubation is calculated (from the amount of hemoglobin in the unheated and heated samples).

PROCEDURE

1. Place 2 to 4 mL of patient's fresh whole blood into a 15-mL centrifuge tube and 2 to 4 mL of normal control blood into a second centrifuge tube.
2. Fill both test tubes with 0.85% sodium chloride to wash the red blood cells. Centrifuge at 1200 to 1500 g for 5 minutes. Remove the supernatant.
3. Wash the red blood cells two more times as described in step 2 above, and remove the final supernatant.
4. Remove a measured amount of washed red blood cells from the patient's tube and place in a 13 × 100-mm test tube. Repeat this procedure for the normal control.
5. Add a volume of distilled water to each tube which is 5 times the volume of the red blood cells in the tube. Stopper tube and mix by inverting several times. The red blood cells should completely hemolyze and the resultant solution should be crystal clear. Any turbidity present indicates incomplete hemolysis of the red blood cells.
6. Add a volume of tris buffer that is equal to the amount of distilled water added to the tube (5 times the red cell volume). Cap tube and mix well.
7. Centrifuge tubes at 1200 to 1500 g for 10 minutes.
8. Remove at least 4.5 mL of the supernatant from each tube and place in a second labeled test tube.
9. Label two 10 × 55 mm test tubes for each patient and control. Label one tube with an 'H' (heat) and one tube with an 'R' (refrigerate).
10. Place 2 mL of the patient's buffered

hemolysate into each of the two above test tubes. Stopper tube. Repeat, for each patient and control. Place all of the tubes marked 'H' in the 50°C waterbath. Incubate tubes for 2 hours. Place the 'R' tubes in the refrigerator for 2 hours.

11. At the end of the 2-hour incubation, remove tubes from the waterbath and refrigerator. Centrifuge all tubes at 1200 to 1500 g for 10 minutes.
12. While the above tubes are centrifuging, label one 13 × 100 mm-test tube for each of the tubes. Pipet 9.5 mL of cyanmethemoglobin reagent into each tube.
13. Add 0.5 mL of supernatant into the appropriately labeled tubes (step 12 above). Mix and allow tubes to stand for 10 minutes.
14. Centrifuge tubes at 1200 to 1500 g for 10 minutes.
15. Carefully remove the supernatant and read the absorbance in a spectrophotometer at a wavelength of 540 nm, using a blank prepared by adding 0.5 mL of tris buffer to 9.5 mL of cyanmethemoglobin reagent.
16. Calculate the results for the patient and the normal control as shown below:

$$\text{Percent unstable hgb} = \frac{\text{Absorbance of 'R'} - \text{Absorbance of 'H'}}{\text{Absorbance of 'R'}} \times 100$$

17. Report results as the percent of unstable (precipitated) hemoglobin.

DISCUSSION

1. Tris buffer is more sensitive to unstable hemoglobins than the phosphate buffer as described in some procedures.
2. The diagnosis of an unstable hemoglobin should be confirmed by other tests such as the Isopropanol Precipitation test, tests for inclusion bodies, etc.

3. Blood specimens for this test should be less than 72 hours old and should be refrigerated until use.
4. Increased waterbath temperatures over 50°C will cause false positive results.

ISOPROPANOL PRECIPITATION TEST

The isopropanol precipitation test detects unstable hemoglobins. According to the following procedure, normal hemoglobins will begin to show precipitation in a 17% isopropanol solution after about 40 minutes, whereas unstable hemoglobins will begin to precipitate after 5 minutes and show heavier flocculation at 20 minutes.

REFERENCES

Carrell, R.W., and Kay, R.: A simple method for the detection of unstable haemoglobins, Br. J. Haematol., 23, 615, 1972.
Division of Host Factors, Center for Infectious Diseases: Laboratory Methods for Detecting Hemoglobinopathies, Atlanta, Centers for Disease Control, 1984.

REAGENTS AND EQUIPMENT

1. Isopropanol-tris buffer, pH 7.4.
   Tris (hydroxymethyl) aminomethane 12.11 g
   Isopropyl alcohol, 100% 170 mL
   Dilute to 1 liter with distilled water. Adjust to pH 7.4 using concentrated HCl. Store at room temperature. This solution may be used for approximately 1 month.
2. Water bath, 37°C.
3. Test tubes, 10 × 75 mm, with caps.
4. Centrifuge tubes, polypropylene, 15 mL.
5. Sodium chloride, 0.85%, w/v.
6. Distilled water.
7. Carbon tetrachloride (CCl_4).
8. Pasteur pipets.
9. Pipets, 0.2 mL and 2.0 mL.
10. Vortex mixer.
11. Parafilm.
12. Timer.

SPECIMEN

Whole, anticoagulated blood. The type of anticoagulant used is not critical. A normal control blood should be collected at the same time the patient's blood is obtained. A cord blood specimen may be used as a positive control if it is available.

PRINCIPLE

A red blood cell hemolysate is prepared. This hemolysate is then added to a 17% solution of isopropanol and incubated at 37°C. The specimens are examined at 5 minutes and 20 minutes for precipitation of unstable hemoglobin. The isopropanol solution weakens the internal bonding of hemoglobin, causing a faster rate of precipitation of unstable hemoglobins than normal hemoglobin.

PROCEDURE

1. Preparation of hemolysate.
   a. Place 2 to 3 mL of patient's whole blood into a graduated, polypropylene centrifuge tube. Place 2 to 3 mL of normal control blood into a second tube.
   b. Fill both tubes with 0.85% sodium chloride to wash the red blood cells. Centrifuge at 1200 to 1500 g for 5 minutes. Remove the supernatant.
   c. Wash the red blood cells two more times by repeating step b above.
   d. Remove 1 mL of washed red blood cells from each tube and place in a clean, labeled, polypropylene centrifuge tube. Add 1 mL of distillled water to each tube. Mix. Add 0.5 mL of CCl_4 to each tube. Stopper each tube.
   e. Vortex, or vigorously shake, each tube for 5 minutes.
   f. Centrifuge the tubes at 1500 g for 25 to 30 minutes. Carefully remove tubes from the centrifuge.
   g. Remove the upper hemolysate layer from each tube, being careful not to disturb the lower stroma and CCl_4 layers.
   h. The final hemoglobin concentration of each hemolysate should be between 9 and 12 g/dL.
   i. Continue with the following procedure at once.

2. For each patient and control to be tested, place 2.0 mL of the isopropanol-tris buffer solution into a 10 × 75 mm test tube. Stopper each tube and place in the 37°C water bath for 10 minutes in order to pre-warm. Be certain the liquid in the tubes is completely immersed in the water of the incubator. (To save time, place the test tubes in the water bath just prior to the last centrifugation in the preparation of the hemolysate.)

3. Add 0.2 mL of each hemolysate to the appropriately labeled test tubes of buffer in the water bath. Stopper each tube and gently invert 2 times to mix.

4. Check each test tube at 5, 20, and 45 minutes for evidence of precipitation or flocculation. When reading the test tubes, extreme care must be taken not to mix the solution too much. (The precipitate will quickly break up if the solution is physically mixed.) Carefully remove the test tube from the water bath, tilt the tube horizontally, and examine the solution for precipitation against a light source.

5. Interpretation of results.
   a. Negative for unstable hemoglobin: No precipitation or flocculation at 5 minutes or 20 minutes. Precipitation should begin to appear at 45 minutes.
   b. Positive for unstable hemoglobin: Precipitation present at the 5 minute reading, with definite flocculation at 20 minutes.
   c. The normal control should be negative for hemoglobin precipitation at 5 and 20 minutes. To en-

sure that the buffer solution is effective, precipitation should begin appearing at 45 minutes. If these results are not obtained for the normal control, fresh buffer reagent should be prepared and the entire test repeated.

DISCUSSION

1. A cord blood may be used as a positive control and should be prepared and tested in the same manner as that described above for the patient.

2. Toluene and chloroform should not be used in the preparation of hemolysates for unstable hemoglobin testing.

3. Blood that is several days old may be used for this test. The hemolysate, however, must be prepared immediately prior to the performance of the test.

4. The concentration of isopropanol (17%) in the buffer solution is critical as is the temperature of the 37°C water bath.

5. The pH of the buffer solution is not critical but must be at least 7.2.

6. The presence of any red cell stroma in the hemolysate will give false positive results.

7. Small amounts of an unstable hemoglobin may be lost in the hemolysate preparation. This may lead to some falsely negative results in patients having only a small amount of an unstable hemoglobin.

8. Specimens containing large amounts of hemoglobin F, and old samples containing an increase in methemoglobin, may give false-positive results by the above procedure. The addition of 0.05 mL of 2% potassium cyanide (w/v) to 2.5 mL of hemolysate, prior to testing, should eliminate the false-positive results.

9. The diagnosis of an unstable hemoglobin should be confirmed by other tests such as the heat precipitation test, tests for inclusion bodies, etc.

METHEMOGLOBIN TEST

Methemoglobin (Hi) is a form of hemoglobin in which the ferrous ion has been oxidized to the ferric state and is, therefore, incapable of combining with or transporting the oxygen molecule. A small amount of methemoglobin is continuously being formed in the red blood cell but, in turn, is reduced by the red blood cell enzyme systems. Methemoglobin is normally present in the blood in a concentration of 1 to 3%, with slightly higher levels present in infants and heavy smokers. Increased amounts may be found in both hereditary and acquired disorders. The hereditary form of methemoglobinemia is found in disorders in which (1) the red blood cell reducing systems are abnormal and unable to reduce the methemoglobin back to oxyhemoglobin, or (2) in the presence of hemoglobin M, where the structure of the polypeptide chains making up the hemoglobin molecule is abnormal, there is a tendency toward oxidation, and a decreased ability to be reduced back to oxyhemoglobin. The acquired causes of methemoglobinemia are mainly due to certain drugs and chemicals, such as aniline, nitrates, nitrites, and some sulfonamides.

REFERENCE

Dacie, J.V., and Lewis, S.M.: *Practical Haematology,* New York, Churchill Livingstone, Inc., 1984.

REAGENTS AND EQUIPMENT

1. Phosphate buffer, pH 6.8.
   Solution 1

Monobasic potassium phosphate (KH_2PO_4)	9.1 g
Distilled water	1 liter

   Solution 2

Dibasic sodium phosphate (Na_2HPO_4)	9.5 g
Distilled water	1 liter

   For the phosphate buffer, pH 6.8, mix:

Solution 1　　　　　　50.8 mL
Solution 2　　　　　　49.2 mL
2. Potassium cyanide solution.
　　Potassium cyanide　　　5 g
　　Distilled water　　　100 mL
3. Potassium ferricyanide solution.
　　Potassium ferricyanide　5 g
　　Distilled water　　　100 mL
4. Sterox SE solution.
　　Sterox SE　　　　　1 mL
　　Distilled water　　　99 mL
5. Test tubes, 13 × 125 mm.
6. Spectrophotometer.
7. Pipets, 10, 5, and 0.2 mL.

SPECIMEN

Fresh whole blood or anticoagulated whole blood, using EDTA or heparin as the anticoagulant.

PRINCIPLE

Whole blood is diluted with phosphate buffer solution and sterox SE to prevent turbidity. Methemoglobin has a maximum absorbance on the spectrophotometer at a wavelength of 630 nm. The diluted blood is read at this wavelength, and the reading is noted (D_1). Potassium cyanide is added to this solution, converting the methemoglobin to cyanmethemoglobin, and read on the spectrophotometer (D_2). The change in optical density is proportional to the amount of methemoglobin present. Potassium ferricyanide, which converts hemoglobin to methemoglobin, is added to a second dilution of the blood, and its spectrophotometer reading is noted (D_3). Potassium cyanide is added, which converts the methemoglobin to cyanmethemoglobin, and the spectrophotometer reading is noted (D_4). The percentage of methemoglobin present in the blood is then calculated.

PROCEDURE

1. Pipet 4 mL of phosphate buffer solution and 6 mL of sterox SE solution into a test tube and label with the patient's name or sample #.

2. Add 0.2 ml of whole blood and mix well. Label test tube #1.
3. Place 5.0 mL of the diluted blood solution from test tube #1 into a second test tube and label #2.
4. Prepare a blank solution by mixing 2 mL of phosphate buffer with 3 mL of sterox SE solution.
5. Read test tube #1 in a spectrophotometer at a wavelength of 630 nm, using the blank solution to set optical density at 0. Record the optical density of the solution (D_1).
6. Add 1 drop of potassium cyanide solution to test tube #1, mix, and read, as in step 5. Record the optical density (D_2).
7. Add 1 drop of potassium ferricyanide solution to test tube #2, mix, and allow to sit for 5 minutes. Read on the spectrophotometer, as in step 5. Record the optical density (D_3).
8. Add 1 drop of potassium cyanide solution to test tube #2, mix, and read, as in step 5. Record the optical density (D_4).
9. Calculation of results:

$$\text{Percent Methemoglobin} = \frac{D_1 - D_2}{D_3 - D_4} \times 100$$

DISCUSSION

1. Sulfhemoglobin is not measured at any time during this procedure. Therefore, if an appreciable amount of sulfhemoglobin is present, the total hemoglobin reading will be low.
2. This test should be performed within 1 hour of blood collection due to the fact that methemoglobin will convert to hemoglobin in stored blood samples. However, once the blood has been diluted in the buffer reagent, it is stable up to 24 hours at refrigerator temperatures.

SERUM HAPTOGLOBIN TEST

The major breakdown, or hemolysis, of red blood cells occurs in the reticuloendothelial system. Approximately 10% of red blood cell destruction, however, occurs intravascularly. In this circumstance, free hemoglobin is released directly into the blood and undergoes dissociation into α, β dimers, which are then bound to a serum globulin called *haptoglobin*. The binding of the hemoglobin to the haptoglobin prevents renal excretion of the pigment. This complex is then removed from the plasma by the reticuloendothelial system. In normal plasma, the haptoglobin is present in amounts sufficient to bind 30 to 200 mg of hemoglobin per dL of plasma. Haptoglobin decreases and begins to disappear when hemolysis is increased to twice the normal rate. Increased amounts of haptoglobin are found in pregnancy, chronic infections, malignancy, Hodgkin's disease, rheumatoid arthritis, tissue damage, and systemic lupus erythematosus.

REFERENCES

Colfs, B., and Vekeyden, J.: A rapid method for the determination of serum haptoglobin. Clin. Chem. Acta, *12*, 470, 1965.

Dacie, J.V., and Lewis, S.M.: *Practical Haematology.* New York, Churchill Livingstone, 1984.

Lathem, W., and Worley, W.E.: The distribution of extracorpuscular hemoglobin in circulating plasma. J. Clin. Invest., *38*, 474, 1959.

REAGENTS AND EQUIPMENT

1. Phosphate buffer, 0.05 M, pH 7.0.
   Solution 1
   Dibasic sodium phosphate   7.1 g
   (Na_2HPO_4)
   Dilute to 1 L with distilled water.
   Solution 2
   Monobasic sodium
   phosphate   3.45 g
   ($NaH_2PO_4 \cdot H_2O$)
   Dilute to 500 mL with distilled water.
   For phosphate buffer, 0.05 M, pH 7.0, mix:
   Solution 1   1 L
   Solution 2   500 mL
   Store in the refrigerator.

2. O-dianisidine reagent. Prepare just before using.
   O-dianisidine   0.5 g
   Ethyl alcohol, 95% (v/v)   70 mL

3. Acetate buffer, pH 4.7
   Sodium acetate ($Na_2C_2H_3O_2 \cdot 3H_2O$) (27.22 g/L of distilled water) 53.5 mL
   Acetic acid (11.3 mL of glacial acetic acid diluted to 1 L with distilled water)   46.5 mL

4. Hydrogen peroxide, 3% (v/v).

5. Staining reagent. Prepare just before using.
   O-dianisidine reagent   70 mL
   Acetate buffer   10 mL
   Hydrogen peroxide, 3% (v/v) 2.5 mL
   Dilute to 100 mL with distilled water.

6. Tweezers, one pair.

7. Microzone electrophoresis cell, model #R-101 (obtainable from Beckman Instruments, Palo Alto, Calif.).

8. Cellulose acetate membranes, #324330 (Beckman Instruments).

9. Sample applicator, #324399 (Beckman Instruments).

10. DC-regulated power supply.

11. Drying oven, capable of reaching 100 to 110°C.

12. Glass drying plates (same size as the cellulose acetate membranes).

13. Acetic acid, 5% (v/v).

14. Ethyl alcohol, 95% (v/v).

15. Clearing solution. Prepare immediately before using.
    Ethyl alcohol, 95% (v/v)   75 mL
    Glacial acetic acid   25 mL
    It may be necessary to vary the amounts of glacial acetic acid and ethyl alcohol depending on the membranes used.

16. Triton-X wetting agent.

17. Sodium chloride, 0.85% (w/v).

18. Chloroform.

19. Glycerin.

20. Graduated centrifuge tubes, 15 mL.

21. Parafilm.

22. Hemoglobin solutions of 0.25, 0.50, 1.0, and 2.0 g/dL.
    a. Preparation of the hemolysate
       1) Place 3 to 4 mL of normal, whole anticoagulated (EDTA) blood in a 15-mL graduated centrifuge tube.
       2) Centrifuge at 1000 × g for 5 minutes. Remove plasma and discard.
       3) Fill the tube to the 15-mL mark with 0.85% sodium chloride, mix, and centrifuge at 1000 × g for 5 minutes. Remove the supernatant sodium chloride.
       4) Wash the red blood cells two more times.
       5) Add one drop of Triton-X wetting agent, mix tube well, and allow to stand for 15 minutes to ensure complete hemolysis of the red blood cells.
       6) Add a volume of chloroform equal to one-half the volume of the red blood cells. Use stopper and shake the tube vigorously for 1 minute.
       7) Centrifuge for 5 minutes at 1000 × g.
       8) Carefully remove the upper layer of the hemolysate.
       9) Add an equal volume of glycerin to the hemolysate and mix. One may use a stopper and place the mixture in the freezer until ready for use.
    b. Determine the exact hemoglobin concentration of the hemolysate (cyanmethemoglobin method). Using distilled water, adjust the hemoglobin concentration to 10 g/dL.
    c. Prepare the following dilutions as indicated:
       1) Hemoglobin solution of 2.0 g/dL: 2.0 mL of hemolysate (10 g/dL) plus 8.0 mL of distilled water.
       2) Hemoglobin solution of 1.0 g/dL: 2.0 mL of hemoglobin solution (2.0 g/dL) plus 2.0 mL of distilled water.
       3) Hemoglobin solution of 0.5 g/dL: 2.0 mL of hemoglobin solution (1.0 g/dL) plus 2.0 mL of distilled water.
       4) Hemoglobin solution of 0.25 g/dL: 2.0 mL of hemoglobin solution (0.5 g/dL) plus 2.0 mL of distilled water.

SPECIMEN

Clotted blood, 6 mL. Collect a blood specimen from a normal control at the same time the patient's blood is obtained.

PRINCIPLE

The patient and control serums are incubated with varying concentrations of hemoglobin solutions. During this time, the haptoglobin present in the serum binds the hemoglobin, depending on the amount of haptoglobin available. An electrophoretic pattern of the serum-hemoglobin samples is then obtained and stained, and the cellulose acetate strips are examined. One may ascertain the approximate amount of haptoglobin present in the serum by noting at which hemoglobin concentration a second band of free hemoglobin appears.

PROCEDURE

1. Collect 5 to 6 mL of whole blood from both the patient and the normal control. Incubate at 37°C until the clot begins to retract. Remove the serum and centrifuge at 1500 × g for 10 minutes. Remove the supernatant serum and place in clean test tubes. If the test will not be performed at this time, freeze the serum. (If either of the samples is hemolyzed, the blood must be recollected.)
2. Number eight test tubes (#1 through #8) and set up the following serum–hemolysate dilutions.
   a. #1: 0.2 mL of normal control

serum plus 0.02 mL of 0.25 g/dL hemoglobin solution.

b. #2: 0.2 mL of normal control serum plus 0.02 mL of 0.5 g/dL hemoglobin solution.

c. #3: 0.2 mL of normal control serum plus 0.02 mL of 1.0 g/dL hemoglobin solution.

d. #4: 0.2 mL of normal control serum plus 0.02 mL of 2.0 g/dL hemoglobin solution.

e. #5: Same as tube #1, using patient's serum in place of normal control serum.

f. #6: Same as tube #2, using patient's serum in place of normal control serum.

g. #7: Same as tube #3, using patient's serum in place of normal control serum.

h. #8: Same as tube #4, using patient's serum in place of normal control serum.

3. Incubate the above eight tubes at 37°C for 30 minutes.

4. Fill both sides of the microzone cell with phosphate buffer.

5. Fill a small tray (of a size to accommodate one cellulose acetate membrane) with approximately 40 mL of buffer solution.

6. Using tweezers, place a cellulose acetate membrane in the tray of buffer. The membrane should be allowed to float on the surface of the buffer to allow capillary action to draw the buffer up evenly through the membrane. As soon as the entire membrane has become wet, immerse it completely in the buffer by carefully agitating the tray. Immediately remove the membrane from the buffer using the tweezers. Carefully blot the membrane between two pieces of filter paper or blotters by passing a hand lightly over the top blotter once.

7. Immediately suspend and mount the wet membrane on the bridge of the electrophoresis cell, ensuring that the membrane lies evenly and that each end hangs freely in opposite chambers containing the buffer.

8. Replace the upper lid of the microzone cell to guard against drying of the membrane.

9. Attach the connecting cables of the power supply to the electrode terminal pins. Do not turn on the power supply yet.

10. Allow the membrane to equilibrate for about 2 minutes before applying the blood samples. (The serum-hemolysates are inoculated on the cathode side.)

11. Place a small drop of each of the eight serum-hemolysates on a strip of Parafilm.

12. Using the applicator, depress the white button on the top to extend the applicator tip. Without breaking the surface tension of the serum-hemolysate drop, carefully and slowly move the applicator tip across the top surface. In this way, a 0.25-μL sample is picked up by the applicator tip. Retract the applicator tip by carefully depressing the red button.

13. Remove the lid of the microzone cell and place the applicator in the appropriate grooves. Remove your hand from the applicator. Touch the white button carefully. Allow the applicator tip to remain in contact with the membrane for 10 to 15 seconds. Press the red button gently causing the applicator tip to retract. Remove the applicator and replace the lid on the microzone cell.

14. Repeat steps 12 and 13 two more times, using the same serum-hemolysate dilution and inoculating the cellulose acetate membrane in the same place. This gives a 0.75-μL sample.

15. Rinse the applicator tip with a thin stream of distilled water and blot dry.

16. Repeat steps 12 through 15, applying each serum-hemolysate sample in one of the eight positions on the cellulose acetate membrane.

17. As soon as all samples have been applied to the membrane, turn on the power supply to 150 V for 40 minutes.

18. At the end of 40 minutes, turn off the power supply and remove the plugs from the electrode terminal pins.

19. Carefully remove the membrane from the bridge without allowing any buffer to splash or run over the membrane.

20. Immediately immerse the membrane in a pan containing the freshly prepared stain for 5 minutes.

21. Remove the membrane from the stain and wash in distilled water.

22. Place the membrane in a pan containing 5% acetic acid for approximately 5 minutes.

23. Allow the excess acetic acid to drain from the membrane and place it in 95% ethyl alcohol for exactly 1 minute.

24. Drain the excess ethyl alcohol from the membrane and place it in the clearing solution for exactly 30 seconds. While the membrane is immersed in the clearing solution, place the glass drying plate directly over the membrane. As soon as 30 seconds have elapsed, hold the membrane and glass together at one end. Lift this end from the clearing solution first, allowing the membrane to become positioned on the glass plate. Make certain the membrane lies flat on the glass plate and contains no air bubbles.

25. Place the glass plate holding the membrane in the drying oven at 100 to 110°C for 10 to 15 minutes.

26. Carefully remove the glass plate and membrane from the oven and allow to cool. The membrane should be completely transparent when removed from the oven.

27. When the glass plate has cooled sufficiently, loosen one corner of the membrane and carefully peel it from the glass, taking care that it does not tear.

28. The membrane may then be placed in a storage envelope (in between two pieces of plastic) to preserve it and avoid curling at the edges.

29. Interpretation: the free hemoglobin and hemoglobin bound to haptoglobin migrate as shown in Figure 144. The serum-hemolysate dilution containing the greatest amount of hemoglobin determines the amount of haptoglobin present in the serum. For example, if the serum-hemolysate mixture from tube #8 does show a free hemoglobin band, 100 to 200 mg/dL of haptoglobin is reported present in the serum.

DISCUSSION

1. If the freshly incubated serum sample is allowed to stand, methemalbumin is formed. In this situation, the methemalbumin will be present on the membrane as a band located on the right of the hemoglobin-haptoglobin band.

2. This same general procedure may be used to quantitate the amount of haptoglobin present in the serum more accurately, if a densitometer (Beckman R-110 Microzone Densitometer) is available. For this method, incubate the patient's serum with a hemoglobin solution (1 volume hemolysate with 9 volumes of serum). Determine the exact concentration of the hemolysate (it should be 3.5 to 4.0 g/dL). Perform the procedure as described earlier beginning with step 3, and electrophorese one sample/patient or control. Using the densitometer, scan the dried membrane at 450

CATHODE   ANODE

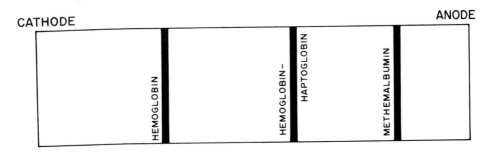

Fig. 144. Electrophoretic migration of free hemoglobin, hemoglobin-haptoglobin, and methemalbumin.

mµ and a 0.3-mm slit width. The haptoglobin is calculated as follows:

Haptoglobin (mg/dL)

$$= \frac{\% \text{ Haptoglobin} \times \text{hemoglobin concentrate}}{10} \times 1000$$

Dilution of hemoglobin = 10
Conversion factor (g/dL to mg/dL) = 1000

SERUM VISCOSITY TEST

Viscosity is the property of a fluid which resists the force causing it to flow. In a protein solution, the viscosity depends on the concentration of the protein. The relative viscosity of serum is determined by comparing it with the viscosity of distilled water and is normally in the range of 1.4 to 1.8. In certain pathologic states associated with qualitative and/or quantitative protein disorders, the serum viscosity is increased. This increase is found most often in Waldenström's macroglobuline-mia, less often in multiple myeloma, and rarely in other disorders. The severity of the clinical abnormalities are often better correlated with the viscosity of the serum than with the level of the protein involved. Therefore, therapy may be followed by serum viscosity measurements.

REFERENCE

Fahey, J.L., Barth, W.F., and Solomon, A.: Serum hyperviscosity syndrome, JAMA, *192*, 464, 1965.

REAGENTS AND EQUIPMENT

1. Water bath, 37°C.
2. Vacuum tubing.
3. Aspirator.
4. Laboratory stand with clamp.
5. Sodium chloride, 0.85% (w/v).
6. Distilled water.
7. Ostwald viscometer (Fig. 145).
8. Stopwatch.

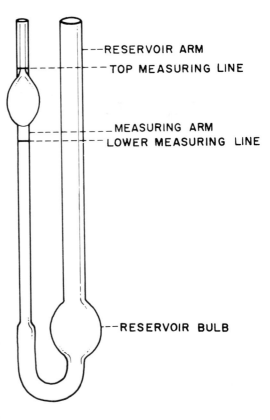

---RESERVOIR ARM
---TOP MEASURING LINE

_MEASURING ARM
--LOWER MEASURING LINE

---RESERVOIR BULB

Fig. 145. Ostwald viscometer.

SPECIMEN

Collect approximately 12 ml of whole blood and allow it to clot. This test requires 5 ml of serum.

PRINCIPLE

The patient's serum is placed in a viscometer and the time required for the serum to flow from one mark to a second mark is measured. This time is then compared with the time required for distilled water to flow the same distance in the viscometer.

PROCEDURE

1. Centrifuge the clotted blood at 3000 × g for 10 minutes. Remove the serum and centrifuge a second time. Place the serum in a test tube.
2. Rinse the Ostwald viscometer well with 0.85% sodium chloride.
3. Suspend the viscometer in a 37°C water bath by means of a laboratory stand.
4. Place 5 ml of patient's serum into the reservoir bulb through the reservoir arm.
5. Allow several minutes for the serum to reach 37°C. At this time, remove any air bubbles in the serum by gently blowing through the aspirator attached to the top of the measuring arm.
6. Using suction, draw the serum up into the measuring arm above the highest line. Release the suction.
7. As the serum flows down through the measuring arm, start the stopwatch as soon as the top of the serum is even with the top measuring line.
8. Time the passage of serum between the two measuring lines: as soon as the upper border of the serum is even with the lower measuring line, stop the watch. Record the flow time of the serum.
9. Repeat steps 6 through 8 two more times and average the three readings.
10. Remove the serum and rinse the vis-

cometer several times with 0.85% sodium chloride followed by two rinses with distilled water.
11. Repeat steps 3 through 9, using 5 ml of distilled water in place of the patient's serum.
12. Calculate the results as shown below:

$$\text{Relative serum viscosity} = \frac{\text{Flow time of serum}}{\text{Flow time of distilled water}}$$

DISCUSSION

1. The flow time of distilled water through the viscometer is generally about 59 seconds.
2. The viscometer, when it is not in use, should be sealed with Parafilm.
3. This procedure may be performed at room temperature if a 37°C water bath is not available.
4. Alternatively, a red cell pipet or a 1-mL volumetric pipet may be used in place of the Ostwald viscometer. The pipet must be supported in a vertical position and the test may be performed at room temperature.
5. Symptoms of the hyperviscosity syndrome are generally present in the patient when the relative serum viscosity is between 6 and 7, but may also be present with a test result as low as 4.

MALARIA SMEARS

Exactly when blood smears should be taken from patients suspected of having malaria is somewhat controversial. It is probably not necessary to wait until the patient has fever and chills to obtain the first specimen for determining a diagnosis of malaria. Specimens obtained during the period of fever and chills will generally contain numerous parasites in the young stages (ring forms). Halfway between the attacks (paroxysms), smears usually contain the parasites in more advanced stages, when they show more identifying characteristics. For these reasons it is probably advisable to obtain most specimens at the time of fever and chills and again midway between paroxysms.

REFERENCE

Hall, R., and Malia, R.G.: *Medical Laboratory Haematology*, Boston, Butterworths, 1984.

REAGENTS AND EQUIPMENT

1. Buffered distilled water, pH 7.2.

   Anhydrous dibasic sodium phosphate (Na_2HPO_4)   3.0 g

   Anhydrous monobasic potassium phosphate (KH_2PO_4)   0.6 g

   Dissolve in 1 liter of distilled water.
2. Giemsa staining solution.

   Liquid Giemsa stain   10 mL

   Buffered distilled water, pH 7.2   90 mL
3. Glass slides.
4. Coplin jar.

SPECIMEN

Several thick and thin blood smears.

PROCEDURE

1. Make two or three routine blood smears from fingertip blood or blood anticoagulated with EDTA. Air dry smears.
2. Make two or three thick smears by placing one large drop of blood on a glass slide. Using the corner of a second slide, carefully spread the drop of blood over an area the size of a dime. Allow the smears to air dry for several hours (2 to 4) or overnight. (To determine the correct thickness of the blood smear, place the slide on a piece of newspaper. Spread the blood until the small newsprint is just visible through the smear.
3. Fix the thin smears with methanol for a few seconds. Do not fix the thick smears.
4. Place the smears in a coplin jar containing Giemsa staining solution for 30 minutes.

5. At the end of 30 minutes, rinse the smears in running tap water and allow to air dry.
6. Examine the smears microscopically, using the oil immersion objective (100×). The red blood cells on the thick, unfixed smears will be destroyed, making examination easier. It is important to identify correctly the species of malaria *(Plasmodium malariae, vivax, falciparum,* or *ovale)* when present so that proper medication can be given (Fig. 146 and Plate VIII).

DISCUSSION

1. The thick blood film is used for the detection of the blood parasite and consists of white cell nuclei and platelet debris. Differentiation of the different types of malaria is made using the thin blood smear.
2. The concentration of malaria parasites in the blood may be as low as 1 parasite/100,000 red blood cells, or 1 parasite/400 high oil immersion fields on a thin blood smear, which could take about 1 hour to examine. However, this same volume of blood may be examined on a thick blood smear in 5 minutes.
3. Mixed infections of malaria are found and are much more difficult to diagnose. The most common mixed infection currently found is Plasmodium falciparum and vivax.
4. The identification of a species of malaria requires the consideration of three factors: the appearance of infected erythrocytes, the appearance of the parasites, and the stages found.
5. *Plasmodium vivax* generally shows all stages of development present in the blood simultaneously. The ring forms are usually large, and there may be two or more rings present in a red blood cell. The red chromatin dot in the early trophozoite may appear singly or, at times, two may be

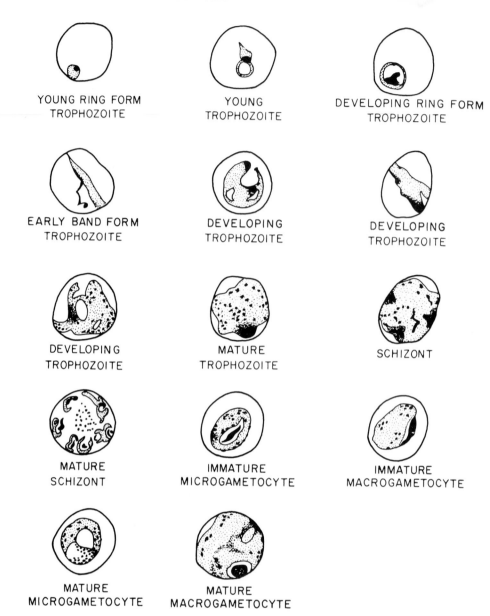

Fig. 146. *Plasmodium malariae.* (Modified from Seiverd, C.E.: Hematology for Medical Technologists, 5th Ed., Philadelphia, Lea & Febiger, 1983.)

present. The trophozoites are frequently quite ameboid, which is a characteristic of this type of malaria. There may be 12 to 24 merozoites present in the mature schizont with an average of 16. The infected red blood cells are usually enlarged and may be irregularly shaped. Schüffner's stippling may also be found. These granules, which fill the red blood cell, appear as orange to pink colored stippling. (These granules may not be visible when normal staining times are used. To detect these granules, allow the smears to stain for 3 hours.)

6. In *Plasmodium falciparum* infections, ring forms and gametocytes are generally the only stages seen on the peripheral blood smear. The ring forms present are generally smaller and more delicate than found in other types of malaria and one or two chromatin dots are common. Multiple ring forms in a single red blood cell is a common finding. The gametocytes in this type of malaria are characteristic, showing a crescent or sausage shape with a golden brown pigment. The red blood cells are normal in size and may show Maurer's spots, which are irregular, orange to pink staining granules that may be present in varying numbers.

7. In *Plasmodium malariae*, all stages of development may be found on the peripheral blood smear, but usually not simultaneously. The ring forms are small and compact, generally contain only one chromatin dot, and only one ring form is usually found in the red blood cell. Most often, the schizont will contain 6 to 12 merozoites. Generally, an abundant amount of hematin granules are present, and the red blood cells are of normal size and may contain a fine stippling (Ziemann's dots).

8. *Plasmodium ovale* infection is rarely encountered. All stages of development may be present on the peripheral blood smear. Like P. malariae, usually only one ring form per red blood cell is present, and these ring forms contain only one chromatin dot. The growing trophozoites are small and compact. There are 6 to 12 merozoites present in the schizont, with an average of 8. The infected red blood cells may be enlarged, and over 20% are oval shaped and fimbriated (irregular border). Hematin granules are generally present and the red cells may also contain Schüffner's dots.

9. Other parasites found in the blood of infected patients are babesia, trypanosomes, and certain microfilaria. Leishmania is not found in the blood but may be found in the bone marrow. These organisms can be studied in more detail in courses on Parasitology.

REAGENTS

SPECIAL HEMATOLOGY-REAGENTS

Acetate Buffer, 0.1 N, pH 5.0

Sodium acetate   4.797 g
  ($CH_3COONa \cdot 3H_2O$)
Acetic Acid, 1 N   14.75 mL
Dissolve the sodium acetate in 1 N acetic acid and dilute to 1 liter with distilled water. Refrigerate.

Acetic acid, 1 N

Glacial acetic acid   6 mL
Dilute to 1 liter with distilled water.

Barbital Buffered Saline Solution, pH 7.35

Sodium diethylbarbiturate   5.875 g
Sodium chloride   7.335 g
Distilled water   785 mL
Hydrochloric acid, 0.1 N   215 mL
Store in the refrigerator.

Buffered Methyl Green, 1% w/v, in Acetate Buffer
(0.1 N, pH 5.0)

Methyl green   1.0 g
Acetate buffer, 0.1 N, pH 5.0   100 mL
Adjust the pH from 4.2 to 4.5 with 1 N sodium hydroxide or 1 N hydrochloric acid. Filter.
Store at room temperature.

Buffered Neutral Red, 1% w/v in Acetate Buffer
(0.1 N, pH 5.0)

Neutral red   1.0 g
Acetate buffer, 0.1 N, pH 5.0   100 mL

Warm the above solution and mix until the stain is dissolved. Filter when cooled to room temperature.

Hydrochloric Acid, 1 N

Hydrochloric acid, concentrated (37.25% purity) 97.85 mL
Dilute to 1 liter with distilled water.

Mayer's Hematoxylin

Hematoxylin 1 g
Aluminum ammonium sulfate (ammonium alum) 50 g
Chloral hydrate 50 g
Dilute to 1 liter with distilled water. Add 0.2 g of sodium iodate (ripening agent) and mix well. Store reagent at room temperature for 7 days in order to ripen before use.

Pararosanilin, 4% w/v in 20% (v/v) Hydrochloric Acid

Pararosanilin hydrochloride 1.0 g
Distilled water 20 mL
Hydrochloric acid, concentrated 5 mL
Gently warm the above while mixing in order to dissolve as much pararosanilin as possible. Allow the mixture to cool, filter, and store in a brown bottle at room temperature.

Phosphate Buffered Formalin Acetone Fixative, pH 6.6 to 6.8

Dibasic sodium phosphate (Na_2HPO_4) 0.1 g
Monobasic potassium phosphate (KH_2PO_4) 0.5 g
Dissolve the above in 150 mL of distilled water and add:
Acetone 225 mL
Formaldehyde, 37% 125 mL
Store in the refrigerator.

Sodium Hydroxide, 1 N

Sodium hydroxide 40 g
Dilute to 1 liter with distilled water.

Sodium Nitrite, 4% w/v

Sodium nitrite 4.0 g
Dilute to 100 mL with distilled water. Prepare immediately before use.

Tris buffer, 0.1 M, pH 7.4

Tris-(2-amino-2-[hydroxymethyl]1,3-propandiol) 12.1g
Dissolve reagent in 800 mL of distilled water. Adjust pH to 7.4 using 0.1 N hydrochloric acid. Dilute to 1 liter with distilled water. Store in the refrigerator. Warm to room temperature before using.

5

Coagulation

HEMOSTASIS, COAGULATION, AND FIBRINOLYSIS

Hemostasis is the process which retains the blood within the vascular system. It basically consists of two steps: primary hemostasis and secondary hemostasis. The hemostatic process involves the interaction of at least five components: blood vessels, platelets, coagulation factors, inhibitors, and fibrinolysis. Each of these will be described in relatively basic terms on the following pages. Hemostasis and coagulation are highly complex mechanisms, which, even today are not completely understood. A basic knowledge of this subject is a necessary tool before carrying out coagulation procedures.

During primary hemostasis there is constriction of the damaged blood vessels, which decreases the blood flow through the injured blood vessel. Platelets clump together and adhere to the injured vessel in this area to form a plug and further inhibit bleeding. When secondary hemostasis takes place, the coagulation factors present in the blood interact, forming a fibrin meshwork, or clot, to completely stop the bleeding. During this process, naturally occurring inhibitors present in the blood will inactivate the activated coagulation factors so that widespread coagulation does not occur. When the clot has formed, slow lysis of the clot begins, and final repair to the injured site takes place.

The blood coagulation mechanism and fibrinolysis will be described first, to acquaint the reader with the numerous substances in these two systems. A short section on primary hemostasis (blood vessels and platelets) follows.

Coagulation System

The complexity of the coagulation process has been made more difficult by the large number of different names given to the 12 coagulation factors. To avoid this confusion, the International Committee on Nomenclature of Blood Clotting Factors established a nomenclature for these clotting factors. Each of the 12 factors has been given a Roman numeral. Listed in Table 7 are the numbers assigned by this committee, along with their most commonly used names. Most of the factors, except fibrinogen, prothrombin, tissue thromboplastin, and calcium are referred to by their number. There are several new factors (prekallikrein and high molecular weight kininogen) which have no numbers. Factor VI, accelerin, is no longer considered one of the coagulation factors.

The interaction of these coagulation factors is shown in Figure 147. For teaching purposes and for testing in the laboratory, the coagulation process may be divided into two systems: the *intrinsic system* and the *extrinsic system*. All factors required for the intrinsic system are contained within the blood. The extrinsic system uses thromboplastin (factor III), which is

195

TABLE 7. COAGULATION FACTORS

FACTOR	NAME
I	Fibrinogen
II	Prothrombin
III	Tissue thromboplastin, tissue factor
IV	Calcium
V	Proaccelerin, labile factor
VII	Proconvertin, stable factor
VIII	Antihemophilic A factor (AHF), antihemophilic globulin (AHG)
IX	Antihemophilic B factor (AHB), plasma thromboplastin component (PTC), Christmas factor
X	Stuart factor, Stuart-Prower factor
XI	Plasma thromboplastin antecedent (PTA)
XII	Hageman factor, contact factor
XIII	Fibrin stabilizing factor
---	Fletcher factor, prekallikrein
---	High molecular weight kininogen, HMWK, Fitzgerald factor

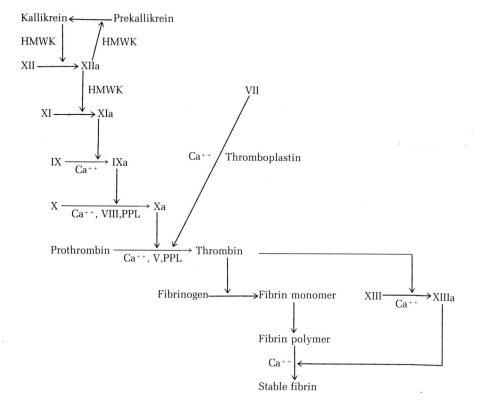

PPL = Platelet phospholipid

Fig. 147. Intrinsic and extrinsic coagulation process.

released from the damaged cells and tissues.

With the exception of calcium and platelet phospholipid, the coagulation factors are proteins. The process of coagulation is a series of biochemical reactions in which an inactive proenzyme is converted to an active enzyme, which, in turn, activates another proenzyme. All of the factors are serine proteases except for factor XIII which is a transpeptidase.

INTRINSIC AND EXTRINSIC COAGULATION PATHWAYS

In the intrinsic system, the exact stimulus which activates the coagulation mechanism is unknown but is thought to be associated with endothelial injury. Activation of the clotting sequence in vitro is brought about by surface contact with glass, kaolin, celite, or other negatively charged substances. Initially, a small amount of factor XII is activated. (When factor XII comes in contact with negatively charged surfaces such as glass or endothelial cells there is a change in the molecular configuration of the molecule. This may be what triggers the activation of small amounts of the factor.) Together with activated factor XII and high molecular weight kininogen (HMWK), prekallikrein is converted into kallikrein and factor XII is further activated. This is thought to be the major pathway for the activation of factor XII. Activated factor XII (XIIa) with HMWK then brings about the activation of factor XI. Factor IX is activated by the enzymatic action of XIa and calcium ions to form IXa. Factor IXa then forms a complex with factor VIII, phospholipid (from platelets), and calcium ions to convert factor X to factor Xa. In the extrinsic system, factor VII together with tissue thromboplastin and calcium ions will also convert factor X to Xa. (This complex is also capable of activating factor IX to IXa.) (It is thought that part or all of factor VII circulates in the blood in the activated form but is unable to activate factor X without tissue factor.)

The conversion of prothrombin to thrombin can occur by way of either the intrinsic or the extrinsic system by the complex formed between factor Xa, factor V, platelet phospholipid, and calcium ions. This begins the *common pathway.* The conversion of prothrombin to thrombin is complex and is accomplished in several steps. One simplified aspect of this reaction shows prethrombin 2 being formed along with fragment 1·2 in the first step. Prethrombin 2 is then converted to thrombin. In turn, the thrombin formed acts on fragment 1·2 to form fragment 1 which will compete with prothrombin for the Xa complex and, therefore, have a slight inhibitory effect on the prothrombin to thrombin conversion.

Fibrin formation occurs by the action of thrombin on fibrinogen. The fibrinogen molecule consists of three polypeptide chains. Thrombin splits off two small peptides on each side of the fibrinogen molecule (Fig. 148). Fibrinopeptide A is released from the alpha chain first, by the action of thrombin. Next, fibrinopeptide B is released from the beta chain (by the action of thrombin) to produce the fibrin monomer. These fibrin monomers then polymerize end to end and laterally to form a fibrin polymer which is soluble in 5 M urea. (Fibrinopeptides A and B are negatively charged and must be removed from the fibrinogen molecule for polymerization to take place; otherwise, the molecules would repel each other. Once fibrinopeptide A is removed, the molecule is able to polymerize end to end. When fibrinopeptide B is removed, the molecules are able to join laterally.) Factor XIII, activated by thrombin and calcium ions, converts the fibrin polymer to an insoluble fibrin clot by changing the hydrogen bonds to covalent bonds. The resulting fibrin is insoluble in 5 M urea.

It should be noted that the extrinsic and intrinsic systems as described are separated only for the purpose of evaluation. In vivo, both the extrinsic and intrinsic

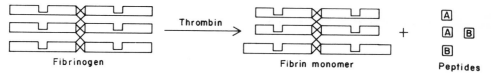

Fig. 148. Action of thrombin on fibrinogen.

mechanisms are involved in activating factor X. The conversion of prothrombin to thrombin is the major event in the coagulation mechanism. In the extrinsic system, only 10 to 20 seconds are required for clotting. A period of 2 to 3 minutes is needed for the formation of thrombin in the intrinsic system.

The Coagulation Factors

The coagulation factors may be divided into three groups based on their properties. The *fibrinogen (thrombin sensitive) group* consists of factors I, V, VIII, and XIII. They are consumed during the process of coagulation and are, therefore, absent in serum and present in plasma. These factors are not adsorbed out by barium sulfate. Factors V and VIII are susceptible to denaturation and are reduced in quantity in stored plasma. Vitamin K is not necessary for the synthesis of these factors. There is an increased concentration of the factors in this group during an inflammatory response and in pregnancy. The *prothrombin (vitamin K dependent) group* includes factors II, VII, IX, and X. Vitamin K is necesssary for their synthesis in the liver. Coumarin drugs, which inhibit vitamin K, cause a decrease in these factors. Factors VII, IX, and X are not consumed during the coagulation process and are, therefore, present in serum as well as plasma. All four factors are adsorbed out of plasma by barium sulfate. They are stable and are well preserved in stored plasma. The *contact group* is composed of factors XI, XII, prekallikrein, and high molecular weight kininogen. These factors are not consumed during coagulation, do not depend on vitamin K for their synthesis, and are not adsorbed out of the plasma by barium sulfate. They are relatively stable. Prekallikrein and HMWK also function in the activation of plasminogen (in the fibrinolytic process).

Factor I (fibrinogen) is synthesized in the liver but does not need vitamin K for its production. It is a plasma protein with a molecular weight of 340,000. The normal plasma level is approximately 200 to 400 mg/dL, depending on the procedure used. A minimum of 60 to 100 mg/dL are required for normal coagulation. Fibrinogen has a half-life of 3 to 4 days. It is relatively stable to heat and storage but may be irreversibly precipitated at 56°C. A fraction of fibrinogen, cryofibrinogen, may precipitate at 4°C but goes back into solution upon warming.

Factor II (prothrombin) is synthesized in the liver and needs vitamin K for its maintenance. It is almost entirely consumed in the coagulation process so that little remains in the serum. It is an alpha-2 globulin with a molecular weight of approximately 69,000. Prothrombin is heat stable and has a half-life of about 60 hours. It readily forms thrombin in the presence of the Xa complex (Xa, V, Ca^{++}, phospholipid).

Factor III (tissue thromboplastin) is a high molecular weight lipoprotein found in most of the body tissues, with increased concentrations in the lungs and brain. It is not, however, found in platelets.

Factor IV (calcium), in the ionized state, is necessary for coagulation. The exact mechanism by which calcium acts in the coagulation process is not known. The fact that it is essential for coagulation makes possible the use of anticoagulants, which merely bind up the calcium and, therefore, completely inhibit coagulation. It is un-

gen is not completely understood. It depends upon the activation of factor XII, and kallikrein is thought to be able to directly activate plasminogen.

c. Therapeutic activation of plasminogen is currently accomplished by the administration of urokinase or streptokinase.

FIBRINOLYTIC PROCESS

In vivo, when a clot forms, 20 to 30% of the circulating plasminogen is trapped in the blood clot. Plasminogen activators adsorb onto and diffuse into the clot and activate the plasminogen to plasmin. The fibrin clot is then broken down by the plasmin in a stepwise fashion. The fibrin is initially broken down into one large fragment (fragment X) and several smaller peptides (fragments A, B, and C). (When streptokinase or urokinase are administered therapeutically, fibrinogen is broken down in the same manner; Fig. 150.) Further action by plasmin breaks fragment X into fragment Y and fragment D. Fragment

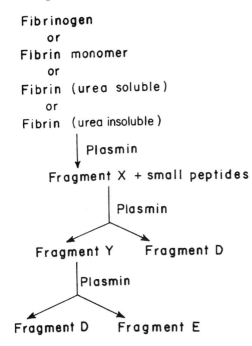

Fig. 150. Degradation of fibrinogen and fibrin by plasmin.

Y is further degraded to fragment E and a second fragment D. Fragments D and E are relatively resistant to further breakdown by plasmin.

Fibrin degradation products are removed from the blood by the liver, kidney, and reticuloendothelial system and have half-lives of about 9 hours. Fragments X and Y and fibrin monomers may form soluble complexes *(soluble fibrin monomer complexes)* which will form precipitates and gels in vitro in the presence of protamine sulfate and alcohol. This has been termed *paracoagulation* and is the basis for certain coagulation tests.

There is much evidence that both the coagulation and fibrinolytic systems are in equilibrium. As a general rule, fibrinolysis increases whenever coagulation increases.

Limiting Mechanisms of Coagulation and Fibrinolysis

Under normal physiologic conditions, coagulation does not occur. When injury does occur, it is imperative that blood coagulation remain localized at the site of injury. The fact that blood is flowing through the circulation has a limiting effect on the development of blood clots. In the area of injury, the flowing blood will move any coagulants present away from the site of injury. These coagulants will be diluted in the blood and can be inactivated by inhibitors present in the plasma or removed from the circulation by the liver. When injury occurs, the platelets localize at the site. The coagulation factors tend to adsorb onto the platelet surface. As fibrin forms, it tends to encapsulate the clot, thus restricting the coagulants to the inside of the clot. As soon as the coagulation process is begun, fibrinolysis is initiated to ultimately break down the clot which is formed. As in coagulation, there are specific inhibitors present in the fibrinolytic system as a means of also limiting this mechanism.

INHIBITORS OF COAGULATION

1. Small amounts of thrombin will ac-

tivate factors V and VIII:C. However, larger concentrations of thrombin will degrade these two factors. During the coagulation process, large amounts of thrombin can be adsorbed onto the fibrin which has formed, neutralizing thrombin and making it unavailable for the fibrinogen to fibrin conversion.

2. *Protein C* is a glycoprotein, produced in the liver, and present in both serum and plasma. When thrombin is complexed with *thrombomodulin* (an endothelial cofactor) it will activate protein C which, in turn, inactivates factors V and VIII:C and inhibits prothrombin activation.

3. *Protein S* is produced in the liver and is present in the serum. It is thought to be a cofactor in speeding up the activity of activated protein C.

4. *Fragment 1,* formed in the conversion of prothrombin to thrombin, has a slight inhibitory effect on this reaction.

5. Originally, there were six antithrombins described and designated with Roman numerals. Of these, only *antithrombin III* is currently considered to have physiologic significance. Antithrombin III is an alpha-2 glycoprotein which is produced in the liver. When thrombin is present, it attaches to the thrombin, forming a complex, and progressively inactivates the thrombin. Heparin, when present, also forms a complex with antithrombin III and increases its inhibitory characteristics. In this way, the anticoagulant action of heparin in normal blood is brought about by activation of antithrombin III. Heparin serves as the catalyst, increasing the rate of thrombin neutralization by antithrombin III. Decreased amounts of antithrombin III present in the blood will cause a failure to respond to heparin therapy and will also cause hypercoagulation of the blood.

Antithrombin III also inactivates factor Xa and, to a lesser degree, factors IXa, XIa, XIIa, kallikrein, and plasmin.

6. *Alpha-2 macroglobulin* is also considered an antithrombin. It is a glycoprotein whose site of production is unknown. It acts progressively to inhibit thrombin and has a slower action than antithrombin III. It is an antiplasmin and also inactivates kallikrein.

7. *Alpha-1 antitrypsin* is an alpha globulin. It inhibits factor XIa and also inhibits plasmin.

8. *C1-inactivator* is an alpha-2 glycoprotein found in plasma which inhibits factors XIIa and XIa, and also kallikrein.

INHIBITORS OF FIBRINOLYSIS

1. *Alpha-2 antiplasmin* is a single chain glycoprotein which forms a complex with, and inactivates, plasmin.

2. *Alpha-2 macroglobulin* reacts very slowly with plasmin. It is currently thought that alpha-2 macroglobulin inhibits that plasmin formed in excess which does not bind to alpha-2 antiplasmin.

3. Antithrombin III, *C1 esterase,* and *alpha-1 antitrypsin* will also inhibit plasmin. Tissues and platelets also contain inhibitors of plasmin.

Primary Hemostasis

BLOOD VESSELS

The endothelial cell in the blood vessels plays an active role in hemostasis. It manufactures and secretes at least three substances which are used in the formation and localization of the hemostatic process: (1) *Prostacyclin* (generated from arachidonic acid via prostaglandin endoperoxides) prevents platelet aggregation on normal uninjured vascular endothelium. (2) Small amounts of the von Willebrand portion of factor VIII are responsible for causing the platelets to adhere to the vascular endothelium. (3) *Plasminogen activator* is an enzyme which converts plasminogen to plasmin, which, in turn, lyses the fibrin clot.

When injury to a blood vessel first occurs, the blood vessels contract, thus limiting the blood flow through the injured area. *Thromboxane A₂* is a vasoconstrictor and most probably assists in this process. It is released from the platelets during the process of platelet adhesion and aggregation.

PLATELETS

Platelets play a central role in primary hemostasis. They contain and release, among other substances, ADP, ATP, platelet factor 4, von Willebrand factor, fibrinogen, factor V, factor Xa, fibronectin, β-thromboglobulin, platelet-derived growth factor, serotonin, calcium, and phosphates. Prostaglandins and thromboxanes are both involved in the platelet response. When arachidonic acid is released from the cellular membranes, it is acted upon by cyclooxygenase from the platelets, with the resultant formation of prostaglandins and thromboxanes. Thromboxane A_2 causes platelet aggregation, stimulates the platelet release reaction, and is a vasoconstrictor. Prostaglandins, however, are strong inhibitors of platelet aggregation and help to limit deposition of the platelet mass. There is a balance between the production of prostaglandins by the tissues and thromboxanes by the platelets. A number of receptor sites have been identified on the platelet membrane for such substances as ADP, epinephrine, collagen, thrombin, fibrinogen, serotonin, factor V, factor Xa, and von Willebrand factor.

Upon injury to the endothelium, the platelets come in contact with the injured tissue. (1) They change from a disk-like shape to a spheroid with the extrusion of many pseudopods. (2) They adhere to the exposed collagen, basement membrane,

and microfibrils. The von Willebrand factor from the endothelial cells and plasma is involved in the adhesion of the platelets to the damaged tissues. Specific binding sites for the von Willebrand factor have been detected on the platelet surface. Thrombin also stimulates adhesion of platelets to the endothelial tissues. This property of the platelets to adhere to the endothelial tissues is termed *platelet adhesiveness.* (3) Following platelet adhesion, the platelets release the contents of the alpha granules, lysosomes, and dense bodies. For this reaction, the microtubules of the platelet fuse with the platelet granules (dense bodies, lysosomes, alpha granules), enabling the contents of the granules to be secreted to the outside *(exocytosis)* through openings in the membrane. (4) As a result of ADP and other substances secreted by the platelet, and in the presence of calcium ions, *platelet aggregation* takes place (the platelets attach to one another). Initial, primary platelet aggregation is reversible. This is followed by a second wave of aggregation caused by higher concentrations of the aggregating substances (ADP, thromboxane A_2) and is irreversible. (5) During the process of coagulation, which probably takes place on the platelet membranes, the platelet contributes phospholipid for activation of factor X and for conversion of prothrombin to thrombin. (6) Once a clot has formed, the platelets, activated by thrombin and in the presence of calcium, act to cause retraction of the clot. This response is thought to depend on a reaction between ATP and *thrombosthenin,* a contractile protein from the platelet.

COAGULATION SCREENING PROCEDURES

The first, and probably the most important, screening procedure for the detection of bleeding disorders is the clinical history of the patient and his family, and is generally performed by the physician. At this time, if a bleeding disorder is suspected, a clue as to the type of disorder may be determined. An abnormality of primary hemostasis may present with easy bruisability and/or bleeding of the mucous membranes. Patients with factor deficiencies generally exhibit bleeding from the larger blood vessels. A family history of bleeding disorders may be helpful in the diagnosis of a hereditary abnormality. There are numerous drugs which may induce bleeding. Aspirin affects the function of platelets and there are, today, over 500 drug preparations which contain aspirin. Also, chlorpromazine hydrochloride, procainamide, and penicillin have been found to adversely affect blood coagulation.

The screening procedures most often performed in the laboratory are an examination of the blood smear, platelet count, bleeding time, prothrombin time (PT), activated partial thromboplastin time (APTT), and a quantitative test for functional fibrinogen (quantitative fibrinogen or thrombin time). Examination of the peripheral blood smear allows for review of platelet morphology (the presence of giant platelets, lack of granules in the platelets, platelet satellitosis, clumping of platelets), and the detection of schistocytes or target cells. The blood smear should also be used as a verification of the whole blood platelet count. The bleeding time is the best procedure available for evaluating primary hemostasis but should probably not be carried out on patients with a platelet count of less than 50,000/μL. The PT evaluates the extrinsic system of coagulation, while the APTT measures the intrinsic system. The APTT is generally sensitive to factor deficiencies of less than 30% activity. In this procedure, the type of activator and source of phospholipid greatly influence the sensitivity of the test. Either one or both of these tests are generally prolonged in the presence of a circulating anticoagulant. The quantitative fibrinogen or thrombin time tests for functional fibrinogen and the conversion of fibrinogen to fibrin. This test may also be abnormal in the presence of a circulating anticoagulant.

If a factor deficiency is suspected, it is very important that the test for circulating anticoagulants be performed first in order to rule out the presence of an inhibitor. If this test is negative, the APTT (or PT) substitution test may then be performed to identify the exact factor deficiency. A factor assay may be done to determine the activity of the deficient factor.

The presence of fibrin(ogen) degradation products may be detected by use of this test. Circulating fibrin monomer-fibrinogen complexes may be detected using the ethanol gel and protamine sulfate procedures. Functional platelet abnormalities may be further studied using platelet aggregation procedures.

In monitoring oral anticoagulant therapy the prothrombin time is generally employed. Heparin therapy is usually followed by use of the activated partial thromboplastin time.

REQUIREMENTS FOR ACCURATE COAGULATION TESTS

To obtain consistently accurate results in coagulation studies, certain procedures should be adhered to.

Collection of the Specimen

1. The anticoagulant of choice for coagulation studies is 0.109 M sodium citrate (buffered or nonbuffered). The usual ratio of blood to anticoagulant is 9 parts blood to 1 part sodium citrate. It is critical that the proper amount of blood ($\pm 10\%$) be added to the anticoagulant.

2. Patient blood that has a high hematocrit will contain less plasma. As a result, when the blood has been centrifuged, the plasma fraction will contain an increased concentration of anticoagulant (sodium citrate), leading to prolonged clotting time results in patients with hematocrits of

55% or higher. (During testing, as calcium is added to the test plasma, it will combine with the excess anticoagulant present instead of being available for the coagulation process.) Therefore, whenever a patient's hematocrit is greater than 55% or less than 20%, the amount of sodium citrate in the collection tube should be decreased (or increased) according to the hematocrit reading. The following formula may be followed for determining the proper amount of sodium citrate to use (when the final volume in the tube is 5.0 mL, and 0.5 mL of 0.109 M sodium citrate is normally used).

$$\text{Amount of sodium citrate} = \frac{\text{Pt. plasma volume } (100 - \text{Hct.}) \times 0.5}{\text{Normal plasma vol. (60)}}$$

For example, when a patient has a hematocrit of 60%, 0.33 mL of 0.109 M sodium citrate should be placed in the tube and blood added to give a final volume of 5.0 mL.

3. A clean venipuncture is absolutely necessary. If there is any contamination of the blood with tissue thromboplastin, false results will occur. For routine coagulation procedures, the Vacutainer blood collection system is adequate. When this system is used, the coagulation tube should be the second or third tube filled. When obtaining a blood specimen for nonroutine, special coagulation procedures, a two-syringe technique may be applied. Using two plastic syringes, withdraw approximately 2 mL of blood into the first syringe. Quickly and carefully disconnect this syringe from the needle (leaving the needle in the patient's vein) and connect the second syringe to the needle. Proceed with the venipuncture, discarding the blood in the first syringe. (Prior to performing the two-syringe venipuncture, make certain the first syringe is easily removed from the needle but fits snugly enough so that the blood will not leak out at the connection.) When testing for 'contact' abnormalities (factors XI and XII and platelet function studies), plastic syringes should be used.

Preparation of the Plasma Sample

1. Before centrifuging the blood specimen, check each tube with applicator sticks (two) for the presence of clots. Because the tubes should be centrifuged with their tops on, an alternative method is to check the cell layer for clots after the plasma has been removed.

2. Unless otherwise noted, coagulation testing should be completed within 4 hours of obtaining the specimen from the patient. The specimen should be centrifuged within 1 hour of collection. The plasma should be removed from the tube using a plastic pipet or one with a nonwettable surface. Once the plasma is removed from the cells, it should be placed in a stoppered test tube having a nonwettable surface. Exposure of the plasma to air results in a pH change of plasma, which may result in invalidly prolonged clotting times.

3. To preserve the labile factors, the blood specimen should be placed on ice immediately after it is withdrawn from the patient. One inexpensive, commercially available ice bath for use in the laboratory is the Kryorack (Streck Laboratories, Inc., Omaha, Nebraska), which contains an aqueous solution within a sealed unit (see Fig. 151) (available in various sizes). This unit, when placed at freezer temperatures ($-18°C$) for 8 hours, maintains a temperature of less than 8°C for 8 hours at room temperature. The tubes do not come in

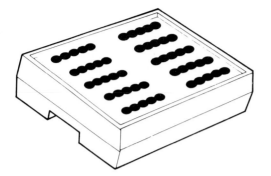

Fig. 151.   Kryorack ice bath.

contact with water or ice, affording a more convenient method of refrigerating plasma than the conventional cup or tray of crushed ice.

4. Hemolyzed plasma should not be used for coagulation studies. It tends to give shortened clotting times. Also, lipemic or icteric plasma samples should, in general, not be tested on instruments designed to detect clots by optical density methods.

Performance of Coagulation Tests

1. As a general rule, all coagulation tests should be performed as soon as possible after the patient specimen has been received in the laboratory.
2. Pipets used for coagulation studies should have a large bore, permitting complete and rapid pipetting. Automatic pipets, of which numerous different types are available, are recommended.
3. Most coagulation studies are carried out at 37°C. It should be noted that specimens incubated in dry heat take slightly longer to reach 37°C than those incubated in a water bath. It is essential, when required, that the specimens and reagents reach the proper temperature of 37°C before proceeding with the test. Overheating or prolonged heating at 37°C, however, may lead to destruction of some of the coagulation factors and,

therefore, a prolonged clotting time. The temperature of the incubator should not fluctuate more than ±0.5°C.

4. Timing of the tests is extremely important. Many of the procedures are timed to within one tenth of a second, so that the initial starting and stopping of the stopwatch must be done precisely.
5. The majority of coagulation procedures use control plasmas, which are generally purchased in the dried form. When the control plasma is reconstituted with distilled water, it should be allowed to sit for approximately 30 minutes (or according to the manufacturer's directions) and then be gently rotated for adequate mixing. The control plasma should never be shaken vigorously. Generally, a normal and abnormal control should be performed at a minimum of once every 20 samples.
6. There are four general techniques in widespread use for reading the end point of most coagulation procedures. The tilt tube method requires gentle tilting of the tube back and forth at the rate of about once per second until a fibrin web is formed. The Nichrome wire loop technique employs the use of a wire loop which is passed through the mixture at the rate of two sweeps per second until a formed clot adheres to the loop. (In these first two techniques, a light source without glare is important. A black background also facilitates the end point readings.) The third and fourth procedures employ the use of automation. In these methods, a clot is detected either by use of a moving probe immersed in the mixture which is triggered by clot formation or by the change in optical density of the mixture when a clot forms.

BLEEDING TIME

The bleeding time is used primarily as a screening test for platelet function since the intrinsic and extrinsic coagulation mechanisms play only a minor role in this test. The number of platelets present (platelet count) and their ability to form a platelet plug directly affect the bleeding time. Prolonged bleeding times are generally found when the platelet count is below 50,000/μL, and where there is platelet dysfunction. The bleeding time may also be affected by the thickness and vascularity of the skin and may be slightly prolonged in diseases which affect the ability of the blood vessels to constrict and retract. The original bleeding time utilized the Duke method and is included here for historic purposes only. This test is difficult to standardize and does not give as reliable results as the Ivy method, or the more widely used template procedures (Mielke or Simplate). Normally, aspirin prolongs the bleeding time by as much as a few minutes except in patient's with von Willebrand's disease where the effect is much more marked.

Duke Method

The earlobe is cleansed with an alcohol sponge and allowed to dry. A standardized puncture of the earlobe is then made, using a sterile blood lancet. The stopwatch is started at the moment of the puncture. Using circular filter paper, the blood is blotted every 30 seconds (without allowing the filter paper to touch the wound). When bleeding ceases, the stopwatch is halted and the bleeding time recorded. The normal bleeding time by this method is 1 to 3 minutes and borderline is 3 to 6 minutes. An alternative procedure uses a glass slide held behind the earlobe for support, or the tip of the third or fourth finger, as the puncture site.

Ivy Method

REFERENCE
Ivy, A.C., Nelson, D., and Beecher, G.: The standardization of certain factors in the cutaneous "venostasis" bleeding time technique, J. Lab. Clin. Med., 26, 1812, 1940.

REAGENTS AND EQUIPMENT
1. Blood pressure cuff.
2. Sterile, disposable blood lancet, capable of making a wound 1 mm wide and 3 mm deep.
3. Stopwatch.
4. Circular test paper.
5. Alcohol prep pads.

PRINCIPLE
A blood pressure cuff is placed on the patient's arm above the elbow, inflated, and maintained at a constant pressure throughout the procedure. Two standardized punctures of the forearm are made, and the length of time required for bleeding to stop is recorded.

PROCEDURE
1. Place a blood pressure cuff on the patient's arm above the elbow. Increase the pressure to 40 mm Hg and hold this exact pressure for the entire procedure.
2. Cleanse an area on the volar surface of the forearm with an alcohol sponge and allow to dry.
3. Choose an area approximately three finger widths below the bend in the elbow. Hold the skin tightly by grasping the underside of the arm firmly. Make two skin punctures, 3 mm deep, avoiding any subcutaneous veins. Start the stopwatch.
4. Blot the blood from each puncture site on a piece of circular filter paper every 30 seconds. The filter paper should not touch the wound at any time.
5. When bleeding ceases, stop the watch and release the blood pressure cuff.
6. Record the bleeding times of the two puncture sites and report the average of the two results. The normal bleeding time is in the range of 1 to 7 minutes, with bleeding times of 7 to 11 minutes considered borderline.

DISCUSSION

1. If bleeding continues for more than 15 minutes, the procedure should be discontinued and pressure applied to the wound sites. The bleeding time should be repeated on the other arm. If bleeding has again not stopped within 15 minutes, the results are reported as greater than 15 minutes.

2. The greatest source of variation in this test is largely due to difficulty in performing a standardized puncture. This usually leads to erroneously low results. On the other hand, if a small vein is punctured, the bleeding time will be prolonged. Therefore, if the bleeding time is less than 1 minute or greater than 7 minutes, the procedure should be repeated using the other arm.

Mielke Method

A modification of the Ivy bleeding time has been described by Mielke and associates (Mielke, C.H., Kaneshiro, I.A., Maher, J.M., Weiner, J.M., and Rapaport, S.I.: The standardized normal Ivy bleeding time and its prolongation by aspirin, Blood, *34*, 204, 1969). In this procedure, a Bard-Parker or similar disposable blade is employed, along with a rectangular polystyrene or plastic template which contains a standardized slit. The blade is placed in a special handle containing a gauge to standardize the depth of the incision. The slit in the template will standardize the length of the incision. The same procedure that was described for the Ivy bleeding time is employed, utilizing the blood pressure cuff inflated to 40 mm Hg. Two incisions, 9 mm long and 1 mm deep, are made. The average of the two bleeding times is reported. Normal values for this procedure are generally 2.5 to 10 minutes. It should be noted, however, that small scars may be caused by this method.

Simplate Method

The bleeding time, utilizing the Simplate bleeding time device (manufactured by Organon Teknika Corp.), is a modification of the Ivy procedure and gives results similar to those obtained in the Mielke test. The Simplate contains a spring-loaded blade within a white plastic case. When the tear away tab (Fig. 152) is removed and the trigger depressed, the edge of the blade (5 mm in length) will spring 1 mm forward out from the housing. The incision made is 5 mm long and 1 mm deep. A Simplate bleeding time device is also available in the form of two blades in one housing (for duplicate testing).

REFERENCES

Organon Teknika Corp.: Simplate bleeding time device., pkg. insert, Durham, N.C., Organon Teknika Corp., 1985.
Sirridge, M.S., and Shannon, R.: *Laboratory Evaluation of Hemostasis and Thrombosis*, 3rd Ed., Philadelphia, Lea & Febiger, 1983.

REAGENTS AND EQUIPMENT

1. Blood pressure cuff.
2. Simplate bleeding time device.
3. Stopwatch.
4. Circular filter paper.
5. Alcohol prep pads.
6. Butterfly bandage.

PRINCIPLE

A blood pressure cuff is placed on the patient's arm above the elbow, inflated, and maintained at a constant pressure throughout the procedure. A uniform incision, 5 mm long and 1 mm deep, is made

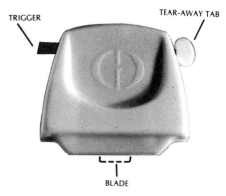

TRIGGER

TEAR-AWAY TAB

BLADE

Fig. 152.   Simplate bleeding time device.

on the forearm, and the length of time required for bleeding to stop is recorded.

PROCEDURE

1. Place a blood pressure cuff on the patient's arm above the elbow. Increase the pressure to 40 mm Hg and hold this exact pressure for the entire procedure.
2. Locate the area for the bleeding time: The patient's arm should be extended, palm down. Beginning at the middle finger move up the arm in a straight line to 5 cm below the fold of the elbow. This area, in the muscular portion of the volar surface of the forearm, 5 cm below the fold in the elbow, is the standardized test site for the puncture.
3. Shave the area if excessive hair is present. Cleanse the site with an alcohol sponge and allow to dry.
4. Remove the tear away tab on the Simplate and place it firmly on the puncture area, either perpendicular or parallel to the fold of the elbow. (Make certain the area is free of scars, surface veins, and bruises.)
5. Depress the trigger and start the stopwatch. Remove the device approximately 1 second after making the incision. (The incision should be made within 30 to 60 seconds after the blood pressure cuff has been inflated to 40 mm Hg.)
6. Blot the blood from the puncture site on a clean section of circular filter paper every 30 seconds. The filter paper should not touch the wound at any time.
7. When bleeding ceases, stop the watch and release the blood pressure cuff. Record the results. The normal range for this procedure is 2.3 to 9.5 minutes.
8. Place a butterfly bandage over the puncture site, and advise the patient to keep the bandage in place for 24 hours.

DISCUSSION

1. Some patients may receive slight scarring at the incision site and should be so informed prior to performing this procedure.
2. The aspirin tolerance test may be used to help distinguish functionally abnormal platelets from normal platelets. In this procedure, bleeding times are performed before and after the ingestion of aspirin. Normally the bleeding time after aspirin ingestion is slightly longer. In von Willebrand's disease, however, the bleeding time after aspirin ingestion will be more markedly prolonged.
3. When performing a bleeding time on infants the blood pressure cuff may be maintained at 30 mm Hg for infants weighing over 5 pounds and for all small children.
4. The incision must be made consistently in the same direction, either parallel or perpendicular to the elbow. Horizontal incisions may give longer bleeding times so vertical incisions may be desired for routine screening purposes.

COAGULATION TIME OF WHOLE BLOOD

In the past, the Lee and White clotting time was used as a screening test to measure all stages in the intrinsic coagulation system and to monitor heparin therapy. It is, however, a time-consuming test, has poor reproducibility, is sensitive to only severe factor deficiencies, and is insensitive to high doses of heparin. It is, therefore, of limited use in today's laboratory. In the coagulation of blood in this procedure, most of the time is consumed in the production of the prothrombin activator (plasma thromboplastin). It requires only a matter of seconds to convert prothrombin to thrombin and fibrinogen to fibrin. Therefore, moderate deficiencies in stages 2 and 3 of the coagulation process do not significantly prolong the clotting time.

The coagulation time is influenced mainly by defects in stage 1 of the clotting process. Severe hemophilia, afibrinogenemia, and severe fibrinolytic states cause a prolonged clotting time, as does circulating anticoagulants (inhibitors), and heparin.

There are a number of modifications of the in vitro test for the coagulation time of whole blood. The use of an activator, the size of the tubes, amount of blood used, and the temperature at which the determination is performed are the main variables between the different modifications employed.

The normal values for the test described below are generally about 5 to 15 minutes, however, each laboratory should determine its own normal range.

Lee and White Method

REFERENCE

Lee, R.I., and White, P.D.: A clinical study of the coagulation time of whole blood, Am. J. Med. Sci., *145*, 495, 1913.

REAGENTS AND EQUIPMENT

1. Water bath, 37°C.
2. Glass test tubes, 13 × 100 mm.
3. Stopwatch.
4. Plastic syringe (10 mL) and 20-gauge needle.

SPECIMEN

Fresh whole blood, 4 mL.

PRINCIPLE

The coagulation time of whole blood is the length of time required for a measured amount of blood to clot under certain specified conditions.

PROCEDURE

1. Label three 13 × 100 mm test tubes with the patient's name, and number them, #1, #2, and #3.
2. Perform a clean, untraumatic venipuncture using a 20-gauge needle and withdraw 4 mL of blood.
3. After obtaining 4 mL of blood from the patient, remove the needle from the syringe, and carefully place 1 mL of the blood in test tube #3, then 1 mL in tube #2, and lastly, 1 mL in tube #1. The last 1 mL of blood may be discarded. Start the stopwatch as soon as the blood is placed in tube #3.
4. Place the three test tubes in a 37°C water bath.
5. At exactly 5 minutes, tilt test tube #1 gently to a 45° angle. Repeat this procedure every 30 seconds, until the test tube can be completely inverted without spilling the contents (that is, until the blood is completely clotted).
6. Record the time it took the blood in test tube #1 to clot.
7. Thirty seconds after the blood in test tube #1 is clotted, proceed with tube #2, and repeat the preceding procedure, tilting the test tube every 30 seconds, until a clot is formed. Record the results. Repeat this procedure for test tube #3.
8. Since agitation and handling speed up coagulation, the coagulation time of test tube #3 is the reported result.

DISCUSSION

1. Whole blood clotting times using an activator, as briefly described below, are faster, much less affected by external factors, are more sensitive to factor deficiencies, and may also be used for monitoring heparin therapy.
   a. The ground glass clotting time is performed by adding ground glass to cover the bottom of the tubes. After the addition of 1 mL of blood to each of the three tubes they are incubated at 37°C and rapidly inverted in sequence until the blood in all three tubes is clotted. Normally, the blood clots within 140 seconds.
   b. The activated clotting time uses 2 mL of whole blood drawn into a

gray stoppered B-D Vacutainer tube containing diatomaceous earth. (At least 1 mL of blood should be drawn and discarded, or used for other tests, prior to drawing blood for this test.) The procedure is carried out at 37°C and the tube tilted after the first 1 minute, and, thereafter at 5-second intervals until the clot forms. Using this procedure a clot will normally form in less than 101 seconds.

2. Poor venipuncture technique, causing hemolysis or tissue thromboplastin to mix with the blood, shortens the clotting time.

3. Incubation at 37°C is important if the normal values for the test have been determined using this technique. Temperatures lower than 37°C retard the clotting time.

4. Bubbles entering the syringe when the blood sample is being obtained increase the rate of coagulation. Unnecessary agitation of the blood shortens the coagulation time.

5. At the completion of the Lee and White clotting time, it is suggested that 1 test tube remain in the 37°C water bath to be checked after 2 and 4 hours for clot retraction. Also, the same tube may be allowed to remain in the water bath overnight and checked the next day for clot lysis.

PROTHROMBIN TIME

The prothrombin time (PT) is a useful screening procedure for deficiencies in factors II, V, VII, and X. Also, the PT will generally be prolonged when the fibrinogen concentration is less than 80 mg/dL and in cases of dysfibrinogenemia. As a general rule, only a 30% concentration of factors V, VII, and X are needed for a normal PT. This test is least sensitive to deficiencies in factor II. The PT is frequently used to follow the course of anticoagulant therapy in patients receiving coumarin drugs. Factors II, VII, IX, and X are inhibited by the coumarin drugs, with factor VII showing decreased activity first. Common causes of a prolonged prothrombin time are vitamin K deficiency, certain liver diseases, specific coagulation deficiencies, disseminated intravascular coagulation, circulating anticoagulants, presence of fibrin(ogen) split products, in some dysproteinemias, and in coumarin drug therapy. The normal prothrombin time is generally 10 to 12 seconds. These values, however, differ according to the method and reagents used in the performance of the test. Therefore, each laboratory should determine its normal range.

REFERENCE

Quick, A.J.: *Bleeding Problems in Clinical Medicine,* Philadelphia, W. B. Saunders Co., 1970.

REAGENTS AND EQUIPMENT

1. Water bath, 37°C.
2. Thromboplastin-calcium chloride reagent. Keep refrigerated when not in use.
3. Normal and abnormal plasma controls.
4. Test tubes, 13 × 100 mm.
5. Stopwatch.
6. Ice bath.

SPECIMEN

Citrated plasma: 1 part 0.109 M sodium citrate to 9 parts whole blood. Testing should be performed within 2 hours after specimen is drawn when the plasma is maintained at room temperature, within 6 to 8 hours when refrigerated, and within 2 to 5 days when the plasma is stored at −20°C.

PRINCIPLE

The calcium in whole blood is bound by sodium citrate, thus preventing coagulation. Tissue thromboplastin, to which calcium has been added, is mixed with the plasma, and the clotting time is noted.

PROCEDURE

1. Centrifuge anticoagulated blood at 1200 to 1500 g for 15 minutes as soon as possible after blood collection.
2. Remove the plasma from the cells immediately and place on ice.
3. Pipet 0.2 mL of thromboplastin-calcium reagent into the appropriate number of 13 × 100 mm test tubes. Warm the test tubes in the water bath for at least 1 minute, until they have reached 37°C. The incubation period for this mixture is not critical once it reaches 37°C.
4. Incubate the plasma for approximately 2 to 3 minutes, until it reaches 37°C. Plasma should be incubated for no longer than 5 minutes after reaching 37°C.
5. Forcibly pipet 0.1 mL of patient's plasma into the test tube containing 0.2 mL of thromboplastin-calcium mixture and simultaneously start the stopwatch.
6. Mix the contents of the tube, remove the tube from the water bath, and wipe dry. Gently tilt the tube back and forth until a clot forms, at which point the timing is stopped.
7. Each test and control plasma should be performed in duplicate. The results should agree with each other within ± 0.5 seconds when the prothrombin time is below 30 seconds. Duplicate tests on a prothrombin time above 30 seconds should agree within 2 to 4 seconds depending on how elevated the clotting time is.
8. Average the two results and report the patient's results along with the normal range for the test as performed in your laboratory.

DISCUSSION

1. The prothrombin time may also be performed by a semiautomated method using the fibrometer or by a more completely automated method employing optical density readings.
2. A control plasma should be run with each group of tests performed. A normal and an abnormal plasma control should be run each time a new lot number of thromboplastin-calcium mixture is opened and at least once per day. The abnormal control should be in the range of about 25 seconds (20 to 30 seconds) or in the same range as the majority of patients on oral anticoagulant therapy.
3. When reconstituting the thromboplastin-calcium reagent, mix well. Excessive shaking does not affect this mixture.
4. Some thromboplastin-calcium reagents are a suspension and not a homogeneous solution, so it is imperative that the suspension be well mixed whenever used.
5. Patients receiving coumarin drugs for thromboembolic disorders generally have prothrombin times of 20 to 30 seconds, or 1.5 to 2.5 times their normal prothrombin time.
6. Normal plasma control values must fall within the laboratory's normal range. If the control results fall outside of this range, there is something wrong with the equipment, reagents, or techniques used, and the test must be repeated.
7. If the patient is receiving heparin, the prothrombin must be drawn at least 6 hours after the last injection, or the results obtained for the prothrombin time may be affected by the heparin.

ACTIVATED PARTIAL THROMBOPLASTIN TIME

The activated partial thromboplastin time (APTT) is the single most useful procedure for routine screening of coagulation disorders in the intrinsic system. It measures those coagulation factors present in the intrinsic system except for platelets and factor XIII. (Factor VII is not measured because it is in the extrinsic system.) The APTT is also the method of choice for monitoring heparin therapy. The normal range for the APTT may vary widely from one laboratory to another and is dependent on the reagents used and the clot detection method employed. It is, therefore, important that each laboratory determine its own normal range for the specific lot number, instrumentation, and the type of reagents used. Generally speaking the normal mean value for the APTT will usually fall between 25 and 35 seconds.

REFERENCE

Proctor, R.R., and Rapaport, S.I.: The partial thromboplastin time with kaolin, Am. J. Clin. Path., *36*, 212, 1961.

REAGENTS AND EQUIPMENT

1. Water bath, 37°C.
2. Calcium chloride, 0.025 M.
3. Partial thromboplastin containing an activator (commercially available).
4. Normal and abnormal control plasmas.
5. Test tubes, 13 × 100 mm.
6. Stopwatch.
7. Ice bath.

SPECIMEN

Citrated plasma: 1 part 0.109 M sodium citrate to 9 parts whole blood. Immediately after collection, place the tube of blood in a cup of crushed ice and deliver to the laboratory.

PRINCIPLE

The calcium in whole blood is bound by the anticoagulant to prevent coagulation. The plasma, after centrifugation, contains all intrinsic coagulation factors except calcium and platelets. Calcium, a phospholipid substitute for platelets (partial thromboplastin), and an activator (to ensure maximal activation), are added to the plasma. The time required for the plasma to clot is the activated partial thromboplastin time.

PROCEDURE

1. Centrifuge the anticoagulated blood at 1200 to 1500 g for 15 minutes as soon as possible after the blood has been collected.
2. Remove the plasma from the cells immediately and place on ice.
3. Incubate a sufficient amount of 0.025 M calcium chloride at 37°C.
4. Pipet 0.2 mL of normal control plasma (or patient's plasma) into a 13 × 100 mm test tube.
5. Pipet 0.2 mL of the partial thromboplastin (containing activator) into the test tube containing the control (or patient's) plasma.
6. Mix the contents of the tube quickly and place in a 37°C water bath for 3 minutes.
7. After exactly 3 minutes, forcibly pipet in 0.2 mL of the prewarmed calcium chloride into the tube, and simultaneously start the stopwatch.
8. Mix the test tube once, immediately after adding the calcium chloride. Allow the test tube to remain in the water bath while gently tilting the tube every 5 seconds. At the end of 20 seconds, remove the test tube from the water bath. Quickly wipe off the outside of the test tube with a clean gauze so that the contents of the tube can be clearly seen.
9. Gently tilt the test tube back and forth until a clot forms, at which point the timing is stopped.
10. Control and patient's plasma specimens should be run in duplicate, and the two results averaged to obtain the final value. The two results should check within ±1.5 seconds of each other when the APTT is less than 45 seconds, within 5 seconds when the results are between 50 and 100 seconds, and within 8 to 10 seconds when the APTT is above 100 seconds. If the formation of the clot has not started by the end of 2 minutes, the test may be stopped and the results reported as greater than 2 minutes.

11. Report the patient's results along with the normal range for the test as determined for your laboratory. (Normal control results must always fall within the normal range, otherwise, something is wrong with reagents, equipment, or the technique being used, and the entire test must be repeated.)

DISCUSSION

1. When the APTT is abnormally prolonged, there may be a deficiency in one of the coagulation factors, or there may be an inhibitor(s) present in the patient's plasma. To differentiate between these two abnormal states, perform, in duplicate, as described previously, an APTT, mixing 0.1 mL of normal control plasma with 0.1 mL of patient's plasma (in place of the usual 0.2 mL of patient's plasma). If the results are closer to the value received for the normal plasma control, the problem is probably due to a deficiency of one of the coagulation factors. (The APTT gives normal results when there is a 50% concentration of the coagulation factors present.) If, however, the results received are closer to the original results (using 0.2 mL of the patient's plasma), the defect is thought to be due to an inhibitor(s) present in the patient's plasma.

2. The partial thromboplastin time (without an activator) is performed in exactly the same manner as the APTT, using partial thromboplastin without an activator. The normal results for the PTT performed in this way are in the range of 40 to 100 seconds, with a result of 120 seconds or longer being considered abnormal. The activator in the APTT allows for maximum activation of the contact factors and gives more consistent and reproducible results.

3. The APTT does not test for factor VII or platelets. It detects deficiencies in factors I, II, V, VIII, IX, X, and is also sensitive to circulating anticoagulants (inhibitors). The test is somewhat insensitive to deficiencies in factors XI and XII, the contact factors.

4. The PTT and APTT are much more sensitive to coagulation factor deficiencies than is the whole blood clotting time.

5. If there are sufficient stopwatches available, it is possible to do more than one test at a time by starting each of the 3 minute incubations at 2-minute intervals.

6. The APTT should be performed within 2 hours of blood collection to avoid invalidly prolonged results. Also, incubation of the plasma at 37°C for more than 5 minutes will cause a decrease in factors V and VIII, and therefore, invalidly prolonged clotting times.

7. An abnormally shortened APTT may be caused by partial clotting of the blood as a result of difficulty in obtaining the blood sample. There may or may not be a clot present in the tube of blood. In circumstances such as this, it is advisable to obtain a new blood sample.

8. A normal plasma control should be run with each group of tests performed. In addition, a normal and an abnormal plasma control should be run each time a new lot # of reagent is opened and at least once per day. The abnormal control should generally be in a range somewhere between 50 and 70 seconds.

PLASMA RECALCIFICATION TIME

(Plasma Clotting Time)

The plasma recalcification time is a measure of the overall intrinsic coagulation process. In the procedure outlined here, a deficiency in platelets or platelet activity is not detected. The normal plasma recalcification time on platelet poor plasma is in the range of 90 to 250 seconds. A decrease in any of the clotting factors present in the intrinsic system will cause a prolonged clotting time.

REFERENCE

Sirridge, M.S., and Shannon, R.: *Laboratory Evaluation of Hemostasis and Thrombosis,* 3rd Ed. Philadelphia, Lea & Febiger, 1983.

REAGENTS AND EQUIPMENT

1. Water bath, 37°C.
2. Calcium chloride, 0.025 M.
3. Test tubes, 13 × 100 mm.
4. Stopwatch.
5. Pipets, 0.2 mL.

SPECIMEN

Citrated plasma: 1 part 0.109 M sodium citrate to 9 parts whole blood. Obtain blood for use as a normal control at the same time the patient's specimen is obtained.

PRINCIPLE

Platelet poor plasma is mixed with sufficient calcium chloride to neutralize the effects of the anticoagulant, and the clotting time is determined.

PROCEDURE

1. Immediately after collection, centrifuge blood at 1500 × g for at least 20 minutes in order to obtain platelet poor plasma.
2. Place a tube of calcium chloride into the 37°C water bath and warm to temperature.
3. Place four 13 × 100 mm test tubes into the 37°C water bath (two tubes for each patient and control).
4. Pipet 0.2 mL of patient's plasma into the first tube. Add 0.2 mL of calcium chloride and simultaneously start a stopwatch. Gently mix the tube.
5. Allow the tube to remain in the 37°C water bath for 90 seconds, gently tilting the test tube every 30 seconds.
6. After 90 seconds, remove the test tube from the water bath and gently tilt at a rate of once per second. Stop the watch as soon as a clot forms, and record the results.
7. Repeat steps 4, 5, and 6 for each patient and control. It is recommended that all testing be performed in duplicate and the results averaged.

DISCUSSION

1. The plasma recalcification time varies according to the number of platelets present in the plasma. As the number of platelets increases, the plasma recalcification time shortens. Therefore, it is important to centrifuge the blood in the prescribed manner.
2. The plasma recalcification time may be performed on platelet rich plasma, in which case the normal range is about 90 to 160 seconds. Using this procedure, remove the tube from the water bath 60 seconds after the calcium chloride has been added. Plasma specimens containing a standard number of platelets, however, are difficult to obtain. This procedure is thought to be quite sensitive to inhibition by the lupus anticoagulant.
3. A modification of the plasma clotting time is called the *activated recalcification time* and employs the use of 0.1 mL of platelet rich plasma, 0.1 mL of 0.025 M calcium chloride, and 0.1 mL of 1% Celite as an activator. The normal clotting time in this procedure is less than 50 seconds.
4. The APTT is more sensitive and reproducible than this test when looking for coagulation factor deficiencies.
5. Testing should be completed within 2 hours of blood collection.

STYPVEN TIME

The Stypven time is capable of detecting deficiencies in prothrombin, fibrinogen, and factors V and X. It, therefore, differs from the prothrombin time in that deficiencies in factor VII are not detected. The normal Stypven time is generally in the range of 6 to 10 seconds when performed by the following procedure. Each laboratory, however, should determine their own normal range.

REFERENCES

Wellcome Research Laboratories, Russell Viper Venom, pkg. insert, Beckenham, England, Wellcome Research Laboratories, 1977.

Triplett, D.A., Harms, C.S.: *Procedures for the Coagulation Laboratory*, Chicago, American Society of Clinical Pathologists, 1981.

REAGENTS AND EQUIPMENT

1. Russell viper venom. (Obtainable from Burroughs Wellcome Co., Research Triangle Park, N. C.) Reconstitute with 2.0 mL of distilled water. Reagent may be used for 1 week after reconstitution if stored in the refrigerator.
2. Platelin. (Obtainable from Organon Teknika Corp., Durham, N. C.) Reconstitute according to directions on vial. Reagent may be used for 1 week after reconstitution if stored in the refrigerator.
3. Calcium chloride, 0.025 M.
4. Water bath, 37°C.
5. Normal control plasma.
6. Test tubes, 12 × 75 mm.
7. Pipets, 0.1 mL.
8. Stopwatch.

SPECIMEN

Citrated plasma: 1 part 0.109 M sodium citrate to 9 parts whole blood. Immediately after blood collection, place the tube of blood in a cup of crushed ice and deliver to the laboratory.

PRINCIPLE

Russell viper venom (Stypven) is a thromboplastin-like substance which activates factor X. When this reagent is added to plasma, along with platelets (Platelin), and calcium chloride, the coagulation process is begun at the point of conversion of prothrombin to thrombin in the coagulation mechanism. Therefore, deficiencies in factors V, X, prothrombin and fibrinogen may be detected.

PROCEDURE

1. Centrifuge specimen at 1200 to 1500 g for 15 minutes as soon as possible after the blood has been collected.
2. Remove the plasma from the cells immediately and place in an ice bath.
3. Combine equal volumes of Platelin and 0.025 calcium chloride in a 12 × 75 mm test tube. Mix gently. (Each test requires 0.2 mL of this mixture.) Incubate mixture at 37°C for a minimum of 5 minutes but for no longer than 30 minutes.
4. Warm the Stypven reagent to 37°C.
5. Incubate the patient's plasma at 37°C for about 3 minutes.
6. Into a 12 × 75 mm test tube in the 37°C water bath, pipet 0.1 mL of patient's plasma and 0.1 mL of Stypven reagent. Mix and allow the tube to incubate for 30 seconds.
7. At the end of 30 seconds, add 0.2 mL of the prewarmed Platelin-calcium chloride mixture to the tube and simultaneously start a stopwatch.
8. Record the clotting time.
9. Each patient and control sample should be tested in the above manner in duplicate.

DISCUSSION

1. If the prothrombin time is normal, the Stypven time need not be performed.
2. In a factor VII deficiency, the prothrombin time would be prolonged and the Stypven time normal.
3. The above procedure as described for the Stypven time may also be used to assay for factors V and X. Make dilutions of the reference, control, and patient's plasma as outlined in

the Factor VII Assay procedure. Perform the Stypven time on each dilution. Draw the reference curve and calculate the control and patient results as outlined for the Factor VII Assay. The Stypven time is sensitive to factors V and X and generally gives reproducible results by this procedure.

REPTILASE TIME

Reptilase is an enzyme found in the venom of the Bothrops atrox snake. It is capable of converting fibrinogen to fibrin and is unaffected by heparin. This test is, therefore, helpful in testing for fibrinogen when a patient is receiving heparin. The normal range for the test outlined below is approximately 10 to 15 seconds, but should be determined for each laboratory.

REFERENCES

Sigma Diagnostics: Atroxin® (Bothrops atrox venom) Determination of Plasma Clotting Time, pkg. insert, St. Louis, Sigma Chemical Co., 1984.

Funk, C., Gmür, J., Herold, R., and Straub, P.W.: Reptilase®-R—A new reagent in blood coagulation, Br. J. Haem., 21, 43, 1971.

REAGENTS AND EQUIPMENT

1. Atroxin® (buffered Bothrops atrox venom). (Available from Sigma Chemical Co.) Reconstitute with 1.0 mL of distilled water. Mix well. Stable in the refrigerator for 1 month after reconstitution.
2. Test tubes, 12 × 75 mm.
3. Pipets, 0.2 mL and 0.1 mL.
4. Water bath, 37°C.
5. Ice bath.
6. Stopwatch.

SPECIMEN

Citrated plasma: 1 part 0.109 M sodium citrate to 9 parts whole blood.

PRINCIPLE

When Atroxin® (Reptilase) is added to plasma, it acts by releasing fibrinopeptides A and AP from the fibrinogen molecule (thrombin splits off fibrinopeptides A, B, and AP). The resultant monomers then polymerize end-to-end, forming a clot. The action of Atroxin® and, therefore, the clotting time, is not affected by heparin.

PROCEDURE

1. Centrifuge specimen at 1200 to 1500 g for 15 minutes.
2. Pipet 0.1 mL of Atroxin® into enough 12 × 75 mm test tubes to perform the test, in duplicate, on all specimens and a normal control. Place tubes in an ice bath.
3. Incubate patient plasma at 37°C for 3 to 5 minutes. Prewarm two tubes containing the Atroxin® at 37°C for 3 minutes.
4. Add 0.2 mL of the prewarmed patient's plasma to the tube containing 0.1 mL of prewarmed Atroxin®. Simultaneously start the stopwatch.
5. Mix the contents of the tube and record the clotting time. Test the duplicate specimens in the same manner.
6. Repeat steps 3, 4, and 5 above for each specimen and control.
7. Average duplicate results and record.

DISCUSSION

1. Patients receiving heparin will generally show a prolonged thrombin time and a normal Reptilase time.
2. Fibrin(ogen) split products in a concentration of 40 µg/mL or higher will interfere with the above test results and give prolonged clotting times using Atroxin®.
3. In cases of a decreased concentration of fibrinogen or dysfibrinogenemia, both the thrombin time and the Reptilase time will be prolonged (when Atroxin® is used). Also, in streptokinase therapy, both test results are abnormally long.
4. Plasma for this test may be stored in the refrigerator for up to 24 hours, or

in the freezer ($-20°C$) for several weeks, without the results being affected.

THROMBIN TIME

The thrombin time tests the third stage of coagulation, the conversion of fibrinogen to fibrin. It measures the availability of functional fibrinogen. The normal thrombin time for this procedure is 15 to 20 seconds. Prolonged times are found when the fibrinogen level is below 100 mg/dL, when the function of fibrinogen is impaired, and in the presence of thrombin inhibitors such as heparin or fibrin degradation products. The thrombin time is a sensitive test in detecting heparin inhibition. It may be normally prolonged in the newborn and in multiple myeloma (the abnormal globulin interferes with the polymerization of fibrin).

REFERENCES

Rapaport, S.I., and Ames, S.B.: Clotting factor assay on plasma from patients receiving intramuscular or subcutaneous heparin, Am. J. Med. Sci., *234*, 678, 1957.
Sirridge, M.S., and Shannon, R.: *Laboratory Evaluation of Hemostasis and Thrombosis*, 3rd Ed., Philadelphia, Lea & Febiger, 1983.

REAGENTS AND EQUIPMENT

1. Barbital buffered saline, pH 7.35.
2. Stock thrombin (100 units/mL). Reconstitute one vial of Bovine Thrombin, Topical, 5,000 NIH units (Parke, Davis & Co.) with 25 mL of barbital buffered saline solution (pH 7.35) and 25 mL of glycerol. Freeze in small aliquots. This mixture, stored at 0°C, is stable for several months.
3. Normal control plasma.
4. Water bath, 37°C.
5. Nichrome wire loop.
6. Stopwatch.
7. Plastic test tubes, 13 × 100 mm.

SPECIMEN

Citrated plasma: 1 part 0.109 M sodium citrate to 9 parts whole blood.

PRINCIPLE

A measured amount of thrombin is added to plasma. The length of time for a fibrin clot to form is recorded as the thrombin time.

PROCEDURE

1. Centrifuge blood at 1500 × g for 10 minutes to obtain platelet poor plasma.
2. Immediately before use, prepare working thrombin solution by diluting 0.1 mL of stock thrombin with 0.9 mL of barbital buffered saline. Incubate at 37°C. (This solution is stable for 20 minutes at 37°C.)
3. Incubate a sufficient amount of barbital buffered saline solution at 37°C (0.4 mL/patient or control).
4. Place 0.2 mL of patient's plasma or normal control into a 13 × 100 mm test tube.
5. Add 0.2 mL of barbital buffered saline solution to the tube, mix, and allow to incubate for 1 minute.
6. At the end of 1 minute, pipet 0.2 mL of working thrombin solution into the tube, simultaneously starting the stopwatch.
7. With a Nichrome wire loop, sweep through the mixture, 2 times per second, until a clot is formed. Stop the watch and record the thrombin time.
8. Run a normal control with each series of thrombin times. Each specimen should be tested in duplicate.

DISCUSSION

1. Duplicate tests performed on the same plasma sample should check within ±1.5 seconds of each other.
2. Whenever thrombin is used, plastic or siliconized pipets should be employed to pipet the thrombin.
3. The concentration of thrombin in the working thrombin solution should be at a concentration which gives a clotting time of 15 to 20 seconds on normal plasma. When the stock throm-

bin solution is first prepared, it may be necessary to use a 1:12 or greater dilution when preparing the working thrombin mixture. As the stock solution ages, the reverse is true, and a dilution of 1:8 or less with barbital buffered saline solution may be required.

4. If the thrombin time is greater than 25 seconds, repeat the procedure, using a 1:1 mixture of the patient's plasma and normal control to test for heparin or other inhibitors. If inhibitors are present, the thrombin time will not be shortened.

QUANTITATIVE FIBRINOGEN

A deficiency in fibrinogen may occur as a result of numerous causes. When it does occur, it may produce severe hemorrhage, and little time should be lost in diagnosing the problem. A lack of fibrinogen may be caused by a congenital defect. Dysfibrinogenemia shows up as a congenital deficiency of clottable fibrinogen. Acquired deficiencies of fibrinogen occur in disseminated intravascular coagulation, systemic fibrinolysis, in pancreatitis, and in some obstetric and surgical cases. A chronic deficiency of fibrinogen may occur in such cases as liver disease, where production may be defective. Elevated fibrinogen levels are normally found in pregnancy, near term or after delivery, and may also be found in patients in a pre-thrombotic or hypercoagulable state as in patients with a thrombosis. Normally, spontaneous bleeding does not occur in patients with fibrinogen levels above 50 mg/dL, but under traumatic conditions such as surgical procedure, a level of 100 mg/dL may be necessary to prevent bleeding.

The normal value for this test is about 150 to 400 mg/dL, but each laboratory should determine its own normal range.

REFERENCE

Organon Teknika Corp., *Fibriquik,* Durham, N.C., Organon Teknika Corp., 1983.

REAGENTS AND EQUIPMENT

1. The following reagents are obtainable from Organon Teknika Corp.:
   a. Thrombin reagent, 100 NIH units/ mL. Available in a 1.0 or 3.0 mL size. Reconstitute with distilled water. Mix gently. Once reconstituted, the thrombin reagent may be stored in the refrigerator for up to 3 days.
   b. Owren's veronal buffer, pH 7.35. Contains sodium barbital (0.028 M). Store in the refrigerator. Discard if the solution becomes cloudy.
   c. Fibrinogen calibration reference plasma, 1.0 mL, for use in preparing the fibrinogen calibration curve. Reconstitute with 1.0 mL of distilled water, allow to stand for 30 minutes, and gently mix. Once reconstituted this reagent may be stored in the refrigerator for up to 24 hours.
2. Pipets, plastic, 0.1, 0.5, 1.0, and 2.0 mL.
3. Test tubes, plastic, 10 × 75 mm.
4. 2 × 2 cycle logarithmic graph paper.
5. Fibrometer. (Manual methods, or any coagulation instrument capable of performing this test, may be used.)
6. Normal and abnormal control plasma.

SPECIMEN

Citrated plasma: 1 part 0.109 M sodium citrate to 9 parts whole blood. It is recommended that plasma be placed on ice and tested within 4 hours of obtaining the specimen.

PRINCIPLE

An excess amount of thrombin is added to a specimen of diluted plasma and the clotting time noted. This result is compared with clotting times of plasmas containing known amounts of fibrinogen. From this information, the amount of fibrinogen in mg/dL in the unknown sample is determined. The clotting time of the plasma in this test is inversely proportional to the concentration of fibrinogen in the specimen.

PROCEDURE

1. Preparation of calibration curve. When this procedure is first set up and each time a different lot # of thrombin is used, a new calibration curve must be run as outlined below.
    a. Reconstitute the fibrinogen calibration standard and thrombin reagent as indicated above.
    b. Label four 10 × 75 mm test tubes # 1 through #4.
    c. Add the appropriate amount of buffer to each tube as indicated in Table 8.
    d. When the calibration standard is ready, add the amount indicated in Table 8 to tube #1. Mix tube well (gently), and transfer 0.5 mL to tube #2 as indicated. Transfer the appropriate mixtures to each tube as indicated in Table 8, being careful to mix each tube well after adding the calibration standard.
    e. Perform the quantitative fibrinogen procedure on each dilution as described below (steps 2 through 8). Each test should be run in duplicate and the results averaged.
    f. Using 2 × 2 cycle logarithmic graph paper draw a fibrinogen curve by plotting the clotting time (in seconds) on the Y (vertical) axis and the fibrinogen concentration in mg/dL (assay value × the dilution factor from Table 8)

on the X (horizontal) axis. Draw a straight line which best fits all 4 data points (Fig. 153).
    g. Check the validity of the above fibrinogen curve by running normal and abnormal fibrinogen controls. Results must check within ± 15% of the assay value of the controls. If they do not, the fibrinogen curve may have to be repeated.

2. Centrifuge the blood specimens at 1200 to 1500 g for 15 minutes to obtain platelet-poor plasma.

3. Remove Owren's veronal buffer from the refrigerator and allow to warm to room temperature.

4. Reconstitute thrombin with the appropriate amount of distilled water. Mix gently and label bottle with the time and date of reconstitution.

5. Make a 1:10 dilution of each plasma specimen and control: place 0.9 mL of Owren's veronal buffer into appropriately labeled 10 × 75 mm test tubes (one tube for each plasma and control specimen). Add 0.1 mL of plasma to each of the appropriately labeled test tubes. Mix carefully.

6. Pipet 0.2 mL of the first plasma dilution to be tested into each of 2 Fibrometer cups. Allow plasma to reach 37°C (3 minutes). Set a clock for 6 minutes. At 30-second intervals, pipet 0.2 mL of diluted plasma into each of two more Fibrometer cups. (All plasmas and controls should be run in duplicate.)

7. When there is exactly 3 minutes left on the clock, place the first plasma

TABLE 8. DILUTIONS FOR FIBRINOGEN CALIBRATION CURVE

TUBE #	FIBRINOGEN CALIBRATION REFERENCE	OWREN'S VERONAL BUFFER	DILUTION	DILUTION FACTOR
1	0.5 mL	2.0 mL	1:5	2
2	0.5 mL of mixture from tube #1	0.5 mL	1:10	1
3	0.5 mL of mixture from tube #2	0.5 mL	1:20	0.5
4	0.5 mL of mixture from tube #3	0.5 mL	1:40	0.25

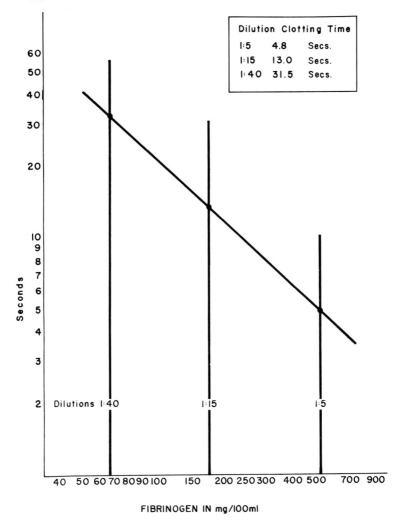

Dilution	Clotting Time	
1:5	4.8	Secs.
1:15	13.0	Secs.
1:40	31.5	Secs.

Fig. 153. Curve for quantitative fibrinogen procedure.

dilution in the Fibrometer test well. Add 0.1 mL of thrombin reagent (unheated) to the test cup and start the timer. When clotting has occurred, record the results. Repeat this step for each diluted plasma or control, beginning each test 3 minutes after incubation was started.

8. Duplicate results should agree within ± 0.5 seconds. If results exceed 15 seconds, results should agree within ± 1.0 second, and within ± 1.5 seconds if the results are above 20 seconds.

9. Average the duplicate results and determine the fibrinogen concentration for each control and patient specimen by referring to the previously prepared fibrinogen curve. Control results must agree within ± 15% of the assay value. If they do not, the cause must be determined and the test repeated.

DISCUSSION

1. If the test cannot be run within 4 hours of obtaining the specimen, the

plasma may be frozen and stored at −20°C.

2. When the fibrinogen value is below 50 mg/dL, the plasma should be diluted 1:5 (0.2 mL of plasma added to 0.8 mL of buffer) or 1:3 (0.3 mL of plasma added to 0.6 mL of buffer). Perform the fibrinogen in duplicate as outlined above, average the results, and determine the fibrinogen value from the curve. Divide these results by 2 (for the 1:5 dilution) or by 3 (for the 1:3 dilution). If no clot forms with the 1:3 dilution, report a result of less than the lowest value on the curve divided by 3.

3. When the fibrinogen value is above 800 mg/dL, the plasma should be diluted 1:20 (0.1 mL of plasma added to 1.9 mL of buffer). Perform the fibrinogen, in duplicate, as outlined above, average the results, and determine the fibrinogen value from the curve. Multiply these results by 2.

4. A 1:3 dilution of the plasma is the lowest dilution which may be used in this test. Inaccurate results may occur if a smaller dilution is used due to the presence of inhibitors in the plasma.

5. In the presence of significant levels of fibrin degradation products (above 100 μg/mL) or heparin (above 0.6 USP units/mL), the test results will be invalidly low.

6. Most manufacturers of coagulation reagents also produce a fibrinogen kit similar to the one described above.

FACTOR IDENTIFICATION (PT AND APTT SUBSTITUTION TEST)

A specific factor deficiency can be identified by mixing correction reagents with a patient's plasma and then performing the prothrombin time (PT) and/or the activated partial thromboplastin time (APTT).

REFERENCE

Proctor, R.R., and Rapaport, S.I.: The partial thromboplastin time with kaolin, Am. J. Clin. Path., 36, 212, 1961.

REAGENTS AND EQUIPMENT

1. Water bath, 37°C.
2. Reagents for the APTT.
   a. Calcium chloride, 0.025 M.
   b. Partial thromboplastin with activator.
3. Reagent for the PT.
   a. Tissue thromboplastin reagent.
4. Normal control plasma.
5. Sodium chloride, 0.85% (w/v).
6. Test tubes, 12 × 75 mm.
7. Pipets, 1.0, 0.1, and 0.2 mL.
8. Stopwatch.
9. Adsorbed plasma (rich in factors V, VIII, XI, and XII). Obtainable commercially.
10. Aged serum (rich in factors VII, IX, X, XI, and XII). Obtainable commercially.

SPECIMEN

Citrated plasma: 1 part 0.109 M sodium citrate to 9 parts whole blood.

PRINCIPLE

An APTT and/or a PT is performed on the patient's plasma diluted 1:1 with:

1. Adsorbed plasma (factors V, VIII, XI, and XII).
2. Aged serum (Factors VII, IX, X, XI, and XII).
3. Sodium chloride, 0.85%.
4. Normal control plasma.

The patient's undiluted plasma is also tested in the same manner. The specific coagulation defect may be obtained by noting which reagent, adsorbed plasma, or aged serum corrects the APTT and/or the PT. (The APTT [or PT] may then be repeated, diluting the patient's plasma 1:1 with a plasma specimen deficient in the specific factor identified as the deficiency. The factor deficient plasma, unable to correct the APTT [or PT], is a further check as to the exact coagulation deficiency.)

PROCEDURE

1. Centrifuge the patient's citrated blood at 1200 to 1500 g for 15 minutes immediately after the blood has been collected.
2. Remove the plasma from the cells immediately and place on ice.
3. Perform a PT and an APTT on the patient's plasma. If both test results fall within the normal range, a factor deficiency probably does not exist. If either, or both, of the tests are abnormal, proceed to the next step, performing the substitution test on the procedure (PT and/or APTT) which gave abnormal results.
4. If there is a possibility of a circulating anticoagulant being present, this test should first be performed to rule out the presence of inhibitors.
5. Reconstitute the aged serum and adsorbed plasma according to manufacturer's directions. Keep these reagents, along with the patient plasma and normal control plasma, in crushed ice.
6. Perform an APTT and/or PT, in duplicate, on the following mixtures:
    a. 0.1 mL patient's plasma + 0.1 mL adsorbed plasma.
    b. 0.1 mL normal control plasma + 0.1 mL adsorbed plasma.
    c. 0.1 mL patient's plasma + 0.1 mL aged serum.
    d. 0.1 mL normal control plasma + 0.1 mL aged serum.
    e. 0.1 mL patient's plasma + 0.1 mL 0.85% sodium chloride.
    f. 0.1 mL normal control plasma + 0.1 mL 0.85% sodium chloride.
7. Average results and record.
8. For interpretation of results, see Table 9.

DISCUSSION

1. If a factor deficiency is noted, the PT or APTT may be performed, using the specific factor-deficient plasma indicated, in a 1:1 dilution with the patient's plasma. When the deficient factor(s) has been positively identified, appropriate specific factor assays should then be performed.
2. For the patient's PT or APTT to be considered as corrected, the corrected values must fall close to the normal plasma control value, but will not necessarily fall within the normal range because the plasma has been diluted. The plasma diluted with sodium chloride will give an example of uncorrected test results.
3. A factor identification may be difficult to determine in cases of a mild deficiency, since this is a qualitative test and a significant correction (by adsorbed plasma or aged serum) is needed for interpretation of the results.

THROMBOPLASTIN GENERATION TEST

The thromboplastin generation test is included here primarily for teaching purposes. The test is not generally used in today's laboratory due to the commercial availability of factor deficient plasmas. Historically, this test was used to measure the efficiency with which plasma thromboplastin is formed. It detects factor VIII and factor IX deficiencies and is able to distinguish between the two disorders. Factor XI and XII deficiencies may be detected but cannot be differentiated from each other. If the patient's platelets are used in the test, a platelet abnormality may also be detected. The primary problem with this procedure is that it is complicated and time consuming. In addition, it is not always sensitive enough to detect mild deficiencies of a factor (>10% but <50% activity).

REFERENCE

Biggs, R., and Douglas, A.S.: The thromboplastin generation test, J. Clin. Path., 6, 23, 1953.

REAGENTS AND EQUIPMENT

1. Barium sulfate, powdered.

TABLE 9. PROBABLE COAGULATION DEFICIENCIES BASED ON THE APTT AND PT SUBSTITUTION TEST RESULTS

| APTT | PT | ADSORBED PLASMA | | AGED SERUM | | PROBABLE DEFICIENCY |
		APTT	PT	APTT	PT	
N	N	—	—	—	—	No deficiency
A	N	C	—	C	—	XI or XII
A	N	NC	—	C	—	IX
A	A	NC	NC	C	C	X
A	A	C	C	NC	NC	V
N	A	—	NC	—	C	VII
A	N	C	—	NC	—	VIII
A	A	NC	NC	NC	NC	II

N = Normal result. A = Abnormal (prolonged result). C = Corrected result, NC = Not corrected.

2. Water bath, 37°C.
3. Calcium chloride, 0.025 M.
4. Thromboplastin-calcium chloride mixture.
5. Sodium chloride, 0.85% (w/v).
6. Partial thromboplastin (platelet substitute). (Commercially available.)
7. Ice bath (crushed ice).
8. Test tubes, 13 × 100 mm.
9. Stopwatch.

SPECIMEN

One test tube of clotted blood and one test tube of oxalated blood (1 part 0.1 M sodium oxalate to 9 parts whole blood) from both a normal patient (to be used as control) and from the patient to be tested.

PRINCIPLE

The patient's diluted serum and adsorbed plasma are mixed with calcium chloride and a substitute platelet factor. This constitutes the patient's thromboplastin generation mixture. The amount of plasma thromboplastin formed by the patient's coagulation factors is measured by the ability of this mixture to clot a normal plasma (which primarily supplies prothrombin and fibrinogen). The patient's generation mixture is incubated for a total of 6 minutes. At 1-minute intervals during this time, samples of the generation mixture are added to a normal plasma, and the clotting time is determined. Normally, there will be enough thromboplastin generated during these 6 minutes to clot normal plasma in 12 seconds or less. When an abnormal result is obtained, normal adsorbed plasma (source of factors I, V, VIII, XI, XII) and normal serum (source of factors VII, IX, X, XI, XII) are substituted, one at a time, to determine which corrects the patient's defect. If the prothrombin time is normal, factors I, II, V, VII, and X are assumed to be normal. Therefore, deficiencies in factors VIII, IX, XI, or XII may be detected.

PROCEDURE

1. Preparation of patient and normal control plasma. (Source of factor VIII.)

   a. Centrifuge the normal control and patient's anticoagulated blood specimens at 1500 × g for 10 minutes within 15 minutes of collection.

   b. Remove the plasma and pipet 1.0 mL of each plasma into a separate 13 × 100 mm test tube containing 100 mg of barium sulfate. Place the remaining patient's plasma in the refrigerator in case it is needed for future tests. Refrigerate the remaining control plasma for use as the plasma substrate.

   c. Stir the plasma-barium sulfate mixtures with a glass rod for 10 minutes. Refrigerate for 10 minutes.

   d. Centrifuge the two mixtures at 1500 × g for 10 minutes. Remove the adsorbed plasma specimens and place in respective test tubes in crushed ice.

e. Perform a prothrombin time on each of the adsorbed plasma specimens. The prothrombin times should be greater than 3 minutes. If not, readsorb the plasma.

f. Refrigerate the adsorbed plasma specimens.

2. Preparation of the patient and normal control serums. (Source of factor IX.)

a. When the patient's and normal control blood specimens have clotted, place the test tubes in a 37°C water bath for 2 hours.

b. At the end of 2 hours, centrifuge the clotted blood specimens at 1800 × g for 5 minutes. Remove the serum specimens and place in respective test tubes in crushed ice.

3. Test.

a. Dilute the normal control and patient's adsorbed plasma 1:5 with 0.85% sodium chloride (0.1 mL of adsorbed plasma and 0.4 mL of 0.85% sodium chloride). Place in respective test tubes in crushed ice.

b. Dilute the normal control and patient's serum 1:10 with 0.85% sodium chloride (0.1 mL of serum and 0.9 mL of 0.85% sodium chloride). Place the respective test tubes in crushed ice.

c. Pipet approximately 5 mL of 0.025 M calcium chloride into a 13 × 100 mm test tube and place in the 37°C water bath.

d. Place six 13 × 100 mm test tubes in the 37°C water bath and pipet exactly 0.1 mL of plasma substrate (unadsorbed and undiluted control plasma) into each test tube.

e. Prepare the control generation mixture. Add the following solutions to a 13 × 100 mm test tube in the 37°C water bath:

(1) 0.3 mL of diluted adsorbed control plasma.

(2) 0.3 mL of partial thromboplastin.

(3) 0.3 mL of diluted control serum.

(4) 0.3 mL of 0.025 M calcium chloride.

Start a stopwatch at exactly the same time the last reagent (calcium chloride) is added to the mixture. If a clot forms in this generation mixture at any time, it should be removed so that it will not interfere with pipetting.

f. When 55 seconds have elapsed on the stopwatch, pipet 0.1 mL of the generation mixture. With the other hand, pipet 0.1 mL of 0.025 M calcium chloride.

g. When 1 minute has elapsed on the stopwatch, add the 0.1 mL of generation mixture into one of the test tubes containing 0.1 mL of plasma substrate. Immediately add the 0.1 mL of calcium chloride into the same test tube and simultaneously start a second stopwatch.

h. Determine the clotting time of this mixture by the tilt tube method. If clotting has not occurred within 40 to 45 seconds, have a second person continue tilting the test tube until clotting occurs. Record the results. If the clotting time is greater than 60 seconds, record as over 60 seconds.

i. Repeat steps f, g, and h at 1-minute intervals for all 6 test tubes containing the 0.1 mL of plasma substrate. (Start the second clotting time when 1 minute and 55 seconds have elapsed on the first stopwatch.) Do not stop the first stopwatch at any time during this procedure.

j. If any of the six test tubes has a clotting time of 12 seconds or less within the 6-minute incubation period of the generation mixture, the test is considered to be normal. If the control test performed on the plasma substrate is abnormal, the entire test must be repeated.

k. Place six 13 × 100 mm test tubes in the 37°C water bath and pipet exactly 0.1 mL of plasma substrate (unadsorbed and undiluted control plasma) into each tube.

l. Prepare the patient's generation mixture. Add the following solutions to a 13 × 100 mm test tube in the 37°C water bath:

(1) 0.3 mL of diluted adsorbed patient's plasma.

(2) 0.3 mL of partial thromboplastin.

(3) 0.3 mL of diluted patient's serum.

(4) 0.3 mL of 0.025 M calcium chloride.

Start a stopwatch at exactly the same time the last reagent (calcium chloride) is added to the mixture. If a clot forms in this generation mixture at any time, it should be removed so that it will not interfere with pipetting.

m. Repeat steps f through j.

n. If none of the test tubes has clotted in less than 12 seconds using the patient's generation mixture, proceed to step 4, Substitutions. If any of the preceding six test tubes has a clotting time of 12 seconds or less, the results for this test are normal, and step 4 of this procedure may be omitted.

4. Substitutions.

a. Pipet 0.1 mL of plasma substrate into each of six 13 × 100 mm test

tubes and place in a 37°C water bath.

b. Prepare a generation mixture. Add the following solutions to a 13 × 100 mm test tube in the 37°C water bath:

(1) 0.3 mL of diluted adsorbed control plasma.

(2) 0.3 mL of partial thromboplastin.

(3) 0.3 mL of diluted patient's serum.

(4) 0.3 mL of 0.025 M calcium chloride.

Start a stopwatch at exactly the same time the last reagent (calcium chloride) is added to the mixture. Remove the clot, if formed.

c. Repeat steps f through j, as described previously in step 3, Test, and record results.

d. Repeat step a and prepare another generation mixture as follows:

(1) 0.3 mL of diluted adsorbed patient's plasma.

(2) 0.3 mL of partial thromboplastin.

(3) 0.3 mL of diluted control serum.

(4) 0.3 mL of 0.025 M calcium chloride.

Start the stopwatch. Remove the clot, if formed.

e. Repeat steps f through j, as described previously in step 3, Test, and record results.

5. Interpretation of results. See Table 10.

DISCUSSION

1. Abnormal platelet activity may be detected using the patient's platelets in place of partial thromboplastin in the patient's generation mixture. If this procedure is employed, a prolonged clotting time, using the patient's serum, platelets, and adsorbed plasma, must be followed up by a

TABLE 10.   INTERPRETATION OF THE THROMBOPLASTIN GENERATION TEST

FACTOR DEFICIENCY	CLOTTING TIME CORRECTED BY		PROTHROMBIN TIME
	ADSORBED PLASMA	NORMAL SERUM	
VIII	Yes	No	Normal
IX	No	Yes	Normal
XI or XII	Yes	Yes	Normal
Anticoagulant	No	No	May be normal

substitution test, using partial thromboplastin in the patient's generation mixture. Correction of the generation clotting time by partial thromboplastin indicates defective platelet activity. The patient's platelets for this procedure may be prepared as follows:

a. Centrifuge oxalated blood for 10 minutes at 150 to 200 × g immediately after collection.

b. Transfer the platelet rich plasma to a siliconized or plastic test tube and note the volume of the plasma.

c. Centrifuge the platelet rich plasma at 1500 × g for 15 minutes. A platelet button will be formed.

d. Note the total plasma volume. Pour off the supernatant plasma and refrigerate until 20 minutes before use.

e. Resuspend the platelets in 0.85% sodium chloride and centrifuge at 1500 × g for 15 minutes.

f. Pour off the supernatant sodium chloride and resuspend the platelets in a volume of 0.85% sodium chloride equal to ⅓ of the original plasma volume.

2. The presence of circulating anticoagulants may give abnormal results in this test.

3. Oxalated plasma must be used if the plasma is to be adsorbed by barium sulfate. If citrated plasma is employed, aluminum hydroxide must be used as the adsorbing agent.

4. The thromboplastin generation test may also be performed on the fibrometer.

PROTHROMBIN CONSUMPTION TEST

The prothrombin consumption test is merely a prothrombin time carried out on serum. It tests primarily for the coagulation factors present in stage 1 of the intrinsic system, namely, factors VIII, IX, and platelet factor 3, which are necessary for plasma thromboplastin formation. The normal prothrombin consumption for the procedure outlined below is above 20 seconds. Clotting times of 18 to 20 seconds are borderline, and abnormal results show a clotting time of less than 18 seconds. The normal range, however, should be determined for each laboratory. An abnormal prothrombin consumption is found in factors VIII, IX, and platelet factor 3 deficiencies. If the blood is allowed to clot before performing the test, factor XI and XII deficiencies will not be detected, other than by a prolonged clotting time.

REFERENCE

Lenahan, J.G., and Smith, K.: *Hemostasis,* Durham, N.C., Organon Teknika Corp., 1985.

REAGENTS AND EQUIPMENT

1. Water bath, 37°C.

2. Simplastin-A. (This reagent supplies fibrinogen, thromboplastin, calcium and an optimum amount of factor V. It is available from Organon Teknika Corp.) Reconstitute according to the directions in the package insert.

3. Test tubes, 13 × 100 mm.

4. Stopwatch.

SPECIMEN

Whole blood, 1 to 3 mL, placed in a plain glass test tube (unsiliconized). A normal control blood sample should be obtained at the same time the patient's blood is collected.

PRINCIPLE

When the formation of plasma thromboplastin is normal, all but trace amounts of prothrombin are converted to thrombin. If a prothrombin time is then performed on the serum, with the addition of fibrinogen (and thromboplastin-calcium reagent), the resulting prothrombin time should be prolonged due to decreased amounts of prothrombin. When plasma thromboplastin formation is defective, however, prothrombin conversion to thrombin is decreased, and there is an excess of prothrombin present in the serum. When fibrinogen, thromboplastin, and calcium are added to this serum, therefore, a shortened clotting time results.

PROCEDURE

1. As soon as the patient's and control blood specimens are drawn, place them in a 37°C water bath and observe for clotting.
2. Incubate the blood at 37°C for 2 hours after the blood has clotted.
3. Centrifuge the blood at 1500 × g for 10 minutes.
4. Remove the serum from the clot. At this point, the serum may be refrigerated for a maximum of 2 hours.
5. Pipet 0.2 mL of Simplastin-A into each of four 13 × 100 mm test tubes and place in the 37°C water bath for 2 minutes.
6. Pipet 0.1 mL of control or patient's serum into one of the preceding test tubes, simultaneously starting the stopwatch.
7. Remove the tube from the water bath and gently tilt. As soon as a fine web or clot forms, stop the watch and record the results.

8. Repeat steps 6 and 7, performing duplicate clotting times on the patient and control serum specimens. Results on the normal control serum must be within the normal range for the test to be considered valid.

DISCUSSION

1. In drawing blood, contamination with tissue thromboplastin must be avoided. If this occurs or serum is hemolyzed, the specimen must be redrawn.
2. In place of Simplastin-A, fibrinogen reagent (1.0 mL) may be mixed with thromboplastin-calcium reagent (2.0 mL). The normal results obtained when using these reagents will generally be slightly longer than when the Simplastin-A is used.
3. A severe deficiency in prothrombin yields a normal prothrombin consumption time. Also, a normal result is obtained when there are deficiencies present in more than one factor, such as in Owren's disease (factor V and VIII deficiencies), when one of the decreased factors is present in stage 2 of the coagulation process. Therefore, if the prothrombin time is abnormal, a prothrombin consumption should not be performed.
4. In the presence of thrombocytopenia (decreased platelet count) or abnormally functioning platelets, the results of the prothrombin consumption test will be abnormal.

FACTOR V (II, VII, X) ASSAY

The prothrombin time (PT) is commonly used to determine the plasma concentration of factors II, V, VII, and X. The normal plasma concentration of each of these factors is in the range of 50 to 150% activity; however, each laboratory should determine its own normal values.

The factor V assay is described below. For a factor II, VII, or X assay, substitute factor II, VII, or X deficient substrate in place of factor V deficient substrate and use a factor II, VII, or X assayed reference plasma instead of the factor V reference plasma. Factor V may also be assayed using the Stypven time test since Russell's viper venom is quite sensitive to this factor.

REFERENCES

Biggs, R., and MacFarlane, R.G.: *Human Blood Coagulation and Its Disorders,* Oxford, Blackwell Scientific Publications, 1962.

Hardisty, R.M., and Ingram, C.I.C.: *Bleeding Disorders, Investigation and Management,* Oxford, Blackwell Scientific Publications, 1965.

Lenahan, J.G., and Smith, K.: *Hemostasis,* Durham, N.C., Organon Teknika Corp., 1985.

REAGENTS AND EQUIPMENT

1. Thromboplastin-calcium chloride mixture.
2. Water bath, 37°C.
3. Factor V deficient substrate. Obtainable commercially.
4. Reference plasma with known factor V assay. Obtainable commercially.
5. Normal control plasma assayed for factor V.
6. Owren's veronal buffer, pH 7.40.
7. Ice bath.
8. Pipets, 1.0, 0.2, and 0.1 mL.
9. Stopwatch.
10. Test tubes, 12 × 75 mm.
11. Two-cycle log-log graph paper.

SPECIMEN

Citrated plasma: 1 part 0.109 M sodium citrate to 9 parts whole blood. Place the tube of blood in a cup of ice immediately after collection.

PRINCIPLE

A prothrombin time is performed on factor V-deficient substrates (plasmas) containing varying dilutions of the patient's plasma (Table 11), which is used to correct the prothrombin time. The amount of correction by the patient's plasma is compared with the results of the prothrombin time performed on a known reference plasma in place of the patient's plasma.

The factor V content of the patient's plasma is expressed as the percentage of normal.

PROCEDURE

1. Centrifuge the patient's blood at 1200 to 1500 g for 15 minutes immediately after collection. Remove the plasma and place in a cup containing crushed ice.
2. Warm sufficient thromboplastin-calcium reagent to 37°C.
3. Reconstitute the factor V-deficient substrate and the reference plasma according to manufacturer's directions and place on ice.
4. Label six 12 × 75 mm test tubes and add Owren's veronal buffer in the amounts listed in Table 11. (At least two separately prepared dilutions [e.g., 1:10 and 1:20] should be made. If this is not done, and an error is made in the original dilution, the serial dilutions will be incorrect, but will not reflect this.)
5. Place several 12 × 75 mm empty test tubes in the 37°C water bath. (All testing should be performed in duplicate.)
6. Prepare the dilutions of the reference plasma as indicated in Table 11.
7. To one of the 12 × 75 mm test tubes in the water bath, add:
   a. 0.1 mL of factor V-deficient substrate.
   b. 0.1 mL of the first diluted (reference) plasma.
8. Add 0.2 mL of thromboplastin-calcium reagent to the test tube and simultaneously start a stopwatch.
9. Remove the test tube from the water bath and gently tilt the tube at a rate of about once per second. Stop the watch at the first indication of clot formation. Record results.
10. Repeat steps 7, 8, and 9 for each of the reference plasma dilutions.
11. Prepare 1:10 and 1:20 dilutions of the patient's and normal control plasmas

TABLE 11.   DILUTIONS FOR FACTOR V (II, VII, and X)

TUBE (#)	BUFFER (mL)	PLASMA (mL)	ACTIVITY (%)	DILUTION
1	0.9	0.1	100	1:10
2	1.9	0.1	50	1:20
3	0.5	0.5 mL from tube #2	25	1:40
4	0.5	0.5 mL from tube #3	12.5	1:80
5	0.5	0.5 mL from tube #4	6.3	1:160
6	0.5	0.5 mL from tube #5	3.2	1:320

(see Table 11 for amounts) immediately before use and repeat steps 7 through 9, above, for each of the dilutions. Test each dilution in duplicate.

12. Calculation of results:

   a. Using 2-cycle log-log graph paper and the results obtained on the reference plasma, plot each average clotting time in seconds (on the Y-axis) against the plasma concentration in percent (on the X-axis). There will be six points plotted (Fig. 154).

   b. Draw a straight line that best connects the six points of the reference plasma. This represents the normal activity curve.

   c. Using the average clotting times of each patient and control plasma dilution, determine from the graph the percent of factor V present in each dilution. The 1:10 dilution represents the percent activity present in undiluted plasma. The results of the 1:20 dilution should be multiplied by 2 in order to arrive at the percent

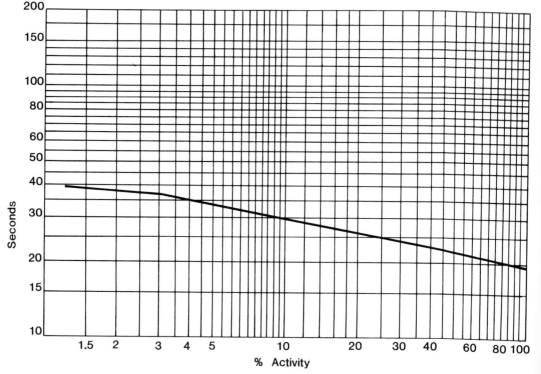

Fig. 154.   Factor V activity curve.

activity present in undiluted plasma. Average these two values for the percent of factor V activity present in the patient and control plasmas.

DISCUSSION

1. Pooled normal plasma may be used in place of reference plasma for the activity curve. The advantage of using assayed reference plasma is that it contains a known concentration of the factor. Different lots of pooled plasma will vary in the concentration of the factor.
2. Factor V-deficient plasma may be used in place of the factor V-deficient substrate. If this is employed, a prothrombin time greater than 60 seconds should be obtained on the factor V-deficient plasma before it is used. (Factor V-deficient plasma may be prepared by incubating normal plasma at 37°C for 24 hours or by refrigerating the normal plasma at 4 to 10°C for 2 weeks.)
3. Samples must be tested within 30 minutes of diluting in Owren's veronal buffer. Testing should be complete within 2 hours of obtaining the plasma sample from the patient.
4. It is advisable to run a new curve each time the assay is performed. As more experience is gained, the curve may be made from tubes #1, 2, 3, and 5.
5. When drawing the factor activity curve, do not extend the curve below the upper and lower concentration limits of the reference plasma.
6. As indicated in the factor VIII procedure, this assay may also be performed on the Fibrometer and on most automated coagulation systems.

FACTOR VIII (VIII:C) (IX, XI, XII) ASSAY

The activated partial thromboplastin time (APTT) is generally used to deter-mine the plasma concentration of factors VIII, IX, XI, and XII. The normal plasma concentration of each of these factors is in the range of 50 to 150% activity; however, each laboratory should determine its own normal values.

The factor VIII assay is described below. For a factor IX, XI, or XII assay, substitute factor IX, XI, or XII deficient substrate in place of factor VIII deficient substrate and use a factor IX, XI, or XII assayed reference plasma instead of the factor VIII reference plasma. Assays for prekallikrein and high molecular weight kininogen (HMWK) may also be performed by this procedure if the respective factor deficient substrates and assayed reference plasmas are available.

REFERENCES

Hardisty, R.M., and MacPherson, J.C.: A one-stage factor VIII assay and its use on venous and capillary plasma. Thromb. Diath. Haemorrh., 7, 215, 1962.
Lenahan, J.G., and Smith, K.: Hemostasis, Durham, N.C., Organon Teknika Corp., 1985.

REAGENTS AND EQUIPMENT

1. Partial thromboplastin containing an activator (platelet substitute with activator). Obtainable commercially.
2. Water bath, 37°C.
3. Calcium chloride, 0.025 M.
4. Factor VIII deficient substrate. Obtainable commercially.
5. Reference plasma with known factor VIII assay. Obtainable commercially.
6. Normal control plasma assayed for factor VIII.
7. Owren's veronal buffer, pH 7.40 (± 0.1).
8. Ice bath.
9. Pipets, 1.0, 0.2, and 0.1 mL.
10. Stopwatch.
11. Timers, 2.
12. Test tubes, 12 × 75 mm.
13. Two-cycle log-log graph paper.

SPECIMEN

Citrated plasma: 1 part 0.109 M sodium citrate to 9 parts whole blood. Place specimen in a cup of ice immediately after collection.

PRINCIPLE

An APTT is performed on factor VIII-deficient substrates (plasmas) containing varying dilutions of the patient's plasma (Table 12). The patient's plasma is used to correct the APTT. The amount of correction by the patient's plasma is then compared with results of the APTT using a known reference plasma in place of the patient's plasma. The factor VIII content of the patient's plasma is expressed as the percentage of normal.

PROCEDURE

1. Centrifuge the patient's blood at 1200 to 1500 g for 15 minutes immediately after collection. Remove the plasma and place on ice. Proceed with the test immediately.
2. Maintain the partial thromboplastin at room temperature.
3. Incubate sufficient 0.025 M calcium chloride at 37°C.
4. Reconstitute the factor VIII-deficient substrate and the reference plasma according to manufacturer's directions and place on ice.
5. Label seven 12 × 75 mm test tubes and add Owren's veronal buffer in the amounts listed in Table 12. (At least two separately prepared dilutions [e.g., 1:5 and 1:10] should be made. If this is not done, and an error is made in the original dilution, the

serial dilutions will be incorrect, but will not reflect this error.)
6. Place several 12 × 75 mm test tubes in the 37°C water bath. (All testing should be performed in duplicate.)
7. Prepare the dilutions of the reference plasma as indicated in Table 12.
8. To one of the 12 × 75 mm test tubes in the water bath add:
   a. 0.1 mL of partial thromboplastin.
   b. 0.1 mL of factor-VIII deficient substrate.
   c. 0.1 mL of the first diluted (reference) plasma.
9. Quickly mix the contents of the test tube and set clock #1 for 3 minutes.
10. When 1 minute has elapsed on clock #1, repeat steps 8 and 9 for the duplicate sample, setting clock #2.
11. When 3 minutes have elapsed on clock #1, quickly pipet 0.1 mL of 0.025 M calcium chloride into the first test tube, simultaneously starting a stopwatch. Gently mix the contents of the tube and leave it in the 37°C water bath for 30 seconds.
12. After 30 seconds have elapsed on the stopwatch, remove the test tube from the water bath and gently tilt the tube at a rate no faster than once per second.
13. When clotting occurs, stop the watch. This is the end point.
14. Repeat steps 11, 12, and 13 for clock #2 and the duplicate specimen.
15. Average the preceding two results and record the clotting time for that dilution.

TABLE 12. DILUTIONS FOR FACTOR VIII (IX, XI, and XII)

TUBE (#)	BUFFER (mL)	PLASMA (mL)	ACTIVITY (%)	DILUTION
1	0.4	0.1	100	1:5
2	0.9	0.1	50	1:10
3	0.5	0.5 mL from tube #2	25	1:20
4	0.5	0.5 mL from tube #3	12.5	1:40
5	0.5	0.5 mL from tube #4	6.3	1:80
6	0.5	0.5 mL from tube #5	3.2	1:160
7	0.5	0.5 mL from tube #6	1.6	1:320

16. Repeat steps 8 through 15 for each of the reference plasma dilutions.

17. Prepare 1:5 and 1:10 dilutions of the patient's and normal control plasmas (see Table 12 for amounts) immediately before use and repeat steps 8 through 15 for each of the dilutions. Test each dilution in duplicate.

18. Calculation of results.
    a. Using 2-cycle log-log graph paper and the results obtained on the reference plasma, plot each average clotting time in seconds (on the Y-axis) against the plasma concentration in percent (on the X-axis). There will be 7 points plotted.
    b. Draw a straight line that best connects the 7 points of the reference plasma. This represents the normal activity curve.
    c. Using the average clotting times of each patient and control plasma dilution, determine from the graph the percent of factor VIII present in each dilution. The 1:5 dilution represents the percent activity present in undiluted plasma. The results of the 1:10 dilution should be multiplied by 2 in order to arrive at the percent activity present in undiluted plasma. Average these two values for the percent of factor VIII activity present in the patient and control plasmas.

DISCUSSION

1. Pooled normal plasma may be used in place of reference plasma for the activity curve. However, the advantage of using assayed reference plasma is that it contains a known concentration of the factor. Different pools of normal plasma differ from each other in the concentration of the factor.

2. Factor VIII-deficient substrate may be replaced by plasma known to be deficient in factor VIII. This plasma may be stored at $-20°C$ and thawed immediately before use. A plasma to be used as factor VIII-deficient, however, must have a concentration no higher than 0 to 1% of normal activity of the factor before it is acceptable. Also, even though the plasma is stored at $-20°C$, it may gradually become deficient in additional clotting factors, particularly factor V.

3. The 3-minute activation time in this procedure is critical for accurate results.

4. Excessive mixing of the tubes during the procedure may cause prolonged clotting times.

5. Samples must be tested within 30 minutes of diluting in Owren's veronal buffer. Testing should be complete within 2 hours of obtaining the plasma sample from the patient.

6. A new curve should be run each time an assay is performed. As more experience is gained, the curve may be made from tubes #1 through 5, or, tubes #1, 2, 4, 6, and 7.

7. The reference plasma curve will generally flatten out at a dilution of 1 to 2%, indicating a lack of sensitivity at these concentrations.

8. When drawing the factor activity curve, do not extend the curve beyond the concentration (upper and lower) of the reference plasma.

9. Due to the slope of the curve, a 1-second variation in clotting time will cause a relatively large difference in percent activity. Therefore, a CV of 10 or 15% is not unusual for this procedure.

10. Factor assays may also be performed on the Fibrometer and on most automated coagulation systems. On the newer automated instruments, a built in computer will automatically determine the activity curve and calculate the control and patient results.

von WILLEBRAND FACTOR (RISTOCETIN COFACTOR) ASSAY

The von Willebrand factor (ristocetin cofactor [VIII:R:RCo]) is that property of the factor VIII protein which is responsible for in vitro platelet agglutination in the presence of ristocetin. Decreased amounts or abnormalities of this factor are associated with the von Willebrand syndrome.

REFERENCE

Bio/Data Corporation, vW Factor Assay™ for the Quantitation of von Willebrand Factor, pkg. insert, Hatboro, Pa., Bio/Data Corporation, 1986.

REAGENTS AND EQUIPMENT

1. vW Factor Assay™ Kit (obtainable from Bio/Data Corp.).
    a. Lypholized platelets. Reconstitute with 4.0 mL of Tris buffered saline solution before use. Once reconstituted the platelets may be refrigerated for up to 60 days. Resuspend platelets gently by mixing, immediately before use.
    b. Ristocetin reagent. Reconstitute with 0.5 mL of distilled water before use. This gives a concentration of 10 mg/mL. Invert vial gently and allow to stand at room temperature for 10 minutes prior to use. Once reconstituted this reagent is stable for 7 days stored in the refrigerator.
    c. Normal reference plasma (von Willebrand factor). Reconstitute with 0.5 mL of distilled water and let stand at room temperature for 10 minutes prior to use. Stable for 8 hours after reconstitution when stored in the refrigerator.
    d. Abnormal control plasma (von Willebrand factor deficient). Reconstitute with 0.5 mL of distilled water and allow to stand at room temperature for 10 minutes prior to use. Stable for 8 hours after reconstitution when stored in the refrigerator.
    e. Tris buffered saline solution, pH 7.5, 10.0 mL. Store reagents a through e (above) at 2 to 8°C prior to use. These reagents may also be purchased separately.
2. Platelet aggregometer capable of stir speeds between 900 and 1200 rpm.
3. Platelet aggregometer cuvets.
4. Stir bars.
5. Pipets, 5.0, 1.0, 0.5, 0.2, 0.1, and 0.05 mL.
6. Plastic test tubes, 10 × 75 mm.
7. Distilled water.
8. Log-log graph paper.
9. Slope reader.

SPECIMEN

Citrated plasma: 1 part 0.109 M sodium citrate to 9 parts whole blood.

PRINCIPLE

Patient's plasma (source of ristocetin cofactor) is added to a standardized mixture of platelets and ristocetin reagent. The degree of resultant platelet aggregation is measured using the platelet aggregometer. This result is then compared to a curve prepared from a normal reference plasma, and the % concentration of ristocetin cofactor (von Willebrand factor) is determined.

PROCEDURE

1. Preparation of specimen. Centrifuge citrated plasma at 1500 g for 15 minutes. Remove plasma from cells, making certain the plasma is free of red cells, white cells, and platelets. Cap the plasma tube and refrigerate if testing is not to proceed immediately. (Plasma may be refrigerated for up to 8 hours prior to testing, or frozen at −20°C or lower for up to 8 weeks.)
2. Preparation of normal reference plasma dilutions (1:2, 1:4, and 1:8).
    a. Label three 10 × 75 mm test tubes: 100%, 50%, and 25%.
    b. Pipet 0.1 mL of tris buffered sa-

line solution into the tube labeled 100%, 0.3 mL of tris buffered saline solution into the 50% tube, and 0.2 mL into the 25% tube.

c. Pipet 0.1 mL of the normal reference plasma into the 100% and 50% tubes. Mix each tube thoroughly. Transfer 0.2 mL of the mixture from the 50% tube to the 25% tube and mix well.

3. Preparation of patient dilutions (1:2, 1:4, and 1:8). For each plasma to be tested, pipet 0.1 mL, 0.3 mL, and 0.7 mL of tris buffered saline solution into appropriately labeled 10 × 75 mm test tubes. Add 0.1 mL of each patient's plasma to each tube. Mix well. Prepare the abnormal control dilution (1:2) as described above.

4. Preparation of the aggregometer blank. Pipet 0.25 mL of reconstituted platelets into an aggregometer cuvet and add 0.25 mL of tris buffered saline solution. Mix well. This blank is used to set the baseline in the aggregometer.

5. Pipet 0.4 mL of reconstituted platelets into an aggregometer cuvet. Add 0.05 mL of ristocetin to the tube (no air bubbles) and mix by tapping the cuvet gently. Allow the mixture to equilibrate at room temperature for 2 minutes.

6. Set the baseline using the aggregometer blank prepared in step 4 above.

7. Add a stir bar to the test mixture and place in the aggregometer.

8. As soon as the 0% baseline is stable, add 0.05 mL of the first reference plasma dilution directly into the test mixture in the cuvet. (Do not allow the reagent to touch the sides of the cuvet.)

9. Watch the pattern of aggregation as it prints out on the chart recorder. Stop the instrument when the reaction is complete.

10. Repeat steps 5 through 9 above for each dilution of the reference plasma

and for each patient dilution and abnormal control.

11. Determine the slope value for each agglutination curve.

a. Draw a straight line along the steepest portion of the curve that is linear (immediately following the lag phase resulting from the addition of the diluted plasma). Extend the line to the bottom of the graph paper.

b. Line up the slope reader so that the slope line bisects the slope reader scale at the bottom right of the base line.

c. Read the slope value at the point on the left scale of the reader where the slope line intersects it.

d. If the slope line is printed in the opposite direction, reverse the above procedure, lining up the baseline of the reader on the left side and reading the slope value from the right side.

12. Preparation of standard curve. Using log-log graph paper, plot the slope values for the reference plasma dilutions on the vertical axis against the percent activity on the horizontal axis. Draw a straight line which best fits these 3 points. If the points do not approximate a straight line, the test should be repeated.

13. Determine the percent von Willebrand activity of each plasma and control dilution by looking up the slope value on the reference curve and reading the corresponding percent von Willebrand factor activity from the horizontal axis. Multiply the results of the 1:4 dilutions by 2 and the 1:8 dilutions by 4 in order to obtain the correct test result. The 1:2, 1:4, and 1:8 dilutions should give results which agree closely. If the 1:2 dilution is above 100%, obtain the results from the 1:4 and 1:8 dilutions.

DISCUSSION

1. If the test results show less than 25% von Willebrand activity, the test should be repeated on the specimen, performing the test on undiluted plasma. The final result would then be divided by 2.
2. Each time this test procedure is performed a standard curve should be prepared.
3. Normally, von Willebrand factor activity should be above 40% and is generally in the range of 60 to 180%. A normal range should be determined by each laboratory.
4. In order to conserve reagents, the above procedure may be performed using micro methods if micro cuvets are available. In this modification, the test mixture should contain 0.2 mL of platelet suspension, 0.025 mL of ristocetin, and 0.025 mL of diluted plasma.

FLETCHER FACTOR (PREKALLIKREIN) SCREENING TEST

A deficiency of Fletcher factor may be determined by use of a modification of the activated partial thromboplastin time (APTT).

REFERENCE

Hattersley, P.G., and Hayse, D.: The effect of increased contact activation time on the activated partial thromboplastin time, Am. J. Clin. Path., *66*, 479, 1976.

REAGENTS AND EQUIPMENT

1. Water bath, 37°C.
2. Calcium chloride, 0.025 M.
3. Activated partial thromboplastin (APTT) reagent, containing kaolin, silica, or celite as the activator. Ellagic acid cannot be used as an activator in this test since it will not correct the APTT in a Fletcher factor deficiency.
4. Normal control plasma.
5. Test tubes, 12 × 75 mm.
6. Stopwatch.

SPECIMEN

Citrated plasma: 1 part 0.109 M sodium citrate to 9 parts whole blood. Immediately after blood collection, place the tube of blood in a cup of crushed ice and deliver to the laboratory.

PRINCIPLE

Patients with a Fletcher factor deficiency will have a prolonged APTT. If the plasma + APTT reagent mixture is incubated for 10 minutes (instead of the routine 3 or 5 minutes) the prolonged APTT will be shortened to normal, or almost normal, if the deficiency is due to Fletcher factor.

PROCEDURE

1. Centrifuge the patient's blood at 1200 to 1500 g for 15 minutes. Remove the plasma from the cells immediately and place on ice.
2. Perform an APTT on the patient and normal control plasma specimens as outlined previously in the section entitled Activated Partial Thromboplastin Time. If the patient results are normal, a Fletcher factor deficiency is not considered to be present. If the patient results are prolonged, proceed with step 3.
3. Perform an APTT on the patient and normal control plasma specimens, incubating the plasma + APTT reagent mixture for 10 minutes (instead of the routine 3 or 5 minutes). Add calcium chloride and determine the clotting time.
4. Interpretation of results. The APTT performed in step 3 (with the 10 minute incubation) should correct to a normal, or almost normal, clotting time in the presence of a Fletcher factor deficiency. If the APTT is not corrected by the increased incubation time, a problem other than a Fletcher factor deficiency is assumed to be present. The normal plasma control should remain within or near the

normal range with the 10 minute incubation period.

DISCUSSION

1. Normal clotting occurs with concentrations of Fletcher factor of 1.5 to 2.0% and above.
2. To confirm a Fletcher factor deficiency, an APTT may be performed on a 1:1 dilution of patient's plasma with Fletcher factor deficient substrate. The APTT should not correct using this substrate. If it does correct, a Fletcher factor deficiency does not exist.

FACTOR XIII SCREENING TEST

Factor XIII, known as the fibrin stabilizing factor, is responsible for converting the fibrin clot to a more stable form. It is thought to exist in the plasma in an inactive form and is activated by thrombin during the fibrinogen-to-fibrin conversion. Activated factor XIII causes the formation of covalent bonds between the fibrin monomers, thus stabilising the fibrin polymer. When factor XIII is present, the fibrin clot formed is insoluble in 5 M urea and 1% monochloroacetic acid when left standing for 24 hours. A deficiency in this factor is rare. Generally, a 1% level of factor XIII is sufficient to make a clot insoluble in 5 M urea.

REFERENCE

Losowsky, M.S., Hall, R., and Goldie, W.: Congenital deficiency of fibrin-stabilising factor, Lancet, *2*, 156, 1965.

REAGENTS AND EQUIPMENT

1. Urea, 5.0 M.
   Urea   30 g
   Dissolve urea and dilute to 100 mL with distilled water. Stable at room temperature for several months.
2. Calcium chloride, 0.025 M.
3. Normal control plasma.
4. Test tubes, 13 × 100 mm.
5. Pipets, 0.2 and 5.0 mL.
6. Water bath, 37°C.

SPECIMEN

Citrated plasma: 1 part 0.109 M sodium citrate to 9 parts whole blood.

PRINCIPLE

The patient's plasma is clotted by the addition of calcium chloride. Urea (5 M) is added to the clot. If factor XIII is absent in the patient's plasma, the clot is dissolved in less than 24 hours by the urea.

PROCEDURE

1. Centrifuge patient specimen at 1200 to 1500 g for 15 minutes.
2. Label two tubes for each patient and control.
3. Pipet 0.2 mL of patient's plasma into each of two test tubes. Repeat, pipetting 0.2 mL of normal control plasma into each of two additional test tubes.
4. Add 0.2 mL of 0.025 M calcium chloride to each tube. Mix. A clot should form in each tube.
5. Incubate the fibrin clots at 37°C for 30 minutes.
6. Loosen the clots from the sides of the test tubes by gently tapping the sides of the tube.
7. Transfer one of the patient's clots and one of the normal control clots to respectively labeled test tubes containing 5 mL of 5 M urea. To a third tube labeled 'patient/control', and containing 5 mL of 5 M urea, transfer both the remaining patient clot and the normal control clot.
8. Allow all tubes to incubate at room temperature for the next 24 hours. Examine the tubes at 1, 2, 3, and 24 hours and note if the clots have dissolved.
9. Report the length of time it took for the patient's clot to dissolve after urea was added. If the clot is still present at the end of 24 hours, report

that the clot was insoluble after 24 hours.

10. If the patient's clot dissolves within the 24-hour period, this is indicative of a factor XIII level of less than 1 to 2%. In this instance, the patient/control clot should not dissolve. If this clot does dissolve, this may indicate the presence of a fibrinolytic process rather than a factor XIII deficiency.

DISCUSSION

1. As an alternate procedure, 2% acetic acid or 1% monochloroacetic acid may be used. These reagents may, however, give an occasional false result.

2. A positive control (a clot that will dissolve in 5 M urea) may also be tested along with the patient, using thrombin and EDTA plasma. Add 10 NIH units of thrombin (0.5 mL of 20 NIH units/mL of thrombin) to 0.5 mL of EDTA plasma. Place the resultant clot in 5 mL of 5 M urea. This clot should be dissolved within 24 hours, due to the lack of calcium which is necessary for the action of factor XIII.

CIRCULATING ANTICOAGULANTS (INHIBITORS)

Some coagulation deficiencies are caused by inhibitors of specific factors rather than by a decreased concentration of a factor. These coagulation problems are generally termed 'circulating anticoagulants' and can act at any stage in the coagulation process. They may be fast-acting or may progressively destroy the factor. The two most common inhibitors are those specific for factor VIII, whose action increases with time, and lupus inhibitors which tend to act immediately. The factor VIII inhibitor is most commonly found in some cases of classic hemophilia, immunologic disorders, following pregnancy, and in the elderly where there is no underlying disease. The lupus inhibitor rarely causes abnormal bleeding and will occur in some cases of systemic lupus erythematosus, carcinoma, myeloma, gynecologic disorders, rheumatoid arthritis, and rarely in antibiotic therapy. Less commonly found are factor IX inhibitors which tend to act immediately, and factor V inhibitors.

The APTT (or PT) is generally the test employed for detecting circulating anticoagulants, using that test which yields abnormal results in the routine procedure.

REFERENCES

Hardisty, R.M., and Ingram, C.I.C.: *Bleeding Disorders, Investigation and Management,* Oxford, Blackwell Scientific Publications, 1965.

Lenahan, J.G., and Smith, K.: *Hemostasis,* Durham, N.C., Organon Teknika Corp., 1985.

REAGENTS AND EQUIPMENT

1. Water bath, 37°C.
2. If the APTT procedure is performed:
   a. Calcium chloride, 0.025 M.
   b. Partial thromboplastin with activator.
3. If the PT procedure is performed:
   a. Tissue thromboplastin reagent.
4. Owren's veronal buffer.
5. Normal control plasma.
6. Test tubes, 12 × 100 mm.
7. Pipets, 1.0 and 0.1 mL.
8. Stopwatch.

SPECIMEN

Citrated plasma: 1 part 0.109 M sodium citrate to 9 parts whole blood.

PRINCIPLE

Circulating anticoagulants are generally detected by performing the APTT procedure on patient plasma, normal control plasma, and on different ratios of patient and normal control plasma, at specifically timed intervals. (If the routine APTT is normal and the PT is abnormal, this test is performed using the PT procedure.) All results are recorded as indicated on a worksheet similar to the format shown in Table 13. In the presence of an inhibitor, there will be little to no correction of the clotting time when the patient's plasma is mixed with normal plasma. If a factor deficiency exists, since only 50% of plasma factors are necessary for normal coagulation times, the clotting time of the patient's plasma will show significant correction when mixed with normal plasma.

PROCEDURE

1. Place the test tube of blood in a cup containing crushed ice immediately after the blood is drawn.
2. Centrifuge the blood at 1200 to 1500 g for 15 minutes. Immediately remove the plasma and place the test tube in a cup containing crushed ice.
3. Perform an APTT (or PT) on the patient's plasma and on a normal control plasma.
4. Label four 10 × 75 mm test tubes and prepare the following mixtures (keep tubes covered when not in use):
   a. 0.9 mL patient plasma + 0.1 mL normal control plasma.
   b. 0.5 mL patient plasma + 0.5 mL normal control plasma.
   c. 0.1 mL patient plasma + 0.9 mL normal control plasma.
   d. 0.5 mL Owren's veronal buffer + 0.5 mL normal control plasma. (This mixture serves as the control.)
5. Place the four mixtures in step 3 above, in a 37°C water bath and note the beginning time of incubation.
6. Perform an APTT (or PT), in duplicate, on the four mixtures after 10, 30, 60, and 120 minutes of incubation. Average results and record.
7. Interpretation of results. To interpret the results of this procedure, compare the clotting times at the different time intervals. It must be kept in mind, however, that as the plasmas incubate, there is normally a slight increase in the clotting times because of some loss of labile components in the plasma. For this reason, attention must be paid to the clotting times of the normal control plasma. Before the clotting times of the patient's plasma and the patient-control mixture are considered prolonged, the degree of prolongation from the previously run test must be greater than that shown by the normal control plasma. See Table 13 for an example of a circulating anticoagulant and a factor deficiency.
   a. Circulating anticoagulant. If an inhibitor is present, the clotting times of the patient's plasma will not be corrected (shortened) appreciably by the addition of normal plasma. Generally, in the presence of an inhibitor, the 9:1 mixture of the patient's plasma and normal control shows no significant correction of the clotting time; the 1:1 mixture may show slight correction; and the 1:9 mixture slightly more correction. It must be kept in mind, however, that some inhibitors act progressively, and it may be a while before the clotting time of the patient plasma-normal control mixtures show the effects of the inhibitor (a prolonged clotting time). It is, therefore, important to incubate the plasma samples for 60 and 120 minutes and note these results.
   b. Factor deficiency. In the presence of a factor deficiency, the clotting time of the patient plasma samples should be corrected by the addition of normal control plasma.
8. Report results as positive or negative for circulating anticoagulants.

DISCUSSION

1. If the patient's APTT is within 10 seconds of normal (or the PT within 3 seconds of normal) the results of the test may be difficult to interpret.
2. In cases where the circulating anti-

TABLE 13. EXAMPLES OF A CIRCULATING ANTICOAGULANT AND A [FACTOR DEFICIENCY] USING THE APTT PROCEDURE

TIME (min)	PATIENT'S PLASMA (sec)	NORMAL CONT. PLASMA (sec)	1:1 PATIENT'S PLASMA AND NL. CONTROL (sec)	1:1 BUFFER AND NORMAL CONTROL (sec)	9:1 PATIENT'S PLASMA AND NL. CONTROL (sec)	1:9 PATIENT'S PLASMA AND NL. CONTROL (sec)
0	75	29				
10			83 [35]	39	89 [41]	64 [31]
30			95 [37]	40	102 [42]	78 [31]
60			99 [36]	41	114 [42]	92 [33]
120			120 [42]	44	142 [48]	115 [37]

coagulant increases with time, the APTT coagulation time may show normal or near normal results on a fresh blood specimen.

PLATELET NEUTRALIZATION PROCEDURE

The platelet neutralization procedure is used for the detection of the lupus inhibitor (anticoagulant). This procedure is more specific and sensitive for this inhibitor than the tissue thromboplastin inhibition test. The lupus inhibitor was first recognized in patients having systemic lupus erythematosus, and was thus named the 'lupus anticoagulant'. Subsequently, this inhibitor has been associated with a number of other disorders such as thrombotic conditions, recurrent fetal loss, and acquired prothrombin deficiency. The lupus anticoagulant appears to be an IgG or IgM antibody which has a specificity for negatively charged phospholipids.

REFERENCES

Triplett, D.A., Brandt, J.T., Kaczor, D., and Schaeffer, J.: Laboratory diagnosis of lupus inhibitors: A comparison of the tissue thromboplastin inhibition procedure with a new platelet neutralization procedure, Am. J. Clin. Path., 79, 678, 1983.

Lenahan, J., and Smith, K., (eds): Clotters' Corner, Durham, N.C., Organon Teknika Corp., 43, 1986.

REAGENTS AND EQUIPMENT

1. Expired platelet concentrate (obtain from the blood bank).
2. Tris buffered saline solution, pH 7.3-7.5.

   Sodium chloride   8.766 g

   Tris(hydroxymethyl) aminomethane   6.055 g

   Dilute to 1 liter with distilled water. (Also obtainable from Sigma Chemical Co.) Store in refrigerator.
3. Calcium chloride, 0.025 M.
4. APTT reagent (partial thromboplastin reagent containing activator).
5. Sodium chloride, 0.85%, w/v.
6. Centrifuge tubes, plastic, 50 mL and 15 mL.
7. Test tubes, 12 × 75 mm.
8. Pipets, 0.1 mL.
9. Stopwatch.
10. Waterbath, 37°C.

SPECIMEN

Citrated plasma: 1 part 0.109 M sodium citrate to 9 parts whole blood.

PRINCIPLE

The patient's platelet poor plasma is mixed with a suspension of ruptured platelets (source of phospholipid), APTT reagent, and calcium chloride. The clotting time is noted and compared with the clotting times of: (1) a similar mixture substituting sodium chloride for the platelets, and (2) an APTT performed on the same plasma sample. If a lupus inhibitor is present, the effects of the anticoagulant will be decreased or bypassed by the freeze-thawed platelets and the clotting time of the patient's mixture (containing the platelet suspension) will be shorter than the clotting times of both the mixture containing the saline and the original APTT.

PROCEDURE

1. Preparation of the platelet concentrate.
   a. Obtain a newly expired unit of platelet concentrate from the blood bank.
   b. Place 15 mL aliquots of the platelet concentrate into 50 mL plastic centrifuge tubes.
   c. Add 15 mL of cold tris buffered saline solution to each tube. Mix.
   d. Centrifuge each tube at 197 $\times$ g for 15 minutes to remove any red blood cells present.
   e. Remove the supernatant platelet rich plasma from each tube and transfer to 15 mL plastic centrifuge tubes. Centrifuge at 2500 $\times$ g for 10 minutes.
   f. Discard supernatant and resuspend platelets in 5 to 10 mL of tris buffered saline solution.
   g. Centrifuge at 2500 $\times$ g for 10 minutes.
   h. Repeat steps f and g above 2 more times so that the platelets have been washed three times.
   i. Remove the supernatant from the final wash and resuspend the platelets in an amount of tris buffered saline sufficient to give a platelet count between 200,000 and 300,000/μL.
   j. Place 1 mL aliquots of the platelet suspension into test tubes, stopper, and place in a freezer at a temperature of $-20°C$ or below. (These platelet suspensions are stable for approximately 3 months stored at this temperature.)

2. Centrifuge patient's plasma at 2500 $\times$ g for 10 minutes in order to obtain platelet poor plasma.

3. Remove one tube of the frozen platelet suspension from the freezer and allow to thaw at room temperature.

4. Perform a routine APTT on the patient's plasma. It should be at least 5 to 10 seconds above the normal range.

5. Prewarm a sufficient volume of 0.025 M calcium chloride at 37°C.

6. Place 0.1 mL of APTT reagent into a 12 $\times$ 75 mm test tube and place in the 37°C water bath. Add 0.1 mL of patient plasma to the tube. Mix. Add 0.1 mL of the thawed platelet suspension and start a stopwatch. Mix the contents of the tube well and allow to incubate for 5 minutes at 37°C.

7. At the end of exactly 5 minutes, add 0.1 mL of calcium chloride to the tube, simultaneously starting a stopwatch. Tilt the tube back and forth and stop the watch as soon as clotting is detected.

8. Perform the test in duplicate.

9. Repeat steps 5, 6, 7, and 8, for the patient control, substituting 0.1 mL of sodium chloride for the 0.1 mL of thawed platelet suspension.

10. A positive and negative control should also be run with this test. Pooled normal plasma may be used as the normal control.

11. Interpretation of results. In the presence of a lupus inhibitor, the clotting time of the patient's plasma mixed with the thawed platelet suspension should be at least 5 seconds shorter than the patient's control mixture (containing the saline solution in place of the thawed platelet suspension) and also shorter than the original APTT. It may not necessarily completely correct the APTT, however. Generally, the more prolonged the original APTT is, the greater will be the shortening of the clotting time with the thawed platelet suspension. False-positive results may be encountered in patients who are receiving heparin and in patients with factor V inhibitors.

DISCUSSION

1. If the patient's plasma is frozen prior

to performing this test, it is imperative that there be no platelets present in the plasma prior to freezing.

2. The prepared platelet suspension must be frozen before use. The freezing and thawing of the platelet suspension causes the platelets to rupture, freeing the phospholipid from the platelet.

3. If a lupus inhibitor is present, it can interfere with the action of heparin in open heart surgery.

4. Use of a positive control is necessary in order to monitor the effectiveness of the thawed platelet suspension.

5. This test may be performed manually, on the Fibrometer or similar instrument, or by use of a photo-optical detection instrument. For interpretation of results all tests (including the APTT) should be performed using the same method.

ANTITHROMBIN III

Antithrombin III slowly and progressively destroys the activated forms of factors XII, XI, IX, X, and kallikrein, and most importantly, it destroys thrombin. It is also thought of as a heparin cofactor in that heparin, when present, forms a complex with antithrombin III. The anticoagulant effect of heparin is catalytic, dramatically increasing the inhibitory effects of the antithrombin III. A deficiency may be inherited or acquired. It will be decreased in thrombotic disease, disseminated intravascular coagulation, and in women taking oral contraceptives. Antithrombin III may be measured by electroimmunoassay, radial immunodiffusion, by the neutralization of thrombin (described below), and by chromogenic methods (described below).

Neutralization of Thrombin Method

REFERENCES

Lenahan, J.G., and Smith, K.: *Hemostasis,* Durham, N.C., Organon Teknika Corp., 1985.
Zuck, T.F., Bergin, J.J., Raymond, J.M., and Dwyre,

W.R.: Implications of depressed antithrombin III activity associated with oral contraceptives, Surg., Gynecol. Obstet., *133*, 609, 1971.

REAGENTS AND EQUIPMENT

1. Barbital acetate buffer, pH 7.32 to 7.52.

Solution A

Sodium acetate	9.714 g
Sodium barbital	14.714 g

Dilute to 500 ml with distilled water.

Solution B

Hydrochloric acid, 0.1 N	5.0 mL
Sodium chloride, 0.85%, w/v	2.0 mL
Distilled water	15.0 mL
Solution A	5.0 mL

Working barbital acetate buffer, pH 7.32 to 7.52.

Solution B	1 part
Sodium chloride, 0.85%. w/v	4 parts

2. Stock thrombin (200 U/mL). Reconstitute 1 vial of Bovine Thrombin, Topical, 1,000 NIH units (Parke, Davis and Co.) with 5.0 mL of 50% glycerol (v/v).

3. Working thrombin reagent (100 U/mL). Mix equal parts of the stock thrombin with barbital acetate buffer.

4. Bovine fibrinogen. (May be obtained from Sigma Chemical Co., St. Louis, Mo.) Reconstitute according to manufacturer's directions.

5. Glass test tubes, 12 × 75mm.

6. Water bath, 37°C.

7. Pipets, 1.0, 0.1, and 0.2 mL.

8. Stopwatch.

SPECIMEN

Whole blood, 5 mL, placed in a plain test tube, 13 × 100 mm in size. A normal control blood from a male donor should be obtained at the same time the patient's blood is collected.

PRINCIPLE

Whole blood is allowed to clot and then incubated at 37°C for 2 hours during which time, 20 to 30% of the antithrombin III present in the blood will be consumed. The serum is then incubated with a specific amount of thrombin for 6 minutes. During this period, the antithrombin III present will neutralize the added thrombin. Fibrinogen is then added to the serum-thrombin mixture, and the clotting time is noted. The lower the concentration of antithrombin III originally present in the patient's plasma, the less thrombin will be neutralized and the shorter will be the clotting time when fibrinogen is added.

PROCEDURE

1. Allow the patient's and control blood specimens to clot. Incubate at 37°C for 2 hours.
2. Centrifuge the blood specimens at 1500 × g for 10 minutes. Remove the serums and place in appropriately labeled test tubes.
3. Label 12 × 75 mm test tubes: one for each patient, normal control, and abnormal control.
4. Place 0.6 mL of normal control and patient's serums into appropriately labeled test tubes. Pipet 0.6 mL of 0.85% sodium chloride into the abnormal control test tube.
5. Incubate the patient's serum test tube at 37°C for 1 minute.
6. Add 0.15 mL of the working thrombin reagent to the patient's serum test tube. Mix. Start the stopwatch.
7. When 5 minutes have elapsed on the stopwatch, place 0.1 mL of the fibrinogen solution in a 12 × 75 mm test tube and place in the 37°C water bath.
8. When exactly 6 minutes have elapsed on the stopwatch, add 0.2 mL of the patient's serum-thrombin mixture to the 0.1 mL of fibrinogen. Start the stopwatch. Gently tilt the test tube backward and forward until a clot forms, at which point the timing is stopped. Record the results.
9. Repeat steps 5 through 8 for the normal and abnormal control specimens.
10. Interpretation of results. The abnormal control should yield a clotting time between 4 and 8 seconds. (This control measures the activity of the thrombin solution.) The normal control should give a result greater than 30 seconds, but this result will depend on the normal range for the test as determined for your particular laboratory. Patient results of less than 30 seconds generally indicate a decreased concentration of antithrombin III.

DISCUSSION

1. If hemolysis is present in the patient or normal control serum, the specimen should be recollected. Hemolysis or the presence of red blood cells will cause an increased consumption of prothrombin, causing lower antithrombin III activity in the serum.
2. Following the 2-hour incubation period, the serum may be frozen for up to 24 hours with little loss in antithrombin III activity.
3. The 2-hour incubation period is critical for closely standardizing the loss of antithrombin III activity.
4. The 6-minute incubation period for the serum-thrombin mixture is critical. Excessive incubation will inactivate the added thrombin.
5. The thrombin solution may have to be adjusted to yield a clotting time of 4 to 8 seconds for the abnormal control when a new lot of thrombin or fibrinogen is used.

Chromogenic Assay

REFERENCE

Organon Teknika Corp.: Chromostrate® Antithrombin III Assay, pkg. insert, Durham, N.C., Organon Teknika Corp., 1986.

REAGENTS AND EQUIPMENT

1. Chromostrate® assay kit (Organon Teknika Corp.).
   a. Substrate reagent (H-D-cyclo-hexyl tyrosyl-L-alpha amino bu-tyryl-L-arginine-paranitroanilide). Reconstitute according to directions. May be stored in the refrigerator for 30 days after reconstitution.
   b. Thrombin reagent. Reconstitute according to directions. May be stored in the refrigerator for 7 days after reconstitution.
   c. Buffer concentrate (contains sodium azide as preservative). Dilute 1:10 with distilled water for working buffer solution. Store in refrigerator for up to 30 days after dilution.
2. Chromostrate reference plasma (Organon Teknika Corp.). Reconstitute according to directions.
3. Acetic acid, 50% (v/v).
4. Plastic test tubes, 12 × 75 mm.
5. Plastic pipets, 2.0, 1.0, 0.05, and 0.2 mL.
6. Stopwatch.
7. Verify normal citrate control (Organon Teknika Corp.).
8. Linear graph paper.
9. Water bath, 37°C.
10. Spectrophotometer, wavelength of 405 nm.

SPECIMEN

Citrated plasma: 1 part 0.109 M sodium citrate or buffered sodium citrate to 9 parts whole blood.

PRINCIPLE

Plasma is incubated with an excess amount of thrombin. During this time, the antithrombin III present will neutralize the thrombin. Upon addition of the substrate, the remaining thrombin will catalyze the release of paranitroanilide (from the substrate). The amount of paranitroanilide released is then measured by the spectrophotometer and the reading compared to the calibration curve to determine the amount of antithrombin III present. The concentration of antithrombin III is inversely proportional to the amount of paranitroanilide released.

PROCEDURE

1. Centrifuge the patient's specimen at 1500 × g for 10 minutes to obtain platelet poor plasma.
2. Preparation of the calibration curve.
   a. Reconstitute Chromostrate reference plasma according to directions on the vial.
   b. Prepare a 1:40 dilution (100%) by adding 0.05 mL of reference plasma to 1.95 mL of working buffer. Prepare a 1:80 dilution (50%) by mixing 1.0 mL of the 1:40 dilution with 1.0 mL of working buffer. Prepare a 1:160 dilution (25%) by adding 1.0 mL of the 1:80 dilution to 1.0 mL of working buffer.
3. Prepare 1:40 dilutions (in duplicate) of the patient and control plasmas: Add 0.05 mL of the plasma to be tested to 1.95 mL of working buffer solution.
4. Label three 12 × 75 mm test tubes for each plasma dilution. Two tubes will be used for the test (to be performed in duplicate) and the third tube will be used as the blank.
5. Add 0.2 mL of the plasma dilution to the first test tube and incubate at 37°C for 3 to 5 minutes.
6. Add 0.2 mL of thrombin to the tube, mix, and incubate at 37°C for exactly 60 seconds.
7. Add 0.2 mL of substrate reagent, mix, and incubate at 37°C for exactly 30 seconds.
8. Add 0.2 mL of 50% acetic acid to the tube and immediately mix well.
9. Repeat steps 5 through 8 above for each plasma dilution, performing the test in duplicate.

10. Prepare the blank for each dilution by mixing together 0.2 mL of the plasma dilution, 0.4 mL distilled water, and 0.2 mL of 50% acetic acid.

11. Read the absorbance of all samples in the spectrophotometer at a wavelength of 405 nm, against a water blank, using a semi-micro cuvet with a 1-cm light path. Average the absorbance readings for the duplicate samples and subtract the reading of the blank. To determine the percent activity of the reference dilution, multiply the percent (1.0, 0.50, or 0.25) by the assay value as assigned for that lot of reference plasma. Plot the 3 points on linear graph paper (O.D. vs. % activity) and draw a straight line which best fits all 3 points.

12. To determine the % activity of antithrombin III for each plasma, refer to the calibration curve.

DISCUSSION

1. Addition of the 50% acetic acid stops the reaction. It is therefore imperative that the tube be mixed well as soon as the acetic acid is added. Once added, the color remains stable for several hours.

2. This test measures the functional potential of antithrombin III. The test results will therefore not always correlate with immunochemical assays.

3. Each laboratory should determine its own normal range. The normal range given with this procedure (to be used as a guide) is 85 to 111% activity.

4. As soon as the blood specimen is obtained, the plasma should be removed and placed at refrigerator temperatures. Testing should be performed within 4 hours after sample collection. The plasma may be frozen rapidly and stored for up to 30 days without loss of antithrombin III activity.

5. This procedure may be adapted to kinetic analysis. See the package insert for an outline of this method.

HEPARIN ASSAY

Heparin binds with antithrombin III. When this occurs there is an immediate anticoagulant effect. The procedure described below is a chromogenic method for assaying the amount of heparin present in plasma.

REFERENCE

Organon Teknika Corp.: Chromostrate™ Heparin Assay, pkg. insert, Durham, N.C., Organon Teknika Corp., 1986.

REAGENTS AND EQUIPMENT

1. Chromostrate™ heparin assay kit (obtainable from Organon Teknika Corp.).

   a. Substrate reagent (H-D-cyclohexyl tyrosyl-L-alpha amino butyryl-L-arginine-paranitroanilide). Reconstitute according to directions. May be stored in the refrigerator for 30 days after reconstitution.

   b. Thrombin reagent. Reconstitute according to directions. May be stored in refrigerator for up to 72 hours after reconstitution.

   c. Antithrombin III reagent. Reconstitute as directed. May be stored in the refrigerator for 7 days after reconstitution.

   d. Buffer concentrate (contains sodium azide as a preservative). Dilute 1:10 with distilled water for working buffer solution. Store in refrigerator for up to 30 days after dilution.

2. Acetic acid, 50% (v/v).

3. Heparin (same source as used in the patient's therapy).

4. Plastic test tubes, 12 × 75 mm.

5. Plastic pipets, 5.0, 1.0, 0.1, and 0.2 mL.

6. Stopwatch.

7. Verify H control plasma (Organon Teknika).

8. Normal (platelet poor) plasma pool.
9. Linear graph paper,.
10. Water bath, 37°C.
11. Spectrophotometer, wavelength of 405 nm.

SPECIMEN

Citrated plasma: 1 part 0.109 sodium citrate to 9 parts whole blood.

PRINCIPLE

The patient's plasma (containing heparin) is incubated with measured amounts of antithrombin III and thrombin (in excess). A complex of heparin, antithrombin III, and thrombin is then formed. Substrate reagent is added to the mixture and during incubation the remaining (excess) thrombin catalyzes the release of paranitroanilide from the chromogenic substrate. The amount of paranitroanilide (pNA) released is then measured by the spectrophotometer and the reading compared to the calibration curve to determine the amount of heparin present. The heparin concentration is inversely proportional to the amount of paranitroanilide released. (The more heparin present, the more thrombin neutralized and the less thrombin available to release pNA from the substrate reagent.)

PROCEDURE

1. Centrifuge the patient's specimen at 1800 × g for 15 minutes to obtain platelet poor plasma.
2. Preparation of calibration curve.
   a. Prepare a stock solution of heparin, 5 U/mL. Dilute the stock solution 1:50 with working buffer solution (0.1 mL of stock heparin + 4.9 mL of working buffer) for a concentration of 0.1 U/mL.
   b. Prepare standards for the calibration curve using the volumes shown in Table 14. (Equivalent heparin levels correspond to the patient and control samples being diluted 1:10 for testing.) (Anti-

thrombin III is added in case there is any deficiency of this factor in the normal pooled plasma.)
   c. Test each standard, in duplicate, as described below (steps 5 through 8) for the patient and control plasmas.
3. Prepare a 1:10 dilution of the patient and control plasmas: 0.1 mL of plasma to be tested + 0.8 mL working buffer + 0.1 mL of antithrombin III reagent. Mix.
4. Label three 12 × 75 mm test tubes for each patient, control, and standard to be tested. (Two tubes are for the test [to be performed in duplicate] and the third tube is for the blank.)
5. Add 0.2 mL of the plasma dilution to the first tube and incubate at 37°C for 3 to 5 minutes.
6. Add 0.2 mL of thrombin to the tube, mix, and incubate at 37°C for exactly 30 seconds.
7. Add 0.2 mL of substrate reagent, mix, and incubate at 37°C for exactly 30 seconds.
8. Add 0.2 mL of 50% acetic acid to the tube and immediately mix well.
9. Repeat steps 5 through 8 for each sample dilution, performing each test in duplicate.
10. Prepare the blank for each dilution by mixing together 0.2 mL of the plasma dilution, 0.4 mL distilled water, and 0.2 mL of 50% acetic acid.
11. Read the absorbance of all samples in the spectrophotometer at a wavelength of 405 nm, against a water blank, using a semi-micro cuvet with a 1-cm light path. Average the absorbance readings for the duplicate samples and subtract the reading of the blank.
12. Plot the 4 points of the heparin standards on linear graph paper (O.D. vs. heparin concentration [U/mL]) and connect the points by a straight line which best fits all points.

TABLE 14. DILUTIONS FOR HEPARIN ASSAY CURVE

EQUIVALENT HEPARIN LEVEL U/mL	PPP POOL (mL)	HEPARIN SOLUTION (0.1 U/mL) (mL)	WORKING BUFFER (mL)	ANTITHROMBIN III REAGENT (mL)
0.1	0.1	0.1	0.7	0.1
0.2	0.1	0.2	0.6	0.1
0.4	0.1	0.4	0.4	0.1
0.6	0.1	0.6	0.2	0.2

13. To determine the U/mL of heparin in each plasma and control, refer to the calibration curve.

DISCUSSION

1. To measure the actual heparin effect in the patient's plasma, substitute 0.1 mL of working buffer for the 0.1 mL of antithrombin III reagent in the plasma dilution. (Patient's plasma would be diluted: 0.1 mL patient's plasma + 0.9 mL working buffer.)
2. This procedure may be adapted to kinetic analysis. See the procedure as outlined in the package insert.
3. Once the acetic acid is added to the test mixture the color is stable for several hours.
4. The blood specimen should be centrifuged within 1 hour of collection and should not sit for more than 2 hours at 2° to 8°C. The plasma may be frozen rapidly and stored for up to 30 days.

PROTAMINE SULFATE TITRATION FOR HEPARIN NEUTRALIZATION

The effects of heparin in vivo may be neutralized by the administration of protamine sulfate. In excess, however, protamine sulfate is capable of interfering with factor IX activity and with thromboplastin generation. The protamine titration, therefore, is used to estimate the minimum required dose which will neutralize the effects of the heparin present.

REFERENCE

Sirridge, M.S., and Shannon, R.: *Laboratory Evaluation of Hemostasis and Thrombosis*, 3rd Ed., Philadelphia, Lea & Febiger, 1983.

REAGENTS AND EQUIPMENT

1. Barbital buffered saline solution, pH 7.35.
2. Protamine sulfate, 1%. Obtain from the hospital pharmacy. (This should be the same protamine sulfate which is used by the patient.) Store at 4°C.
3. Thrombin solution. Prepare as directed for the Thrombin Time procedure.
4. Test tubes, 12 × 75 mm.
5. Pipets, 2.0, 1.0, and 0.1 mL.
6. Normal plasma control.
7. Water bath, 37°C.
8. Stopwatch.

SPECIMEN

Citrated plasma: 1 part 0.109 M buffered sodium citrate to 9 parts whole blood.

PRINCIPLE

Varying concentrations of protamine sulfate are added to the patient's plasma. Thrombin is added to this mixture and the clotting time noted. The lowest concentration of protamine sulfate needed to clot the patient's plasma in the same time as the normal control plasma, is used to calculate the amount of protamine sulfate needed to neutralize the effects of heparin in the patient.

PROCEDURE

1. Centrifuge blood at 1500 × g for 10 minutes to obtain platelet poor plasma.
2. Prepare a stock protamine solution of 100 μg/mL by diluting 1 mL of 1% protamine sulfate to 100 mL with barbital buffered saline solution.

3. Label 10 tubes #1 through #10 for the protamine dilutions, and prepare as shown in Table 15.

4. Immediately before use, prepare thrombin as described for the Thrombin Time procedure. (A clotting time of 10 to 15 seconds should be obtained using the normal control plasma.)

5. Perform a thrombin time on the normal control plasma and the patient's plasma mixing 0.1 mL of the plasma, 0.1 mL of barbital buffered saline solution, and 0.1 mL of thrombin. If the clotting time of the patient is within 1 second of the normal control, there is no demonstrable heparin in the patient's specimen and the test may be stopped at this point. If the patient's clotting time is prolonged, proceed with this test.

6. Label ten 12 × 75 mm test tubes for each patient to be tested. Place 0.1 mL of patient plasma into each tube. Transfer 0.1 mL of protamine sulfate dilution into the appropriately numbered tube.

7. Testing each plasma-protamine sulfate mixture separately, incubate the tube in the water bath for 1 minute. Add 0.1 mL of thrombin simultaneously starting the stopwatch. Record the clotting time.

8. Determine the lowest dilution of protamine sulfate which gives a clotting time within 1 second of the normal control. Report this concentration of protamine sulfate in μg/mL. This figure is then multiplied by the patient's estimated plasma volume to determine the total dose of protamine sulfate needed to neutralize the effects of the heparin.

FIBRINOGEN DEGRADATION PRODUCTS

Fibrinogen degradation products (FDP) may be demonstrated in the blood of patients with primary fibrinolysis and during the process of disseminated intravascular coagulation with secondary fibrinolysis. This test will also be elevated in any kind of a thrombotic state including postoperative deep vein thrombosis, myocardial infarction, and in certain disorders of pregnancy. Slight to moderate increases of FDP will also be seen in alcoholic cirrhosis of the liver and during late pregnancy.

The Thrombo-Wellcotest procedure described here is a rapid, sensitive test for fibrinogen degradation products present in the blood. The normal level of serum FDP in the adult is less than 8 μg/mL.

Thrombo-Wellcotest Procedure

REFERENCE

Wellcome Diagnostics: Thrombo-Wellcotest. Rapid latex test for detection of fibrinogen degradation products, Dartford, England, The Wellcome Foundation Ltd., 1986.

REAGENTS AND EQUIPMENT

1. The following reagents are available

TABLE 15.   PROTAMINE SULFATE DILUTIONS

SOLUTION	TUBE									
	1	2	3	4	5	6	7	8	9	10
Barbital buffered saline solution (mL)	1.0	1.1	1.2	1.3	1.4	1.5	1.6	1.7	1.8	1.9
Protamine sulfate (100 μg/mL) (mL)	1.0	0.9	0.8	0.7	0.6	0.5	0.4	0.3	0.2	0.1
Final conc. protamine sulfate (μg/mL)	50	45	40	35	30	25	20	15	10	5

from Burroughs Wellcome Co., Research Triangle Park, N. C. All reagents must be refrigerated when not in use.

a. Sample collection tubes (contain thrombin to cause rapid and complete clotting and soya bean enzyme inhibitors to prevent the breakdown of fibrin).

b. Glycine saline buffer.

c. Latex suspension. (The latex particles have been sensitized with an anti-fibrinogen degradation product globulin.)

d. Positive and negative control serums.

e. Glass test slide.

f. Disposable pipet droppers.

g. Disposable mixing rods.

2. Test tubes, 10 × 75 mm.

SPECIMEN

Using a clean, dry syringe, obtain 2.0 mL of blood from the patient and transfer immediately to the sample collection tube. These tubes may also be used with a Vacutainer system and will draw 2 mL of blood. As soon as the blood is in the tube, mix well by inverting several times. (A minimum of 0.5 mL of whole blood may be added to the collection tube if larger volumes are not available.)

PRINCIPLE

Whole blood is added to thrombin (to ensure complete clotting) and soya bean enzyme inhibitors (to prevent breakdown of fibrin). After complete clotting, the patient's serum is diluted and mixed with latex particles coated with anti-FDP. If fibrinogen degradation products are present, agglutination of the latex particles will occur.

PROCEDURE

1. As soon as the blood sample arrives in the laboratory, ring the clot with an applicator stick to allow for clot retraction. Incubate the tube at room temperature for 30 to 60 minutes. (If the patient is receiving heparin, Reptilase-R should be added to the patient's blood in the sample collection tube in order for complete clotting to occur. Reconstitute the Reptilase-R with 1.0 mL of distilled water. Add 0.1 mL of the reconstituted Reptilase-R to each 1.0 mL of whole blood in the tube.)

2. At the end of the incubation period, centrifuge the specimen for 5 minutes at 1500 × g. (The blood must be completely clotted before centrifuging.)

3. Carefully remove the serum and place in 10 × 75 mm test tube. No red blood cells should be present.

4. Label two 10 × 75 mm test tubes 1:5 and 1:10 for each specimen and control to be tested. Using the graduated dropper from the test kit, place 0.75 mL of the glycine buffer into the test tube labeled 1:5. Using a disposable dropper from the test kit, add 5 drops of the patient's serum to this test tube. Mix. Using a disposable dropper from the test kit, place 4 drops of glycine buffer into the test tube labeled 1:10. Transfer 4 drops of diluted serum from the test tube labeled 1:5 to the test tube labeled 1:10.

5. Label rings on the glass slide: positive, negative, 1:5, and 1:10.

6. Place 1 drop of each control serum in the appropriate ring. Transfer 1 drop of the 1:5 dilution and 1 drop of the 1:10 dilution to the appropriate rings on the glass slide. (Allow all drops to fall freely from the pipet. Do not touch the pipet to the glass slide during this process.)

7. Mix the latex suspension of the anti-fibrinogen degradation products globulin vigorously. Immediately add 1 drop to each of the serum dilutions and control specimens.

8. Using a separate applicator stick for each sample, quickly stir each mix-

ture, spreading over the entire area of the ring. Immediately set a clock for 2 minutes.

9. Rotate the slide for exactly 2 minutes, using a backward and forward motion. Examine each mixture for macroscopic agglutination. Determine the presence or absence of agglutination immediately after the 2-minute mixing period. False positive results may occur after the 2-minute period because of drying effects. The appearance of graininess must not be interpreted as macroscopic agglutination.

10. Interpretation of results (see Table 16). The negative and positive control specimens must show no agglutination and agglutination, respectively.

11. If the 1:10 dilution of the patient's plasma shows agglutination, further dilutions of the patient's plasma should be made as described below. If qualitative results only are desired, the result may be reported as >20 μg/mL. If semi-quantitative results are desired, continue with this procedure.

12. Label four 10 × 75 mm test tubes 1:20, 1:40, 1:80, and 1:160. Using the disposable pipet, place 4 drops of glycine buffer into each of the test tubes. Transfer 4 drops of the patient's 1:10 dilution into the test tube labeled 1:20. Mix and transfer 4 drops of the 1:20 dilution to the test tube labeled 1:40. Mix and transfer 4 drops of the 1:40 mixture to the test tube labeled 1:80. Mix and transfer 4 drops of the 1:80 dilution to the test tube labeled 1:160.

13. Label the rings on the glass slide for each of the above dilutions and for the negative and positive control specimens.

14. Place 1 drop of each control serum and 1 drop from each patient dilution onto the appropriate ring on the glass slide. Repeat steps 7, 8, and 9 above and interpret the results as shown in Table 16.

DISCUSSION

1. This procedure may also be performed using a urine sample. For the exact procedure, the reader is referred to the Thrombo-Wellcotest package insert.

2. The centrifuged serum sample may be refrigerated for up to 1 week or stored at −20°C for longer periods before performing the test.

3. False-positive results may occur in patients with rheumatoid arthritis (patients positive for the rheumatoid factor).

4. It is suggested that a positive and negative control be run on each slide. When interpreting the results, compare the patient's sample with the positive and negative controls to de-

TABLE 16.   FIBRINOGEN-DEGRADATION PRODUCTS
(Interpretation of Results)

PLASMA DILUTION	PATIENT RESULTS (− = no agglutination, + = agglutination)						
1:5	−	+	+	+	+	+	+
1:10	−	−	+	+	+	+	+
1:20			−	+	+	+	+
1:40				−	−	+	+	+
1:80					−	−	+	+
1:160					−	−	−	+
Results (μg/mL)	<10	10− 20	20− 40	40− 80	80− 160	160− 320	>320

termine the presence of agglutination.

ETHANOL GELATION TEST

The ethanol gelation test is designed to detect the presence of fibrin monomers in the plasma. It is a screening procedure to be utilized as an aid in the diagnosis of disseminated intravascular coagulation and in distinguishing this condition from primary fibrinolysis.

REFERENCE

Breen, F.A., Jr., and Tullis, J.L.: Ethanol gelation: A rapid screening test for intravascular coagulation, Ann. Intern. Med., 69, 1197, 1968.

REAGENTS AND EQUIPMENT

1. Buffered sodium citrate
   Sodium citrate, 0.11 M   3 parts
   Citric acid, 0.1 M   2 parts
   (19.2 g dissolved in
   1 liter of distilled water.)
2. Plastic test tubes, 10 × 75 mm.
3. Disposable dropper pipets.
4. Sodium hydroxide, 0.1 N.
5. Ethyl alcohol, 50%, v/v.
6. Plastic dropper pipets.

SPECIMEN

Citrated plasma: 1 part 0.11 M buffered sodium citrate to 9 parts whole blood. Obtain blood for a normal control at the same time the patient's specimen is drawn.

PRINCIPLE

During the process of disseminated intravascular coagulation, the level of fibrin monomer (intermediate product of fibrinogen breakdown to fibrin) in the blood increases. Sodium hydroxide is added to the plasma to increase the pH to above pH 7.70. Ethyl alcohol, then added to the plasma, causes precipitation of any fibrin monomers which may be present.

PROCEDURE

1. Centrifuge the patient's blood at 1200 to 1500 g for 15 minutes in order to obtain platelet poor plasma.
2. Into two appropriately labeled 10 × 75 mm test tubes, place 9 drops of patient's plasma and normal control plasma.
3. Add 1 drop of 0.1 N sodium hydroxide and mix tubes gently.
4. Add 3 drops of 50% ethyl alcohol to each tube. Mix gently and place in a test tube rack at room temperature.
5. At the end of 1 minute, inspect tubes for the presence of a precipitate. Precipitation or gel formation, at this time, generally constitutes a positive test.
6. If the test is negative after 1 minute, allow the test tubes to sit for 9 additional minutes. At the end of this time, if a precipitate or gel forms, add 1 more drop of 0.1 N sodium hydroxide to the tube and gently mix. If the precipitate formed is nonspecific, it will disappear. Persistence of the precipitate or gel constitutes a positive test.

DISCUSSION

1. A positive control may be prepared and used with this test. Dilute 1,000 NIH units of thrombin (Parke, Davis, and Co. may be used) with 10.0 mL of 0.85% sodium chloride. Add 1.2 μL of diluted thrombin to 4.0 mL of normal plasma for a final concentration of thrombin (in the plasma-thrombin mixture) of 0.03 NIH units/mL. Incubate mixture at 37°C for 30 minutes. After incubation, carefully remove the fibrin strands present in the mixture, using two applicator sticks. (If there are no fibrin strands present, this most probably indicates that the concentration of the thrombin was not sufficient to begin clotting the fibrinogen and there will, therefore, be no fibrin monomers present.) The resultant plasma should test positive for fibrin monomers according to the above procedure.

2. This test must be performed at room temperature. Temperatures of 37°C inhibit gel formation.
3. The final concentration of ethyl alcohol in the final test mixture should be between 10 and 15%.
4. If the pH of the plasma is below 7.70, precipitation of fibrinogen may occur when the ethyl alcohol is added.
5. Perform test as soon as possible after collection. Storage of blood at 4°C for 24 hours does not appear to affect results.
6. The presence of heparin, or contamination with red blood cells, does not alter the results of this test.

PROTAMINE SULFATE

The protamine sulfate procedure is used to detect the presence of fibrin monomers. During the process of coagulation, when thrombin acts on fibrinogen, fibrinopeptides A and B are removed from the fibrinogen molecule, leaving fibrin monomers (which are then free to polymerize and form fibrin). Protamine sulfate detects the presence of fibrin monomers by causing the formation of fibrin strands or gel-like clots (this process is also termed paracoagulation). Early fibrin(ogen) degradation products (fragments X and Y) will also form fibrin strands and/or a gel clot in the presence of protamine sulfate.

Under certain pathologic conditions, intravascular coagulation may be stimulated and there will be widespread appearance of fibrin clots in the blood vessels of the microcirculation. Fibrin monomers are, therefore, present in the plasma. Because of the presence of coagulation, there is stimulation of the fibrinolytic system and the formation of fibrin(ogen) split products. Rapid detection of the presence of fibrin monomers is an important aid in the diagnosis of disseminated intravascular coagulation. The presence of fibrin monomers is also associated with pulmonary embolism, cirrhosis of the liver, deep vein thrombosis, and acute thromboembolism.

Normally, there should be no fibrin monomers present in the plasma.

REFERENCES

American Dade: Data-Fi protamine sulfate reagents, pkg. insert, Aguada, Puerto Rico, American Hospital Supply, 1985.
Niewiarowski, S., and Gurewich, V.: Laboratory identification of intravascular coagulation, J. Lab. Clin. Med., *77*, 665, 1971.

REAGENTS AND EQUIPMENT

1. The following reagents are available from American Dade, American Hospital Supply:
   a. Data-Fi protamine sulfate reagent 0.2% (w/v). Store at 2° to 8°C. Reconstitute with 3.0 mL of distilled water. Once reconstituted, this reagent is stable for 8 hours at 2° to 8°C.
   b. Data-Fi positive monomer control plasma. Store at 2° to 8°C. Reconstitute with 1.5 mL of distilled water while constantly agitating the vial. If the control is not correctly reconstituted, the fibrin monomers may polymerize and form fibrin strands. If no more than one or two strands form, they may be removed with applicator sticks and the control should not be affected. Reconstituted reagent is stable for 4 hours at 2° to 8°C.
2. Test tubes, 13 × 100 mm and 10 × 75 mm.
3. Pipets, 1.0 and 0.2 mL.
4. Timer.
5. Sodium chloride, 0.85% (w/v).
6. Ice bath.

SPECIMEN

Citrated plasma: 1 part 0.11 M sodium citrate to 9 parts whole blood. Place specimen in crushed ice as soon as it is collected. Obtain a normal control plasma at the same time the patient sample is obtained. The test should be set up immediately after collection.

PRINCIPLE

Patient and control plasmas are mixed with varying dilutions of protamine sulfate. Each tube is incubated at room temperature for 30 minutes and then observed for fibrin strand or gel formation. The protamine sulfate causes gel formation of fibrin monomers and/or early fibrin split products when they are present in the plasma.

PROCEDURE

1. Centrifuge the patient's blood specimen immediately after collection at 1200 to 1500 g for 15 minutes.
2. Label five 13 × 100 mm test tubes 1:5, 1:10, 1:20, 1:40, and 1:80. Add 1.0 mL of 0.85% sodium chloride to each tube except the tube labeled 1:5.
3. Reconstitute the Data-Fi protamine sulfate reagent and the Dati-Fi positive monomer control as outlined previously.
4. Pour the entire contents of the vial of protamine sulfate reagent into the tube labeled 1:5. Transfer 1.0 mL of protamine sulfate from the 1:5 tube into the tube labeled 1:10. Mix contents of tube well and transfer 1.0 mL of the diluted reagent to the next tube (1:20). Continue to dilute the protamine sulfate reagent in this manner (transfer 1 mL of mixture from 1:20 tube to the 1:40 tube, mix, etc.) in order to obtain the 1:40 and 1:80 dilutions.
5. Label one set of 10 × 75 mm test tubes 1:5, 1:10, 1:20, 1:40, and 1:80 for each patient and control to be tested. Label each set with the patient's name and/or control type.
6. Pipet 0.2 mL of patient plasma into each tube in the appropriately labeled set. Repeat for the normal and abnormal control.
7. Add 0.2 mL of the appropriate protamine sulfate reagent dilution to each tube of the patient, normal control, and abnormal control. Use a

clean pipet for each tube, and mix by forcefully expelling the reagent into the plasma. Do not agitate or mix the tubes any further.

8. Incubate all tubes at room temperature for 30 minutes. Do not disturb the tubes during this period.
9. At the end of 30 minutes, tilt each tube several times and observe for fibrin strands or gel formation. Use of a bright light against a dark background is helpful for reading the results. Report the test as positive or negative for fibrin monomers.
10. The positive fibrin monomer control should show clot or strand formation in the tubes labeled 1:5, 1:10, and 1:20. If it does not, repeat the test, reconstituting another vial of fibrin monomer control and another vial of protamine sulfate.
11. The normal control should show no fibrin strands or gel formation.

DISCUSSION

1. Fibrinogen may at times be precipitated by the protamine sulfate especially in the 1:5 and 1:10 dilutions. This shows up as an amorphous, whitish precipitate which will usually clear upon shaking the tube. Continued tilting of the tubes will cause the precipitate to break up. This should not be interpreted as clot or fibrin strand formation.
2. With positive results, continued tilting of the tubes with fibrin strand formation will cause the strands to accumulate into larger fibrin clots, while the plasma becomes clear.
3. Due to the sensitivity of this test, a positive result should be evaluated in light of other clinical findings. However, a negative result for this test does not automatically rule out intravascular coagulation since fibrin monomers and early fibrin(ogen) split products may not al-

ways be present at all stages of the process.

4. This test procedure is not affected by therapeutic levels of heparin.

5. The ethanol gelation test is easier to perform than the protamine sulfate procedure but may not be quite as sensitive to small quantities of fibrin monomers and early fibrin(ogen) split products. The protamine sulfate test is somewhat quantitative in that the more dilute the protamine sulfate tube showing positive results, the higher the concentration of fibrin monomers and/or early fibrin(ogen) split products.

EUGLOBULIN CLOT LYSIS TIME

The euglobulin clot lysis time is a screening procedure for the measurement of fibrinolytic activity. It is a more sensitive test than the clot lysis time. The euglobulin fraction of plasma contains plasminogen, plasminogen activator, and fibrinogen. Once a clot is formed in the euglobulin portion of the plasma, clot lysis occurs more quickly than in whole blood. Increased fibrinolytic activity has been associated with circulatory collapse, adrenalin injections, sudden death, pulmonary surgery, pyrogen reactions, and obstetric complications. Normally, clot lysis does not occur in less than 1 hour using the following procedure. Clot lysis in less than 60 minutes is indicative of abnormal fibrinolytic activity.

REFERENCES

Chakrabarti, M., Bielawiec, J.F., Evans, J.F., and Fearnley, G.R.: Methodological study and a recommended technique for determining the euglobulin lysis time, J. Clin. Path., *21*, 698, 1968.
American Dade: Data-Fi euglobulin lysis reagents, Aguada, Puerto Rico, American Hospital Supply, 1985.

REAGENTS AND EQUIPMENT

1. The following reagents are available from American Dade, American Hospital Supply:

   a. Phosphate buffered saline, pH 7.2. Store at 2 to 8°C.

   b. Acetic acid, 1% (v/v). Store at 2 to 8°C.

   c. Buffered bovine thrombin, 100 NIH units/vial. Store at 2 to 8°C. Reconstitute with 2.0 mL distilled water. Solution is stable at 2° to 8°C for 8 hours once it is reconstituted.

   d. Pipets, 25 μL, disposable.

   e. Positive control. Store both reagents at 2° to 8°C. Very unstable once prepared. Reconstitute and prepare immediately before use.

   (1) Plasminogen activator. Approximately 12 USP units of streptokinase/vial. Reconstitute with 1.0 mL of distilled water immediately before use.

   (2) Plasmin control plasma. Reconstitute with 1.0 mL of plasminogen activator immediately before use.

2. Test tubes, 12 × 100 mm.
3. Pipets, 0.1, 1.0, and 10 mL.
4. Water bath, 37°C.
5. Ice bath.
6. Distilled water, 2 to 8°C.
7. Stopwatch.

SPECIMEN

Citrated plasma: 1 part 0.109 M sodium citrate to 9 parts whole blood. Place specimen in crushed ice as soon as it is collected. Obtain a normal control plasma at the same time the patient sample is obtained.

PRINCIPLE

The plasma is diluted. Addition of 1% acetic acid causes the euglobulin portion of the plasma to precipitate. After removing the supernatant, the euglobulins are dissolved in a buffer solution. Thrombin is added in order to clot the euglobulins. The clot is incubated at 37°C and the time of complete clot lysis is noted.

PROCEDURE

1. Centrifuge the blood specimen at 1200 to 1500 g for 15 minutes in order to obtain platelet poor plasma. The test must be set up within 30 minutes after collection.
2. Prepare sufficient distilled water (6 mL/sample) at a temperature of 2° to 8°C.
3. Label one 12 × 100 mm test tube for each patient specimen and control to be tested.
4. Add 0.5 mL of patient sample and normal control to the appropriately labeled tube. Prepare the positive control and place 0.5 mL of the plasma into the appropriately labeled tube. Proceed to step 5 immediately.
5. Add 6 mL of cold (2° to 8°C) distilled water to each of the above tubes. Add 0.1 mL of 1% acetic acid to each tube. Mix each tube well, by inversion.
6. Place all tubes in the refrigerator (2° to 8°C) for 10 minutes to allow for complete precipitation of the euglobulins.
7. Centrifuge tubes at 1200 to 1500 g for 3 minutes. Do not over-centrifuge. Excessive packing of the euglobulin precipitate makes it difficult to dissolve (step 9) and may prolong the lysis time.
8. Carefully pour off the supernatant from each tube and discard. Invert tubes onto filter paper in a test tube rack. Working with one tube at a time, blot the excess supernatant on gauze several times. Remove all liquid from the inside walls of the test tube with cotton tipped applicators. (The supernatant contains inhibitors to fibrinolysis so it is important to remove all traces of the supernatant.)
9. Add 0.35 mL of phosphate buffered saline solution to each tube. Mix each tube gently. All precipitate must go into solution.
10. Reconstitute the thrombin with 2.0 mL of distilled water. Mix gently.
11. Add 25 μL of thrombin reagent to each tube. Mix the tubes immediately by gentle shaking and place in the 37°C water bath, simultaneously starting a stopwatch. After 30 seconds, verify clot formation by gently tilting the tubes.
12. Check each tube in the incubator at 10-minute intervals for lysis of the clot. When clot lysis begins, check the tube every 5 minutes until the lysis is complete.
13. Report results as the time for complete lysis to occur. If the clot has not lysed within 1 hour, report results as greater than 60 minutes. The positive control will completely lyse within about 35 minutes. The normal control should not lyse until after 60 minutes.

DISCUSSION

1. If the patient sample has a fibrinogen concentration of less than 80 mg/dL, fibrinolytic activity will be difficult to measure due to the small size of the clot. In these instances, perform the test making a 1:1 dilution with a normal plasma (at the beginning of the test in step #4).
2. When removing plasma from the top of the red cell layer, do not pipet too close to the buffy coat. The presence of platelets will prolong the lysis time due to the antiplasmin activity of the platelets.
3. This test should be set up immediately after collection. The plasma should be kept on ice at all indicated times in the procedure. Plasminogen activator is very labile, and at room temperature, will decrease in concentration quite rapidly.

CLOT LYSIS

The whole blood clot lysis procedure tests for increased fibrinolysis: the total activity of plasminogen activator, inhibitors, plasmin, plasminogen, and fibrinogen. The tubes used for the Lee and White clotting time may also be used to detect abnormal clot lysis. Leave 1 of the tubes from the Lee and White clotting time in the 37°C incubator and inspect at the end of 8, 24, and 48 hours for disappearance or degeneration of the clot. One tube used in the Lee and White clotting time should be placed in the refrigerator as soon as it has clotted, to serve as a control. If the incubated clot becomes fluid in less than 48 hours, pour the blood out onto a piece of filter paper to be certain the clot has disappeared. Examine the refrigerated clot. If this clot is still intact, if may be assumed that clot lysis has taken place in the incubated tube. If the refrigerated clot has also disappeared, it may be assumed that the disappearance of the clot in both tubes was due to a fibrinogen deficiency rather than clot lysis. If no lysis occurred in either tube, the results may be reported as "no clot lysis after 48 hours."

PLASMINOGEN ASSAY

Plasminogen is the precursor of plasmin in the fibrinolytic system. Its concentration in the blood is decreased during disseminated intravascular coagulation (DIC), and may be increased in liver disorders, thrombolytic therapy, and fibrinolytic disorders.

REFERENCE

Organon Teknika Corp.: Chromostrate® Plasminogen Assay, pkg. insert, Durham, N.C., Organon Teknika Corp., 1985.

REAGENTS AND EQUIPMENT

1. Chromostrate® plasminogen assay kit (obtainable from Organon Teknika Corp.) contains the following reagents.
   a. Substrate reagent, 8 μmoles/vial (H-D-valyl-L-cyclohexyl tyrosyl-L-lysine-paranitroanilide). Reconstitute with 2.0 mL distilled water, swirl gently to mix, and allow to stand at room temperature for 5 minutes before use. Once reconstituted the reagent may be refrigerated for up to 30 days at 2° to 6°C.
   b. Streptokinase reagent, approximately 10,000 IU/vial. Reconstitute with 2.0 mL of distilled water, swirl gently to mix, and allow to sit at room temperature for 5 minutes before use. Once reconstituted the reagent may be stored at 2° to 6°C for 7 days.
   c. Buffer concentrate (substrate specific), pH 7.4. (Caution: contains sodium azide.) Prior to use dilute buffer 1:10 (mix 1 volume of buffer with 9 volumes of distilled water). Once diluted, the buffer may be stored at 2° to 6°C for up to 30 days.
2. Chromostrate reference plasma (obtainable from Organon Teknika Corp.).
3. Acetic acid, 50% (v/v).
4. Verify normal citrate control plasma (Organon Teknika Corp.).
5. Stopwatch.
6. Plastic test tubes, 12 × 75 mm.
7. Pipets, 0.4 and 0.2 mL.
8. Water bath, 37°C.
9. Spectrophotometer (wavelength of 405 nm).
10. Linear graph paper.

SPECIMEN

Citrated plasma: 1 part 0.109 M sodium citrate to 9 parts whole blood. Deliver to laboratory immediately.

PRINCIPLE

The patients plasma is incubated with an excess of streptokinase reagent. The plasminogen present in the plasma specimen forms a plasminogen-streptokinase complex which possesses plasmin-like activity. When the substrate is added to the plasma-streptokinase mixture, the plasmin-like activity present will release par-anitroanilide (pNA) from the substrate. The pNA released may be measured spectrophotometrically and is directly proportional to the amount of plasminogen present in the plasma.

PROCEDURE

1. As soon as the patient specimen is received in the laboratory, centrifuge at 1500 × g for 10 minutes. Place the sample in a capped test tube and place at 2° to 8°C until the test is to be performed. (Testing should be performed within 4 hours of obtaining the specimen from the patient.)
2. Preparation of the calibration curve.
   a. Reconstitute Chromostrate reference plasma according to directions on the vial.
   b. Prepare a 1:20 dilution (100% activity) by adding 0.1 mL of the reference plasma to 1.9 mL of working buffer. Prepare a 1:40 dilution (50%) by mixing 0.05 mL of the reference plasma with 1.95 mL of working buffer. Prepare a 1:80 dilution (25%) by adding 1.0 mL of the 1:40 dilution to 1.0 mL of working buffer.
3. Prepare 1:20 dilutions (in duplicate) of the patient and control plasmas: Add 0.1 mL of the plasma to be tested to 1.9 mL of working buffer solution.
4. Label three 12 × 75 mm test tubes for each plasma dilution (patient, control, and reference plasmas) to be tested. Two tubes will be used for the test (to be performed in duplicate) and the third tube will be used as the blank.
5. Add 0.2 mL of the plasma dilution to the first test tube and incubate at 37°C for 3 to 5 minutes.
6. Add 0.2 mL of streptokinase reagent to the tube, mix, and incubate at 37°C for exactly 3 minutes.
7. Add 0.2 mL of substrate reagent to the tube, mix, and incubate for exactly 1 minute.
8. Add 0.2 mL of 50% acetic acid to the tube and immediately mix.
9. Repeat steps 5 through 8 above for each plasma dilution, performing the test in duplicate.
10. Prepare the blank for each dilution by mixing together 0.2 mL of the plasma dilution, 0.4 mL of distilled water, and 0.2 mL of 50% acetic acid. Mix well.
11. Read the absorbance of all samples in the spectrophotometer at a wavelength of 405 nm, against a water blank, using a semi-micro cuvet with a 1-cm light path. Average the absorbance readings for the duplicate samples and subtract the reading of the respective blank. To determine the percent activity of the reference dilutions, multiply the percent (1.0, 0.50, or 0.25) by the assay value as assigned for that lot of reference plasma. Plot the 3 points on linear graph paper (O.D. vs percent activity) and draw a straight line which best fits all three points.
12. To determine the % activity of plasminogen for each plasma, refer to the calibration curve.

DISCUSSION

1. Addition of the 50% acetic acid stops the reaction. It is imperative that the tube be mixed well as soon as the acetic acid is added. Once added, the color remains stable for several hours.
2. This test measures the functional potential of plasminogen. The test results will, therefore, not always correlate with immunochemical assays.
3. Each laboratory should determine its own normal range. The normal range given with this procedure (to be used as a guide) is 75 to 128% activity.
4. If the test cannot be performed within 4 hours of obtaining the spec-

imen, the plasma should be frozen rapidly and may be stored for up to 30 days without loss of plasminogen activity.

5. This procedure may be adapted to kinetic analysis. See the package insert for an outline of this method.

CLOT RETRACTION

When blood coagulation is complete, the clot normally undergoes contraction, where serum is expressed from the clot, and the clot becomes denser. Thrombosthenin, released by the platelets, is responsible for clot retraction. The number of platelets present also affects the clot retraction time, and, if the platelet count is below 100,000 per μL, poor clot retraction may occur. In rare instances where the platelet count is normal, there may be poor clot retraction due to an abnormality present in the platelets. Normally, clot retraction begins within 30 seconds after the blood has clotted. At the end of 1 hour, there should be appreciable clot retraction and almost complete retraction by the end of 4 hours. Clot retraction should be complete within 24 hours. An abnormal clot retraction time is found in Glanzmann's thrombasthenia.

REFERENCE

Cartwright, G.E.: *Diagnostic Laboratory Hematology,* New York, Grune & Stratton, Inc., 1963.

REAGENTS AND EQUIPMENT

1. Water bath, 37°C.
2. Glass test tubes, 13 × 100 mm.

SPECIMEN

One of the tubes containing 1 mL of whole blood, used in the Lee and White clotting time, or 3 mL of whole fresh blood, placed in a 13 × 100 mm glass test tube.

PRINCIPLE

Fresh whole clotted blood is placed in a 37°C water bath and inspected at 1, 2, 4, and 24 hours for the presence of a retracted clot.

PROCEDURE

1. If a Lee and White clotting time was not performed, obtain 3 mL of blood and dispense carefully into a 13 × 100 mm glass test tube.
2. Place the test tube of blood in the 37°C water bath and allow the blood to clot. If a Lee and White clotting time was performed, use one of the three tubes of blood.
3. As soon as the blood has clotted, inspect the clot at 1, 2, 4, and 24 hours for the formation of a retracted clot. The clot should be firm and retracted from the sides of the tube. It generally occupies a little more than half of the original volume.
4. Results are reported as the length of time it took for the clotted blood to retract. As an alternative method, the results may be reported as normal, if clot retraction has occurred at 2 to 4 hours; poor, if retraction occurs after 4 hours and within 24 hours; and none, if no retraction occurs after 24 hours.

DISCUSSION

1. Clot retraction should be almost complete within 4 hours. Normally, the clot will retract from the walls of the test tube until the red blood cell mass occupies approximately 50% of the total volume of blood in the tube. In abnormal states, there may be variable degrees of retraction or no retraction at all.
2. Shaking or jarring of the test tube of blood should be avoided. This may lead to a falsely shortened clot retraction time.
3. Clot retraction varies inversely with the plasma fibrinogen concentration. That is, if the plasma fibrinogen level is elevated, clot retraction may be poor.

4. Clot retraction may be affected by the red blood cell mass. In blood containing a high red cell count, the degree of retraction is limited because of the large volume of red blood cells within the clot. In anemic states, the reverse occurs, and the degree of clot retraction is increased.

5. Generally, there is a small amount of *red blood cell fallout* during clot retraction. This is seen as a few red blood cells at the bottom of the tube that have fallen from the clot. The significance of an increased amount of red blood cell fallout is not known. When the fibrinogen level is slightly decreased, however, there will be an increased number of free red blood cells at the bottom of the tube. Whenever red blood cell fallout is increased, a notation on the patient's report should be made.

PLATELET AGGREGATION

During the coagulation process platelets clump (aggregate) at the site of injury. Adenosine diphosphate (ADP), derived from injured tissues, red blood cells, or the platelets themselves are responsible for platelet aggregation. There are various reagents which will normally cause the platelets to aggregate and/or release ADP. When platelet dysfunction is suspected, platelet aggregation studies should be performed in which the platelets are exposed to various aggregating reagents and the platelet response noted.

REFERENCE

Bio/Data Corp.: *Operating Instructions and Methods Manual, Platelet Aggregation Profiler® Model PAP-4,* Hatboro, Pa., Bio/Data Corp., 1985.

REAGENTS AND EQUIPMENT

1. Platelet aggregation reagents: ADP, epinephrine, collagen, arachidonic acid, and ristocetin. (Available from Bio/Data Corp. individually, or, as Par/Pak II [contains only ADP, epi- nephrine, and collagen].) Reconstitute vials according to manufacturer's directions.

2. Bio/Data Platelet Aggregation Profiler Model PAP-4.

3. Cuvets, 8.75 mm × 50 mm (Bio/Data Corp.).

4. Plastic pipets, 1.0, 0.5, and 0.05 mL.

5. Plastic test tubes, 12 × 75 mm with caps.

6. Magnetic stir rods (Bio/Data Corp.).

SPECIMEN

All specimens must be drawn using a plastic syringe. Obtain 9 mL of whole blood and immediately transfer to a plastic test tube containing 1.0 mL of 0.109 M sodium citrate. Mix contents of tube well. Collect a specimen of blood from a normal control in the same manner and at the same time the patient's blood is obtained.

PRINCIPLE

Platelet rich plasma (PRP) is placed in the test well of the platelet aggregometer. An aggregation reagent is added to the PRP and, at the same time, the optical density of the sample is monitored. As the platelets in the plasma clump (aggregate) the plasma becomes more clear and light transmittance through the specimen increases. These changes in optical density are recorded by the instrument in the form of a graph. The aggregometer also calculates the slope of the aggregation curve and the amount (%) of platelet aggregation.

PROCEDURE

1. Turn the instrument on. When the instrument is first turned on, the display will read INSTRUMENT NOT READY. In 8 to 10 minutes the incubation block will reach 37°C, and the temperature indicator will light. The display will then read READY for each of the four channels.

2. Preparation of the platelet rich plasma (PRP) and platelet poor plasma (PPP) specimens.

a. Prepare the patient and control plasmas in the same manner.

b. Centrifuge each specimen at 150 × g for 5 minutes (at room temperature). Examine the platelet rich plasma. If any red blood cells are present, recentrifuge the specimen at the same speed for an additional 5 minutes.

c. Remove the supernatant PRP and place in a covered plastic tube at room temperature. (Specimens should be capped at all times to prevent pH changes due to loss of CO_2.)

d. Centrifuge the original blood specimen at 1500 × g for 15 minutes. Transfer the PPP to a test tube and cover.

e. Perform a platelet count on the PRP. The count should be between 200,000 and 300,000/μL. Using the PPP adjust the platelet count of the PRP to this level.

f. The PRP specimen should be at room temperature for at least 30 minutes prior to testing.

3. Prepare the aggregating reagents (ADP, epinephrine, collagen, ristocetin, and/or arachidonic acid) according to the manufacturer's directions.

4. Pipet 0.5 mL of PPP into a 8.75 × 50 mm aggregometer cuvet. Pipet 0.45 mL of PRP into 1 to 4 aggregometer cuvets, depending on how many channels and aggregation reagents are to be utilized for testing.

5. Place one or more of the PRP cuvets into the wells of the incubation block for approximately 2 minutes. Place a magnetic stir bar into each cuvet.

6. Set the 100% baseline: Place the PPP cuvet into the first test well. Depress the appropriate channel operation switch one time. When the display reads PPP SET, remove the cuvet. Repeat this procedure for the other three channels if they are to be used.

7. Set the 0% baseline: Insert the patient's PRP cuvet into each test well to be used. Depress each channel operation switch one time. The display should read 0%. (If the display reads LO RANGE or HI RANGE, however, this indicates that the difference in the optical densities of the PRP and PPP are not greater than 5% and/or less than 95%, respectively. The platelet count on the plasma specimens should be rechecked and/or the specimens reprepared. The procedure must then be repeated beginning with step 4 above.) (If the display reads STIR BAR, after the channel operation switch was pressed, add the stir bar and repeat the procedure beginning with step 4 above.)

8. Perform the platelet aggregation test: Add 0.05 mL of the reagent directly into the PRP cuvet in the first test well. At the termination of the test, press the appropriate channel operation switch. Repeat this step for each channel being used. When testing has been terminated in each channel, the printer will print the percent aggregation and slope for each channel.

9. Interpretation of results.

a. Description of printout from aggregometer.

(1) One-minute intervals are printed along the bottom of the paper. Each 1 minute is divided into 15-second intervals by dotted lines. Each dot represents 5 seconds.

(2) Every 30 seconds the appropriate test channel number is printed out on the form.

(3) Every 4 minutes the 0 to 100% aggregation scale is printed. Each dotted line represents 10% while each dot represents 2%.

(4) At the conclusion of each test,

the percent aggregation and slope are calculated by the instrument and printed out as part of the report. A section is also made available for comments.

b. *Primary phase aggregation* is the initial response of the platelets to the aggregation reagent. *Secondary phase aggregation* is additional platelet aggregation caused by the release of ADP from the platelets themselves. The *slope* is a number which represents the rate at which platelet aggregation occurs. The *percent aggregation* is a measurement of the extent of platelet aggregation.

c. Patterns of platelet aggregation (Figs. 216 and 217).

(1) Using optimal concentrations of ADP (2×10^{-5} M), normal platelet aggregation occurs in two waves. The primary wave is caused by the addition of the ADP reagent and the secondary wave by ADP released from the platelets themselves. The secondary wave, however, begins prior to completion of the first wave and the resultant pattern appears as one large wave of aggregation. Abnormalities in ADP induced platelet aggregation will be found in aspirin-like release defects, uremia, storage pool disease, and thrombasthenia.

(2) Epinephrine normally causes two waves of irreversible platelet aggregation. However, a small percent of normal people will show only a single wave of aggregation with this reagent. Abnormalities in platelet response to epinephrine will be found in patients with thrombasthenia, uremia, and storage pool disease.

(3) Collagen will normally cause a single wave of aggregation following a short lag and shape change period (as the platelets adhere to the soluble collagen fibrils). Abnormal collagen induced aggregation is found in aspirin-like release defects, storage pool disease, thrombasthenia, and uremia.

(4) Arachidonic acid will normally produce a single wave of platelet aggregation. Aspirin is a strong inhibitor of this reagent and its effects on platelet aggregation will last up to 8 days after ingestion. If a patient's platelets show no aggregation with this reagent, the drug status of the patient should be closely examined. In the absence of aspirin effects, abnormal platelet aggregation with this reagent will be found in thrombasthenia.

(5) Ristocetin induced platelet aggregation normally occurs rapidly with no visible distinction shown between primary and secondary waves. (This is the basis of the von Willebrand Factor Assay procedure [Bio/Data Corp.].) Large platelet clumps are generally formed during the aggregation process. Platelet aggregation with ristocetin is decreased in patients with von Willebrand's syndrome and Bernard-Soulier syndrome.

DISCUSSION

1. To stop a test before its conclusion, press the channel operation switch. Only that channel will be affected.

2. For micro volume testing, 0.2 mL PPP and PRP samples are used in

place of the routine 0.5 and 0.45 mL volumes and 0.02 mL of reagent is utilized (instead of the 0.05 mL volume). The test is performed in the same manner as previously described, except that a micro volume adapter is used in the test well, 7.5 × 55 mm cuvets are needed, and a micro magnetic stir bar is used.

3. To recall the previously run results from the instrument's memory, all channels must be in the READY position, as shown on the display. Press the memory switch. NO PRINT should appear on the display in each channel. Press the channel operation switch for each channel to be recalled. PRINT should appear on each channel's display. (If the oscillations are to be filtered out, press the appropriate trace filter switches.) Press the memory switch a second time. The printer will automatically begin printing and will label the form PRINT FROM MEMORY. The percent aggregation and slope will be printed for each channel activated.

4. This instrument has a diagnostic mode, which is used to determine proper functioning of the instrument. The procedure for entering this mode and performing the tests is clearly outlined in the instrument's operations manual.

5. The magnetic stir motor in each channel turns on when PPP SET appears on the display. It shuts off at the end of the aggregation step. If the test is left unattended for a period of time, the stir bar motor will automatically shut off after 2 hours.

6. The normal range for platelet aggregation should be established by each laboratory. Studies have shown that ADP, arachidonic acid, epinephrine, collagen, and ristocetin normally cause 60 to 90% platelet aggregation in normal donors. The lag phase using collagen is about 1 minute, but when arachidonic acid is used, platelet aggregation should begin within the first 30 seconds.

7. The platelet aggregation procedure should not be performed on any patient who has ingested aspirin within 8 days prior to the test. Aspirin inhibits platelet aggregation and would, therefore, mask any qualitative platelet defect present. Other compounds which inhibit platelet aggregation are antihistamines, alcohol, cocaine, tricyclic antidepressants, dipyridamole, and nonsteroidal anti-inflammatory agents.

8. In most cases of von Willebrand's disease, the platelets fail to show aggregation with ristocetin but do aggregate with the other reagents.

9. Testing must be complete within 3 hours of blood collection. Hemolysis or excessive lipemia will interfere with test results.

PLATELET ADHESIVENESS TEST

One of the functions of platelets is their participation in hemostasis, where they adhere to each other and to the walls of damaged blood vessels to form a hemostatic plug. The adhesiveness of blood platelets is measured in vitro by their ability to adhere to glass surfaces. The normal values for this test as described below is 26 to 60% platelet adhesiveness; however, each laboratory should determine its own normal range. Decreased values, using the procedure to be described, are found in thrombasthenia, where there is a qualitative disorder in platelets, von Willebrand's disease, and in some cases of myeloid metaplasia and thrombocythemia. Increased platelet adhesiveness has been reported in venous thrombosis, pulmonary embolism, coronary disease, following splenectomy, and diabetes mellitus.

Salzman Method

REFERENCES

Lenahan, J.G., and Smith, K.: *Hemostasis,* Durham, N.C., Organon Teknika Corp., 1985.

Salzman, E.W.: Measurement of platelet adhesiveness, a simple in vitro technique demonstrating an abnormality in von Willebrand's disease., J. Lab. Clin. Med., *62,* 724, 1963.

REAGENTS AND EQUIPMENT

1. A double ended, 20 gauge, Vacutainer needle.
2. Hypodermic needle, 20 gauge.
3. Vacutainer holder.
4. Vacutainer tubes (2) containing EDTA anticoagulant.
5. Siliconized ML-ML adapter, obtainable from Becton-Dickinson Co. (#3113).
6. Siliconized 3200 A adapter, obtainable from Becton-Dickinson Co.
7. Polyvinyl tubing (inner diameter of 0.113 inch). (Obtainable from Insultab, Inc., 252 Mishawuum Rd., Woburn, Ma., 01802.)
8. Glass beads, obtainable from Potter's Industries, Hasbrouck Heights, N. J. (#P-0170).
9. Siliconized nylon mesh, with openings of 0.002 inch. (Nylon stocking material may be used, but must first be washed in 10% silicone solution and allowed to dry.)
10. Duco cement.
11. Materials necessary for two platelet counts.
12. Glass bead filter.
    a. Cut two pieces of siliconized nylon mesh to fit exactly over the ends of the two siliconized adapters.
    b. Using Duco cement, glue a piece of the nylon mesh to one end of each of the adapters.
    c. Attach one end of the polyvinyl tubing to that end of the adapter to which the nylon mesh is glued (Fig. 155).
    d. Fill the polyvinyl tubing with 3.3 g of glass beads.

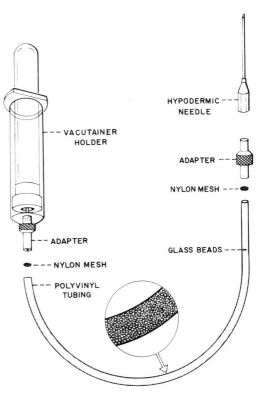

Fig. 155. Salzman glass bead collecting system.

    e. After packing the glass beads into the tube, cut the tubing. Allow a little extra unfilled tubing to remain to fit over that end of the second adapter which contains the nylon mesh. (The degree of packing of the glass beads and, therefore, the length of the polyvinyl tubing should be such that it takes 40 to 50 seconds for the blood to be collected through this system.)

SPECIMEN

One tube of whole blood collected by routine procedure, using the Vacutainer assembly with a 20-gauge needle and drawing the blood directly into an EDTA vacuum tube. A second specimen of blood is collected through the glass bead collecting system directly into an EDTA vacuum tube.

PRINCIPLE

A platelet count is performed on both specimens of blood. The number of platelets in the blood, collected through the glass bead collecting system, will be lower than the number obtained by routine venipuncture. This is because platelets have adhered to the column of glass beads due to their adhesive characteristics. The results of this procedure are expressed as the percentage of platelets retained in the glass bead column.

PROCEDURE

1. Perform two clean venipunctures at separate sites, with and without the use of the glass bead collecting system. (The blood collection rate through the glass bead column should be 6 to 10 mL/minute.)
2. Perform a platelet count on both blood samples.
3. Calculate the percent of platelet adhesiveness as shown below:

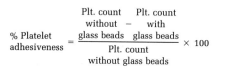

$$\% \text{ Platelet adhesiveness} = \frac{\text{Plt. count without glass beads} - \text{Plt. count with glass beads}}{\text{Plt. count without glass beads}} \times 100$$

DISCUSSION

1. If the glass beads are siliconized, there will be no platelet adhesion.
2. There is no correlation between the patient's platelet count and platelet adhesion.
3. Heparin therapy does not interfere with platelet adhesiveness.
4. It is recommended that each laboratory determine its own set of normal values. Slight differences in technique and the length of the polyvinyl tubes are important factors.
5. If is felt that calcium ions are necessary for platelet adhesion under the conditions of this test. For this reason, the blood passes through the filter system prior to being anticoagulated.

6. This test is difficult to standardize and the results are affected by the rate at which the blood flows through the glass bead column, the length of this column, the size of the glass beads, the hematocrit, and the fragility of the red blood cells.
7. A modification of this procedure may be utilized to produce more standardized and reproducible results. Use of a constant flow syringe pump provides a constant rate of blood flow through the column. Whole blood is collected and anticoagulated with heparin. Part of this whole blood is then drawn through the glass bead column at a constant preset rate by means of an infusion pump and is collected in a tube containing EDTA. Platelet counts are then determined on the whole blood sample drawn through the glass bead column and on the blood sample not drawn through the column. The percent of platelet adhesiveness is calculated as previously outlined. (An infusion pump, Model #901, is obtainable from Harvard Apparatus Company, South Natick, Ma.)

TEST FOR PLATELET FACTOR 3 AVAILABILITY

Platelets activated during the coagulation process liberate platelet factor 3, a phospholipid, which is essential for normal blood coagulation. Normal values for this method are determined by the correlation of patient and control results. The patient's platelet rich plasma should give a clotting time similar in length to that of the normal platelet rich control plasma. Increased clotting times occur in thrombocytopenia and in defects in platelet factor 3 availability, as found in thromboasthenia and some uremic patients.

REFERENCES

Hardisty, R.M., and Ingram, C.I.C.: *Bleeding Disorders, Investigations and Management,* Oxford, Blackwell Scientific Publications, 1965.

Dacie, J.V., and Lewis, S.M.: *Practical Haematology,* New York, Churchill Livingstone, Inc., 1984.

REAGENTS AND EQUIPMENT

1. All glassware in this test must be siliconized or plastic because platelets adhere to glass.
2. Water bath, 37°C.
3. Calcium chloride, 0.025 M.
4. Light kaolin suspension.

Kaolin	0.50 g
Barbital buffered saline solution, pH 7.35	100 mL

(Celite 505, a 1% suspension in sodium chloride, 0.85%, w/v, may be used in place of the kaolin. This is obtainable from Johns-Manville Products Corporation, New York.)
5. Normal platelet poor control plasma.
6. Normal platelet rich control plasma.
7. Reagents and equipment as used for the platelet count.
8. Test tubes, 13 × 100 mm.
9. Stopwatch.

SPECIMEN

Platelet rich and platelet poor patient and normal control plasma specimens. Collect blood using a plastic syringe. Mix 1 part 0.109 M sodium citrate with 9 parts whole blood and place in a plastic test tube. Collect two tubes of blood from both the patient and the normal control.

PRINCIPLE

Equal parts of patient's platelet rich plasma (PRP) are mixed with normal control platelet poor plasma (PPP). A second mixture of equal parts of patient's PPP and normal control PRP is made. Kaolin is added to activate the platelets and subsequently cause the release of platelet factor 3. Calcium chloride is added, and the clotting time of the mixtures is recorded. Platelet counts are performed on the PRP specimens of both the patient and normal control.

PROCEDURE

1. For PRP, centrifuge one test tube each of the patient's and normal control blood at 150 to 200 × g for 10 minutes. Remove the plasma from the cells using a plastic transfer pipet. For PPP, centrifuge both the patient's and normal control blood at 1500 × g for at least 20 minutes. Remove the plasma from the cells.
2. Label eight 13 × 100 mm test tubes as shown in Table 17 and pipet the indicated plasma specimens into each test tube.
3. Place test tube #1 in the water bath. Add 0.2 mL of the well-mixed kaolin suspension.
4. Set a clock for 27 minutes. (This mixture is to be incubated for 20 minutes.)
5. At 1-minute intervals, repeat step 3 starting with test tube #2, then test tube #3, and so forth until the kaolin suspension has been added to all eight test tubes in the water bath.
6. When the clock has 7 minutes remaining (20 minutes after kaolin was added to test tube #1), add 0.2 mL of 0.025 M calcium chloride to test tube #1 and simultaneously start a stopwatch.
7. Using the tilt tube method, determine the clotting time. It should be approximately 30 seconds.
8. Continue to add 0.2 mL of 0.025 M calcium chloride to each succeeding tube at 1-minute intervals. That is, when the clock has 6 minutes remaining, add calcium chloride to test tube #2 and so forth, so that calcium chloride is added to each test tube

TABLE 17. MIXTURES FOR PLATELET FACTOR 3 AVAILABILITY TEST

TEST TUBE #	PRP	PPP
1, 8	0.1 mL control	0.1 mL control
2, 7	0.1 mL control	0.1 mL patient
3, 6	0.1 mL patient	0.1 mL control
4, 5	0.1 mL patient	0.1 mL patient

exactly 20 minutes after the kaolin was added.

9. Average the duplicate results and record.

10. Perform a platelet count on the patient's PRP and the normal control PRP.

11. Interpretation of results: the plasma mixtures in test tubes #2 and #7, and in #3 and #6 differ only in their source of platelets. If the average clotting times of these 2 groups agree within 2 to 3 seconds of each other and the platelet counts on the patient's and normal control PRP specimens are within 100,000 to 300,000/μL, the patient has no significant defect in platelet factor 3 availability. If, however, the clotting times in test tubes #3 and #6 are more prolonged and differ more widely from test tubes #2 and #7, this may be due to decreased platelets (thrombocytopenia) in the patient or to defective platelet factor 3 availability. If the platelet count performed on the patient's PRP is within the range of 100,000 to 300,000/μL, the prolonged clotting time is probably due to defective platelet factor 3 availability. A patient with abnormal platelet function generally has a clotting time about 15 seconds longer than the control.

TOURNIQUET TEST (CAPILLARY FRAGILITY TEST)

The tourniquet test is a crude measure of capillary fragility. Because platelets function to maintain capillary integrity, the degree of thrombocytopenia will correlate with the tourniquet test, as will the bleeding time. In normal patients, none to very few petechiae are formed during this test. (Petechiae are minute hemorrhages under the skin and appear as small bruises.) A positive tourniquet test (presence of numerous petechiae) will be found in thrombocytopenia, decreased fibrinogen and in vascular purpura.

REFERENCES
Cartwright, G.E.: *Diagnostic Laboratory Hematology*, New York, Grune & Stratton, Inc., 1963.

Sirridge, M.S., and Shannon, R.: *Laboratory Evaluation of Hemostasis*, 3rd Ed., Philadelphia, Lea & Febiger, 1983.

REAGENTS AND EQUIPMENT

1. Stethoscope.
2. Blood pressure cuff.

PRINCIPLE

An inflated blood pressure cuff on the upper arm is used to apply pressure to the capillaries for 5 minutes. The arm is then examined for petechiae.

PROCEDURE

1. Apply a blood pressure cuff on the upper arm above the elbow, and take a blood pressure reading.

2. Inflate the blood pressure cuff to a point halfway between the systolic and diastolic pressures. (However, never exceed a pressure of 100 mm Hg.) Maintain this pressure for 5 minutes.

3. Remove the blood pressure cuff and wait 5 to 10 minutes before proceeding.

4. Examine the forearm, hands, and fingers for petechiae. Disregard any petechiae within ½ inch of the blood pressure cuff because this may be due to pinching of the skin by the cuff.

5. The test results may be graded roughly as follows:

1+ = A few petechiae on the anterior part of the forearm.

2+ = Many petechiae on the anterior part of the forearm.

3+ = Multiple petechiae over the whole arm and back of the hand.

4+ = Confluent petechiae on the arm and back of the hand.

DISCUSSION

1. An alternative procedure uses the inflated blood pressure cuff at a pressure of 80 mm Hg, regardless of the patient's blood pressure.
2. The test should not be repeated on the same arm within 7 days.
3. Normally, there will be 0 to occasional petechiae present.

REAGENTS

Adsorbed Plasma (Rich in Factors V, VIII, XI, and XII)

1. Add 100 mg of barium sulfate to each 1 mL of fresh oxalated (sodium oxalate) normal plasma.
2. Stir this mixture for 10 minutes at room temperature and refrigerate (or place on ice) for an additional 10 minutes.
3. Centrifuge at 2500 RPM for 10 minutes and remove the supernatant plasma.
4. Dilute the adsorbed plasma 1:5 with 0.85% sodium chloride (1 part adsorbed plasma to 4 parts 0.85% sodium chloride).

Aged Serum (Rich in Factors VII, IX, X, XI, and XII)

1. Incubate a tube of clotted normal blood at 37°C for 3 hours.
2. Add 1 part 0.109 M sodium citrate to 9 parts whole blood to the preceding test tube.
3. Allow the test tube to incubate for 2 additional hours at 37°C.
4. Centrifuge for 10 minutes and remove the serum.
5. The serum may be used immediately, or stored at −20°C.
6. Prior to use, dilute the aged serum 1:5 with 0.85% sodium chloride (1 part aged serum to 4 parts 0.85% sodium chloride).

Calcium Chloride, 0.025 M

Anhydrous calcium chloride	1.38 g

Dilute to 500 mL with distilled water.

Owren's Veronal Buffer, pH 7.40

Sodium barbital	5.9 g
Sodium chloride	7.1 g
Hydrochloric acid	215 mL

Dilute to 1 liter with distilled water.

6

Diseases

ANEMIA

Anemia signifies a decreased amount of hemoglobin in the blood and, therefore, a decreased amount of oxygen reaching the tissues and organs of the body. This is responsible for many of the symptoms in an anemic person. Anemia has many different causes, and before effective treatment can be initiated, the exact cause must be found. Numerous tests have been devised and are used in conjunction with the clinical findings to differentiate the various types of anemia.

The medical history of the patient is a source of information and can give important clues which may assist in the diagnosis: an anemia of long duration may indicate an inherited disorder, the racial origin or ethnic background may be of assistance in pointing to red cell enzyme deficiencies or abnormal hemoglobins, and exposure to toxic chemicals or the use of various medications should be noted.

To detect anemia in the laboratory, the two most important tests are the hemoglobin and hematocrit. An accurate red blood cell count is also most helpful in calculating the red blood cell indices. The anemia may then be classified as normocytic, microcytic, or macrocytic, depending on the values obtained for the mean corpuscular volume (MCV). The presence or absence of hypochromia, as shown by the mean corpuscular hemoglobin concentration (MCHC), is also valuable in diagnosis.

The MCH closely parallels the MCV and generally increases or decreases with the MCV. Most anemias are normocytic-normochromic, macrocytic-normochromic, or microcytic-hypochromic, depending on the cause.

Examination of the red blood cell morphology on a stained blood smear is a basic tool in evaluating anemia, and it is an opportunity to double check the results obtained for the red blood cell indices. Further examination of the red blood cell may be made: The shape of the red blood cell may be determined and the presence or absence of nucleated red blood cells, schistocytes, sickle cells, spherocytes, target cells, and inclusion bodies noted. In addition, white blood cell and platelet numbers and morphology should be examined. In certain cases, a clue to the cause of the anemia may rest with these cells, as in cases of leukemia. In some anemias, there are specific abnormalities present in the white blood cells or platelets in addition to those found in the red blood cells.

The reticulocyte count, most specifically, the reticulocyte production index, is a test performed routinely for anemia diagnosis. It is a relatively accurate reflection of the amount of effective red blood cell production taking place in the bone marrow. In cases where the reticulocyte count is decreased, this may point to defective hemoglobin synthesis, replacement of the normal marrow by tumor cells, or failure of the bone marrow to produce the normal number of cells. On the other hand, increased reticulocyte counts in the presence of anemia may indicate such conditions as increased red blood cell destruction or blood loss. It must be remembered, however, that if effective erythropoiesis is taking place, the reticulocyte count is slightly elevated in proportion to the degree of anemia present.

Examination of bone marrow smears may prove helpful in estimating the relative number and morphology of red blood cells and their precursors being produced by the marrow. Normally, 20 to 35% of the nucleated cells present in the marrow are erythroid cells. This figure may be written as the myeloid:erythroid ratio (M/E), which normally is 3:1, or as the erythroid: granulocyte ratio (E/G), which is, therefore, 1:3 in a normal marrow. This figure may then be studied in conjunction with the reticulocyte count. For example, if the relative number of erythroid cells in the marrow is increased, but the reticulocyte count is normal or decreased, there may be a defect in the maturation of the erythroid cells (since the red blood cells are obviously not reaching the peripheral blood). Ineffective erythropoiesis may be said to be occurring. It is also important to note the morphology of the erythroid cells (as well as other cellular elements) and the presence of any tumor cells.

When a bone marrow biopsy is performed in cases of anemia, an iron stain should be done on a marrow concentrate smear to determine the percentage of sideroblasts. The presence or absence of ringed sideroblasts should also be noted. An estimation of the marrow iron stores may be determined from a marrow particle smear stained with the Prussian-blue iron stain.

The serum lactic dehydrogenase (LDH) test is less specific than the previously discussed procedures but may be of some help. Increased levels are present in he-

molytic anemias especially when there is intravascular hemolysis, and also in some cases of ineffective erythropoiesis (such as megaloblastic anemias).

The serum iron and iron binding capacity (tests usually performed by the chemistry department) are helpful aids in differentiating anemias. The high incidence of iron deficiency anemia increases the usefulness of this procedure. The serum ferritin level may be measured by various immunoassay techniques. Generally, the amount of circulating ferritin is proportional to the amount of storage iron so that the body iron stores may be evaluated with this procedure.

A test for the determination of fecal urobilinogen (usually performed by the urinalysis or chemistry department) measures the total excretion of the breakdown products of heme. Increased amounts of urobilinogen are generally found in hemolytic anemias and in those anemias in which ineffective red blood cell production is present.

The zinc erythrocyte protoporphyrin test may be performed to determine the amount of protoporphyrin present which was not used for hemoglobin synthesis. Elevated levels are seen in iron deficient erythropoiesis, lead poisoning, and rare disorders of porphyrin metabolism.

The serum bilirubin (performed in the chemistry department) indicates increased destruction of red blood cells, as found in hemolytic anemias.

In addition to the aforementioned laboratory procedures, other tests concerned with red blood cell production, although not employed routinely, deserve mention here. The plasma iron turnover is a procedure employing the use of radioactive iron (^{59}Fe). A known amount of this isotope is injected into the patient intravenously and its rate of disappearance from the blood is measured. In anemias in which total red blood cell production is decreased, the ^{59}Fe remains in the blood longer. The red cell turnover (or red blood cell utilization of iron) is a measure of effective erythropoiesis. After injection of the ^{59}Fe (as described above), blood samples are collected for a period of 2 to 3 weeks and the radioactivity in the samples is measured to determine how much of the ^{59}Fe was incorporated into the red cells. The life span of the red blood cell may also be determined by the use of radioisotopes. The patient's red blood cells may be tagged with radioactive chromium (^{51}Cr). Blood samples are then measured for radioactivity over a period of time and a red blood cell survival curve plotted.

In summary, total erythropoiesis refers to the total production of red blood cells and is measured by the erythroid:granulocytic ratio, the fecal urobilinogen, and the plasma iron turnover. Effective erythropoiesis is the production of red blood cells that reach the circulation or peripheral blood and is measured by the red blood cell iron turnover (utilization of iron), the reticulocyte production index, and the red blood cell life span. In addition, more specific tests have been devised for diagnosing anemias. Many of these procedures have been outlined in Chapter 4, Special Hematology Procedures, and include, among others, hemoglobin electrophoresis, osmotic fragility, autohemolysis, acid serum test, and Heinz body preparation.

Anemia basically results from 1 of 2 causes: (1) decreased red blood cell production or (2) increased red blood cell destruction. In addition, in circumstances where there is an increased plasma volume, laboratory test results (hemoglobin, hematocrit, and red blood cell count) may also show a state of anemia even though the red blood cell mass is normal.

Several classifications of anemia have been devised. None of these is completely satisfactory but will be of some help in learning the basics of anemia. A brief outline of the anemias classified according to morphology and according to cause are given in the following section. These are not complete lists and contain only the more common anemias and causes.

Morphologic Classification of Anemias

1. Macrocytic, normochromic red blood cells.
   A. Vitamin B_{12} deficiency, folic acid deficiency.
      (1) Pernicious anemia
      (2) Sprue
      (3) Following gastrectomy
   B. Disease of the liver.
2. Normocytic, normochromic red blood cells.
   A. Defective formation of the blood cells or the presence of tumor cells in the bone marrow.
      (1) Aplastic anemia
      (2) Leukemia
      (3) Hodgkin's disease
      (4) Multiple myeloma
      (5) Leukoerythroblastosis
      (6) Metastatic cancer
      (7) Anemia associated with renal disease
      (8) Anemia associated with inflammatory disease
   B. Abnormal hemoglobin, increased destruction of red blood cells.
      (1) Certain acquired hemolytic anemias
      (2) Paroxysmal nocturnal hemoglobinuria
      (3) Sickle cell anemia
      (4) Hemolytic disease of the newborn
3. Microcytic, hypochromic red blood cells.
   A. Iron deficiency anemia.
   B. Thalassemia.
   C. Sideroblastic anemias.

Classification of Anemias According to Cause

1. Decreased production of red blood cells.
   A. Bone marrow damage, infiltration, atrophy.
      (1) Leukemia

(2) Leukoerythroblastosis
(3) Aplastic anemia
(4) Lymphoma
(5) Multiple myeloma
(6) Myelofibrosis
B. Decreased erythropoietin.
(1) Inflammatory process
(2) Renal disease
(3) Hypothyroidism
C. Deficiency of substances.
(1) Iron deficiency
(2) Vitamin B_{12} deficiency, folic acid deficiency
(3) Vitamin C deficiency
D. Defect in globin synthesis.
(1) Thalassemia
E. Defect in heme sythesis.
(1) Sideroblastic anemia
F. Cirrhosis of the liver.
2. Increased red blood cell destruction or loss.
A. Acute blood loss.
B. Intrinsic defects within the red blood cell.
(1) Hereditary
a. Spherocytosis, ovalocytosis
b. Hemoglobinopathies such as sickle cell disease, hemoglobin C disease
c. Enzyme defects such as G-6-PD deficiency, pyruvate kinase deficiency
(2) Acquired
a. Paroxysmal nocturnal hemoglobinuria
C. Extracorpuscular causes.
(1) Drugs or chemicals
(2) Physical trauma to the red blood cells such as thermal injury
(3) Infection (malaria)
(4) Antibodies
3. Increased plasma volume.
A. Last trimester of pregnancy.
B. Hyperproteinemia.

MEGALOBLASTIC ANEMIAS

There are a variety of megaloblastic anemias due to deficiencies of vitamin B_{12} and folic acid. The major abnormality is the decreased synthesis of DNA. Megaloblastic marrow cells have both a prolonged intermitotic resting phase and a block in early mitosis. This results in enlarged red cells, granulocytes, and megakaryocytes. Pernicious anemia is a classic example of this form of anemia.

Pernicious Anemia

Pernicious anemia is most often found in people above 60 years of age and rarely in patients below 40 years of age. This disease is caused by a deficiency in vitamin B_{12} caused by an inability of the gastric mucosa to secrete the intrinsic factor that is necessary for the absorption of vitamin B_{12}. There is strong evidence at present that this disorder may be an inherited autoimmune disease. Antibodies to intrinsic factor have been found in over half of the cases of pernicious anemia, and antibodies to the parietal cells of the stomach have been found to be present in over 85% of the patients having pernicious anemia. The clinical symptoms evolve slowly over a period of several months. Generally, the person shows weakness and shortness of breath, and the skin takes on a lemon yellow pallor. Characteristically, the tongue may be raw and red or, more commonly, may be sore, pale and smooth. Gastrointestinal symptoms are usually present in the form of abdominal pain, diarrhea, nausea, and vomiting. There are central nervous system disorders in the degeneration of the white matter in parts of the spinal cord. This is the cause of several neurologic symptoms such as numbness and tingling of the extremities, loss of position sense, muscle weakness, and decreased tendon reflexes. In more advanced cases, the brain may be affected, and the patient may become emotionally unstable or show personality changes, commonly known as "megaloblastic madness."

The peripheral blood smear shows characteristic changes. Pancytopenia is the usual finding, with white blood cell counts usually in the range of 4000 to 5000/μL. The majority of red blood cells are macrocytic-normochromic, with some oval macrocytes present. There may be a few microcytes and teardrop-shaped red blood cells, and moderate to marked anisocytosis and poikilocytosis is commonly found. Basophilic stippling, Howell-Jolly bodies, and nucleated red blood cells exhibiting karyorrhexis are usually seen. Neutrophils showing hypersegmentation are commonly encountered, many with 6 to 10 lobes. These cells may be larger in size than the normal neutrophil. The nuclear chromatin pattern of the erythrocytic and granulocytic cells often gives a much looser or more open appearance than normal. A patient with severe, untreated anemia usually shows thrombocytopenia, with giant platelets found on the blood smear. The bone marrow contains an increased number of erythroid cells that are characteristically megaloblastic, and the developing granulocytic cells are often larger in size than normal. The giant metamyelocyte is a characteristic cell present. The absolute reticulocyte count is low, but there are an increased number of reticulocytes in the bone marrow.

One of the more consistent findings in pernicious anemia is the lack of free hydrochloric acid in the gastric secretions (achlorhydria) after histamine stimulation. The Schilling test (usually performed by the radiology department) is positive in pernicious anemia. (The Schilling test involves giving a standard dose of radioactive vitamin B_{12} orally and measuring the amount excreted in the urine.) The serum vitamin B_{12} level is decreased. The serum iron level may be normal to elevated, and the serum bilirubin level may show a slight increase due to decreased erythrocyte survival.

Other Conditions Caused by Vitamin B_{12} Deficiency

A megaloblastic anemia will result following a total *gastrectomy* because all of the intrinsic factor-secreting cells have been removed. Vitamin therapy is used to treat this condition. A partial gastrectomy or surgery for a gastric ulcer may or may not leave the patient with a megaloblastic anemia, which, again, is treatable with vitamin therapy.

A *dietary deficiency of vitamin B_{12}* is rare but may be found in vegetarians who also avoid consuming milk and egg products.

One case of megaloblastic anemia has been reported in a patient who was found to have an *abnormal intrinsic factor.*

Various *diseases of the small intestine,* such as the 'blind loop syndrome', may cause a megaloblastic anemia. Normally, vitamin B_{12} is absorbed in the lower ileum, which contains little or no bacteria. When bacteria are present, they compete for the vitamin B_{12} thus making it unavailable for absorption. Treatment involves aggressive administration of broad spectrum antibiotics.

Reversible malabsorption of vitamin B_{12} has occurred in patients taking para-aminosalicylic acid (PAS), colchicine, neomycin, and a few other drugs.

Imerslund's syndrome is inherited as an autosomal recessive trait and manifests itself during the first 2 years of life. These patients are not able to absorb vitamin B_{12}, regardless of whether it is bound to intrinsic factor, since there is a deficiency of the receptor site in the terminal ileum. They also have persistent proteinuria. The megaloblastic anemia is treated with vitamin B_{12}.

In *Zollinger-Ellison syndrome*, there is impaired vitamin B_{12} absorption but no megaloblastic anemia. This disease is characterized by the hypersecretion of gastric juice, which results in a low intestinal pH. This interferes with the binding of vitamin B_{12} to intrinsic factor.

Patients on *hemodialysis* will have decreased vitamin B_{12} concentrations that are treatable with the administration of vitamin B_{12}.

In *Crohn's disease,* or regional enteritis,

there is a vitamin B_{12} deficiency and megaloblastic anemia since the disease affects the terminal ileum where vitamin B_{12} absorption normally occurs.

Vitamin B_{12} deficiency will also be found in carriers of the fish tapeworm, *Diphyllobothrium latum,* because the organism lodges in the ileum and takes up the host's vitamin B_{12}. Treatment consists of expulsion of the organism and vitamin B_{12} therapy. This disorder is common in Finland.

Folate Deficiency

Folic acid deficiency manifests itself in a manner similar to vitamin B_{12} deficiency, except that neurologic symptoms are absent.

Dietary deficiencies of folic acid are relatively rare in this country and are found primarily in chronic alcoholics and people with peculiar dietary habits, where relatively few fresh green vegetables or little animal protein is consumed.

The most common cause of folate deficiency occurs during pregnancy, due to increased fetal requirements for folate. The laboratory findings are generally less abnormal than those found in pernicious anemia, and this condition is treated with folic acid.

Megaloblastic anemia may be found during infancy, occurring most often between 6 and 12 months of age, and is caused by a folic acid deficiency that may be accompanied by a vitamin C deficiency. Laboratory test results show macrocytosis, anisocytosis, and poikilocytosis but in a less severe state than is found in pernicious anemia. The bone marrow shows mild to severe megaloblastic changes and includes the granulocytic alterations. Treatment consists of administration of vitamin C and folic acid.

Megaloblastic anemia is also found in patients with alcoholic cirrhosis of the liver and is almost always due to folic acid deficiency. This is due in part to lack of dietary folic acid and also to abnormal folate metabolism.

Some contraceptive drugs and anticonvulsants such as phenobarbital, diphenylhydantoin (Dilantin), and primidone (Mysoline) will cause a folate deficiency and mild hematologic changes.

Disorders Affecting DNA Synthesis

A number of disorders affect DNA synthesis and produce a megaloblastic anemia. Transcobalamin II deficiency, foramino-transferase deficiency, N-methyl tetrahydrofolate transferase deficiency, and dihydrofolate reductase deficiency are all inherited disorders, in addition to orotic aciduria (disorder of pyrimidine metabolism) and Lesch-Nyhan syndrome (disorder of purine metabolism). There are also acquired drug induced disorders caused by a variety of drugs, including those used in chemotherapy which act by inhibiting DNA synthesis.

Steatorrheas

Three malabsorption disorders have been classified as steatorrheas: *tropical sprue, nontropical sprue, (idiopathic steatorrhea),* and *celiac disease.* The last two disorders are now called *gluten-sensitive enteropathies* because they are caused by an abnormal reaction to gluten.

The exact cause of tropical sprue is unknown. At the onset of the disease, there is diarrhea, anorexia, and marked weakness. After several weeks to months, there is a depletion of nutrients, and malabsorption takes place. Following this phase a macrocytic anemia develops, most likely caused by a lack of absorption of folic acid in the beginning and an ensuing lack of vitamin B_{12} as the disease becomes more chronic. Administration of folic acid is used for treatment of the anemia and also appears to improve the intestinal problems.

The gluten-sensitive enteropathies may be inherited and represent an abnormal reaction to gluten, a component of wheat and other grains. In these enteropathies, there is an abnormal small bowel mucosa with a resultant malabsorption of vitamin B_{12}. These patients show chronic diarrhea and weight loss, with possible hypocalcemia, demineralization of bones, and possible deficiency of vitamin K dependent coagulation factors. Children with celiac disease generally show an iron deficiency anemia, with about 30% having a folic acid deficiency. Adults usually have a folic acid deficiency. About 40% of adults will also show malabsorption of vitamin B_{12}. Iron absorption is decreased, and iron stores may be low. Treatment includes folate and/or vitamin B_{12}, in addition to iron therapy and a gluten free diet.

IRON-DEFICIENCY ANEMIA

Iron-deficiency anemia results when the iron stores of the body have been depleted, and there is no longer sufficient iron available for normal hemoglobin production. The iron stores become depleted over time when iron utilization or loss exceeds iron intake.

The normal adult body contains approximately 4,000 mg of iron. About 60% of this total iron is present in the circulating blood, where 1 mL of red blood cells contains approximately 1 mg of iron. The remaining iron is stored as ferritin or hemosiderin, mainly in the liver and reticuloendothelial cells of the bone marrow. Each day, 20 to 25 mL of red blood cells are broken down as a result of normal red blood cell aging. During this process, approximately 1 mg of iron is lost and excreted through the urine, bile, and other secretions. The remaining 19 to 24 mg of iron are reutilized for production of more hemoglobin in the formation of new red blood cells. The normal adult absorbs 5 to 10% of the iron in his diet. This provides 1 to 2 mg per day and compensates for the normal daily losses due to red cell turnover. From this discussion, it can be seen that unless there is an increased need for iron, as in childhood, pregnancy, or excessive blood loss, iron-deficiency anemia will not occur. When iron deficiency does occur, it develops in three stages: (1) In the first step, there is iron depletion, where iron is being utilized by the red blood cells at a faster rate (as during infancy or bleeding) and the dietary intake of iron is not sufficient to keep up with the increased use. The iron stores will then be utilized. (2) Iron deficient erythropoiesis then takes place, where the iron stores become exhausted and anemia may not yet be present. (3) Iron-deficiency anemia then results, where intake does not meet demand, stores are depleted and anemia is detectable.

An increased amount of dietary iron is needed during infancy, childhood, pregnancy, and in women during the childbearing years. The adult male has no increased demands for iron and could live without dietary iron for approximately 3 to 4 years before iron-deficiency anemia developed. Therefore, when this anemia is found in men, it is almost always due to chronic blood loss.

Iron-deficiency anemia is characterized by microcytosis, hypochromia, and poikilocytosis of the red blood cells, as seen on the stained blood smear. The reticulocyte count is within the normal range, except following hemorrhage or iron therapy, when it is increased. The platelet count is normal. Frequently, the platelets may appear smaller in size than usual. When the iron stain is employed on bone marrow concentrate smears, the number of sideroblasts is decreased and storage iron is absent. The serum iron is decreased, whereas the total iron binding capacity is increased.

Treatment for iron deficiency involves replacement therapy with amounts of iron sufficient to correct the anemia and replenish the iron stores. Ferrous iron is given orally in preparations which provide 20 to 40 mg per day. Reticulocytosis will develop within 1 to 2 weeks and the hemoglobin usually increases by 1 to 2 g per week. After the hemoglobin returns to normal, treatment should continue for several weeks in order to replace the iron stores.

ANEMIA OF CHRONIC DISORDERS

Anemia associated with chronic disease is present in disorders such as chronic infections, rheumatoid arthritis, and malignancy. It is the most common form of anemia among hospitalized patients and is second to iron deficiency as the most common of all the anemias.

Anemia of chronic disorders is generally a mild to moderate anemia that develops during the first or second month of illness. The hematocrit rarely falls below 30%. In severe illness, however, the hematocrit level may decrease further. This usually begins as a normocytic-normochromic anemia. Slight hypochromia may develop, and, more rarely, microcytosis may be found, but not to the degree seen in iron-deficiency anemia. Also, microcytosis occurs after hypochromia is present. In iron-deficiency anemia, microcytosis develops before hypochromia. There may be slight anisocytosis and poikilocytosis. The reticulocyte count is generally normal to decreased. The white blood cell and platelet counts are unaffected by the anemia. The serum iron level is decreased, and the total iron binding capacity (TIBC) is normal to decreased. The percent saturation is usually decreased. Three factors which may contribute to the anemia of chronic disorders are: (1) a reduced red blood cell life span, (2) inability of the bone marrow to increase red blood cell production enough to compensate for the decreased red blood cell life span, and (3) a decrease in the transfer of iron from the reticuloendothelial storage sites to the bone marrow. The anemia of chronic disorders shows no improvement with iron therapy and only improves with correction of the primary underlying disorder.

SIDEROBLASTIC ANEMIA

The sideroblastic anemias are a group of disorders characterized by iron loading due to a defect in heme synthesis. These disorders may be classified as inherited or acquired.

Hereditary sideroblastic anemia is inherited as a sex linked recessive trait, and it occurs primarily in males. The anemia usually manifests itself in adolescence, although it may be present at birth or during infancy. The anemia is generally severe, with hematocrit levels of approximately 20%. The blood smear shows a dimorphic population of normochromic-normocytic and hypochromic-microcytic red blood cells. These latter cells show moderate anisocytosis and poikilocytosis. Also, target cells and basophilic stippling are usually present. The white blood cell and platelet counts are generally normal. There is a marked increase of storage iron in the bone marrow, and the serum iron and the % saturation are increased. The bone marrow generally shows erythroid hyperplasia, and 10 to 40% of the late normoblasts are *ringed sideroblasts* (immature red blood cells in which a ring of iron granules surrounds the nucleus).

Primary idiopathic sideroblastic anemia is more common than hereditary sideroblastic anemia and is an acquired disease found in adults above 50 years of age. There is moderate anemia, with hematocrit levels of approximately 25 to 30%. In contrast to the dimorphic population of hereditary sideroblastic anemia, the red blood cells in primary sideroblastic anemia are generally normocytic to slightly macrocytic. A small group of hypochromic-microcytic red blood cells may be found. The white blood cell and platelet counts are normal, and the bone marrow generally shows erythroid hyperplasia along with the presence of large numbers of ringed sideroblasts in all stages of development. Approximately 10% of the patients with this form of sideroblastic anemia develop acute leukemia.

A sideroblastic anemia may also develop secondary to such other diseases as leukemia, hemolytic anemia, neoplastic and inflammatory disease, and uremia. In these circumstances, there are anemia, some hypochromic red blood cells in the peripheral blood, and a few ringed sideroblasts in the bone marrow.

Sideroblastic anemia may also be caused by certain agents or drugs that interfere with heme synthesis. This anemia may be found in alcoholism, lead poisoning, tuberculosis therapy (antituberculosis drugs), and as a result of receiving large doses of chloramphenicol. Drug induced sideroblastic anemia is reversible, in that withdrawal of the drug results in correction of the anemia.

Some patients with sideroblastic anemia respond to treatment with pyridoxine. The response is usually incomplete, although the anemia does improve and iron levels decrease. Patients with the hereditary form of this disease generally respond more satisfactorily than do patients with the acquired forms.

HEMOCHROMATOSIS

Excessive amounts of iron that accumulate in the blood and tissues is classified as *hemosiderosis* if the iron accumulation in the macrophages causes little parenchymal cell injury. In hemochromatosis, however, the iron accumulates in the parenchymal cells and injures the tissues.

Hereditary hemochromatosis is a rare disease and is inherited as an autosomal recessive trait. It is found primarily in middle aged men. It is caused by a disorder in the absorption of iron. The iron contained in food is absorbed into the system irrespective of the body's requirement for iron. This excess iron is stored in the tissues, to their detriment.

These patients generally show hepatomegaly (enlarged liver) and a bronze colored skin pigmentation. In about 50% of the cases, there will be splenomegaly, rheumatoid arthritis type symptoms, and diabetes mellitus (frequently insulin resistant). Weakness and weight loss are commonly found as a result of the diabetes. Cardiac abnormalities and loss of hair may also result.

Laboratory tests show an increased serum iron level, slightly decreased transferrin, and an increased saturation of transferrin. The patient's hemoglobin, hematocrit, and blood smear are generally normal, as is the test for rheumatoid arthritis. The macrophages in the bone marrow generally show many small, stainable particles of iron. A liver biopsy will generally show the parenchymal cells to be overloaded with iron.

Hemochromatosis is generally treated by the use of phlebotomy procedures, removing 500 mL of blood at regular intervals until the accumulated iron is removed. This process may take several months, as the average patient has approximately 20 to 40 g of stored iron.

Iron overload may also be caused: (1) By increased numbers of blood transfusions, where the iron is usually stored in the macrophages and not in the parenchymal cells of the liver. (2) In association with chronic anemias (termed *erythropoietic hemochromatosis*), such as thalassemia major and intermedia, and sideroblastic anemias, where the clinical symptoms are similar to hereditary hemochromatosis. (3) By an increased dietary intake of iron (exceeding 100 mg per day). (4) By contributory factors such as alcohol abuse and liver disease.

CONGENITAL DYSERYTHROPOIETIC ANEMIAS

The congenital dyserythropoietic anemias are so named because the normoblasts in the bone marrow show multinuclearity, karyorrhexis, and bizarre malformations. These anemias are divided into three groups: Type I, Type II (also termed HEMPAS), and Type III.

Type I is rare and thought to be inherited as an autosomal recessive trait. It is a mildly macrocytic anemia and shows marked anisocytosis and poikilocytosis. Cabot rings and basophilic stippling are often present in the red blood cells of the peripheral blood. The bone marrow shows megaloblastic characteristics in the developing red blood cells, along with binucleated and incompletely separated or multilobed cells. Splenomegaly is often present.

Type II is also termed HEMPAS (hereditary erythroblast multinuclearity with positive acidified serum test) and is the most common form of this anemia. It is inherited as an autosomal recessive trait. Hepatosplenomegaly is generally present, and jaundice may or may not occur. There is usually a normocytic anemia, along with anisocytosis, poikilocytosis, and basophilic stippling. The bone marrow shows multinuclearity of the normoblasts but shows no megaloblastic changes. The red blood cells show hemolysis in the acid serum test but do not hemolyze in the sugar water test. The red blood cells in this disorder contain an antigen on them, termed the *HEMPAS antigen.* This disorder generally runs a benign course. A splenectomy is only rarely performed.

Type III is rare and is thought to be inherited as an autosomal dominant trait. It is a normocytic to slightly macrocytic anemia and shows as many as 30% multinucleated red blood cells.

ANEMIA OF BLOOD LOSS

The clinical symptoms associated with anemia due to blood loss depend on the severity of the bleeding. The patient's cardiovascular status, age, and emotional and physical health also play a part in the response to bleeding.

In acute blood loss, when there is a sudden loss of 25 to 30% of the total blood volume (1,000 to 1,500 mL), most healthy patients show light headedness, hypotension, and rapid heart rate when they are in an upright position. A loss of 30 to 40% of the blood volume leads to shortness of breath, sweating, loss of consciousness, and decreased blood pressure. The pulse becomes rapid and weak, and urine volume is reduced. With a sudden loss of 40 to 50% of the total blood volume, the patient goes into a severe state of shock, with the possibility of death.

Immediately after an acute major blood loss, the hemoglobin and hematocrit remain normal due to vasoconstriction. After about 3 to 4 hours, fluid enters the circulation in order to restore the plasma volume. This causes dilution of the blood and is the body's initial defense mechanism to compensate for the lost blood. When this occurs, the hemoglobin, hematocrit, and red blood cell count begin to drop and the platelet count and white blood cell count increase. The peripheral blood smear shows a normocytic-normochromic anemia with slight anisocytosis and poikilocytosis. The white cells show a shift to the left. Following severe bleeding, large polychromatophilic red blood cells and nucleated red blood cells are present in the peripheral blood. The reticulocyte count becomes elevated within 2 to 3 days, peaks in about 6 to 10 days, and remains elevated until the hemoglobin returns to the normal level. This usually occurs about 6 weeks after the episode of blood loss.

In chronic blood loss, when the bleeding occurs in small quantities over a period of time, iron deficiency anemia may develop as a result of the depletion of the iron stores. The white blood cell count is generally low, as is the reticulocyte count, and polychromatophilia is present.

LEUKOERYTHROBLASTOSIS

Leukoerythroblastosis has several synonyms: *leukoerythroblastic anemia, myelophthisic anemia,* and *myelopathic anemia,* to name a few. It is a condition of anemia caused by space occupying disorders of the bone marrow.

The most common cause of leukoerythroblastosis is metastatic carcinoma of the breast, prostate gland, lungs, adrenal gland, or thyroid, due to the tendency of the cancer to spread by vascular channels to bone. The bone marrow becomes infiltrated with fibrotic, granulomatous, or neoplastic cells. It is also found secondary to such diseases as Niemann-Pick disease, Gaucher's disease, Schüller-Christian disease, leukemias, and in some cases of Hodgkin's disease and multiple myeloma.

A normochromic-normocytic anemia of varying degrees is present. One distinguishing characteristic of this condition is the increased presence of nucleated red blood cells in the peripheral blood, quite out of proportion to the degree of anemia. Polychromatophilia, basophilic stippling, and reticulocytosis are usually present. The white blood cell count is generally normal to decreased, with a normal distribution of white blood cells. Frequently, however, a few immature granulocytes may be present. The platelet count is normal to moderately decreased with occasional bizarre forms of the platelet present. Examination of the bone marrow usually shows the cause of leukoerythroblastosis.

ANEMIA OF CHRONIC RENAL INSUFFICIENCY

Patients with chronic renal insufficiency generally show anemia due to failure of the kidneys to produce erythropoietin and to a decreased bone marrow response to erythropoietin. Many times, there is a direct relationship between the blood urea nitrogen levels and the severity of the anemia. Generally, the higher the blood urea nitrogen, the more severe the anemia.

In anemia of chronic renal insufficiency, the red blood cells are normocytic-normochromic, and the hematocrit level is generally 15 to 30%. Hemolysis may be present due to mechanical trauma or to the adverse metabolic environment of the red blood cells. Burr cells and irregularly contracted and fragmented red blood cells are seen on the peripheral blood smear. The reticulocyte count is generally normal but may sometimes be increased. Some macrocytosis may be present in patients in a dialysis program, due to loss of folic acid during dialysis. The white blood cell count is usually normal, with slight neutrophilia. The platelet count is normal to slightly increased. In many cases, however, platelet function is impaired, resulting in bleeding from the genitourinary or gastrointestinal tracts. When this occurs, iron deficiency anemia may develop. The bone marrow generally shows erythroid hyperplasia. When the renal failure becomes acute, however, the bone marrow may show erythroid hypoplasia.

ANEMIA OF ENDOCRINE DISEASES

Anemia is frequently associated with diseases of the thyroid, the pituitary, the adrenals, and the gonads. Many hormones are involved in the regulation of erythropoiesis, and deficiencies of such hormones lead to the development of anemia.

In *hypothyroidism,* there is generally a mild to moderate normochromic-normocytic anemia. The reticulocyte count is normal, as is the red blood cell survival time. This anemia is usually a result of decreased bone marrow production caused by a decrease in the oxygen requirements of the tissues. Hypothyroidism, however, is often complicated by iron deficiency, or a folic acid or vitamin B_{12} deficiency. In such cases, the red blood cells will be microcytic-hypochromic or macrocytic, respectively. The response of the anemia to therapy is generally slow, and it may take 6 months to 1 year for the hemoglobin to become normal. Anemia is uncommon and does not generally occur in *hyperthyroidism.*

In *Addison's disease* (a disorder of the adrenal gland), a mild normocytic-normochromic anemia may be present. Anemia may not be readily apparent in the presence of the reduction in plasma volume which accompanies this condition.

In *hypopituitarism,* there is generally a moderate normocytic-normochromic anemia present. This may be caused by a deficiency of the pituitary hormones or by deficiencies of hormones secreted by glands that are regulated by the pituitary.

Androgens are capable of increasing erythropoietin synthesis. A decrease in testosterone secretion in males will result in decreased red blood cell production, causing a drop in hemoglobin of 1 to 2 g/dL. This is probably due to loss of the erythropoietic effect of the androgen hormone.

A normocytic anemia has been reported in some cases of *hyperparathyroidism.*

ANEMIA OF LIVER DISEASES

Anemia is a common finding in the presence of cirrhosis of the liver and other liver diseases. There is generally a normocytic to slightly macrocytic anemia present. The MCV is rarely greater than 115 fL. This anemia may be caused by folate deficiency, a decreased red blood cell survival, an inability of the bone marrow to respond to the anemia, or an increase in the total blood volume that exaggerates the anemia. In some cases, iron deficiency anemia may result from blood loss. A sideroblastic anemia may develop in cases of chronic alcoholism. The anemia, however, is rarely severe. The bone marrow will show normal cellularity or an increased cellularity with erythroid hyperplasia. The reticulocyte count is often increased but can be decreased as a result of alcohol ingestion. The platelet count may be normal or slightly decreased, as found in cirrhosis of the liver. In hepatitis, obstructive jaundice, and cirrhosis of the liver, there may be changes in the red blood cell membrane lipids. An increase in cholesterol and phospholipid levels leads to an increased red blood cell membrane surface, which gives rise to 'thin' macrocytes or target cells. In some instances, there will be an increase in the red blood cell membrane cholesterol level, but not the phospholipid level. In this circumstance, spur cells are formed, which are red blood cells with thorny projections, similar to acanthocytes.

APLASTIC ANEMIA

The basic defect in aplastic anemia is a failure in the production of the red blood cells, white blood cells, and platelets. Another term used to describe this condition is *pancytopenia,* which is a reduction in all of the formed elements of the blood. Aplastic anemia may be acquired as a result of exposure to chemical or physical agents, in association with other diseases, or as a result of an unknown cause. It may also occur as a congenital defect.

Acquired aplastic anemia occurs as the result of exposure to certain physical and chemical agents. These include ionizing radiation, benzene and its derivatives, heavy metals, and certain chemotherapeutic agents. Other substances may produce a pancytopenia in some persons due to individual sensitivities. Among these agents are anticonvulsants, sedatives and tranquilizers, insecticides, and certain antimicrobials. The clinical course of the disease may show a rapid onset and a rapid progression to death, or it may have a slow onset and a chronic course. Laboratory tests generally show pancytopenia with low white blood cell, red blood cell, and platelet counts. The red blood cells are usually normocytic and normochromic. In rare cases, the red blood cells may be macrocytic. Varying degrees of anisocytosis and poikilocytosis may be present. Basophilic stippling, polychromatophilia, and nucleated red blood cells are absent from the peripheral blood. Reticulocytes are decreased to absent. There is generally a neutropenia along with a relative lymphocytosis. The bone marrow is hypocellular, with an increase in fat. Relative lymphocytosis may also be present in the bone marrow. Occasionally, biopsies show a normal marrow. This is misleading because there may be small areas in the marrow in which there is residual blood cell producing activity. A repeat marrow biopsy at another location gives the typical hypocellular picture. The bleeding time and clot retraction are usually abnormal because of the absence of platelets. The serum iron level is increased, and the iron binding protein is saturated. Erythropoietin levels are greatly increased. Treatment of aplastic anemia involves: (1) removal of the causative agent, if known, (2) red blood cell transfusions to maintain a minimum hemoglobin level, (3) platelet transfusions if necessary, (4) prevention of infection, (5) bone marrrow transplantation for severe forms of the disease, and (6) corticosteroids, androgens, and splenectomy for those patients with less severe forms of the illness or those who cannot undergo bone marrow transplantation.

Aplastic anemia may also develop several months following the onset of viral hepatitis. The prognosis in these cases is not good and may result in death. Aplastic anemia has also been found as a complication of tuberculosis, following pregnancy, in autoimmune diseases, and in paroxysmal nocturnal hemoglobinuria.

Idiopathic aplastic anemia is an acquired condition of unknown cause which accounts for about 50% of the cases of aplastic anemia. The symptoms and laboratory tests are similar to those of the other acquired aplastic anemias.

Fanconi's anemia (familial aplastic anemia) is a congenital form of pancytopenia which occurs in children. Some chromosomal defects have been described, and developmental abnormalities are present. Deposits of melanin are common, which show up as patches of brown pigmentation of the skin. There is generally a normocytic to slightly macrocytic anemia. Target cells may be present, along with nucleated red blood cells and immature white blood cells. The bone marrow may be normocellular to hypercellular in the beginning but will become hypocellular as the disease progresses. Hemoglobin F is generally increased. This disorder is usually treated with androgens and corticosteroids and has about the same prognosis as the acquired form of the disease.

PURE RED BLOOD CELL APLASIA

Pure red blood cell aplasia is a term given to a category of diseases in which red blood cell production is suppressed, with little or no abnormalities found in the white blood cells or platelets.

Congenital erythroid hypoplasia (Diamond-Blackfan syndrome) is a rare disorder that is characterized by a moderate to severe anemia. It generally manifests itself during the first 2 to 3 months of life. Infants with this disorder generally show pallor and may or may not have splenomegaly and/or hepatomegaly. At diagnosis, the hemoglobin is quite low, 2 to 10 g/dL, and the anemia is normochromic and may be slighly macrocytic. Reticulocytes in the peripheral blood are decreased to absent. The bone marrow is generally normal except for a marked decrease in erythroid cells. Corticosteroid therapy is used in the treatment of this disorder. When patients do not respond to this treatment, blood transfusions are used. Hemochromatosis and severe liver damage may develop, however, as a complication of transfusion therapy.

Acute acquired pure red blood cell aplasia (acute acquired erythropoietic hypoplasia) may suddenly occur for a short period during the course of a hemolytic anemia, certain infections, malnutrition, or with various kinds of drug therapy. The erythroblasts in the bone marrow will suddenly disappear, and an anemia soon develops if this condition persists for any length of time. When this condition occurs during drug therapy, removal of the drug is generally followed by a return to normal erythropoiesis.

Chronic acquired pure red blood cell aplasia (chronic acquired erythrocytic hypoplasia) occurs in adults. About one half of the cases of this disorder have been found in patients with a thymoma (thymic tumor). Removal of the tumor, when present, is followed by an improvement in erythropoiesis more than 50% of the time. The anemia of this disorder is generally severe and is normocytic to slightly macrocytic. The white blood cells and platelets are usually normal. Reticulocytes are decreased to absent. The bone marrow shows normal white blood cell and platelet development and a marked decrease in maturing red blood cells. The serum iron level is usually increased, and the iron binding capacity is saturated. Some patients have been treated successfully with corticosteroids and immunosuppressive drugs. Patients with systemic lupus erythematosus and with lymphomas may also develop an acquired pure red cell aplasia.

HEMOLYTIC ANEMIAS

The hemolytic anemias are a group of anemias that are characterized by an increased destruction of red blood cells. In this condition, the bone marrow is able to respond to the red blood cell destruction. These anemias may be divided into those that are inherited and those that are acquired. Generally speaking, the red blood cells in hemolytic anemias that are inherited have intrinsic defects within the red blood cell itself. These intrinsic defects involve membrane disorders, defects in hemoglobin synthesis, and enzyme disorders within the red cell. The acquired hemolytic anemias usually have normal red blood cells that are destroyed by extrinsic factors or agents outside of the red blood cell. Intravascular hemolysis and extravascular hemolysis refer to the site of red blood cell breakdown: within the bloodstream or outside the blood.

Hereditary Spherocytosis

Hereditary spherocytosis, also known as *congenital hemolytic anemia* and *congenital hemolytic jaundice,* is inherited as a non-sex-linked dominant trait. The symptoms of this condition are variable, depending on the severity of the disease. As a general rule, those cases recognized early in the life of the patient are likely to be more severe than those cases where the symptoms appear later in life. Most often, hereditary spherocytosis is diagnosed in childhood, adolescence, or early adult life. The disorder is caused by a defect in the red blood cell membrane. Evidence suggests the primary defect involves the structure of spectrin, a skeletal protein on the internal surface of the red blood cell membrane. The red cells become hyperpermeable to sodium due to the weakened membrane structure. Normally, the osmotic balance of the red cell is maintained with sufficient glucose and ATP to expel sodium at a rate equal to its influx. However, spherocytes consume glucose at a rapid rate. When the amount of glucose is low, there is an increased rate of destruction of the red cells. The water content of the red cell increases and as a result, swelling and hemolysis of the red blood cells occur. As the name of the disease implies, the red cells are spherocytic. The exact defect present, however, is not known. The most consistent physical finding is splenomegaly. Jaundice is commonly present and increases during hemolytic episodes. The liver is usually enlarged, and the patient may also exhibit pallor, depending on the degree of anemia present.

This disease is usually accompanied by a moderate anemia. The most constant finding in the peripheral blood is spherocytes. These cells have a decreased diameter and an increased concentration of hemoglobin. The number of spherocytes varies from a few to many. Polychromatophilia is present, and the reticulocyte count may be increased to 20% or higher. There are usually a few nucleated red blood cells present in the peripheral blood. This number increases, however, as the bone marrow responds during hemolytic episodes. The white blood cell and platelet counts are usually normal, except during periods of hemolysis, when there is thrombocytosis and a slight leukocytosis with a left shift. The osmotic fragility test is increased, and the autohemolysis test usually shows greater than 20% hemolysis after 48 hours' incubation. The serum bilirubin level is elevated, and the urine and stool may contain increased amounts of urobilinogen. Plasma haptoglobin is generally reduced and may be undetectable. The direct Coombs' test is negative. The bone marrow is hypercellular, with an absolute increase in the erythroid cells. These cells usually constitute 25 to 60% of all the marrow cells.

The treatment for this condition is splenectomy. Spherocytosis continues, but the red blood cell survival time is no longer decreased, because the spleen was the organ responsible for the destruction of the red blood cells (extravascular hemolysis). The red blood cell count (also hemoglobin and hematocrit) increases, and the bilirubin level returns to normal. The reticulocyte count decreases, and increased red blood cell production is no longer present. The osmotic fragility and autohemolysis tests continue to be increased.

Hereditary Elliptocytosis

Hereditary elliptocytosis is a red cell membrane disorder and is transmitted as an autosomal dominant gene. This condition is characterized by the presence of variable numbers of elliptical, or oval shaped, mature red cells on the blood smear. The nucleated red blood cells and reticulocytes are normal in shape, however.

Approximately 90% of the individuals showing elliptocytosis have no clinical symptoms other than the presence of elliptical red blood cells. The remaining patients with this condition, however, display a hemolytic anemia and splenomegaly similar to hereditary spherocytosis. In this case, the osmotic fragility and

autohemolysis of the red blood cells are increased. A splenectomy alleviates the hemolytic condition.

Abetalipoproteinemia

Abetalipoproteinemia is characterized by the absence of beta-lipoprotein in the blood. Normally, beta-lipoproteins are major components of the red cell membrane. This disorder manifests itself during the first few months of life with growth failure, abdominal distention, and steatorrhea. Acanthocytosis of the red blood cells, retinitis pigmentosa, and neurologic damage are also present. Laboratory tests show a decreased cholesterol level (usually less than 50 mg/dL) and the absence of beta-lipoprotein in the plasma. The blood smear exhibits large numbers of acanthocytes. The reticulocyte count is normal to increased, and if anemia is present, it is mild. The red blood cell life span may or may not be shortened. There is no definite treatment for this disorder.

Stomatocytosis

Several causes of stomatocytosis have been described: (1) red blood cells contain an increased amount of sodium and a decreased amount of potassium, (2) red blood cells lack the Rh blood group antigens (Rh_{NULL} phenotype), or (3) red blood cells have neither of the above characteristics. Stomatocytes may also be found in acute alcoholism, liver disorders, cardiovascular disease, and in a small percentage of normal individuals.

Stomatocytosis caused by increased sodium and decreased potassium is inherited as an autosomal dominant trait. The hemolytic anemia may be mild to severe. The reticulocyte count may be normal to moderately elevated and is usually 10 to 20%. Approximately 10 to 50% of the red blood cells will appear as stomatocytes. The serum bilirubin level will be increased and the haptoglobin decreased, depending on the amount of hemolysis present. The osmotic fragility may be decreased, normal, or increased. Autohemolysis is increased and is corrected with glucose and ATP. Red blood cell survival is generally slightly shortened. Splenectomy may or may not aid in the treatment of this disorder.

Rh$_{NULL}$ Disease

Rh$_{NULL}$ disease is inherited as a result of gene deletion or suppression. It represents an absence of all Rh-Hr antigens on the red blood cell which results in red cell membrane abnormalities. It is characterized by a mild normocytic-normochromic anemia. The blood smear shows both stomatocytes and spherocytes. The reticulocyte count is generally slightly elevated. The autohemolysis and osmotic fragility are both increased.

High Phosphatidylcholine Hemolytic Anemia

High phosphatidylcholine hemolytic anemia is inherited and represents an imbalance in the membrane phospholipid content of the red blood cell. It usually causes a mild anemia with morphologically normal red blood cells. The anemia may increase in the presence of infection or under conditions of stress.

Glucose-6-Phosphate Dehydrogenase Deficiency

Glucose-6-phosphate dehydrogenase (G-6-PD) deficiency is inherited. It is sex linked, being carried on the X chromosome. The disease becomes fully expressed in the hemizygous male and the homozygous female. It is the most common red cell enzyme abnormality, and it affects about 10% of American black males.

Glucose-6-phosphate dehydrogenase is an enzyme present in the red blood cell. It plays a major role in the hexose monophosphate shunt. It is concerned with the regeneration of TPNH, necessary for the reduction of oxidized glutathione—a mechanism by which hemoglobin is pro-

tected from oxidation. The absence of this enzyme is usually harmless unless the red blood cell is exposed to redox compounds (antimalarial drugs, sulfonamides, nitrofurans, sulfones, analgesics, and antipyretics). When there is a deficiency of G-6-PD, the red blood cell is unable to generate reduced nicotinamide-adenine dinucleotide phosphate (NADP) rapidly enough to combat the effects of oxidizing drugs. Hemoglobin is oxidized to methemoglobin which denatures and precipitates as Heinz bodies. Red cell hemolysis occurs as a result of the increased rigidity of the red cell caused by Heinz body inclusions and membrane damage from the oxidants. There are both quantitatively and qualitatively abnormal forms of the enzyme, which may be due to a decrease in the enzyme activity or to a qualitative abnormality of the enzyme itself. Certain individuals have a type of the deficiency which renders them sensitive to fava beans, resulting in severe hemolytic episodes.

Upon continual ingestion of a redox compound by a patient deficient in G-6-PD, a hemolytic episode will occur. This condition may be divided into three phases: (1) During the acute hemolytic phase, there is destruction of 30 to 50% of the red blood cells. There is Heinz body formation, and basophilic stippling and polychromatophilia are present on the peripheral blood smear. The serum bilirubin is elevated, as is the reticulocyte count. (2) During the recovery phase (tenth to fortieth day), the reticulocyte count reaches a peak of 8 to 12%. Macrocytes are present on the peripheral blood smear, and the hemoglobin and hematocrit levels begin to increase to normal. Haptoglobin is absent in the blood, and methemalbumin is present. Plasma hemoglobin is increased during the first two stages. (3) The resistant phase begins when the anemia disappears and continues as long as the same dose of the drug is administered. If the drug dosage is increased, another hemolytic episode will occur.

A few patients continually show chronic anemia, but the majority are not anemic except during a hemolytic episode after exposure to certain drugs. The autohemolysis test shows increased hemolysis of red blood cells after 48-hour incubation in patients with glucose-6-phosphate dehydrogenase deficiency. The autohemolysis, however, is partially corrected by the addition of glucose or ATP. This deficiency has, therefore, been described as having type I autohemolysis. The ascorbate-cyanide test is positive for patients with this deficiency. Heinz body formation is increased when blood from G-6-PD deficient individuals is incubated with acetylphenylhydrazine. Treatment involves the avoidance of drugs known to induce hemolysis.

Pyruvate Kinase Deficiency

Pyruvate kinase is an enzyme in the Embden-Meyerhof pathway and may be the most common cause of hereditary nonspherocytic hemolytic anemia involving this pathway. Pyruvate kinase catalyzes the formation of pyruvate from phosphoenolpyruvate with subsequent conversion of ADP to ATP. ATP provides the energy required for normal red cell membrane function and other glycolytic reactions. Pyruvate kinase deficient red cells have a decreased life span due to the lack of ATP and their inability to utilize glucose. The red blood cells are removed from the circulation extravascularly by the spleen and liver.

Pyruvate kinase deficiency is inherited as an autosomal recessive trait, with members of both sexes being equally affected. Heterozygous individuals manifest no symptoms (as there is sufficient pyruvate kinase activity to support normal red cell survival), whereas homozygous individuals have the clinical disease. If the disease is present at birth, the newborn is jaundiced and may require transfusions or

exchange transfusions. In most instances of pyruvate kinase deficiency, however, the disease is first found in infancy or childhood, with some cases not appearing until adulthood. Characteristics of this disorder are jaundice, splenomegaly, anemia of varying severity, and occasional dark urine.

The laboratory findings in this disorder show mild to severe anemia with hematocrit levels of approximately 18 to 36%. The red blood cells are normochromic and may be slightly macrocytic. The reticulocyte count is moderately to markedly increased, and the peripheral blood smear shows polychromatophilia and the presence of nucleated red blood cells. There may be slight anisocytosis, and there are generally irregularly contracted red blood cells present. Heinz bodies are not formed. The white blood cell and platelet counts are usually normal. In the autohemolysis test, the type II pattern is found. Mildly affected patients, however, may show a normal autohemolysis test. The bone marrow shows erythroid hyperplasia. The serum bilirubin and fecal urobilinogen levels are increased. The serum haptoglobin is decreased to absent. The red blood cell pyruvate kinase activity is in the range of 5 to 25% of normal.

There is no exact treatment for pyruvate kinase deficiency. Limited use of blood transfusions and splenectomy have been utilized to raise the blood hemoglobin levels.

Other Red Blood Cell Enzyme Deficiencies

Other red blood cell enzyme deficiencies, not as common as G-6-PD and pyruvate kinase deficiencies, can also cause a hemolytic anemia.

Pyrimidine 5-nucleotidase (PN) deficiency causes an abnormality in nucleotide metabolism. Pyrimidine-5-nucleotidase deficiency is inherited as autosomal recessive and is characterized by mild to moderate chronic hemolytic anemia, reticulocytosis of greater than 10%, and splenomegaly. Pyrimidine nucleotides from degraded RNA in the reticulocyte normally cross the red cell membrane and leave the cell aided by pyrimidine-5-nucleotidase. A deficiency results in an accumulation of these pyrimidines in the red cell, impaired degradation of RNA, and pronouced basophilic stippling. The red blood cell autohemolysis is increased and only poorly corrected with glucose.

Glucosephosphate isomerase deficiency causes an abnormality in anaerobic glycolysis and is the third most common red blood cell enzyme deficiency. It causes a moderately severe anemia. The stained blood smear shows anisocytosis, poikilocytosis, and marked polychromatophilia, and nucleated red blood cells may also be present. The reticulocyte count may be significantly increased, and the autohemolysis test is increased with only partial correction by glucose and ATP. *Triosephosphate isomerase, hexokinase,* and *diphosphoglycerate mutase* are other enzyme deficiencies that have been found to occur and are involved in anaerobic glycolysis.

Several deficiencies (in addition to G-6-PD) have been found in enzymes required in the hexose monophosphate shunt. These deficiencies are rare and have been reported only in a few families, but do cause a hemolytic anemia. These deficiencies include *glutathione synthetase, glutathione peroxidase,* and *glutathione reductase.* As with G-6-PD deficiency, hemolysis increases with oxidant drug exposure or infection.

Unstable Hemoglobin Disease

Unstable hemoglobin disease is rare and may be caused by any one of a large number of hemoglobin variants, all of which are less stable than normal hemoglobin. Unstable hemoglobins occur as a result of amino acid substitutions, deletions, or cross-overs in one or several of the four polypeptide chains. They are inherited as autosomal dominant traits and all of the known cases are heterozygous. It has been suggested that homozygosity is incompatible with life. The severity of the disease varies according to the hemoglobin variant, and there may be no clinical symptoms or the disease may produce a mild, moderate, or severe hemolytic anemia. Jaundice is common if the hemolysis is severe. Cyanosis may be present in certain unstable hemoglobin diseases due to the formation of methemoglobin or sulfhemoglobin, or due to a decreased affinity of the hemoglobin molecule for oxygen. Hemoglobins H, Köln, and Zurich are examples of unstable hemoglobins causing hemolysis.

The degree of anemia and reticulocytosis present will depend on the severity of the disease. Heinz bodies are characteristically present in the red blood cells because of the instability of the hemoglobin. These may cause a lower than normal MCHC because the hemoglobin present in Heinz bodies is not measured. The stained blood smear generally shows anisocytosis, poikilocytosis, basophilic stippling, polychromatophilia, and sometimes hypochromia. If the anemia is severe, spherocytes and schistocytes may also be present. If the spleen is enlarged, there may be a thrombocytopenia caused by sequestering of the platelets in the spleen. The reticulocyte count will generally be increased. Much care must be taken when performing the reticulocyte count to distinguish the Heinz bodies from true reticulocytes. The heat denaturation test and the isopropanol precipitation test are both positive. Citrate agar gel electrophoresis at pH 6.2 and cellulose acetate hemoglobin electrophoresis at pH 8.6 are not useful for isolating unstable hemoglobins as most variants migrate with other major hemoglobins. Therapy is generally not necessary in cases of mild anemia. When the anemia is more severe, a splenectomy is generally performed.

Normal Hemoglobins and Hemoglobinopathies

The hemoglobin molecule is composed of two pairs of polypeptide chains, each with a specific amino acid sequence. Each polypeptide chain has a single heme group, consisting of an atom of iron bound within a protoporphyrin-9 ring. The polypeptide chains are twisted around on an axis in a helical arrangement, and are bound together to form the hemoglobin tetramer.

Different types of normal hemoglobins have been described and given specific names based on the number and sequence of amino acids composing each polypeptide chain. On the following pages, the normal and more common abnormal hemoglobin forms are discussed.

NORMAL HEMOGLOBINS

The major portion of normal hemoglobin in adult blood is termed *hemoglobin A*. The globin portion of each hemoglobin A molecule is composed of two alpha chains, containing 141 amino acids, and two beta chains, made up of 146 amino acids. The molecule is ellipsoidal, with the four heme groups (responsible for oxygen transport) at the surface. The formula for hemoglobin A is: $\alpha_2{}^A\beta_2{}^A$, indicating that the molecule is made up of two normal hemoglobin A, alpha chains, and two normal hemoglobin A, beta chains. The concentration of hemoglobin A normally comprises 95% or more of the total adult hemoglobin.

A second type of hemoglobin, hemoglobin A_2, is normally found in the adult in a concentration of 1.5 to 3% of the total hemoglobin. Iron deficiency can cause decreased hemoglobin A_2 synthesis. Hemoglobin A_2 consists of two alpha^A chains, and two other chains that differ from the beta^A chains by the substitution of 10 amino acids. These two chains, since they differ so greatly from beta^A chains, are termed delta, thus giving hemoglobin A_2 the formula: $\alpha_2{}^A\delta_2{}^{A2}$.

Fetal hemoglobin, hemoglobin F, is normally present in high concentrations during fetal life. At birth, at least half of the hemoglobin present in the newborn is hemoglobin F. The concentration of hemoglobin F then falls rapidly and assumes the normal adult level of 2% or less by 1 or 2 years of age. Hemoglobin F is composed of two alpha chains and two other chains that differ from the beta^A chains and are termed gamma. The formula for hemoglobin F is therefore: $\alpha_2{}^A\gamma_2{}^F$.

In early fetal life, three primitive or embryonal hemoglobins are found, namely, *hemoglobin Gower 1,* and *hemoglobin Gower 2,* and *hemoglobin Portland.* These three hemoglobins persist for only a short time in the embryo. Hemoglobin Gower 1 is composed of 2ζ (zeta) and 2ϵ chains, hemoglobin Gower 2 contains 2α and 2ϵ chains, and hemoglobin Portland, 2ζ and 2γ chains.

ABNORMAL HEMOGLOBINS

The structure of abnormal hemoglobins is based on at least four kinds of polypeptide chains, alpha, beta, delta, and gamma, and possibly a fifth chain, epsilon. The synthesis of any given type of chain is under genetic control. The structurally abnormal hemoglobins usually consist of polypeptide chains with a normal number of amino acids but with a single amino acid substitution. For example, if a normal pair of chains has glutamic acid at the sixth position, the abnormal form may have a valine molecule in place of the glutamic acid. In clinically significant disease, either the alpha or beta chains are affected. A large number of hemoglobin variants involving the gamma or delta chains are not clinically significant because of the small amount of hemoglobin involved. Alterations in the amino acid composition of the polypeptide chain usually cause a change in the net charge of the molecule. This property is then employed to detect the presence of different hemoglobins. Using the techniques of electrophoresis, blood is placed on a medium in an electric field in a buffer with a specific pH. The difference in the net charge of the hemoglobin molecule determines its mobility and the speed with which it migrates. Most of the abnormal hemoglobins that have been discovered are now detected by this method.

Hemoglobin S is an abnormal hemoglobin that causes sickling of the red blood cells under conditions of reduced oxygen concentration. It shows an amino acid substitution in the beta chains and is written as $\alpha_2^A\beta_2^{6\ val}$, indicating a substitution of valine for glutamic acid at the sixth position in the normal beta chain. Hemoglobin S is confined to blacks and, in the homozygous state, causes sickle cell anemia. An individual heterozygous for hemoglobin S shows the sickle cell trait.

Hemoglobin C $(\alpha_2^A\beta_2^{6\ lys})$ is found primarily in blacks and only rarely in whites and occurs as a result of the substitution of the amino acid lysine for glutamic acid on the sixth position of the beta chain. It is, many times, inherited in combination with hemoglobin S and may also be found in the homozygous or heterozygous state. When hemoglobin C is present, the red blood cells appear as target cells, or, less often, hemoglobin crystals may be demonstrated within the red blood cell.

Hemoglobin D shows several varieties of abnormal hemoglobin that are indistinguishable from each other by electrophoretic methods using cellulose acetate at a pH of 8.4. The variants with the highest frequency are hemoglobin D Punjab and hemoglobin D-Los Angeles. Both alpha and beta chain abnormalities have been reported. The electrophoretic mobility of hemoglobin D is the same as hemoglobin S, although red blood cells containing hemoglobin D show no sickling at a reduced oxygen concentration.

Hemoglobin E $(\alpha_2^A\beta_2^{26\ lys})$ shows the same electrophoretic mobility on cellulose acetate at a pH of 8.4, as hemoglobin A_2 and is sometimes associated with thalassemia.

Hemoglobins have also been found that contain no alpha chains. For example: *hemoglobin H* consists of four beta chains: β_4^A; and *hemoglobin Bart's* is comprised of four gamma chains: γ_4^F.

HEMOGLOBIN C DISEASE AND TRAIT

In the homozygous condition, there is almost 100% hemoglobin C present in the red blood cells. In some patients, there may also be an increased concentration of hemoglobin F. *Homozygous hemoglobin C disease* is characterized by a mild to moderate normocytic normochromic, hemolytic anemia with splenomegaly. The stained blood smear shows 40 to 90% target cells, a few spherocytes, and slight polychromatophilia. The reticulocyte count is slightly increased. In some instances, rod-shaped crystals (termed *hemoglobin C crystals*) may be seen within the red blood cell in the Wright-stained blood smear, or the crystals may be demonstrated by incubating the red blood cells at 37°C in 3% (w/v) sodium chloride. Hemoglobin electrophoresis shows almost 100% hemoglobin C and less than 7% hemoglobin F. Most patients with hemoglobin C disease live a normal life span. The incidence of hemoglobin C disease is rare in the United States with only about 0.02% of blacks having the disease.

In the heterozygous condition (hemoglobin C trait), there are no clinical symptoms. The blood smear shows about 40% target cells and mild hypochromia. About 2 to 3% of American blacks have hemoglobin C trait. Hemoglobin electrophoresis shows 35 to 45% hemoglobin C and 55 to 65% hemoglobin A.

SICKLE CELL ANEMIA

A person homozygous for hemoglobin S is said to have sickle cell anemia. This disorder occurs chiefly in blacks or persons of black ancestry. Its incidence in the United States is 2.5 to 3.5%. The red blood cells contains 90 to 100% hemoglobin S, with the remainder being hemoglobin F and hemoglobin A_2. There is normal synthesis of the α, γ, and δ chains, but only the characteristic α^S chains are synthesized. The symptoms of sickle cell anemia rarely occur prior to about 6 months of age, because hemoglobin F predominates at birth and for a short time thereafter. This disease is usually fatal by the age of 30. The physical properties of the red blood cells have much to do with the clinical manifestations of the disease. Under decreased oxygen tension, hemoglobin S is much less soluble than hemoglobin A. This forces the red blood cell into a rigid sickle-shaped cell when the oxygen concentration is reduced. As a result, clinical crises occur. There is severe abdominal, bone, and joint pain thought to be due, possibly, to plugging up of some of the small blood vessels by masses of the sickled red blood cells. There may be local thrombus formation as platelets adhere to damaged endothelium, factor XII is activated, and tissue thromboplastin is released. This, in turn, causes infarcts in different organs of the body. The spleen, enlarged during infancy, eventually shrivels up and becomes fibrotic in the adult (autosplenectomy) because of these numerous infarcts. The sickled red blood cells also have an increased mechanical fragility that results in a decreased survival time. There is severe marrow hyperplasia, and changes, such as necrosis and lesions, are produced in the bones.

On a stained blood smear, the red blood cells show moderate anisocytosis, poikilocytosis, and hypochromia. Some sickle cells are generally present. Target cells, Howell-Jolly bodies, and nucleated red blood cells are usually seen. Polychromatophilia is generally present, and an elevated reticulocyte count is found. The platelets are usually increased, and there may be moderate neutrophilia. The osmotic fragility test is decreased, and the erythrocyte sedimentation rate is low. Sic-

kle cell preparations are quickly and strongly positive. Hemoglobin electrophoresis shows a single abnormal band, hemoglobin S, which migrates more slowly than hemoglobin A. The bone marrow is hypercellular due to an increase in the erythroid cells. Cell maturation and morphology in the bone marrow are normal.

Treatment involves the use of antibiotics to combat infections and analgesics for pain, during crises. There are a number of antisickling agents under trial, and papaverine as a vasodilator has been used with good success.

SICKLE CELL TRAIT

The sickle cell trait is found in approximately 10% of American blacks. In this condition, the patient is heterozygous for hemoglobin S. The red blood cells contain 20 to 40% hemoglobin S and 60 to 68% hemoglobin A. Under normal conditions, sickling of the red blood cells does not occur, there are no clinical symptoms of the disease, and the patient lives a normal life span. There is no anemia present, and the red blood cell morphology is normal. An occasional target cell may be found, but no sickle cells are demonstrable in the stained blood smear. The reticulocyte count is normal, and there is no polychromatophilia on the stained blood smear. The sickle cell preparation is always positive, and hemoglobin electrophoresis shows a band of hemoglobin S. Over 50% of the patients with sickle cell trait do not have the ability to concentrate urine (hyposthenuria).

Under certain conditions, such as a respiratory infection, administration of anesthesia, or airplane flight in a nonpressurized cabin, there may be some sickling of the red blood cells with accompanying clinical manifestations.

Persons with sickle cell trait seem resistant to infection with P. falciparum malaria. Various hypotheses have been suggested about why cells containing hemoglobin S are not parasitized, but none are definite.

HEMOGLOBIN SC DISEASE

The combination of two abnormal β chain hemoglobins (S and C) leads to a disease only slightly less severe than the homozygous state of hemoglobin S. There is a high incidence in blacks of hemoglobin SC. This disease shows bone necrosis, splenomegaly, muscular pain, and complications during pregnancy. During pregnancy, crises are more frequent and can lead to fatal infarctions.

The peripheral blood smear shows up to 85% target cells, slight to marked anisocytosis and poikilocytosis, with sickle cells and hemoglobin C crystals often present. The anemia may be mild to moderate.

HEMOGLOBIN SD DISEASE

The combination of hemoglobins S and D is uncommon, but resembles hemoglobin SC disease in severity when found. Only the combination of hemglobins S and D Punjab shows moderate hemolytic anemia.

HEMOGLOBIN D DISEASE AND TRAIT

Hemoglobin D is rare in the United States, with the highest incidence in India or in British people with Indian ancestry. The trait is asymptomatic, with no anemia and a normal blood smear. The homozygous condition is extremely rare, but still asymptomatic with no hemolytic anemia. Hemoglobin D migrates with hemoglobin S on cellulose acetate at pH 8.6.

HEMOGLOBIN E DISEASE AND TRAIT

Hemoglobin E is rare in the United States, but is a common abnormal hemoglobin in southeast Asia. It is seen with increasing frequency in the United States as southeast Asians have emigrated to this country.

The homozygous state is characterized by mild hemolytic anemia and the peripheral smear shows marked hypochromia, many target cells, and microcytosis. The heterozygous state is asymptomatic with slight microcytosis on the blood smear. Hemoglobin E migrates with hemoglobins A_2 and C on cellulose acetate at pH 8.6, but with hemoglobin A on citrate agar gel at pH 6.2.

THALASSEMIA

Thalassemia is an hereditary disease found in people of Mediterranean, Asian, and African ancestry. It is caused by impaired production of one of the polypeptide chains of the hemoglobin molecule. The structural formation of the chains is normal, but the rate of formation is decreased or, the chains may not be synthesized at all. Impaired synthesis of the beta chain is the most common, and the term applied to this abnormality is *beta thalassemia*. In β^0 thalassemia, β chain synthesis is absent. In β^+ thalassemia, β chain synthesis is reduced. Decreased production of alpha chains and delta chains may also be found.

THALASSEMIA MAJOR

Thalassemia major, or *Cooley's anemia*, is a homozygous beta thalassemia. Despite impaired synthesis of the β chains, synthesis of α chains continues at a normal rate. This imbalance results in precipitation of excess α chains in the erythrocyte and membrane damage to the red blood cell. This disease generally has its onset during infancy. The most common physical findings are marked pallor and moderate to marked splenomegaly. Enlargement of the liver is also frequently present. Most of these patients exhibit retarded growth, and their facial features show a mongoloid appearance. Patients with Cooley's anemia rarely live beyond the second decade.

There is severe hemolytic anemia present. The peripheral blood smear shows microcytic, hypochromic red blood cells, probably due to the decreased synthesis of globin. There is marked anisocytosis and poikilocytosis. Basophilic stippling, increased polychromatophilia, numerous target cells, Howell-Jolly bodies, and siderocytes are commonly found in the blood smear. Nucleated red blood cells are present in the peripheral blood and may be as numerous as 200 or more per 100 white blood cells. The reticulocyte count is increased. The white blood cell count may be slightly increased, with occasional immature granulocytes present. A slight increase in platelets may also be found. The osmotic fragility test is decreased. The bone marrow shows an erythroid hyperplasia. Due to chronic hemolysis and frequent blood transfusions, excess iron accumulates in the spleen and liver. The plasma haptoglobin level is generally markedly decreased to absent and serum bilirubin is elevated. Hemoglobin electrophoresis most often shows 40 to 60% hemoglobin F. In some cases, hemoglobin A_2 is also increased.

THALASSEMIA MINOR

Thalassemia minor is a heterozygous beta thalassemia that is also known as Cooley's trait. This condition is characterized by slight splenomegaly and mild anemia. Patients with this trait generally live a normal life span.

The peripheral blood usually shows a hemoglobin of 10 to 11 g/dL. Microcytic, hypochromic red blood cells are found on the blood smear. Target cells, increased polychromatophilia, basophilic stippling, and an occasional nucleated red blood cell are found on the Wright stained smear. The reticulocyte count is slightly elevated. The white blood cell count is normal. The bone marrow shows slight erythroid hyperplasia and increased storage iron. Hemoglobin electrophoresis shows 2 to 6% hemoglobin F and 3 to 7% hemoglobin A_2, with the remainder being hemoglobin A.

SICKLE CELL-β-THALASSEMIA DISEASE

Patients doubly heterozygous for β thalassemia and hemoglobin S show an ane-

mia which may be mild to severe. In severe cases (β^0 thalassemia), the peripheral blood smear shows microcytosis, hypochromia, anisocytosis and poikilocytosis. The reticulocyte count is about 10 to 20%. Hemoglobin electrophoresis shows hemoglobin S in excess of hemoglobin A (which may be absent) and increased hemoglobins A_2 and F. Clinical manifestations are similar to sickle cell anemia, and the spleen is enlarged. Mild cases (β^+ thalassemia) have little or no anemia.

HEREDITARY PERSISTENCE OF FETAL HEMOGLOBIN (HPFH)

Hereditary persistence of fetal hemoglobin is characterized by the persistence of fetal hemoglobin in adult life and is a benign condition with no hematologic abnormalities. There is a suppression of β chain synthesis in a heterozygous state with 20 to 30% hemoglobin F, or, the rarer homozygous state with 100% hemoglobin F. When combined with hemoglobin S, persons exhibit no symptoms or anemia of the sickle cell disease. The presence of hemoglobin F in red cells inhibits in vivo sickling.

ALPHA (α) THALASSEMIAS

An α thalassemia of varying severity results from reduced or absent α-chain synthesis affecting the two pairs of α globin genes (one pair in each chromosome). The degree of abnormality varies in proportion to the number of genes affected. As the capacity to produce α chains decreases, this results in an accumulation of excess γ chains to form hemoglobin Barts (γ_4) and an excess of β chains to form hemoglobin H (β_4).

When there is deletion of only one gene, the resultant microcytosis is slight with no anemia. In a two gene deletion moderate microcytosis with no anemia results and is called α^0 thalassemia trait. A three gene deletion causes hemoglobin H disease with MCV's less than 70 fL and mild to severe anemia caused by hemoglobin H denaturation and red cell destruction. The peripheral blood smear shows hypochromia, microcytosis, anisocytosis, target cells, and basophilic stippling. Since hemoglobin H is unstable, it readily precipitates in the form of H bodies when fresh blood is incubated with brilliant cresyl blue. When α chain production is totally absent, there is no hemoglobin A or F production or oxygen transport, which leads to death in utero (hydrops fetalis).

Acquired Hemolytic Anemias

A hemolytic anemia may develop as a result of exposure to various physical agents such as heat. A substantial amount of third degree burns to the body will damage red blood cells. The blood smear in these cases will show schistocytes, microspherocytes, and irregularly contracted red blood cells. The red blood cells will also show increased osmotic fragility. In cardiac valve disease where the diseased valve has been surgically replaced, mechanical damage to the red blood cells may occur.

Infectious agents, such as Clostridium perfringens, Bartonella bacilliformis, and some staphylococcal and other bacterial infections, have been known to produce a hemolytic anemia by producing toxins.

Some chemicals and drugs are capable of denaturing hemoglobin or causing a hemolytic response. Venom from some spiders and snakes may also cause intravascular hemolysis of the red blood cells.

Isoimmune Hemolytic Anemia

Isoantibodies are antibodies formed by a person who lacks any antigen that would react with this antibody. An example of this would occur if an Rh negative person were transfused with Rh positive blood. Isoimmune hemolytic anemia will occur as a result of hemolytic transfusion reactions and will also be found in hemolytic disease of the newborn.

Hemolytic Disease of the Newborn

Hemolytic disease of the newborn, or *erythroblastosis fetalis,* is a disorder found in the fetus that manifests itself in the infant during the first several days of life. This disease is usually associated with cases of Rh incompatibility where the mother is Rh negative, and the newborn is Rh positive. It is found, with more frequency and less severity, when there is incompatibility within the mother and child's ABO groups. Usually, the mother is type O, and the fetus is type A or B. This disorder may also be caused by other blood group systems such as Kell and Duffy. Transplacental hemorrhage of fetal erythrocytes containing an antigen absent on maternal red blood cells results in antibody production by the mother. Since transplacental hemorrhage usually occurs at the time of delivery, first born infants are usually asymptomatic. In ABO hemolytic disease, first born infants can be affected. IgG antibodies with subsequent pregnancies cross the placental barrier from the maternal to fetal circulation, where they combine with the antigens on fetal erythrocytes to destroy them.

In hemolytic disease of the newborn, the infant's peripheral blood shows a large increase in nucleated red blood cells, usually present in all stages of development. There is very little anisocytosis; however, a marked polychromatophilia is present. The reticulocyte count is increased and may even be as high as 60%. The red blood cells are usually normochromic and macrocytic. When the hemolytic anemia is due to an ABO incompatibility, there may be marked spherocytosis (accompanied by an increase in the osmotic fragility of the red blood cells). The hemoglobin level at birth is generally slightly lower than normal, decreasing rapidly as the disease progresses. At the same time, the nucleated red blood cells decrease in number and may disappear from the peripheral blood. The white blood cell count is generally elevated, and immature forms of the granulocytic cells are usually present. Platelets are normal to decreased in number. If decreased, there may be a prolonged bleeding time, poor clot retraction, and petechiae. The serum bilirubin level of umbilical cord blood will be above 3 mg/dL. After birth, the bilirubin level rises rapidly and may reach 40 to 50 mg/dL by the third day in cases where no treatment has been given. This rise in bilirubin is due to the indirect fraction of bilirubin. Lipid soluble unconjugated bilirubin may be taken up by nervous tissue causing toxic damage (kernicterus). The direct Coombs' test on the baby's red blood cells is positive in all cases except in ABO incompatibility, where the direct Coombs' test is generally negative or weakly positive, becoming negative within 12 hours after birth. The infant with this disorder has an enlarged spleen and liver.

The most common treatment for hemolytic disease of the newborn is the exchange transfusion. If the cord blood bilirubin level at birth is above 4.5 mg/dL, an exchange transfusion is usually carried out immediately. Albumin infusions are also used to bind unconjugated bilirubin, and light treatments are used in milder cases to convert bilirubin to less toxic derivatives. During the first few days of life, the bilirubin level is allowed to rise to 20 mg/dL before an exchange transfusion is performed. More than one exchange transfusion may or may not be required, depending on the severity of the disease.

AUTOIMMUNE HEMOLYTIC ANEMIA

Autoantibodies are antibodies produced by an individual that react with specific antigens on his own red blood cells. Therefore, in autoimmune hemolytic anemia, the antibodies are produced by the patient's immune system. These anemias may be classified as (1) warm reactive, (2) cold reactive, or (3) drug induced.

Autoimmune hemolytic anemia caused by warm reactive antibodies may occur without any obvious cause or may be secondary to or associated with various disease states such as viral infections, malignant tumors, systemic lupus erythematosus, and other autoimmune disorders. These warm-reactive IgG antibodies bind optimally at 37°C and the red cell-antibody complexes are cleared by the spleen. The clinical symptoms will include weakness and dizziness. Fever may be present, and jaundice is a fairly common finding. This anemia may be variable in its severity, ranging from mild to very severe. The blood smear generally shows anisocytosis, polychromatophilia, spherocytosis, and some macrocytosis, and nucleated red blood cells may also be present. The reticulocyte count is variable and may show a marked increase. Siderocytes will be increased. The white blood cell count may be increased during the acute phase of the disease. Generally, the platelet count is normal. The autohemolysis test is increased, and the osmotic fragility will be increased during the acute phase but may be normal during periods of remission. The direct antiglobulin test is generally positive but may be negative in cases of weak red blood cell sensitization. Several methods of treatment are used for this disorder. If the hemolytic anemia is secondary to another disorder, treatment of the primary condition may alleviate the hemolytic anemia. In addition, blood transfusions are used to treat the decreased hemoglobin, although steroids are the therapy of choice. When steroid therapy is ineffective, a splenectomy may be performed. Cytotoxic drugs have also been utilized.

Autoimmune hemolytic anemia due to IgM cold reactive antibodies is caused by antibodies most reactive at temperatures below 32°C. This disease occurs most often in people over 50 years of age and may occur in association with infection, malignancy, or autoimmune disorders. It is most commonly found as a complication of Mycoplasma pneumoniae. The two most common cold agglutinins are anti-I and anti-i. A stained blood film generally shows polychromatophilia, possibly some spherocytosis, and agglutination of the red blood cells (unless measures were taken to maintain the blood and equipment at 37°C during smear preparation). The white blood cell count may or may not be elevated. The direct antiglobulin test will be positive if the reagents used contain anticomplement activity. The cold agglutinin titer is increased. Treatment of the patient includes keeping body temperature above the temperature at which the antibody reacts. Plasmapheresis has been used for the acutely ill patient. Also, treatment of the primary illness may lessen the hemolytic disorder.

Drug-induced autoimmune hemolytic anemia may result from penicillin, stibophen, or an alpha-methyldopa type of drug. The mechanism by which the drug causes hemolysis depends on the type of drug involved. Penicillin and cephalosporin combine with proteins on the red cell membrane and provoke an immune response by the formation of antibodies to these drugs. Stibophen and sulfonamides cause an antibody response with subsequent absorption of the complex to the red cell membrane. Alpha-methyl dopa induces the formation of an antibody specifically directed against normal red blood cell antigens.

Paroxysmal Cold Hemoglobinuria

Paroxysmal cold hemoglobinuria is a rare disorder caused by a complement dependent hemolytic antibody described by Donath and Landsteiner, which has thus been named the *Donath-Landsteiner antibody*. It has classically been found secondary to syphilis but has also been seen in viral infections with no apparent cause. The Donath-Landsteiner antibody is an IgG immunoglobulin. The hemolytic reaction occurs as the antibody is bound to the red blood cell in the presence of complement at low temperatures, followed by hemolysis at body temperature.

This disorder manifests itself following exposure to cold, and the patient will exhibit fever, chills, and back and leg pain, along with hemoglobinuria. The patient generally recovers from the attack quickly and may have no symptoms in between attacks.

Laboratory tests show an anemia, the severity of which depends on the severity of the attacks. The reticulocyte count is usually increased. During attacks, the plasma shows marked hemolysis and will contain methemalbumin. The urine contains hemoglobin and methemoglobin, and the serum bilirubin level is elevated. Treatment consists of improving the primary infection, when present, or having the patient avoid cold temperatures.

Disorders Causing Fragmentation of the Red Blood Cells

There are numerous circumstances during which the red blood cells are subjected to physical trauma causing fragmentation and lysis.

Replacement of cardiac valves by *prosthetic devices* may result in enough damage and destruction to the red blood cell (by the prosthetic device itself) to cause anemia of varying severity. This has been aptly called the 'Waring blender syndrome'. In this situation, the stained blood smear characteristically shows schistocytes. Polychromatophilia and some macrocytosis may also be present. The reticulocyte count will be increased. The bilirubin and plasma hemoglobin may be elevated, depending on the severity of the anemia. Cases where the anemia is severe may indicate a malfunction of the replaced valve, and repeat surgery may be necessary.

Microangiopathic hemolytic anemia is generally a result of fibrin deposits within the small blood vessels, as found in association with thrombotic thrombocytopenia purpura and intravascular coagulation. Blood flowing through fibrin strands results in 'clothesline-like' shearing of the red blood cells. It is also present in malignant hypertension, disseminated carcinoma, and hemolytic uremic syndrome in children. The common denominator in these diseases is the presence of small blood vessel disease or pathologic lesions of the small blood vessels. Red cell contact with damaged endothelial cells of the blood vessels results in fragmentation. In this anemia, red blood cell fragmentation (schistocytes) and irregular contraction of the red blood cells are characteristic findings on the blood smear. Microspherocytes may also be present. The reticulocyte count is generally elevated, and the white blood cell count may be slightly to moderately increased. The platelet count may be normal or decreased, largely depending on the primary disorder. The bone marrow usually shows increased red blood cell hyperplasia and megakaryocyte hyperplasia. The plasma hemoglobin is generally increased, urine hemoglobin is present, and hemosiderin can most often be demonstrated in the urine. Therapy usually consists of treating the primary disease. Blood transfusions have been used to treat the anemia when necessary.

Paroxysmal Nocturnal Hemoglobinuria

Paroxysmal nocturnal hemoglobinuria (PNH) is a rare, chronic, acquired, hemolytic disease. The exact cause of this disorder is unknown. There appears to be an acquired intrinsic defect in the red blood cells that makes the cell sensitive to lysis by heat labile serum factors (complement). Infections and physical stress may result in complement activation and subsequent hemolytic episodes. The severity of the disorder varies from patient to patient and from time to time in the same patient. In cases of severe hemolytic episodes, blood transfusion may be necessary. The transfused red blood cells have normal survival rates. Thrombotic complications are common in these patients.

This disorder is characterized by intravascular hemolysis and hemoglobinuria during and following sleep in the classic case. However, typical sleep related hemoglobinuria is seen in less than 25% of the patients. The peripheral blood shows normocytic-normochromic anemia. The platelet and white blood cell counts are usually decreased. The reticulocyte count is elevated. The bone marrow may be hypercellular with erythroid hyperplasia, or, as occurs in some patients, it may be hypocellular. The leukocyte alkaline phosphatase is decreased, the direct Coombs' test is negative, and the serum haptoglobin is decreased. Diagnosis of this condition may be confirmed by the acid serum test and sugar water test.

POLYCYTHEMIA

Polycythemia is a term used to signify an above normal hemoglobin, hematocrit, and red blood cell count. It may also be referred to as *erythrocytosis.* This condition is classified as relative or absolute. Absolute polycythemia is further subdivided into secondary and primary polycythemia (polycythemia vera).

Relative Polycythemia

Relative polycythemia is caused by a decrease in the fluid (plasma) portion of the blood. Therefore, the actual number of red blood cells in the blood is not increased, but the number of cells per unit volume of blood is increased.

Relative polycythemia is found in association with acute dehydration and in cases of stress or spurious polycythemia. This latter condition occurs primarily in middle aged males and may be associated with smoking, cardiovascular problems, hypertension and diuretic therapy.

The peripheral blood smear shows normocytic-normochromic red blood cells and normal white blood cell, red blood cell, and platelet morphology. The hemoglobin, hematocrit, and red blood cell count are elevated. The white blood cell count may be normal or, in dehydration, slightly elevated. The whole blood volume is decreased, whereas the total red blood cell volume is normal. A normal bone marrow is found in this condition, and the leukocyte alkaline phosphatase is also normal.

Absolute Polycythemia

SECONDARY POLYCYTHEMIA

Secondary polycythemia is caused by an increased level of erythropoietin in the blood. This may occur as a normal response to hypoxia or as the result of inappropriate erythropoietin production. An appropriate response to hypoxia occurs in any disorder or circumstance that decreases the arterial oxygen saturation of the blood or decreases the capacity of the hemoglobin molecule to carry oxygen. Specific causes include: residence at high altitudes, chronic pulmonary disease, chronic congestive heart failure, smoking, abnormal hemoglobins which have a high oxygen affinity and in methemoglobinemia. An inappropriate production of erythropoietin is found in certain tumors of the liver, brain, kidney, and the adrenal and pituitary glands. In this type of secondary polycythemia, the erythropoietin level is elevated, but the arterial oxygen saturation of the blood is normal and no conditions of hypoxia are present.

The peripheral blood smear shows normocytic-normochromic red blood cells, and normal white blood cell, red blood cell, and platelet morphology. The hemoglobin, hematocrit, and red blood cell count are elevated. The white blood cell count is normal. The whole blood volume is increased as a result of the increased total red blood cell mass. The bone marrow shows erythroid hyperplasia, and the leukocyte alkaline phosphatase is normal.

PRIMARY POLYCYTHEMIA (POLYCYTHEMIA VERA)

Polycythemia vera is a myeloproliferative disease of unknown origin that is found most often in patients over 60 years of age. At onset, this disease is characterized by an absolute increase in red blood cells, white blood cells, and platelets. This gives rise to an increased blood volume that may measure 2 to 3 times normal. The plasma volume shows little or no change. Because of the increased red blood cell concentration, the viscosity of the blood becomes increased, and the patient shows increased skin coloration. The blood pressure is usually elevated. Increased platelets, along with the increased blood viscosity, may cause the formation of intravascular thrombi. Splenomegaly is a relatively common finding, and an enlarged liver is found in many cases. The arterial oxygen saturation and erythropoietin level are both normal. There is a marked increase in the incidence of peptic ulcer among patients with this disorder.

The peripheral blood smear shows normocytic-normochromic red blood cells, moderate anisocytosis, and slight polychromatophilia. There may be occasional nucleated red blood cells and immature granulocytes present. Atypical platelets or megakaryocyte fragments may also be seen. The relative and absolute number of eosinophils and basophils may be increased, and neutrophilia is usually present. The red blood cell count, hemoglobin, hematocrit, white blood cell count, and platelet count are increased. The reticulocyte count generally shows a slight elevation, not usually over 4%, however. The erythrocyte sedimentation rate is usually decreased. The bone marrow is hypercellular, showing an increase in the granulocytic, erythroid, and megakaryocytic cells. The distribution, morphology, and maturation of the marrow cells are normal. The leukocyte alkaline phosphatase is usually increased, which aids in distinguishing polycythemia vera from other types of erythrocytosis.

Methods of treatment for polycythemia vera include phlebotomies at regular intervals, radioactive phosphorus, and alkylating agents, as used for treatment in leukemia. If the patient does not die from complications of the disease, the bone marrow may become fibrotic until it reaches an aplastic stage. A mild anemia develops, which later becomes marked. Hemorrhagic problems may develop due to platelets that are decreased or abnormal. Hematopoiesis may begin to occur in the liver and spleen. Nucleated red blood cells, myelocytes, and sometimes even myeloblasts may be found in the peripheral blood. Some cases terminate in acute or chronic myelogenous leukemia or myelofibrosis with myeloid metaplasia.

METHEMOGLOBINEMIA

Methemoglobinemia may be inherited as an autosomal recessive trait caused by a deficiency in NADH-methemoglobin reductase, it may be acquired as a result of exposure to various chemical compounds, or it may be caused by any one of five hemoglobin M variants. Methemoglobin differs from normal oxyhemoglobin in that the iron in the heme molecule is in the ferric state rather than the ferrous state, and the O_2 is replaced by –OH. Normally, less than 1% of the hemoglobin is methemoglobin. Due to decreased affinity of methemoglobin for oxygen, one of the primary characteristics of these disorders is cyanosis, which gives a bluish color to the skin and mucous membranes.

In *hereditary methemoglobinemia,* infants are cyanotic at birth. Mental retardation may be present, but otherwise the disease is usually benign. A mild polycythemia may sometimes be present. The cyanosis is generally only of importance cosmetically. This disease may be treated with methylene blue taken orally to maintain the methemoglobin concentration below 10%. Ascorbic acid is also used in treatment.

Acquired methemoglobinemia is the most common type of this disorder and is usually due to the toxic effect of such drugs as aniline dyes and derivatives, sul-fonamides, nitrates and nitrites, chlorates, nitroglycerin, and some benzenes, among others. The concentration of methemoglobin in the blood will depend on the degree of exposure to the drug. Cyanosis generally appears when the methemoglobin reaches a level of 15%. Concentrations exceeding 60 to 70% are generally associated with coma and even death. Treatment consists of withdrawal of the offending drug, and when symptoms are present, methylene blue or ascorbic acid may be given.

Hemoglobin M disease is characterized by an amino acid substitution in the alpha or beta globin chain. It is genetically inherited as an autosomal dominant. Cyanosis is the only clinical symptom present and is generally not apparent until the infant is 3 to 6 months of age. These individuals lead normal lives and do not respond to methylene blue or ascorbic acid therapy.

SULFHEMOGLOBINEMIA

Sulfhemoglobinemia, when present, is generally the result of exposure to sulfonamides, acetanilid, or phenacetin but may accompany methemoglobinemia. Sulfhemoglobin, once formed, is stable and remains for the life of the red blood cell. Sulfhemoglobinemia is generally a benign disorder, and about the only symptom it causes is cyanosis. Treatment consists of removing the offending drug.

THE PORPHYRIAS

The porphyrias are a group of inherited or acquired disorders caused by specific enzyme defects necessary for the synthesis of the heme molecule (Fig. 156). These disorders are characterized by an increased production and excretion of the porphyrins and/or their precursors above the site of the enzyme defect (Fig. 156). The porphyrias will cause cutaneous photosensitivity and/or neurologic abnormalities, depending on the specific defect. Historically, hereditary porphyria affected many members of the royal houses of

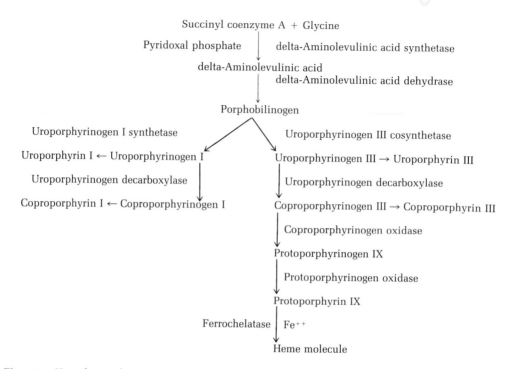

Fig. 156. Heme biosynthesis as related to the porphyrias.

Stuart, Hanover, and Prussia. Traced back to Mary, Queen of Scots, several royal members exhibited classic symptoms of porphyria, and several deaths were attributed to it.

Congenital erythropoietic porphyria (Gunther's disease) causes cutaneous photosensitivity and is one of the rarer types of porphyria. It is inherited as an autosomal recessive trait. In this disorder, there is decreased production of uroporphyrinogen III cosynthetase, which then results in an overproduction of uroporphyrinogen I and, to a lesser extent, an overproduction of coproporphyrinogen I. These excess porphyrins are then excreted in the urine and feces. Exposure to sunlight causes lesions, which heal slowly and eventually lead to scarring and disfigurement. There is generally a mild normocytic-normochromic anemia resulting from red blood cell hemolysis, and there is also ineffective erythropoiesis. Most characteristic is an increased excretion of uroporphyrinogen I in the urine, which

may be pink to deep burgundy in color. Splenectomy may improve the anemia, but the primary concern is to protect the patient from exposure to sunlight.

Porphyria cutanea tarda is inherited as an autosomal dominant trait and is caused by a decreased production of uroporphyrinogen decarboxylase. It is manifested clinically by a skin sensitivity to light and to minor trauma. This disease may only manifest itself in the presence of a liver disorder. The urine is generally reddish or brownish in color and contains increased amounts of uroporphyrin I. Improved liver function may effectively decrease the symptoms of the disease. Phlebotomy has also been used to remove iron stores from the liver. An acquired form of porphyria cutanea tarda has been found that is caused by exposure to halogenated aromatic hydrocarbons.

Erythropoietic protoporphyria is inherited as an autosomal dominant trait. It is caused by a decreased activity of heme ferrochelatase (heme synthetase), resulting in increased concentrations of protoporphyrin IX in the feces. The red blood cells also contain a marked increase in protoporphyrin IX and will show fluorescent cytoplasm. There is generally no anemia present. This disorder is clinically manifested by a mild sensitivity to sunlight but with minimal lesions and scar formation. Several drugs, including beta-carotene beadlets, and cholestyramine have been used effectively for treatment.

Acute intermittent porphyria causes neurologic abnormalities and is inherited as an autosomal dominant trait. It is caused by a deficiency in uroporphyrinogen I synthetase. The symptoms of this disorder are intermittent and may occur as frequently as several times in 1 year or as rarely as 2 or 3 times in the patient's entire life. During the active, or acute, phase, there is usually abdominal pain. Psychologic disturbances and neurologic symptoms may occur. During the active phase, the white blood cell count is usually elevated, and the urine will contain increased amounts of delta-aminolevulinic acid and porphobilinogen. The acute attacks of this disorder have been successfully treated with large amounts of glucose, hematin, and sodium benzoate.

Hereditary coproporphyria resembles acute intermittent porphyria in its clinical picture. It is caused by a decrease in coproporphyrinogen oxidase, which results in increased amounts of coproporphyrin III in the urine and feces. Acute attacks of this disease have been successfully treated with hematin.

Variegate porphyria is inherited as an autosomal dominant trait. The clinical symptoms are similar to acute intermittent porphyria, except that these patients also show a sensitivity to sunlight. Acute attacks of this disorder are generally precipitated by exposure to such drugs as sulfonamides, barbiturates, anesthetics, and alcohol. This disease is thought to be caused by a deficiency in protoporphyrinogen oxidase. The feces contain large amounts of protoporphyrinogen and coproporphyrin. During acute attacks, the urine will contain increased amounts of porphobilinogen and delta-aminolevulinic acid. This disorder is generally treated in the same way as acute intermittent porphyria.

In the *acquired porphyrias,* several of the enzymes controlling heme synthesis are inhibited. In lead poisoning, delta aminolevulinic acid dehydrase and ferrochelatase are inhibited, resulting in increases in excreted delta aminolevulinic acid and coproporphyrin III. Erythrocyte protoporphyrin IX levels are increased. Anemia associated with lead poisoning is mild, with basophilic stippling on the blood smear. Symptoms include abdominal pain, vomiting, and, in advanced cases, neurologic complications such as seizures, coma, and cerebral edema.

Toxic exposure to hexachlorobenzene, a chemical used to prevent mold in wheat, results in inhibition of the enzyme uroporphyrinogen decarboxylase. Uroporphyrin I levels are increased, individuals are photosensitive and have reddish urine.

MALARIA

Parasites that cause malaria in man and other animals belong to the class Sporozoa, suborder Haemosporidia, genus *Plasmodium.* The four species most commonly found in man are *Plasmodium vivax, malariae, falciparum,* and *ovale.*

Malaria is mainly transmitted from person to person through the bite of the female *Anopheles* mosquito. Other means of transmission are through the use of contaminated needles, by congenital means, and through blood transfusions.

The life cycle of the malaria parasite requires two types of hosts: the invertebrate (female Anopheles mosquito), where the parasite reaches maturity and the sexual cycle occurs (*sporogony*), and the vertebrate (e.g., the human), where the immature stages occur and asexual multiplication takes place *(schizogony).* When the infected Anopheles mosquito bites a human, sporozoites are injected into the peripheral blood of the individual. The sporozoites then invade the parenchymal cells of the liver, where preerythrocytic development takes place, ending with the schizont phase. At this time, the parasites rupture the cells, and the merozoites from the schizont penetrate the red blood cells or continue the exoerythrocytic phase by penetrating other liver cells and repeating the cycle, again developing into schizonts.

When the red blood cell has been penetrated by the merozoite, the parasite develops into the trophozoite ring form and thence to a mature schizont. This process takes 48 to 72 hours and is called *schizogony.* The merozoites rupture from the mature schizonts and penetrate other red blood cells. Fever and chills are associated with the rupture of the red blood cells. The merozoites entering the red blood cell then repeat the process of schizogony, forming mature schizonts from which more merozoites emerge. When several of the preceding asexual cycles have occurred, some of the merozoites enter red blood cells and become sexually differentiated into the male microgametocyte or the female macrogametocyte. In this circumstance, the gametocyte remains in the red blood cell as long as the red blood cell lives and does not influence the patient's symptoms.

The gametocyte is the only form of the parasite that is now infective to the Anopheles mosquito. When the mosquito bites the infected person, the gametocytes enter the mosquito and mature in its stomach. The zygote is formed when the microgamete exflagellates and fertilizes the macrogamete. The zygote matures, becoming actively motile, to form an ookinete, which penetrates the stomach wall of the mosquito. It moves to the outside of the stomach wall and becomes an oocyst. The oocyst matures to a sporocyst, which ruptures and gives rise to sporozoites. These sporozoites migrate to the salivary glands of the female Anopheles mosquito, where

they remain until a person is bitten by this mosquito. At this time, the sporozoites enter the peripheral blood and the cycle is repeated (Fig. 157).

It is important, when diagnosing malaria, to be able to identify the infecting species. Occasionally, mixed infections occur, the most common being P. falciparum and P. vivax. This may be accomplished by microscopic examination of thick and thin blood smears stained with Giemsa stain. Care should be taken not to confuse blood platelets with various stages of malarial parasites. Blood films several hours apart may be required to demonstrate the infection or diagnose the species.

Malaria may occur in the chronic, recurrent, or acute form. Parasites of P. vivax and P. ovale can persist within hepatic cells, resulting in relapses from activation of these parasites. The patient has sudden onsets of severe chills, along with fever, weakness, and often, splenomegaly. Generally, mild anemia is present as a result of shortened red blood cell life span due to the parasite invading the red blood cell. The osmotic fragility of the red blood cells is increased, and due to the hemolysis present, the haptoglobin is decreased to absent. *Blackwater fever,* although rarely seen, may occur in P. falciparum infections. As many as 50% of the red blood cells can be parasitized. This condition is characterized by severe, acute intravascular hemolysis, severe anemia, chills, weakness, fever, and vomiting. It has sometimes been found in patients who have been treated for malaria with quinine.

PELGER-HUËT ANOMALY

The Pelger-Huët anomaly is inherited as an autosomal dominant trait and is characterized by decreased segmentation of the nucleus of granulocytes, and coarseness and condensation of the nuclear chromatin in the granulocytes, lymphocytes, and normoblasts. These changes are most

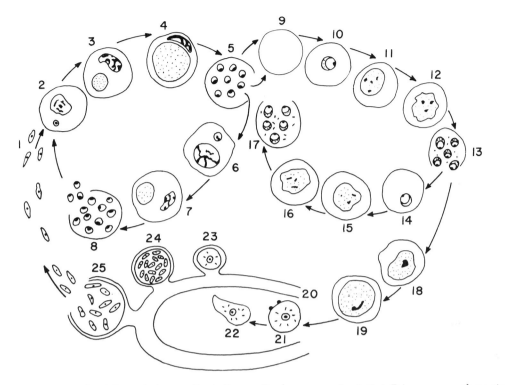

Fig. 157. Life cycle of the malaria parasite. 1, Sporozoites from mosquito. 2, 3, 4, Primary exoerythrocytic parasite in liver cells. 5, Merozoites being released from the ruptured exoerythrocytic schizont. 6, 7, Merozoite of the secondary exoerthrocytic cycle in liver cells. 8, Second generation of merozoites being released from the exoerythrocytic schizont. 9, Red blood cell in peripheral blood. 10, 11, 12, Erythrocytic schizogony in peripheral blood. 13, Erythrocytic merozoites and gametocytes being released from the ruptured erythrocytic schizont. 14, 15, 16, 17, Erythrocytic schizogony. 18, 19, Development of female gametocyte (macrogametocyte) in peripheral blood. 20, Stomach wall of mosquito. 21, Macrogamete. 22, Ookinete. 23, Oocyst. 24, Development of oocyst and production of sporozoites. 25, Sporozoites leaving the ruptured oocyst.

evident in the neutrophil, where the nuclei will appear round, dumbbell-shaped, or peanut-shaped. In the homozygous state, all of the neutrophil nuclei are round or oval. This anomaly, however, is most frequently seen in the heterozygous state, where less than 40% of the neutrophils contain a single-lobed nucleus; the majority of neutrophils contain a bilobed nucleus, and a small percentage of neutrophils have three-lobed nuclei. Pelger Huët cells appear to function normally. A defect in nucleic acid metabolism is thought to be responsible for the abnormal maturation seen in the nuclei of these cells.

Acquired or *pseudo-Pelger-Huët anomaly* is most often seen in chronic myelogenous leukemia and myeloid metaplasia but may also be seen in many other diseased states.

CHÉDIAK-HIGASHI ANOMALY

Chédiak-Higashi syndrome is inherited as an autosomal recessive trait. In this condition there is a defect in the lysosomes (cytoplasmic granules that are involved with the destruction of material ingested by phagocytic cells). Abnormal lysosomes are present in many cells of the body and appear predominately in the white blood cells. The affected patient generally shows albinism, photophobia, and poor resistance to infection. This disorder is generally fatal by early childhood. Death often occurs from recurrent infection or from a lymphoma-like disease. The Wright-stained blood smear is striking in that the granulocytes contain large azurophilic or reddish-purple granules in the cytoplasm. There are often multiple granules in the same cell. The lymphocytes and, less often, the monocytes may also contain one or more of these granules. Cytochemical staining of these cells shows the granules to be peroxidase positive.

MAY-HEGGLIN ANOMALY

The May-Hegglin anomaly is inherited as an autosomal dominant trait. It is characterized by the presence of pale blue-staining inclusions resembling Döhle bodies in the cytoplasm of neutrophils, and by thrombocytopenia with giant and abnormal appearing platelets. The inclusion bodies appear to consist of RNA. They are usually larger and more prominent than Döhle bodies, and may also be found in eosinophils, basophils, monocytes, and occasionally, lymphocytes. Approximately one-third of the patients with this anomaly have a mild to severe bleeding disorder which may result from the decreased platelet count or from a functional abnormality of the platelets.

ALDER-REILLY ANOMALY

Alder-Reilly anomaly is inherited as a recessive trait and is characterized by the presence of azurophilic staining granules in the neutrophils. These granules are similar to those seen in toxic granulation, but they are slightly larger, are unrelated to infection, and are a permanent feature of the cells. The granules may also be seen in the eosinophils, basophils, monocytes, and lymphocytes. These granules are most often seen in conjunction with *Hurler's* or *Hunter's syndromes.* The basic defect in these conditions appears to be a metabolic disorder of mucopolysaccharides. The facial and skeletal abnormalities observed have led to the use of the term gargoylism to describe these syndromes. The granules of Alder-Reilly anomaly have also been observed in otherwise healthy individuals.

STORAGE DISEASES

The storage diseases outlined here represent a group of disorders in which there are deficiencies in the enzymes responsible for the metabolic breakdown of lipids. All tissues of the body are affected and accumulation of lipid is prominent in the cells of the monocyte-macrophage system.

Gaucher's disease is a rare, chronic disorder caused by an inherited deficiency of the enzyme, beta-glucosidase. As a result, there is an accumulation of glycolipids within the cells of the body. Patients with this disorder generally have splenomegaly, hepatomegaly, some skin pigmentation, and a hypochromic anemia. The white blood cell count and platelet count are generally decreased. When this disease is found in infants, it is generally characterized by retarded growth and neurologic signs. The diagnostic cell, termed the *Gaucher cell,* will be present in the bone marrow and in aspirates from the liver, spleen, and lymph nodes. The Gaucher cell is large, 20 to 80 μm, with a small eccentric nucleus. The markedly abundant cytoplasm is filled with lipid, giving it a fibrillar appearance. The periodic acid Schiff reaction of these cells is positive.

Niemann-Pick disease affects primarily infants and is due to a deficiency in sphingomyelinase that causes an accumulation of sphingomyelin. These patients show enlarged livers and spleens. Accumulation of undegraded sphingomyelin leads to neuron (nerve cell) degeneration. Death usually occurs within a few months of diagnosis, and few patients live beyond the age of 20 years, with most patients dying between 2 and 3 years of age. In the stained blood smear, vacuoles may be present in the cytoplasm of the lymphocytes and monocytes. Niemann-Pick cells will be found in the bone marrow and spleen. These cells are similar in size to the Gaucher cell and have an eccentrically placed nucleus. The accumulated sphingomyelin gives the cytoplasm a more globular appearance. These cells are often called foam cells, and their periodic acid Schiff reaction is negative or weakly positive.

Sea-blue histiocytes are occasionally found in the bone marrow of patients with lipid storage diseases. These cells are large (20 to 60 μm in diameter), with an eccentric nucleus containing one nucleolus. The cytoplasm contains varying numbers of granules, which are blue to blue-green in color when stained with Wright stain. These cells contain an accumulation of lipid and are found in association with increased tissue stores of phospholipids and glycolipids.

HISTIOCYTOSIS X

Eosinophilic granuloma of the bone, Letterer-Siwe disease, and Hand-Schüller-Christian disease have all been categorized as histiocytosis X by some hematologists because they all show an abnormal proliferation of histiocytes in various tissues of the body. The cause of this abnormal proliferation is unknown. The process may result in impaired function of certain organs or tissues or it may result in their destruction.

Eosinophilic granuloma of the bone is found primarily in older children and young adults. Biopsy of the bone shows many eosinophils and histiocytes. This is a localized process that produces skeletal lesions.

Letterer-Siwe disease is generally found in young children. It is an acute and disseminated process. Proliferation of histiocytes is found primarily in the lymph nodes, spleen, liver, lungs, and bone marrow.

Hand-Schüller-Christian disease is a chronic and progressive form of histiocytosis found in older children. It affects primarily the bones. Some patients also have abnormal hypothalamic-pituitary function.

The treatment and prognosis for histiocytosis X is a function of the age of the patient, the extent of organ involvement and the degree of organ impairment. Chemotherapy and irradiation are used to treat this disorder.

INFECTIOUS MONONUCLEOSIS

Infectious mononucleosis was first described in the 1880s. One of the names ascribed to it at that time was glandular fever, a term no longer in use today. In the early 1900s, several cases of 'cured leukemia' were reported. These cases are now felt to have been examples of infectious mononucleosis.

Infectious mononucleosis is predominantly a disease of children and young adults and occurs in all races in all parts of the world. As a rule, the symptoms include fatigue, sore throat, moderate fever, and enlargement of the lymph nodes. Some patients may show splenomegaly, hepatomegaly, or jaundice. The causative agent for infectious mononucleosis is the Epstein-Barr (EB) virus, a member of the herpes group of viruses.

In patients with infectious mononucleosis, the red blood cell count and platelet count are usually normal. The white blood cell count may be variable but is usually normal to slightly elevated. Generally, the white blood cell count is lowest in the beginning of the disease and increases slowly during the first 2 to 5 days after onset, not usually going over 20,000/μL. There is a relative and absolute increase in lymphocytes, of which 20 to 90% are atypical. These cells are thought to be transformed T lymphocytes responding to B lymphocytes which are infected with the EB virus. The cells vary in size but are usually equal to or larger than the normal lymphocyte. They are often irregularly shaped and are frequently indented by the surrounding red blood cells. The nucleus of the lymphocyte may be round or oval but is often irregularly shaped. The cytoplasm of the cell is often increased in relative size and appears basophilic. This basophilia may appear throughout the entire cytoplasm but more often appears radially or at the peripheral edge of the cell. It is not uncommon to find a rare to few immature lymphocytes as a result of lymphocyte transformation into blast-like cells in response to stimulation by the virus. Lymphocytes with foamy or vacuolated cytoplasm may also be present. The three types of lymphocytes as suggested by Downey are found in this disorder. Usually, the number of atypical lymphocytes increases for several days and reaches a maximum by the fifth to tenth day. From then on, the number decreases, becoming normal within the next 3 weeks. In some instances, however, some atypical lymphocytes persist for 3 months or more. A serologic procedure, the heterophile antibody test, is positive in 90% or more of the patients with infectious mononucleosis. Generally, relatively high titers are obtained, reaching a peak in the second or third week of the illness and lasting for 2 to 8 weeks. In some cases, a positive test may persist even longer.

The diagnosis of infectious mononucleosis is generally based on the presence of atypical lymphocytes in the peripheral blood, a positive heterophile test, and the patient's clinical symptoms. Other laboratory findings may include abnormal liver enzyme tests (alkaline phosphatase, serum lactic dehydrogenase, and serum glutamic oxaloacetic transaminase levels).

Infectious mononucleosis is a benign, self-limited illness. Treatment is aimed at the symptoms and the condition usually resolves itself over a 4- to 6-week period. Complications occur in a small percentage of patients. These include neurologic, cardiac and liver function abnormalities.

CHRONIC GRANULOMATOUS DISEASE

Chronic granulomatous disease is inherited as a sex-linked recessive trait and is caused by a defect in white blood cell function. The disease is seen primarily in males and is generally fatal during early childhood because of recurring staphylococcal gram-negative or catalase positive bacterial infections. The development of granulomas (sites of chronic inflammation involving primarily large macrophages) in many organ systems is also a characteristic of this disorder. The white blood cells are morphologically and quantitatively normal. The white blood cell count (primarily neutrophils) does increase during periods of infection. The nitroblue-tetrazolium (NBT) test is used to diagnose this disorder. Failure to reduce the NBT dye is indicative of a lack of the oxidative burst which occurs in normal leukocytes during the process of phagocytosis and bacterial killing. Neutrophils and monocytes from chronic granulomatous patients ingest bacteria normally but are unable to kill catalase positive organisms due to a defect in the oxygen-dependent bacteriocidal mechanism of these cells.

WISKOTT-ALDRICH SYNDROME

The Wiskott-Aldrich syndrome is an immune-deficiency disease. It is inherited as a sex-linked recessive trait and is characterized by a moderate to marked thrombocytopenia, eczema, and recurrent infections. Defects in both cellular and humoral immunity are present. During the progress of the disease, there is a decline in the total number of active T lymphocytes. If the patient does not die from infection or bleeding due to the thrombocytopenia, malignant lesions generally form.

LEUKEMIA

Leukemia is an abnormal, uncontrolled proliferation and accumulation of one or more of the hematopoietic cells. Usually, there are qualitative changes in the affected cells, but this does not always have to be true. It is a disease of the blood forming tissues and the bone marrow is always involved. The proliferating cells can infiltrate other organs such as the spleen, liver, and lymph nodes.

Many different factors appear to play a role in the cause of the various leukemias. The ability of ionizing radiation to cause leukemia has been recognized for years; the evidence of this has come from observations regarding nuclear accidents and the atomic explosions in Japan in 1945. An increased frequency of leukemia has been found in patients receiving radiation therapy. It is likely that chemical agents contribute in a major way to leukemia incidence; however, at present benzene represents the only specific chemical. The precise mechanisms by which these factors cause leukemia are not known.

It is now clear that hereditary factors and genetic composition are of importance in the occurrence of leukemia. Statistics indicate that there is a significant tendency for leukemia to cluster in families, particularly in childhood twins. Acute leukemia has long been associated with Down's syndrome, and has occurred with increased frequency in persons with chromosomal breakage. The Philadelphia chromosome (Ph[1]), characterized by the shortening of the long arms of chromosome number 22, is seen in the majority of patients with chronic granulocytic leukemia.

Leukemia occurs at any age. Chronic lymphocytic leukemia, however, is usually found in patients over 50 years of age, whereas acute leukemia is generally found in persons under 20 years of age. Chronic granulocytic leukemia is most often found in the 20- to 50-year age bracket. Cases of acute leukemia are generally more common in males than females, and in whites than blacks.

The major symptoms of leukemia are fever, weight loss, and increased sweating. Enlargement of the liver, spleen, and lymph nodes may occur. The basal metabolic rate is often elevated, and there may be hemorrhagic tendencies if marked thrombocytopenia is present.

The different types of leukemia may be classified according to the duration of the disease, number of white blood cells present in the peripheral blood, and the type of white blood cell involved. (See following outline and Table 18.)

1. Duration of the untreated disease.
    a. Acute leukemia: rapidly progressive disease that lasts several days to 6 months.
    b. Subacute leukemia: 2 to 6 months.
    c. Chronic leukemia: the length of this disease is somewhat variable, depending on the age of the patient and the type of cell involved. Most patients live a minimum of 1 to 2 years or more.
2. Number of white blood cells present in the peripheral blood.
    a. Leukemic leukemia: white blood cell count greater than 15,000/µL.
    b. Subleukemic leukemia: white blood cell count less than 15,000/µL with immature or abnormal forms of white blood cells present in the peripheral blood.
    c. Aleukemic leukemia: white blood cell count less than 15,000/µL with no immature or abnormal white blood cells present in the peripheral blood.

In *acute leukemia,* the onset of the disease is sudden, and almost half of all cases occur in children under 14 years of age. There is generally normocytic-normochromic anemia that increases as the disease progresses with resultant fatigue and weakness. The platelet count is low to markedly decreased. The bleeding time is usually prolonged, and there is poor clot retraction. Occasionally, the clotting time is also prolonged. The white blood cell count is variable, usually showing a moderate to marked elevation. White blood cell counts of 50,000 to 100,000/µL are not uncommon. Frequently, however, the white blood cell count may be normal to

TABLE 18. CELL TYPE INVOLVED IN VARIOUS LEUKEMIAS

TYPE OF LEUKEMIA	TYPE OF CELL INVOLVED
Acute lymphocytic	Lymphoblast
Chronic lymphocytic	Lymphocyte (small)
Acute myelogenous	Myeloblast
Acute promyelocytic	Promyelocyte
Chronic myelogenous	Immature neutrophils
Eosinophilic	Eosinophil
Acute monocytic (Schilling)	Immature monocyte
Acute myelomonocytic (Naegeli)	Myeloblast showing monocytoid nucleus
Di Guglielmo's syndrome	Normoblast (myeloblast)
Plasma cell	Plasma cell
Mast cell	Mast cell
Stem cell	Primitive blast
Leukemic reticuloendotheliosis	"Hairy" cell
Acute megakaryocytic	Megakaryocyte

decreased. Blasts cells are present on the peripheral blood smear and may predominate. The bone marrow is hypercellular, with blast cells usually predominating, typically over 75% of the marrow cell total.

Acute leukemia is generally treated by *chemotherapy* (the use of chemicals that damage the capacity of the cell for reproduction). Combinations of several different drugs are utilized. These drugs may also destroy some normal cells and have toxic side effects. The primary goal of chemotherapy is to prolong life by eliminating the leukemic cells. When the patient becomes asymptomatic and has only normal cells in the blood and bone marrow, the patient is said to be in complete remission. A patient in partial remission shows improvement, but some leukemic cells remain. The period of time a patient remains in remission is variable, as is the number of remissions possible. In addition, general supportive therapy for bone marrow failure due to replacement by leukemic blasts and cytotoxic therapy includes the administration of packed red blood cells to treat anemia. Platelet concentrates are given in cases of severe thrombocytopenia (less than 20,000/μL). Severely neutropenic patients are given leukocyte concentrates to combat infections. Antibiotic therapy is also used to treat bacterial infections as a result of the neutropenia. The cause of death in patients with acute leukemia is most often infection and/or hemorrhage due to thrombocytopenia.

Subacute leukemias are similar to and are usually treated clinically as acute leukemia. The white blood cell count may show elevations up to 50,000/μL or in some instances may be normal to decreased. The predominant cell present in the peripheral blood is usually the blast, although there are not as many present as there are in acute leukemia. Thrombocytopenia and normocytic-normochromic anemia are also present.

Chronic leukemia has an insidious onset, frequently being asymptomatic for a long time. Anemia is not usually present until late in the disease, and hemolytic anemia may develop as the disease progresses. Platelet counts are usually normal and may frequently be increased in myelogenous leukemia. In the late stages of chronic leukemia, however, thrombocytopenia and anemia usually occur. The white blood cell count is most often markedly increased and may be as high as 900,000/μL. However, it is not unusual for the white blood cell count to be normal to decreased. Less than 10% blast cells are found in chronic myelogenous leukemia, whereas a rare blast cell (or none) is seen in chronic lymphocytic leukemia. Eventually, the majority of these patients go into blast crisis, where they present an acute type of myelogenous leukemia. Chemotherapy may or may not induce a remission, and, as in acute leukemia, the main cause of death is hemorrhage and/or infection. Chronic lymphocytic leukemia (CLL) generally has a much longer life span than the other types of leukemia. However, complete remission is generally not attained, and treatment may be used only when complications occur. Death is usually caused by infection, or, because this is a disease found in the elderly, the cause of death may be unrelated to CLL.

In 1976, a system for the classification of acute leukemias was developed and is now termed the *French-American-British (FAB)* classification of acute leukemias. It divides the acute leukemias into lymphoblastic or myeloblastic. These two main groups are subdivided according to morphology, cytochemical staining results, and, more recently, T and B lymphocyte marker study results. The lymphoblastic leukemias have been divided into three types (L1, L2, and L3), whereas the myeloblastic leukemias have been separated into six types (M1, M2, M3, M4, M5, and M6). In 1985, a seventh classification (M7) was added.

The three types, M1, M2, and M3, are predominantly granulocytic in origin. Types M4 and M5 have at least 20% monocytic precursors, and type M6 has a high proportion of erythroblasts. The purpose of the FAB classification is to attain better discrimination in therapy and prognosis by sorting the morphologic variants of leukemias into types. In general, patients in group M1, M5a, and M6 do less well than patients classified as M2, M3, M4, and M5b (see Acute Myelomonocytic Leukemia of Naegeli for M5a and M5b). Also,

the presence of Auer rods is observed to be an important parameter in prognosis with a complete remission rate of 68% in patients with Auer rods. A minimum of 30% blasts is required for the diagnosis of acute myelogenous leukemia (M1 through M6). Type M7 involves megakaryocytes.

Acute Lymphocytic Leukemia

Immunologic cell markers are being used on lymphoblasts in addition to other T and B cell markers, which suggests that acute lymphocytic leukemia may be classified into one of several categories. The lymphoblast may be classified based on membrane cell markers: immunoglobulins bound to the cell membrane, receptors present on the cell membrane, and formation of rosettes with untreated sheep red blood cells.

In the FAB classification, the lymphocytic leukemias have been divided into three types: L1, L2, and L3. In type L1, acute lymphocytic leukemia of childhood, the lymphoblasts are small, vary little in size, have scanty cytoplasm, rare nucleoli, and the nucleus is round and regular in shape. It is the most common type (84%) of childhood ALL (acute lymphocytic leukemia), and has the best prognosis. In type L2, the lymphoblasts are larger and variable in size with abundant, basophilic cytoplasm, and the nuclei are often clefted with nucleoli present. This type accounts for 14% of the cases of childhood ALL, and includes 64% of the adult type of ALL. In type L3, the Burkitt-type, the lymphoblast is large, but varies little in size. The nucleus is rounded with fine chromatin structure and one to three nucleoli. The cytoplasm is moderate in quantity and deeply basophilic, often with prominent vacuoles. The prognosis is poor.

Acute lymphocytic leukemia can also be divided into five subtypes, based on the reaction of the blast cells with lymphocyte cell marker assays. T-cell leukemias (T cell ALL) account for 10 to 20% of the cases of ALL, usually have a high white blood cell count, a high frequency of mediastinal tumor, central nervous system involvement, and a poor prognosis. It affects males more than females and generally occurs in older children. Common cell leukemia accounts for 60 to 70% of ALL cases, and has a good prognosis. Blast cells in this subtype lack the surface features of either B or T cells, so are termed non-T, non-B cells. The rarest subclass is B-cell leukemia, and it represents the L3 variant of the FAB classification (Burkitt-type).

At the time of diagnosis, the white blood cell count is generally elevated, with 60% or more lymphoblasts and immature lymphocytes present. In some cases, the white blood cell count may be normal or decreased, in which case there would be relatively fewer lymphoblasts present. A normocytic-normochromic anemia is present, which is generally quite severe. The reticulocyte count is decreased, and thrombocytopenia is present. Approximately 2% of the cases of ALL have central nervous system involvement at presentation, with blast cells present in the cerebrospinal fluid. It is treated with intrathecal methotrexate and cranial irradiation if the patient is over 2 years of age. The bone marrow shows a predominance of lymphoblasts. The periodic acid-Schiff stain is variable, whereas the leukocyte alkaline phosphatase stain is normal. The sudan black B stain is negative in lymphoblasts, and the acid phosphatase is positive in blasts of the T-cell variant of ALL. Prednisolone, vincristine, and asparaginase have been used to achieve remissions in over 90% of the cases in 4 to 6 weeks. A maintenance therapy of mercaptopurine daily, and weekly methotrexate is given for 2 to 3 years.

Chronic Lymphocytic Leukemia

The majority of cases of chronic lymphocytic leukemia appear to involve the B lymphocyte. The T lymphocyte is less often involved. The white blood cell count is usually 20,000 to 200,000/μL, with the peripheral blood smear showing 60 to 95% lymphocytes. These cells are generally the small type of mature lymphocyte that often show a small cleft or indentation in the shape of the nucleus. Lymphoblasts are generally absent from the peripheral blood, but a rare prolymphocyte may sometimes be found. These lymphocytes are somewhat more fragile than normal, resulting in many of the cells being ruptured during the preparation of the blood smear. Therefore, large numbers of smudge cells are usually seen on the Wright-stained smear. A normocytic, normochromic anemia generally develops as the disease progresses. The platelet count is usually normal or shows only a slight decrease. The bone marrow is hypercellular and contains large numbers of the small mature lymphocytes. An autoimmune hemolytic anemia may develop during the course of this disease in about 10% of the cases, and the patient shows a positive direct Coombs' test.

Chronic lymphocytic leukemia is more than twice as common in men as in women. Lymphadenopathy, fatigue, weight loss, splenomegaly, and hepatomegaly are common clinical features. A system of five stages has been devised to allow clinical categorization of patients into prognostic groups. In stage 0 (zero), there is absolute lymphocytosis (greater than 15,000/μL) in the peripheral blood and bone marrow only. Stage I includes enlargement of the lymph nodes. Stage II also includes an enlarged liver and/or spleen. Stage III includes all of the above clinical symptoms and anemia. In stage IV, there is also thrombocytopenia.

Usually, there is no treatment for the disease in stage 0; however, in the later stages alkylating agents such as chlorambucil are used to reduce the total lymphocyte count. Corticosteroids and radiation of an enlarged spleen are also employed. Patients in stage 0 have a better prognosis (about 10 years) than those in the later stages, with anemia and thrombocytopenia, where the median survival is 1 to 2 years.

Leukemic Reticuloendotheliosis

Leukemic reticuloendotheliosis is also termed *'hairy' cell leukemia* and is characterized by the presence of 2 to 88% of these 'hairy' cells in the blood and bone marrow. These cells are thought to be of lymphocytic origin and show characteristics of B lymphocytes. They are large cells with a diameter of 15 to 30 μm. The nucleus is round to oval in shape with fine chromatin and may contain one to five distinct nucleoli. There is a small to moderate amount of blue-gray cytoplasm that has hairlike projections around the outer border of the cell. Splenomegaly is a common finding, and the white blood cell count is decreased to elevated, depending on the number of 'hairy' cells present in the peripheral blood. The acid phosphatase stain using L(+) tartaric acid will be positive.

This disease usually occurs in males between 40 and 60 years of age. There is generally a mild normocytic, normochromic anemia. The platelet count is usually decreased below 50,000/μL, and the white blood cell count below 3,000/μL, with no previous therapy. Splenectomy is normally the first choice of treatment, with chlorambucil chemotherapy as a follow-up in a small number of cases. Hairy cell leukemia responds well to splenectomy, with a median survival rate between 5 to 6 years.

Acute Myelogenous Leukemia (FAB M1 and M2)

The peripheral white blood cell count usually shows moderate to marked elevation, with 60% or more of the cells being myeloblasts. Auer rods may or may not be present in the cytoplasm of these cells. Some cases of this disease show micromyeloblasts, a much smaller myeloblast than normal. A severe normocytic-normochromic anemia develops, along with thrombocytopenia. Enlargement of the lymph nodes, spleen, and liver is not pronounced. The platelets that are present may be large and bizarre-looking. The bone marrow shows an increased number of myeloblasts. The granulocytes on the blood smear give the following reactions to cytochemical stains: Sudan black B, positive; peroxidase, positive; ASD chloroacetate, positive; leukocyte alkaline phosphatase, decreased; periodic acid-Schiff, faint diffuse granules.

In acute myelogenous leukemia of the M1 FAB classification (myeloblastic leukemia without maturation), the predominant cell is a poorly differentiated myeloblast without any granulation, or only a few fine azurophilic granules. The nuclear chromatin is fine with one or more nucleoli. The cytoplasm is scanty and Auer rods are rare. In type M2, (myeloblastic leukemia with maturation) cells differentiate beyond the promyelocytic stage. There are about 50% blasts and promyelocytes. Myelocytes, metamyelocytes, and mature granulocytes have abundant cytoplasm and may be agranular. Increased numbers of eosinophilic precursors can be found. Auer rods are often present, and about 30% of the cases of acute myelogenous leukemia are of the M2 type.

Treatment involves prophylactic platelet transfusions for thrombocytopenia, broad spectrum antibiotics for infection, and chemotherapy. This is an extremely toxic program involving the use of daunorubicin and cytosine arabinoside; however, there is no universally accepted therapeutic program. In both the M1 and M2 types, the use of both drugs can result in a 60% rate of remission. However, remissions are of short duration and the median survival is 12 to 18 months. Compatible sibling bone marrow transplantation is being used in some cases in patients under 45 years of age in their first remission.

Acute Promyelocytic Leukemia (FAB M3)

In acute promyelocytic leukemia, the predominant cell in the bone marrow and blood is the promyelocyte. Often the nucleus of this cell is more immature than usual, and the cytoplasmic granules may be large and abnormal appearing. There is also an increased incidence of bleeding disorders in this disease. Disseminated intravascular coagulation may occur, which is thought to be due to the release of thromboplastin-like susbstances by the abnormal promyelocytes.

Acute promyelocytic leukemia is classified as type M3. The majority of cells have abundant cytoplasmic granules, and Auer rods are common and often multiple. The nucleus varies in size and shape and may be kidney-bean shaped or bilobed. A variant of type M3 has similar cell morphology, but only a few granules are present. Sudan black B and peroxidase cytochemical stains are strongly positive. The PAS reaction is diffuse and acid phosphate activity is variable.

Treatment involves the same regimen of cytotoxic drugs as types M1 and M2, plus the administration of fresh frozen plasma to provide clotting factors consumed by DIC when present.

Acute Myelomonocytic Leukemia of Naegeli (FAB M4)

At diagnosis, the white blood cell count usually shows moderate to marked elevation. Anemia is commonly found, and thrombocytopenia may also be present. The most common type of abnormal cell found in this disorder has been described as myelomonocytic, because the cell has characteristics of both the myeloblast and the monocyte. The nucleus is monocytoid, with a fine chromatin pattern, and appears convoluted or folded. The cytoplasm is usually more abundant than that of the myeloblast, and the granules present show characteristics of the granulocytic line of cells. These cells are present in the bone marrow and peripheral blood in all stages of development, from the blast stage to the mature monocyte. The monocytic cells must account for 20% but not more than 80% of the white cells in the bone marrow for the leukemia to be classified as M4. Auer rods may be present in the blast cell. Some immature granulocytes are also present in the peripheral blood. In the nonspecific esterase stain, the blasts are negative to weakly positive, whereas the mature monocytoid cells stain positively.

Acute myelomonocytic leukemia (AMML) accounts for about 25% of adult acute myelogenous leukemia. A small percentage of patients have variable numbers of marrow eosinophils (0.5 to 30%).

Acute Monocytic Leukemia of Schilling (FAB M5)

Acute monocytic leukemia (M5) exists in two forms: differentiated (M5b) and poorly differentiated (M5a). In both forms, the white blood cell count is moderately elevated, with the absolute percentage of granulocyte precursors showing less than 20%. The poorly-differentiated type is characterized by large (30 μm or larger) blasts in the bone marrow and in the peripheral blood. The nuclei of the blasts have delicate, lacy chromatin with three to five nucleoli and are folded or indented. The basophilic cytoplasm is abundant with rare granules, and often has pseudopods or buds. The differentiated form has blasts, promonocytes, and monocytes in the bone marrow, and the peripheral blood has a high proportion of monocytes. The predominant cell type in the bone marrow is the promonocyte which has less basophilic cytoplasm with a grayish ground-glass appearance, and fine azurophilic granules.

Anemia and thrombocytopenia are usually present. The monocytic cells stain positively in the nonspecific esterase stain. In this disease, however, the staining is inhibited by the addition of fluoride. Both types (M5a and M5b) account for 10% of the total cases of acute myelogenous leukemia.

Di Guglielmo's Syndrome (FAB M6)

Di Guglielmo's syndrome has been referred to as *erythroleukemia* and *erythremic myelosis* and may occur in the acute or, less commonly, in the chronic form. The white blood cell count may be slightly decreased to moderately elevated, and myeloblasts and immature granulocytic cells are usually found in the peripheral blood. Immature red blood cells including normoblasts may be present in the blood in few to moderate numbers. These cells may appear megaloblastic-like and show bizarre-shaped, fragmented, and multilobed nuclei. Anemia and thrombocytopenia are common findings. The bone marrow is hypercellular and shows a predominance (more than 50%) of erythroid cells. The abnormal erythroid cells will show positive staining in the nonspecific esterase stain.

Abnormal megakaryocytes are present in the bone marrow, including giant forms. Howell-Jolly bodies are present in the peripheral blood. Iron stores of the bone marrow show ringed sideroblasts. This type of leukemia is rare, constituting only 5% of patients with acute myelogenous leukemia. Patients with erythroleukemia have a poor prognosis.

Acute Megakaryocytic Leukemia (FAB M7)

Acute megakaryocytic leukemia (M7) is a systemic and rapidly progressive proliferation of atypical and immature megakaryocytes. Since the proliferation of megakaryocytes is common in the myeloproliferative and preleukemic syndromes, only rarely will a patient be diagnosed with true acute megakaryocytic leukemia.

This form of acute leukemia usually has pancytopenia without lymphadenopathy, splenomegaly, or hepatomegaly. The disease generally occurs in the middle or late years of life, with males affected more than females. The peripheral blood shows unclassifiable blasts, and bleeding is a frequent mode of presentation. The bone marrow shows a predominance of atypical megakaryocytes and their precursors. The blast cells are smaller than normal megakaryocytes with a high nuclear to cytoplasmic ratio, cytoplasmic vacuoles, multiple nucleoli, and may actually be seen shedding platelets. There is also an increase in reticulum fibers in the bone marrow.

Cytochemical staining involves the use of the platelet peroxidase enzyme to identify megakaryoblasts. The clinical course is short and the response to therapy is usually poor. Terminally, the patient has an acute leukemic phase with high blast counts and widespread infiltration of the lymph nodes, spleen, liver, and bone marrow.

Chronic Myelogenous Leukemia

The white blood cell count is usually 100,000 to 300,000/μL at the time of diagnosis. Less than 10% myeloblasts are present in the peripheral blood, and there is a complete spectrum of granulocytic cells from the myeloblast to the mature neutrophil. There is a predominance of neutrophils and myelocytes. Eosinophils and basophils are commonly increased, and the percentage of monocytes may also show an increase. Mild normochromic anemia is generally present. The platelet count is often increased, and large forms of the platelets may be present. The bone marrow is hypercellular and usually shows an increased number of myeloid cells, with a slightly higher percentage of immature granulocytes than is present in the peripheral blood, and megakaryocytes are more numerous than usual. Leukocyte alkaline phosphatase is decreased or absent in this disorder. One arm of the chromosome in pair number 22 is found to be translocated to chromosome 9 in 90% of the cases of this disease. This chromosome is termed the *Philadelphia chromosome* and occurs in the erythroid, granulocytic, monocytic, and megakaryocytic cells. Patients with this disorder who are negative for the Philadelphia chromosome usually have a poorer prognosis and do not respond particularly well to chemotherapy. Splenomegaly is a fairly constant finding.

Cytotoxic drugs are most commonly used to treat chronic myelogenous leukemia (CML) with excellent response. Busulphan (Myleran) is the treatment of choice to reduce the total granulocyte count to give a median survival of 3 to 4 years. However, CML often converts to a terminal acute leukemia called 'blast crisis' in 70% of the cases.

The Myelodysplastic Syndromes (MDSs)

The myelodysplastic syndromes are a group of disorders characterized by a hypercellular bone marrow and abnormalities in the cellular maturation of the erythroid cells, granulocytes, and megakaryocytes. Historically, it has been termed 'preleukemia' as patients may progress to an acute non-lymphocytic leukemia. MDS occurs primarily in persons over the age of 50. Clinically, they present with a macrocytic anemia and thrombocytopenia, and neutropenia may or may not be present. The spleen, liver, and lymph nodes are not usually enlarged. The peripheral blood shows anisocytosis, poikilocytosis, nucleated red blood cells, basophilic stippling, Howell-Jolly bodies, and oval macrocytes. In general, in MDS the blast count is less than 30%.

In the bone marrow and peripheral blood, dyserythropoiesis is indicated by nuclear fragmentation, multinuclearity, lobulated nuclei, basophilic stippling, ringed sideroblasts and megaloblastic maturation of the red cells. Dysgranulopoiesis is indicated by the presence of pseudo-Pelger-Huët forms, retarded nuclear maturation, hypersegmented forms, and abnormal or absent granulation. Dysmegakaryocytopoiesis results in the presence of large megakaryocytes and micromegakaryocytes, decreased numbers of megakaryocytes, giant platelets, and ab-

normal platelet granulation. Due to abnormal platelet structure and function, hemorrhagic complications are common.

The French-American-British (FAB) group has classified this syndrome into five groups (RA, RARS, RAEB, RAEB-T, and CMML) based on the bone marrow and peripheral blood blast count, and the degree of abnormalities in the three cell lines (erythrocytes, leukocytes, and megakaryocytes). These classifications have proved helpful in diagnosis and treatment; however, not all patients fall neatly into one category.

In *refractory anemia* (RA), there is anemia with a decreased reticulocyte count, less than 1% blasts in the peripheral blood, and less than 5% blasts in the bone marrow. Abnormal erythrocytes are found, but abnormal granulocytes are rare. *Refractory anemia with ringed sideroblasts* (RARS) includes the presence of more than 15% ringed sideroblasts in the bone marrow. In *refractory anemia with excess blasts* (RAEB), the peripheral blood shows less than 5% circulating blasts; however, there are 5 to 20% blasts in the bone marrow. The marrow is hypercellular with abnormalities in the three cell lines. *Refractory anemia with excess blasts in transformation* (RAEB-T) shows more than 5% blasts in the blood and 20 to 30% blasts in the bone marrow. This subgroup has a high risk of evolving into acute myelogenous leukemia. *Chronic myelomonocytic leukemia* (CMML) has 5 to 20% blast cells in the bone marrow, and increased promonocytes. The peripheral blood shows a persistent monocytosis and less than 5% circulating blasts.

Median survival rates range from 6 years for RARS to 5 months for RAEB-T. Low dose cytosine arabinoside has been used to treat MDS with varied success, and supportive therapy involves the use of white cell transfusions and antibiotics to combat infections.

Eosinophilic Leukemia

Eosinophilic leukemia is rare. Anemia and thrombocytopenia may or may not be present. Large numbers of immature eosinophils are present in the blood and bone marrow, and the maturation of these cells may be abnormal.

It is difficult to differentiate between eosinophilic leukemia and a non-neoplastic eosinophilia. However, there are greater than 5% blasts in the bone marrow and tissue infiltration by immature eosinophils in eosinophilic leukemia.

Plasma Cell Leukemia

Plasma cell leukemia is a rare disorder generally found only as an acute terminal stage in multiple myeloma. The white blood cell count may be slightly to moderately elevated, and the peripheral blood smear shows up to 90% plasma cells. There is bone marrow failure due to infiltration with abnormal plasma cells and splenomegaly. The malignant cells are poorly differentiated, and patients do not respond well to therapeutic drugs used in multiple myeloma.

Plasma cell leukemia is found in more males than females, with a median age of 50 to 60 years. The clinical picture includes general fatigue, weight loss, hemorrhagic tendencies, and hepatomegaly. Moderate to marked anemia and thrombocytopenia are seen in 70% of the cases. There is widespread infiltration of plasmacytoid cells in various organs and tissues of the body. Remissions are of short duration (1 to 3 months) and the mean survival is about 9 months.

Mast Cell Leukemia

Mast cell leukemia is extremely rare. Up to 50% of the cells in the peripheral blood may be mature and immature forms of the tissue mast cell, which is difficult to distinguish from the basophil.

Stem Cell Leukemia

In stem cell leukemia, the blast cells present are so immature and undifferentiated that they cannot be identified by cytochemical or immunologic methods. As the disease progresses, these cells may change and become identifiable. This disorder is rare, found mainly in children, and is generally present in the acute form.

MYELOFIBROSIS

Myelofibrosis, also called *idiopathic myelofibrosis* or *agnogenic myeloid metaplasia,* is a myeloproliferative disorder that is characterized by fibrosis and granulocytic hyperplasia of the bone marrow, with granulocytic proliferation in the liver and spleen. Its basic cause is unknown, and it is generally found in middle aged or elderly people.

At diagnosis, the patient may show an enlarged liver and spleen, weight loss, a tendency to bruise easily, and a normochromic-normocytic anemia. The anemia becomes more severe as the disease progresses. The stained blood smear characteristically shows teardrop-shaped red cells and nucleated red blood cells in numbers out of proportion to the degree of anemia. Polychromatophilia is present, and the reticulocyte count is increased. The white blood cell count is variable but is increased in the majority of patients. Immature granulocytes are generally present on the stained blood smear and the number of basophils is often increased. Dwarf megakaryocytes or small megakaryoblasts are often present in small numbers in the peripheral blood and, in certain cases, may be present in large numbers. The platelet count is increased in about 50% of the cases at diagnosis but decreases below normal as the disease progresses. Large and bizarre forms of the platelets are usually present on the stained blood smear and most patients demonstrate functional platelet abnormalities. The leukocyte alkaline phosphatase stain is increased in the majority of cases but may be normal or decreased. The bone marrow is usually hypocellular, and it is often impossible to obtain marrow, except by surgical biopsy. In the early stages of the disease, however, the marrow may be hypercellular and contain an increased number of megakary-ocytes, some of which are abnormal. The marrow generally becomes fibrotic, with an abundance of reticulum fibers.

The cause of death is variable and may be due to infection, bleeding, cardiac failure, or a conversion to leukemia. No specific therapy is currently used to treat the basic problem, and patients will generally survive for 1 to 5 years or longer following diagnosis.

MALIGNANT LYMPHOMAS

The term *lymphoma* represents a group of malignant tumors of the lymphoid tissue (excluding lymphocytic leukemia) that vary greatly in degree of malignancy and response to therapy. Various methods for classifying this group of disorders have been suggested. No one classification system, however, has been completely accepted. The lymphomas generally may be divided into two major groups: Hodgkin's disease and the non-Hodgkin's lymphomas.

Non-Hodgkin's Lymphomas

Non-Hodgkin's lymphomas (NHL) are proliferations of lymphocytes that are blocked at certain stages of differentiation. They are primarily neoplasms (new or recent growth of cells) of the B-cell lymphocytes and occur predominantly in the middle and older age groups.

Non-Hodgkin's lymphomas have been classified by the system of Rappaport for the last 20 years. This system separates the non-Hodgkin's lymphomas morphologically by cell type into four categories, each of which shows a nodular or diffuse pattern. (1) In *well-differentiated lymphocytic lymphoma,* the characteristic cell resembles a small lymphocyte. (2) *Poorly-differentiated lymphocytic lymphoma* is characterized by lymphocytic cells that may vary in size. The nuclear chromatin is less clumped than in the mature lymphocyte, may contain a visible nucleolus, and may be indented or clefted. There is

little cytoplasm. (3) The cells in *histiocytic lymphoma* are relatively large, with fine nuclear chromatin and variable amounts of cytoplasm. The nucleus may be eccentric and may or may not show a nucleolus. (4) *Mixed histiocytic-lymphocytic lymphoma* shows equal proportions of poorly-differentiated lymphocytes and histiocytes. (The cells in categories 3 and 4 may not be true histiocytes but are, in fact, lymphoid in an active state of proliferation.)

Due to problems with terminology in the Rappaport classification, the NCI (National Cancer Institute) funded a study of 1175 cases of non-Hodgkin's lymphoma to develop the Working Formulation for clinical usage in 1982. The Formulation is in widespread use today, and it incorporates the older Rappaport system. The Working Formulation confirms the significance of differentiating the nodular (follicular) from the diffuse pattern.

The Working Formulation bases a diagnosis of NHL on cell morphology and recognizes three major groups: low, intermediate, and high grade malignancies. The *low grade malignancies* include three subgroups: (1) malignant lymphoma, small lymphocytic, (2) follicular, small cleaved (indented or clefted nucleus) cell, and (3) follicular, mixed small cleaved and large cell. In the *small lymphocytic type,* the predominant cell is the small lymphocyte with clumped chromatin. Marker studies indicate that these well-differentiated cells are mostly B lymphocytes. There is a diffuse pattern of lymph node and marrow involvement with an elevated blood lymphocyte count. This is synonymous with chronic lymphocytic leukemia. In the *follicular, small cleaved cell type* of lymphoma, the lymphocytes are of the poorly-differentiated type, and are predominantly B cells. In spite of spleen, liver, and bone marrow involvement, these patients have a survival of 7 years. In the *follicular, mixed small cleaved and large cell* type, there are equal numbers of large non-cleaved cells with prominent nucleoli and small cleaved lymphocytes.

The *intermediate grade of malignant lymphomas* include (1) follicular, predominantly large cell, (2) diffuse small cleaved cell, (3) diffuse, mixed small and large cell, and (4) diffuse, large cell. In the *follicular, predominantly large cell type,* there are predominantly large cleaved cells mixed with non-cleaved cells in a follicular pattern. Many mitotic figures are present. The *diffuse small cleaved cell type* of tumor has small cleaved lymphocytes with scanty cytoplasm. The *diffuse, mixed small and large cell* type has a mixture of small cleaved cells and large cells with prominent nucleoli in a diffuse pattern. They may be either B or T cells. The *diffuse, large cell type* of tumor is composed primarily of large cells with fine chromatin, a large prominent nucleolus, and abundant cytoplasm.

The *high grade malignancies* represent lymphomas with an aggressive clinical course. The *large cell, immunoblastic type* consists of several types of cells, including those with eccentric nuclei and cells which resemble activated lymphocytes (immunoblasts) which are 4 times the size of normal lymphocytes with large, round nuclei. The *lymphoblastic type* shares many of the same features of T-cell acute lymphoblastic leukemia. The cells are blast-like with fine chromatin. This type of tumor has widespread involvement of the lymph nodes, peripheral blood, and may disseminate to the bone marrow and cerebrospinal fluid. The *small, non-cleaved cell type* includes the Burkitt's lymphomas. These cells have a high proliferation rate, interspersed with isolated macrophages which results in a 'starry sky' appearance in tissue sections of lymphoma tumors. Marker studies show these cells to be of B cell origin.

At the time of diagnosis, most patients have enlarged lymph nodes, where the disease is primarily located. The liver and spleen are often enlarged. The white blood cell count is normal, but there may be some abnormal lymphocytes (lymphoma cells) present in the peripheral blood. The hemoglobin level is generally normal in the early stages of the disease. Diagnosis is generally made by examining a lymph node biopsy. The lymphoma cells, however, may also be present in the bone marrow. A combination of chemotherapy and radiotherapy are methods of treatment. In some patients, malignant lymphoma will change into leukemia.

The majority of patients with low grade malignant disease with a follicular pattern survive for longer than 5 years, with a 10-year survival rate not uncommon. The low grade lymphomas are managed conservatively, often with no treatment at all if there are few symptoms and the clinical course is non-progressive. With intensive chemotherapy, patients with widespread high grade lymphomas have a 40 to 50% survival rate after 2 years. A basic regimen of COP (cyclophosphamide, vincristine, and prednisone) has been used to treat intermediate and high grade non-Hodgkin's lymphomas. Other drugs such as bleomycin, adriamycin, and procarbazine have been added to the basic protocol to treat more resistant cases.

Miscellaneous Lymphomas

Sézary syndrome and Burkitt's lymphoma are two miscellaneous lymphoma variants. Both are described as lymphomas as they are lymphoproliferative disorders with lymph node infiltration.

Sézary syndrome, a malignant lymphoma, affects the skin and involves primarily the T lymphocytes. The tumor cells (Sézary cells) are quite characteristic. They resemble a medium-sized lymphocyte with a convoluted nucleus, somewhat resembling the monocyte nucleus. (See Plate VII O, P.) These cells have also been found in patients with mycosis fungoides. Sézary syndrome may be the leukemic phase of mycosis fungoides. This disorder may follow a prolonged, chronic course.

However, as the disease infiltrates the lymph nodes and disseminates to the liver and spleen, the prognosis becomes worse. Experimental treatment has included the use of anti-thymocyte globulin (ATG), an antibody to human T cells.

Burkitt's lymphoma is found most often in children in Africa and New Guinea and commonly affects the jaw and facial bones. In American children, a similar tumor has been found that affects the lymph nodes in the abdominal and pelvic areas, and those in the neck. This lymphoma is sensitive to chemotherapy, and a complete remission is relatively common. If relapse occurs after a complete remission, this usually indicates a poor prognosis. The cause of Burkitt's lymphoma is unknown; however, evidence suggests that the Epstein-Barr virus (EBV) plays a role in transforming the B-cell lymphocytes. Therapy consists of combination chemotherapy. Central nervous system treatment with intrathecal methotrexate and cranial irradiation has been used in more advanced cases.

Hodgkin's Disease

Hodgkin's disease is generally regarded as a malignant lymphoma but differs in that the cells reacting to the neoplasm predominate rather than the neoplastic cells themselves. This disorder is distinguished from other lymphomas by the presence of *Reed-Sternberg cells.* This is a large cell, varying in size from 50 to 100 μm or more. There is an abundance of cytoplasm, and the cell usually has irregular margins. The nucleus may be single or multilobed with large nucleoli. These cells are present in the involved tissue.

Hodgkin's disease is most frequent among young and middle-aged adults with a 2:1 male predominance. When a patient is diagnosed as having Hodgkin's disease, his disorder is further classified according to the histologic appearance of the involved tissue from a lymph node biopsy. The universally adopted Rye clas-

sification subdivides Hodgkin's disease into four types. These are not fixed and rigid categories as the patient who has one type may change to another category in time.

(1) The *lymphocytic predominant* form shows predominantly small mature lymphocytes with a varying number of mature histiocytes. The diagnostic Reed-Sternberg cells are rare and few in number. Prognosis is best in this group where the disease tends to be localized in the cervical lymph nodes in young males. The lymphocyte predominant type accounts for about 7% of the cases of Hodgkin's disease.

(2) In the *lymphocyte depleted* form, there are few lymphocytes, but there may be many histiocytes and varying numbers of eosinophils and atypical Reed-Sternberg cells. This type of Hodgkin's disease is seen as a rapidly progressive disease with fever, pancytopenia, and frequently without lymphadenopathy. There is extensive involvement of the liver, spleen, and bone marrow. This type accounts for about 2% of the cases of Hodgkin's disease.

(3) The *mixed cellularity* type shows eosinophils, lymphocytes, histiocytes, neutrophils, and plasma cells which obliterate the basic structure of the lymph node. Diagnostic Reed-Sternberg cells are frequent. The mixed cellularity type accounts for 23% of the cases of Hodgkin's disease.

(4) In *nodular sclerosis,* bands of collagen are present that divide the tissue into islands. This is the most common type (68%) of Hodgkin's disease, and is often first discovered as a mediastinal mass in young women. Classic Reed-Sternberg cells are difficult to find. Large, atypical histiocytes with abundant pale cytoplasm *(lacunar cells)* are found.

A second classification of the patient's disease may also be made based on the location and extent of the involved tissue. This process is termed *staging.* Prognosis for Hodgkin's disease depends on both the histologic type and the extent of tissue involvement, as determined by staging. Staging of the disease is essential in order to initiate an appropriate treatment program. Staging correlates well with prognosis and helps in deciding whether radiotherapy or chemotherapy should be used.

The staging process involves the following procedures: chest x-ray, bone marrow, and liver biopsy, lymphangiography (x-ray of lymph nodes following the injection of a contrast medium), and laparotomy and splenectomy with accompanying node biopsy. Stage I involves a single lymph node region. The stage II disease involves two or more lymph node areas confined to one side of the diaphragm, and stage III involves lymphatic structures on both sides of the diaphragm which may also involve the spleen. Stage IV is disseminated involvement of the bone marrow, liver, and other extranodal sites in addition to lymph node involvement. Each stage is further divided into A or B categories depending on the absence (A) or presence (B) of unexplained fever, night sweats, and unexplained loss of 10% of total body weight.

At diagnosis, the most common finding is an enlarged, painless, cervical lymph node. Recurring fever is also characteristic, and night sweats are a fairly common symptom. A normocytic-normochromic anemia may be present in 50% of the cases, sometimes severe. Increased eosinophils and monocytes may also be present. The most frequent finding is moderate leukocytosis with white blood cell counts ranging from 12,000 to 25,000/μL, generally due to neutrophilia when the lymph nodes are involved. There is usually neutropenia when the bone marrow is involved. As a rule, lymphopenia, when present, is a poor prognosis. Reed-Sternberg cells have been found in the blood occasionally. The platelet count is usually normal, but may be increased or decreased if the bone marrow is involved. The erythrocyte sedimentation rate is commonly elevated.

Generally, the less extensive the disease, the longer the patient will live. In Hodgkin's disease, survival is significantly better in patients less than 40 years of age, and in the earlier stages of the disease. Also, patients with more mature lymphocytes have a better prognosis. However, many patients with active Hodgkin's disease have a defect in cell-mediated immunity, which makes them susceptible to bacterial, viral, and mycotic infections.

Chemotherapy and irradiation are used to treat patients with Hodgkin's disease. New treatment strategies for Hodgkin's disease, which was fatal 20 years ago, have resulted in an 85% survival rate for stages I and II, 70% for IIIA, and 50% for stage IV. Radiotherapy is the treatment of choice in patients with stage I and II disease to treat all lymph node areas. Chemotherapy is used in patients with stages III and IV Hodgkin's disease and a quadruple therapy with mustine, vincristine, procarbazine and prednisolone (MOPP) has proven superior to single agent therapy. Adriamycin, bleomycin, vinblastine, and dacarbazine (ABVD) chemotherapy has also been used to treat a resistant disease, and is now used alternately with MOPP.

MULTIPLE MYELOMA

Multiple myeloma is a malignant proliferation of atypical and immature forms of plasma cells, primarily occurring in the bone marrow. Onset of this disease is usually between the ages of 40 and 70 years. Equal numbers of males and females are affected. The exact cause of multiple myeloma is unknown, and there is no evidence that heredity plays a role. Bone pain is the main clinical finding in more than 60% of these patients. Pathologic fractures of the bone are common. Pain in the bones of the back and, less often, the chest or extremities is common, and multiple bone tumors may be present. Weakness, fever, and weight loss are frequently encountered. Abnormal bleeding may occur. Gastrointestinal symptoms in the form of nausea, diarrhea, and vomiting are also observed in this disease. Renal failure is a common complication.

The plasma proteins are increased, notably in the globulin portion. On protein electrophoresis, this generally appears as an increased gamma and less frequently as an increased alpha or beta band. Such abnormal patterns are said to contain an M-spot or M-component. Further testing of these M-components by immunoelectrophoresis shows them to be monoclonal proteins (proteins involved in the production of a single specific class of immunoglobulin). The protein types most often found, in order of their frequency, are IgG in greater than 50% of cases, IgA in approximately 20% of cases, and IgD in less than 1% of cases. IgM and IgE myelomas are rare. The Bence Jones urine test (for free immunoglobulin light chains) is positive in approximately 50% of the cases of multiple myeloma. Approximately 20% of the patients produce only these light chain portions of the immunoglobulin molecule.

Moderate normocytic-normochromic anemia almost always develops in this condition. The peripheral blood smear shows marked rouleaux formation. There may be a bluish tinge to the Wright-stained blood smear when it is examined macroscopically. This can be attributed to the increased protein content of the plasma. Occasional nucleated red blood cells may be found in the peripheral blood. Polychromatophilia and reticulocytosis may also be present. The white blood cell count is normal to decreased but is seldom increased. A slight increase in eosinophils and lymphocytes may occur, and a few immature granulocytes may be present. Plasma cells may also be found in the peripheral blood of approximately 15% of myeloma patients. The platelet count is generally normal but may be decreased. Coating of platelets by the myeloma protein may result in functional abnormalities of the platelets. The erythrocyte sedimentation rate is usually elevated. Some coagulation tests may be abnormal due to interference with some of the coagulation factors by the abnormal plasma protein. The most frequent cause of coagulation abnormalities is defective fibrin polymerization. Increased serum calcium levels may also be present, and bone x-rays are abnormal in about 90% of the cases of multiple myeloma. The most characteristic finding in the bone marrow is the myeloma cell (a morphologically abnormal plasma cell), which may comprise as much as 95% of all the cells. These cells may be indistinguishable from normal plasma cells but usually show some abnormalities or variations. Generally, the cell is moderately large and contains an eccentric nucleus with one to two nucleoli. The nuclear chromatin is not as fine as in the myeloblast but not as coarse as that found in the plasma cell. The cytoplasm may be basophilic and bright blue or a little lighter in color. Various types of inclusions may be found in the cytoplasm: red-staining crystalline bodies, Russell bodies (eosinophilic globules), and Mott bodies (colorless vacuoles). In some cases of IgA myeloma, the cytoplasm will be pink to red in color (flame cell).

Chemotherapy and radiation therapy are common treatments in multiple myeloma. Severe anemia is treated with transfusions of packed red cells. Bleeding due to interference with coagulation factors may be treated by plasmapheresis.

HEAVY CHAIN DISEASES

The heavy chain diseases are a group of disorders in which there is malignant proliferation of lymphoid cells which produce incomplete immunoglobulins. These cells produce heavy chain fragments without the associated light chains. This may be caused by the deletion of amino acids which code for the synthesis of the area in the heavy chain that is responsible for attaching to the light chains. Four types of heavy chain disease have been found.

Gamma (γ) heavy chain disease resembles lymphoma with atypical lymphocytes and plasma cells present in the peripheral blood. Anemia and leukopenia are generally present, and the platelets are decreased in about 50% of the cases. The bone marrow shows increased plasma cells and lymphocytes. These patients are usually susceptible to infection and have enlarged lymph nodes, spleen, and liver. This disorder is diagnosed by showing the presence of IgG heavy chain fragments in the urine or serum. These chains are reactive on immunoelectrophoresis with antisera to gamma chains but not with antisera to light chains.

Alpha (α) heavy chain disease is the most common form of heavy chain disease. It is a lymphoma with extensive lymphocyte and plasma cell infiltration of the small intestine and the abdominal lymph nodes. These patients have severe malabsorption with weight loss and diarrhea. Small amounts of the alpha chain may be detected by immunoelectrophoresis.

Mu (μ) heavy chain disease is rare and is often found in patients with chronic lymphocytic leukemia. Vacuolated plasma cells are often found in the bone marrow of these patients. Routine electrophoresis generally shows marked hypogammaglobulinemia. The mu heavy chain is detected by serum immunoelectrophoresis.

Delta (δ) heavy chain disease is rare. It has the same clinical features as myeloma. The abnormal protein has been identified as a tetramer of delta heavy chains.

The clinical course of heavy chain diseases is variable. Most cases are progressive and fatal. Remissions have been obtained in some patients. Melphalan or cyclophosphamide and prednisone are the agents which are used to treat these disorders.

WALDENSTRÖM'S MACROGLOBULINEMIA

Waldenström's macroglobulinemia is a disease of the elderly, most often occurring in males between the ages of 60 and 70. It is a lymphoma-like disorder characterized by infiltration of the bone marrow with small, mature B lymphocytes, many of which have plasmacytoid features. These cells produce macroglobulins (monoclonal IgM immunoglobulins of high molecular weight). These increased macroglobulin levels produce a condition called hyperviscosity syndrome. This includes neurologic symptoms, visual impairment, bleeding, and cardiovascular complications. In contrast to multiple myeloma, bone pain is rarely a symptom of this disease.

The blood generally shows normocytic-normochromic anemia that may become severe. The white blood cell count is usually normal. In the terminal stages of the disorder, the peripheral blood may contain large numbers of abnormal lymphocytes. Thrombocytopenia is present in about 30% of these patients. Marked rouleaux is seen on the Wright-stained smear, and the erythrocyte sedimentation rate is elevated. The serum viscosity test is also elevated. The bone marrow usually contains increased numbers of lymphocytes, plasmacytoid lymphocytes, and plasma cells. The periodic acid-Schiff stain is positive and often shows positive inclusions in the cytoplasm and nucleus of the lymphoid cells. This PAS positive material is probably identical with the circulating macroglobulin.

Alkylating agents such as chlorambucil have been used to treat this disorder. The hyperviscosity responds to plasmapheresis. The average life span of patients diagnosed with this disorder is 2 to 4 years.

PLATELET DISORDERS

Thrombocytopenia

Thrombocytopenia is the most common cause of abnormal bleeding and is generally attributed to either decreased platelet production or increased platelet destruction. Other causes of thrombocytopenia are increased platelet sequestration by the spleen and dilution of the platelet count by multiple blood transfusions.

DECREASED PLATELET PRODUCTION

Congenital hypoplasia of the megakaryocytes in the bone marrow is found in a number of clinical conditions: (1) Fanconi's syndrome, where there is pancytopenia and bone marrow hypoplasia, along with various congenital abnormalities. (2) TAR syndrome (thrombocytopenia with absent radii [bone in the arm]) where there is renal, cardiac, and skeletal malformation. (3) In the newborn infected with a virus such as rubella. (4) Intrauterine exposure to certain drugs such as thiazide diuretics, or tolbutamide.

Acquired hypoplasia of the megakaryocytes is generally not caused by replacement of the bone marrow cells by abnormal cells but is, instead, a result of the action of chemicals, toxic drugs, or other physical agents. Exposure to radiation, cytotoxic drugs and cancer chemotherapy, especially where alkylating agents or antimetabolites are used, will cause bone marrow hypoplasia. Usually, the megakaryocytes are the last cell type to return to normal following bone marrow recovery. Occasionally, they do not return to normal, and the thrombocytopenia may persist indefinitely. Some drugs, such as certain thiazides, the estrogen hormone DES (diethylstilbestrol), and alcohol, selectively decrease megakaryocyte production.

Ineffective thrombopoiesis is found in patients with megaloblastic hematopoiesis due to vitamin B_{12} or folic acid deficiency. In this disorder, the bone marrow generally contains an increased number of megakaryocytes despite the decrease in platelet production. This is thought to be because there is impaired DNA synthesis and, therefore, limited nuclear endoreduplication. The normal increase in cytoplasmic volume does not occur as the megakaryocyte matures. In the bone marrow, the megakaryocytes often appear hyperlobulated, and stained smears will show large platelets. The platelets may have a decreased survival time and may also show abnormal function. This condition is also seen in Di Guglielmo's syndrome, paroxysmal nocturnal hemoglobinuria, preleukemia, and leukemia.

Disorders of the control of thrombopoiesis are not common and result from an impairment in the mechanisms that control platelet production. Cyclic thrombocytopenia has been described, a condition in which thrombocytopenia and normal platelet counts alternate at regular intervals.

Infiltration of the bone marrow by malignant cells will generally result in decreased numbers of megakaryocytes. Inhibitors of thrombopoiesis may be produced by these abnormal cells and account for the thrombocytopenia associated with such conditions as metastatic cancer, myeloma, lymphoma and myelofibrosis.

INCREASED PLATELET DESTRUCTION

Increased platelet destruction may occur as a result of immunologic disorders.

Idiopathic thrombocytopenia purpura (ITP) is the most common among the secondary forms of thrombocytopenia and may occur in the acute, chronic, recurrent, or neonatal form. Acute ITP is found predominantly in children and occasionally in young adults. The majority of cases develop after recovery from a viral infection and are self limiting. Spontaneous remissions occur in about 80% of the cases. Chronic ITP is found in patients of all ages, but more often occurs in women between the ages of 20 and 50 years. It is felt that people with this disorder have a platelet autoantibody that is responsible for the destruction of the platelets. In this condition, the bone marrow contains abundant megakaryocytes. The platelet count may be markedly decreased to only slightly decreased, and the platelets usually appear large in size and have an abnormal appearance on a stained blood smear. Those laboratory tests requiring a normal platelet count will be abnormal: prolonged bleeding time, poor clot retraction, positive capillary fragility, and abnormal prothrombin consumption. Petechiae are present in most patients. Effective treatment of this disorder usually consists of corticosteroid therapy or splenectomy because the spleen is most responsible for removing the platelets (coated with the antibodies) from the blood. Recurrent ITP is found in patients who do not experience permanent remission following corticosteroid therapy or splenectomy. Immunosuppressive drugs and plasmapheresis occasionally are utilized to treat these patients. Neonatal ITP is found in newborns of women with ITP. It is caused by transplacental passage of antiplatelet antibodies and occurs most frequently when the mother is thrombocytopenic at the time of delivery. Recovery follows clearance of the antibody from the circulation and treatment is usually unnecessary.

Drug-induced immunologic thrombocytopenia may be caused by any one of many substances such as antibiotics, hypnotics, analgesics, heavy metals, diuretics, chloroquine, digitoxin, quinine, heparin, and tolbutamide, to name a few. The production of antibodies is the result of a reaction that will occur in only a small number of people exposed to a given drug. Generally both the drug and the antibody must be present in the system at the same time for destruction of platelets to occur. Therefore, the treatment of this disorder is to remove the offending drug. Severe thrombocytopenia may occur within 12 hours of ingestion of the drug, or the reaction time may take longer to occur. Bleeding may be severe and begin abruptly. The megakaryocytes in the bone marrow are generally normal in number, whereas those laboratory procedures that depend on platelets will be abnormal.

Immunologic thrombocytopenia, a condition indistinguishable from chronic ITP, is associated with a number of disorders such as autoimmune hemolytic anemias, chronic lymphocytic leukemia, Hodgkin's disease and other lymphomas, systemic lupus erythematosus, and rheumatoid arthritis.

Nonimmunologic thrombocytopenias are varied and are found in disseminated intravascular coagulation, fibrinogenolysis, and other microangiopathic processes. Thrombocytopenia may be present in a number of rickettsial, bacterial, or viral infections as a result of decreased production or increased destruction of platelets.

Thrombotic thrombocytopenic purpura (TTP) is a rare disorder, the exact cause of which is unknown. In addition to thrombocytopenia, it is characterized by hemolytic anemia, changing neurologic symptoms, fever and renal abnormalities. Most of these findings are caused by the formation of platelet thrombi in capillaries and arterioles throughout the body. The vascular defects also give rise to red blood cell fragments and, occasionally, spherocytes in the peripheral blood. The hemolytic anemia probably occurs as a result of the trauma to the red blood cells. TTP affects all ages, although it is most commonly found in women of child bearing age. It is a serious disease, but at present more than 50% of the patients with this disorder will undergo a long-lasting remission following proper therapy. Treatment consists of the administration of antiplatelet agents and plasma exchange transfusions. In some cases, high doses of steroids are used, and splenectomy may also be helpful.

Hemolytic-uremic syndrome resembles TTP. However, it occurs primarily in children and the intravascular clotting is generally confined to the kidney. Hypertension is a common finding, while neurologic symptoms are rare. Treatments include dialysis, exchange transfusion and antihypertensive therapy.

INCREASED PLATELET SEQUESTRATION

An abnormal distribution of platelets may also cause thrombocytopenia. The normal spleen sequesters approximately one third of the total platelet mass. In circumstances where the spleen is enlarged (splenomegaly), an increased percentage of the platelets will be found in the spleen. Increased splenic pooling may complicate such disorders as Gaucher's disease, Hodgkin's disease, sarcoidosis, and lymphomas. The splenomegaly associated with cirrhosis of the liver and portal hypertension is the most common cause of an abnormal distribution of platelets.

DILUTION OF THE PLATELET COUNT

Blood transfusions dilute the platelet count in proportion to the amount of blood given. Multiple transfusions used to treat massive blood loss produce thrombocytopenia because bank blood contains few, if any, viable platelets. The splenic pool of platelets is usually insufficient to keep up with losses and compensation by increased platelet production does not occur as an acute response to hemorrhage. Transfusions with platelet concentrates usually prevents excessive bleeding in patients with dilutional thrombocytopenia.

Thrombocytosis

A platelet count increased above normal will be found as a result of a variety of circumstances. *Reactive thrombocytosis* describes a moderate increase in the platelet count, which is usually short lived and asymptomatic. *Autonomous thrombocytosis* refers to a marked increase in the platelet count, which generally persists, and is associated with thrombotic and/or hemorrhagic complications.

REACTIVE THROMBOCYTOSIS

Reactive thrombocytosis describes a moderately increased platelet count that generally responds when the underlying disorder is treated. Recovery from splenectomy, major surgery and acute blood loss are commonly associated with reactive thrombocytosis. Following splenectomy, the platelet count will generally show an increase above normal on the first to tenth day following the surgical procedure. It will usually peak at 1 to 3 weeks, and begin to decrease in the next 2 to 3 months. In some instances, however, the platelet count may not reach normal levels for a year or more. The platelet count may also show an increase on the third to tenth day following major surgical procedure. In these cases, there may be thrombocytopenia present immediately after surgical procedure. The platelet count generally decreases to normal levels within about 2 weeks following surgical procedure. Within about a day and a half following acute blood loss, a reactive thrombocytosis may also occur. Other conditions showing a reactive increase in the platelet count are (1) iron deficiency anemia, (2) accompanying some malignant diseases such as carcinoma and Hodgkin's disease, (3) following withdrawal of cytotoxic drugs, (4) in association with increased hematopoiesis, as in patients with hemolytic anemia or secondary polycythemia, (5) in association with acute and chronic inflammatory diseases. In all of these conditions, the megakaryocytes are increased in number, platelet production is effective and platelet survival is normal. Generally the platelets are small in size and of uniform shape.

AUTONOMOUS THROMBOCYTOSIS

Autonomous thrombocytosis is a common feature of the myeloproliferative disorders. These include essential thrombocytosis (thrombocythemia), chronic myelogenous leukemia, polycythemia vera, and myeloid metaplasia.

Thrombocythemia is found most often in middle aged patients of both sexes. It is characterized by a marked increase in the platelet count. Patients with this disorder may have periods of bleeding or thrombosis followed by long periods with no symptoms. Gastrointestinal hemorrhage is the most common form of bleeding. Thrombosis in both the venous and arterial circulation may develop, and involvement of the coronary and cerebral vasculature is common. Splenomegaly is a frequent finding. The platelet count is usually greater than 1 million/μL and may be as high as several million/μL. Because of the extremely high number of platelets, it is frequently difficult to obtain an accurate platelet count, and determination of the packed platelet volume is useful. Stained blood smears often show the platelets to be clumped, forming large masses. The platelets also usually show abnormalities of size, shape, and structure. Platelet life span is generally normal. Megakaryocyte fragments are also frequently present. The red blood cells are normal or may be microcytic and hypochromic due to iron deficiency from blood loss. The white blood cell count is usually increased and may be as high as 40,000/μL. The differential will usually show a neutrophilia with a slight shift to the left. In the bone marrow, a marked increase in the size, volume, and number of megakaryocytes is seen and the megakaryocytes often display bizarre morphology. Platelet function tests are usually abnormal. Treatment for this disorder is aimed primarily at controlling the platelet count. In symptomatic patients where the platelet count is elevated above 1 million/μL radioactive phosphorus, alkylating agents and plateletpheresis are used. Inhibitors of platelet function, especially aspirin, are often employed in an attempt to prevent thromboembolic complications.

The other myeloproliferative disorders share the thrombotic and hemorrhagic complications, as well as many of the morphologic features of the platelets and megakaryocytes, seen in thrombocythemia.

Hereditary Qualitative Platelet Disorders

Qualitative or functional platelet disorders may be attributed to defects of platelet aggregation, the release reaction, or platelet adhesion.

GLANZMANN'S THROMBASTHENIA

Glanzmann's thrombasthenia is inherited as an autosomal recessive trait. People who are heterozygous for this trait are asymptomatic carriers. In this disorder, bleeding can be spontaneous and quite severe and will usually begin at an early age. As the patient becomes older, the severity of the bleeding will decrease somewhat. Platelet aggregation studies show a defective primary response in the presence of collagen, epinephrine, ADP, and thrombin. Ristocetin is capable of inducing an initial wave of aggregation. However, this is followed by disaggregation rather than the normal secondary wave response. Platelet retention is markedly decreased. The platelet count is generally normal but may occasionally be slightly decreased. Clot retraction is decreased to absent, and the bleeding time is prolonged. When viewed on a Wright-stained blood smear, the platelets appear morphologically normal. The platelet release reaction varies from normal to decreased depending on the stimulus, and the platelets show a normal shape change in the presence of aggregating agents. The impaired aggregation seen in Glanzmann's thrombasthenia is due to a decrease or absence of the platelet surface proteins which act as fibrinogen binding sites on the platelet membrane. Few treatment options are currently available for this disorder, except for transfusion of platelet concentrates.

STORAGE POOL DISORDERS

The storage pool disorders are a group of hereditaty conditions in which there is a defective platelet release reaction. Patients may lack only dense bodies, both dense bodies and alpha granules, or only alpha granules (gray platelet syndrome). Patients with dense body abnormalities may also display abnormal prostaglandin and thromboxane synthesis. In these disorders, there is a mild to moderate bleeding tendency, and easy bruising is common. Abnormalities of the dense bodies or alpha granules result in reduced concentrations and abnormal release of platelet ADP, serotonin, and calcium. The platelets will show normal aggregation by high concentrations of ADP but not by collagen. Also, the secondary phase of platelet aggregation will not occur with epinephrine. There is decreased platelet retention using the glass bead column. Storage pool disorders may also be found associated with certain congenital abnormalities such as Wiskott-Aldrich, TAR and Chédiak-Higashi syndromes, and May-Hegglin anomaly. At present, there is no specific treatment for this disorder. All drugs which inhibit platelet aggregation should be withheld from these patients.

BERNARD-SOULIER SYNDROME

The Bernard-Soulier syndrome is inherited as an autosomal recessive trait. It is characterized by bruising and moderate to severe bleeding. One of the most striking characteristics of this disorder is the presence of giant platelets, which may range in size up to 20 μm in diameter. The platelets also show coarse granulation and vacuoles. Mild thrombocytopenia is generally present. The megakaryocytes in the bone marrow are normal to slightly increased in number and appear morphologically normal. The platelets lack the membrane glycoprotein which functions as a receptor for the von Willebrand factor and therefore are unable to adhere normally to vascular endothelium. In addition, the platelets do not bind coagulation factor XI normally and bind a decreased amount of thrombin. The bleeding time is prolonged, but clot retraction is normal. Platelet aggregation by ADP, epinephrine, and collagen is normal, but there is abnormal aggregation by ristocetin and thrombin. There is a decreased retention of platelets in the glass bead column procedure. Platelet transfusions have been utilized for the treatment of this disorder.

VARIOUS HEREDITARY FORMS OF PLATELET DYSFUNCTION

Some inherited connective tissue disorders (Ehlers-Danlos syndrome) and mu-

copolysaccharide disorders may show abnormally large platelets and abnormalities in the release of ADP. Patients with *hereditary afibrinogenemia* usually show a prolonged bleeding time and abnormal platelet aggregation with ADP or epinephrine. Patients with defective prostaglandin synthesis display abnormal aggregation patterns with ADP, epinephrine, and collagen. A deficiency of the enzyme cyclooxygenase or thromboxane synthetase may account for this 'aspirin-like' defect. In von Willebrand's disease, an absent, abnormal or inactive form of the von Willebrand factor results in impaired platelet adhesion. Aggregation studies with ADP, epinephrine and collagen are normal, while ristocetin-induced aggregation is usually abnormal. Abnormalities of the platelet release reaction have also been found in patients with factor VIII deficiency and in those with glycogen storage disease.

Acquired Qualitative Platelet Disorders

Acquired disorders of platelet function are associated with a number of conditions and with the ingestion of certain drugs.

In *uremia,* metabolites that are toxic to the platelets accumulate in the plasma. These toxins, and possibly defective prostaglandin synthesis, contribute to the impaired platelet function seen in this disorder. The platelet release reaction, platelet aggregation, and platelet retention are all abnormal and the bleeding time is prolonged. In this condition, bleeding may be severe at times. Dialysis is of temporary therapeutic value, and the administration of cryoprecipitates will aid in controlling major bleeding episodes.

Bleeding disorders will be present in the various *paraproteinemias.* In multiple myeloma and Waldenström's macroglobulinemia there are various abnormalities of platelet aggregation and reduced platelet retention which are thought to be due to the coating of the platelet membrane with abnormal proteins.

In *acute myeloblastic leukemia,* the megakaryocytes in the bone marrow may be small and somewhat abnormal. The resultant platelets are abnormal, showing defective platelet aggregation and a defective release mechanism.

The *myeloproliferative disorders* (polycythemia vera, chronic myelogenous leukemia, myeloid metaplasia, and essential thrombocythemia) display functional abnormalities in addition to thrombocytosis. In myeloid metaplasia and polycythemia vera, there is defective platelet aggregation. In thrombocythemia, the platelets appear large and morphologically abnormal. There is defective platelet retention, and there may also be defective platelet release. There is a deficiency in membrane glycoproteins in chronic myelogenous leukemia, which places it in the category of an acquired storage pool disorder. Micromegakaryocytes are also found in this disorder.

Fibrinogen degradation products present in increased amounts will inhibit ADP induced platelet aggregation. Fragment E will inhibit thrombin induced platelet aggregation.

The *autoantibodies* in idiopathic thrombocytopenic purpura and in certain autoimmune disorders such as systemic lupus erythematosus may cause functional platelet disorders. These patients may have an acquired type of storage pool disorder because of the reaction of the antibody with the platelet membrane.

Many *drugs* have been shown to inhibit platelet function. Aspirin inhibits both the release reaction and the secondary wave of aggregation. This is a direct result of aspirin's ability to inactivate the enzyme cyclooxygenase. The effect of the aspirin lasts for the life of the platelet. In the presence of aspirin, there is defective platelet aggregation with ADP, epinephrine and collagen. Other drugs which induce qualitative platelet abnormalities include some antihistamines, antidepressants and antibiotics, heparin, dextran and other plasma expanders, ethanol and certain local anesthetics.

COAGULATION DISORDERS

Coagulation Factor Deficiencies

Coagulation factor abnormalities may be due to a defect in the synthesis of the factor (leading to a decreased concentration) or may be due to synthesis of a defective factor (leading to normal amounts of an inactive or abnormally functioning factor). Abnormalities may be classified as quantitative or qualitative based on results of immunologic procedures. The results of these tests are expressed as positive (+) or negative (−) for *cross-reacting material (CRM + or CRM −).* A test that is CRM − indicates that a specific factor is not present. CRM − disorders are quantitative abnormalities. On the other hand, a coagulation disease that is CRM + is considered to have the factor present, but it is thought to be functionally abnormal, and it is, therefore, a qualitative disorder.

Factor I Deficiency

A deficiency in fibrinogen is rare, but when it does occur, severe hemorrhaging may result. Congenital deficiencies of fibrinogen may fall into one of three categories: *(1) Afibrinogenemia,* in which there is no measurable fibrinogen except trace amounts when tested immunologically. (2) *Hypofibrinogenemia,* where the plasma levels of fibrinogen are lower than 100 mg/dL. (3) *Dysfibrinogenemia,* where the fibrinogen present is functionally abnormal.

Hereditary afibrinogenemia is an extremely rare disorder. It is inherited as an autosomal recessive trait and appears to be the result of deficient synthesis of fibrinogen. Patients homozygous for this disorder have low levels of fibrinogen. This hemorrhagic disorder is present from birth, and there may be severe bleeding from the umbilical cord. There may be excesive bleeding following surgical procedure or trauma. Subcutaneous hemorrhages and defective wound healing are also seen. These patients may, however, have long periods where they have no bleeding, and the disorder is generally not as debilitating as Hemophilia A. In most cases, the blood will not clot. The PT, APTT, and thrombin time are markedly prolonged, and the bleeding time is abnormal in about 50% of the cases. Because of the total absence of fibrinogen, the erythrocyte sedimentation rate is generally 0.

Hereditary hypofibrinogenemia has been found to be inherited as both an autosomal dominant trait and an autosomal recessive trait. This condition may possibly be the heterozygous expression of afibrinogenemia. Generally the plasma fibrinogen levels are less than 100 mg/dL, and major bleeding is not seen. The laboratory test results are similar to those described for hereditary afibrinogenemia but are not as markedly abnormal.

Hereditary dysfibrinogenemia is usually inherited as an incompletely dominant autosomal trait. More than 55 different qualitatively abnormal fibrinogens have now been found. These fibrinogens have structural variations which result in abnormalities of all three apsects of the thrombin-fibrinogen reaction (release of fibrinopeptides, polymerization of the fibrin monomers, and stabilization of the fibrin clot). Most patients with this disorder show few symptoms other than a mild hemorrhagic tendency and some problems with wound healing. The PT and APTT generally show slightly prolonged results, and the thrombin time is prolonged. Chemical or immunologic assays of the fibrinogen level are generally normal. Procedures testing for clottable fibrinogen (those procedures using a thrombin reagent), however, are abnormal.

Cryoprecipitate and purified fibrinogen may be used to treat the inherited fibrinogen deficiencies.

An *acquired deficiency of fibrinogen* is more commonly found than a congenital deficiency. The acquired deficiency may be caused by impaired fibrinogen production in conditions such as liver disease. It may occur as a result of excess utilization of fibrinogen, or it may be found as a result of fibrinogen destruction. Both of these processes are present in DIC and liver disease. Acquired deficiencies of fibrinogen are most commonly found in abnormal obstetric cases and may also occur as a complication of surgery.

Factor II Deficiency

A *congenital deficiency of prothrombin* is extremely rare, and is inherited as an autosomal recessive trait. It is a relatively mild hemorrhagic disorder, and bleeding is most common following trauma. A few cases of dysfunctional prothrombin have also been found. Laboratory tests show both the PT and APTT to be abnormal. The whole blood clotting time may or may not be abnormal, and the Stypven time is abnormal. The most sensitive test for this abnormality is the two-stage prothrombin time, which will show a marked reduction in prothrombin. Levels of prothrombin are usually less than 10% of normal in this disorder. Stored plasma or Proplex (a purified prothrombin complex) may be administered for treatment.

Prothrombin is produced by the liver and depends on vitamin K for its synthesis. An *acquired deficiency of prothrombin* is commonly found in association with vitamin K deficiency, in which case deficiencies of factors VII, IX, and X are also present. These deficiencies are found in gastrointestinal disease, obstructive jaundice, and coumarin therapy where there is defective absorption or utilization of vitamin K.

Factor V Deficiency

A *congenital deficiency of factor V* has been designated *parahemophilia*. It is inherited as an autosomal recessive trait and manifests itself clinically in those patients who have inherited the defective gene from both parents. This defect is extremely rare. Clinically, these patients may show varying degrees of mucosal membrane bleeding, easy bruising, gastrointestinal bleeding, and excessive bleeding following dental or surgical procedures. The PT, APTT, and Stypven time are abnormal. The whole blood clotting time and the prothrombin consumption may or may not be abnormal. A factor V assay, based on the prothrombin time, should be performed to determine the extent of the deficiency. Fresh or fresh frozen plasma is used when treatment of this disorder is necessary.

A *combined deficiency of factor V and factor VIII* has been described. It is a rare finding and its biochemistry and genetics have not yet been fully described.

Acquired deficiencies of factor V have been found to be associated with DIC, liver disease, and acute leukemia.

Factor VII Deficiency

Congenital factor VII deficiency is a rare disorder and is inherited as an autosomal recessive trait. It produces a severe deficiency (less than 10% of normal concentrations) in the homozygous patient and a moderate deficiency in heterozygous individuals. Patients have also been found with qualitative abnormalities of factor VII. Clinically, homozygous patients show mild mucosal, genitourinary and gastrointestinal bleeding. A high incidence of factor VII deficiency has been found in patients with Dubin-Johnson syndrome (an hereditary disorder of bilirubin metabolism). The PT is significantly prolonged. The APTT, whole blood clotting time, and Stypven time are normal. A prothrombin time with substitutions may be performed to help identify the factor VII deficiency. An assay for factor VII, based on the prothrombin time, may then be performed to determine the level of factor VII present. This disorder may be treated with stored plasma or Proplex (a purified prothrombin complex).

Factor VII is synthesized in the liver and is vitamin K dependent. *Acquired factor VII deficiency* is found in the same conditions that cause acquired deficiency of factor II.

Factor VIII Deficiency

Genetic abnormalities of factor VIII are found in hemophilia A (or *classic hemophilia*) and *von Willebrand's disease.* These are the two most common hereditary coagulation disorders. It is currently accepted that several functions can be attributed to factor VIII: (1) Factor VIII:C refers to the coagulant portion of the molecule and represents the ability of the factor VIII molecule to correct coagulation abnormalities associated with hemophilia A. This clotting activity is measured in the APTT and the factor VIII assay procedure. (2) Factor VIII:C:Ag is the factor VIII:C related antigen which is measured immunologically. (3) Factor VIII:R:RCo refers to that part of the molecule which makes possible platelet aggregation in the presence of ristocetin, and is termed the ristocetin cofactor. (4) Factor VIII:R:vW is also termed the *von Willebrand factor* and is required for normal platelet adhesion in the hemostatic process. (5) Factor VIII:R:Ag is the factor VIII:R related antigen.

HEMOPHILIA A

Hemophilia A is inherited as a sex linked recessive trait and is felt to be the result of a deficiency or dysfunction of the factor VIII:C component of the factor VIII molecule. The condition is transmitted to males by their mothers who have the defective gene on one X chromosome. The female carrier of hemophilia theoretically passes this defect on to half of her sons and half of her daughters. The affected male transmits the defective gene to all of his daughters but to none of his sons because the sons acquire their X chromosome from their mother. Hemophilia has also been found in females, most commonly seen in the heterozygous carrier, where unusually low levels of factor VIII:C activity may be seen. Females who are homozygous for hemophilia have been seen in whom the disorder was passed on from the parents (an affected father and a mother carrying the defective gene). In these cases, the disorder resembles that seen in the affected male.

Except in mild deficiencies, this hemorrhagic disorder appears in infancy and remains as a lifelong affliction. Bleeding may occur in the gastrointestinal tract, the renal tract, or from the nose. Dental extractions are often followed by excessive bleeding. Hemarthrosis (hemorrhaging into the joints) is a common finding. This causes pain and swelling which may progressively impair joint function and lead to chronic arthritis and joint destruction. Intramuscular and intracranial bleeding is seen in some patients.

Patients with severe hemophilia have less than 1% factor VIII:C activity. The laboratory data are usually characteristic. The platelet count, tourniquet test, PT, and bleeding time are normal. The prothrombin consumption and APTT are abnormal. The Lee and White clotting time is most often abnormal. The APTT with substitutions should be performed, followed by a factor VIII:C assay.

Patients with factor VIII:C levels of 2 to 5% are considered to have moderate hemophilia. These individuals will also suffer spontaneous bleeding but less frequently than the more severely deficient patients. Mild hemophilia is characterized by factor VIII:C levels of 5 to 25%. This type is more difficult to diagnose. The patient generally shows a normal Lee and White clotting time and normal prothrombin consumption but may bleed profusely during or following surgery. As a general rule, spontaneous bleeding does not occur unless the factor VIII:C level falls below 20% of normal.

Approximately 10% of severe hemophiliac patients develop circulating anticoagulants, usually in the form of antibodies to factor VIII:C.

Treatment of hemophilia consists of halting any local bleeding by pressure and coagulants and raising the factor VIII:C level in the blood. The level to which the factor VIII:C activity is raised depends on the severity and cause of bleeding. Surgical and post trauma bleeding require that the level be elevated and maintained close to 100% of normal until healing occurs. There are several therapeutic materials now available for raising the factor VIII:C level in the blood, including the cryoprecipitated fraction of plasma, purified factor VIII:C, and fresh or fresh frozen citrated plasma. Administration of DDAVP (a drug which releases endogenous factor VIII:C from the endothelium) is used to raise the level of factor VIII:C in mild bleeding. If anemia is present, fresh whole blood may also be used.

von Willebrand's Disease

von Willebrand's disease is found more frequently than classic hemophilia. It is inherited as both an autosomal dominant and an autosomal recessive trait. Five subtypes of this disorder have been described. These are characterized by differences in inheritance patterns, in levels of factor VIII:C, VIII:R:Ag, and VIII:R:RCo and by structural differences in the factor VIII:R:vW component of the factor VIII molecule.

The clinical manifestations of von Willebrand's disease vary, depending on the severity of the disorder. In Type I von Willebrand's disease, abnormal bleeding usually begins in childhood. Easy bruising, bleeding from the gums, gastrointestinal bleeding, and prolonged bleeding following surgical procedure or injury are commonly found. Deep tissue hemorrhages are rare. It has been suggested that the severity of the disease may decrease slightly with advancing age.

A prolonged bleeding time is characteristic of this disorder, and about half of the affected patients show a positive capillary fragility test. Aspirin, which will slightly prolong normal bleeding times, has a marked effect on these patients. The platelet count is normal to slightly elevated, and the platelets appear morphologically normal, although morphologic abnormalities have been reported using electron microscopy. Platelet adhesiveness, as determined by the Salzman method, is reported to be markedly decreased. Platelet aggregation studies show a decreased aggregation in the presence of ristocetin (and normal aggregation with ADP, epinephrine, and collagen). The level of factor VIII:R:RCo is usually decreased. The APTT may be abnormal, depending on the level of factor VIII:C. The plasma factor VIII:C activity may range from as low as 1% (rarely) to levels of 30%. The majority of patients show factor VIII:C concentrations of 5 to 15%. The PT is normal in this disorder, and the Lee and White clotting time is generally abnormal but may be normal in some cases. The prothrombin consumption and clot retraction are generally normal.

Treatment consists of local measures to control bleeding and the administration of fresh or fresh frozen plasma or cryoprecipitate.

Factor IX Deficiency

Congenital deficiency of factor IX is also known as *Christmas disease* and *hemophilia B.* It appears to be inherited as a sex linked recessive trait in the same manner as classic hemophilia. Factor IX abnormalities may occur in at least two different forms: CRM − and CRM +. The majority of patients show no detectable factor IX by immunologic procedures, whereas a few patients have been shown to have a qualitatively abnormal factor IX.

This disorder is clinically indistinguishable from classic hemophilia. Both mild and severe forms of the disease have been reported, with the milder forms showing few spontaneous bleeding episodes, but profuse bleeding following surgery or trauma.

The laboratory findings in hereditary factor IX deficiency are similar to those found in classic hemophilia, with the exception of the APTT with substitutions. The platelet count, tourniquet test, and PT are normal. The whole blood clotting time, prothrombin consumption, and APTT are abnormal. Before definite diagnosis can be made, a factor IX assay should be performed.

Whole blood, plasma, and a purified prothrombin complex are used to treat this disorder. Because factor IX is stable when stored, the plasma or whole blood used does not have to be fresh.

An *acquired factor IX deficiency* is found in patients receiving coumarin drugs and also in patients with liver disease because factor IX is vitamin K dependent and requires normal hepatic function for its synthesis.

Factor X Deficiency

A *congenital deficiency of factor X* is rare and is inherited as an autosomal recessive trait. Studies have determined that there are both CRM + (functional or qualitative abnormality) and CRM − (quantitative abnormality) variants of inherited factor X deficiency.

Patients who are homozygous for factor X deficiency have hemorrhagic problems which are similar to those seen in hemophilia A. In the heterozygous state, bleeding is usually less severe.

Because factor X participates in both the intrinsic and extrinsic thromboplastin systems, a deficiency in this factor yields abnormal PT and APTT results. The Stypven time and prothrombin consumption are usually abnormal. The APTT with substitutions, the PT with substitutions, and the factor X assay may be performed for positive identification of this deficiency.

When necessary, this disorder may be treated with stored plasma or with a purified prothrombin complex.

An *acquired defect of factor X* is found in liver disease, vitamin K deficiency, and patients treated with coumarin drugs. Factor X depends on vitamin K and a functioning liver for its synthesis.

Factor XI Deficiency

Congenital factor XI deficiency is currently thought to be transmitted as an incompletely recessive autosomal trait. This disorder is common in persons of eastern European Jewish descent.

Bleeding is less severe than in hemophilia A and spontaneous hemorrhages are rare, although they may occur following surgical procedure or trauma.

Laboratory data for factor XI deficiency show a prolonged whole blood clotting time and an abnormal APTT. The PT is normal. Differentiating factor XI deficiency from factor XII may be accomplished by using known factor XI deficient plasma and known factor XII deficient plasma in the APTT substitution test.

When necessary, stored plasma may be used to treat this disorder.

Factor XII Deficiency

Factor XII deficiency is rare and is inherited as an autosomal recessive trait.

It is a unique defect in that there are usually no significant clinical abnormalities. Patients with this disorder show no bleeding or only a minor bleeding tendency, even after trauma or surgical procedure. An increased tendency toward thrombosis is often observed in these patients.

The laboratory findings are similar to those found in factor XI deficiency.

When necessary, stored plasma may be used to treat this disorder.

Factor XIII Deficiency

Factor XIII deficiency has been found to be inherited as an autosomal recessive trait in most instances. Studies have suggested that both a qualitative abnormality

and a quantitative abnormality of factor XIII are present.

Clinical symptoms may occur at birth, with bleeding from the umbilical cord. Spontaneous hemorrhage is rare but may occur following surgical procedure or trauma. Bleeding into the central nervous system has been found to occur more commonly in this disorder than in other hereditary coagulation disorders. Poor wound healing is also characteristic of this factor deficiency.

A simple screening procedure for the fibrin stabilizing factor, employing 5 M urea, is used to diagnose this deficiency in the laboratory. All other routine coagulation screening tests are normal.

When treatment is necessary, administration of plasma is the method of choice.

Prekallikrein Deficiency

Prekallikrein deficiency is thought to be inherited as an autosomal recessive trait. This abnormality has been identified as CRM −, and is, therefore, a quantitative defect.

Like those with a factor XII deficiency, people with prekallikrein deficiency show little to no bleeding tendencies.

Laboratory data show a normal PT, thrombin time, and bleeding time. The whole blood clotting time and APTT are usually moderately prolonged due to the slow contact activation time caused by the deficiency of prekallikrein.

High Molecular Weight Kininogen Deficiency

High molecular weight kininogen deficiency, is thought to be transmitted as an autosomal recessive trait. Patients with this rare deficiency are asymptomatic. This disorder is characterized by a prolonged APTT and whole blood clotting time.

Coagulation Disorders Caused by Vitamin K Deficiencies

Factors II, VII, IX, and X depend on vitamin K for their synthesis and are produced in the liver. Therefore, a *vitamin K deficiency* or liver dysfunction may produce coagulation disorders. In addition, the oral anticoagulant drug, coumarin, acts as an antagonist which impairs the synthesis of the vitamin K dependent coagulation factors.

Hemorrhagic disease of the newborn results from vitamin K deficiency. Normally, the newborn has a moderate deficiency of these factors at birth and for the following 2 to 5 days. Routine administration of vitamin K however, has made this problem relatively rare. This disorder is prevented by administering vitamin K to the mother before delivery and by giving vitamin K to the infant at birth.

Vascular Disorders

Vascular disorders are characterized by bruising or purpura (bleeding into the skin) caused by defects in the structure or function of the walls of the blood vessels. Extravascular or endothelial defects may also lead to vascular disorders.

In *hereditary hemorrhagic telangiectasia,* there is localized dilation of the walls of the small blood vessels of the skin and mucous membranes. These blood vessels form disorganized and tortuous patterns throughout the body. The walls of the affected blood vessels are thin and lack smooth muscle. For this reason they are unable to contract and bleed readily when injured. This disorder is inherited as an autosomal dominant trait and is the most common inherited vascular bleeding disorder.

Extravascular defects result from loss of elasticity of the skin, as in the benign condition *senile purpura* (bruised areas commonly on the forearms of elderly persons), or from more serious *connective tissue abnormalities. Ehlers- Danlos syndrome* and *Marfan's syndrome* are both inherited as autosomal dominant disorders and display abnormal bleeding due to increased vascular fragility. This increased fragility is caused by abnormalities of the collagen and elastin fibers which form the supporting tissues for blood vessels.

Scurvy (deficiency of ascorbic acid) causes acquired defects in the synthesis of collagen and hyaluronic acid, a component of the intercellular cement substance found between endothelial cells. This disorder is eliminated by the administration of ascorbic acid (vitamin C).

Henoch-Schönlein purpura is a disorder in which gastrointestinal hemorrhage and joint swelling occur in association with a purpuric rash. This condition is most common in children and often follows an upper respiratory infection. Immunologic damage to endothelial cells is most probably the cause of the vascular abnormalities seen in this disorder. Certain drugs and infectious agents are also known to cause vascular abnormalities due to endothelial cell damage.

In vascular disorders, there may be spontaneous bleeding or bleeding as a result of minimal trauma. Petechiae (small purpuric spots on the skin) are present, and in some cases, ecchymoses (larger superficial hemorrhages) may appear secondary to mild trauma. Intramuscular bleeding is rare, but nosebleeds are not uncommon. Generally, the platelet count is normal, as are most platelet function tests and coagulation studies. The bleeding time and tourniquet test are usually abnormal.

Liver Disease

A variety of hemostatic defects may be found in liver disease. These include multiple factor deficiencies, abnormalities of fibrinolysis, thrombocytopenia and qualitative platelet abnormalities. Alterations in clearance mechanisms of the liver further compromise the integrity of the hemostatic process. All of the coagulation factors, except factor VIII, are synthesized in the liver. Decreased levels of the vitamin K dependent factors (II, VII, IX, and X) are among the earliest and most important changes seen in liver disease. Factors V and the contact factors (XI, XII, Fletcher factor, and Fitzgerald factor) are also decreased; however, the clinical significance of these deficiencies in patients with liver disease is unclear. Quantitative and/or qualitative abnormalities of fibrinogen are found in most cases of liver disease. For an unknown reason, factor VIII levels are generally increased in disorders of the liver. Abnormal fibrinolysis is seen due to decreased synthesis of plasminogen, decreased levels of plasmin inhibitors and impaired clearance from the circulation of plasminogen activators and fibrin split products. The thrombocytopenia seen in liver disease is usually secondary to splenomegaly, while the qualitative abnormalities of platelets may be attributed to increased levels of fibrin split products or to the intake of alcohol.

Patients with liver disease may have severe hemorrhaging. Gastrointestinal bleeding is most common and generally results from an ulcer, esophageal varices, or gastritis.

Laboratory test results will be extremely variable, depending on the severity of the liver disorder. The PT, APTT, bleeding time and platelet count are often abnormal. Fibrinogen levels may be decreased, normal or increased. Functionally abnormal variants of fibrinogen are common and usually account for a prolonged thrombin time. Treatment of liver disease may take the form of administration of vitamin K or antifibrinolytic agents, or transfusions of fresh frozen plasma (for factor replacement) or platelets, depending on the severity of the disease and the resultant bleeding.

Disseminated Intravascular Coagulation

Disseminated intravascular coagulation *(DIC), defibrination syndrome,* and *consumption coagulopathy* are terms used to refer to the generalized activation of the coagulation and fibrinolytic systems in the circulating blood. The results of this activation are consumption of coagulation factors and platelets, generation of thrombin, widespread deposition of fibrin in small blood vessels and formation of large amounts of fibrinogen degradation products. All of these contribute to the bleeding, shock, and vascular occlusion that develop.

There are two basic causes of an episode of DIC: (1) the release of tissue thromboplastin or thromboplastin-like substances into the circulation, and (2) the activation of coagulation proteins by exposure to damaged endothelium or in association with the intravascular aggregation of platelets. Clinical conditions associated with the release of thromboplastic material include obstetric complications, acute promyelocytic and monocytic leukemias, intravascular hemolysis of various origins, massive trauma, head injury, burns, major surgical procedures, and malignant tumors. Endothelial damage may occur as a result of infections (viral, bacterial, rickettsial, fungal, and protozoal), heat stroke, or shock. Intravascular platelet aggregation may result from the action of toxins, drugs or antigen-antibody complexes. Venoms from various snakes may produce vascular endothelial damage. They may also contain certain thrombin-like enzymes or substances that may activate prothrombin or factor X.

When thromboplastic material or activated coagulation proteins enter the circulating blood, intravascular coagulation occurs, with a resultant decrease in fibrinogen, prothrombin, factor V, and factor VIII. Factors VII, IX, and X and other coagulation proteins, namely antithrombin III, alpha-2 antiplasmin, and plasminogen, may also be decreased. The platelet count is generally low because the platelets are used in the coagulation process, and they also tend to adhere to the damaged tissues. An immediate reaction in DIC is the formation of small fibrin strands and microclots. This will cause injury to the red blood cells in the area, and schistocytes and microspherocytes will form. Fibrinolysis is almost always present in DIC and may be activated by the thromboplastic substances responsible for the DIC, activated factor XII, or from plasminogen activators present in the vascular endothelium. The resultant fibrin degradation products formed act as antithrombins and inhibit fibrin polymerization. This may be a major cause of hemorrhage. The reticuloendothelial system is responsible for removing the procoagulants and coagulation products from the system.

Thrombosis with infarction and necrosis may be the major feature of DIC when fibrinolytic activity is insufficient to remove clots. Hemorrhage predominates as coagulation factors are consumed and clotting becomes minimal. In a typical case of DIC, the PT, APTT, and thrombin time are generally prolonged. These tests, however, may be normal for some unknown reason. A normal APTT, however, may reflect the partial coagulation (activated coagulation factors) present in the blood. The platelet count is decreased, as is the fibrinogen. The protamine sulfate and ethanol gelation tests are usually positive. Antithrombin III is usually decreased in this disorder. Tests for fibrinogen degradation products may show increased levels of these substances. It is not unusual, however, to find normal results in these tests because these fragments form a complex with fibrinogen during serum preparation. The euglobulin clot lysis test may be normal due to depletion of plasminogen.

When DIC occurs, it must be treated as a medical emergency. Because it occurs secondary to another disorder, the most important aspect of therapy is to treat the primary disorder. To halt the intravascular clotting mechanism, heparin is generally given. Replacement therapy using platelets and/or fresh frozen plasma (for coagulation factors) may sometimes be administered if necessary. If the patient is in shock, this must be treated immediately.

Whole blood or packed red blood cells are given when indicated.

Circulating Anticoagulants and Inhibitors

Acquired circulating anticoagulants or coagulation inhibitors can be divided into two separate classes based on how they affect the coagulation process: (1) those which act immediately to inactivate an activated coagulation factor or block the interaction between coagulation factors and platelets, and (2) a class of inhibitors that progressively inactivates individual coagulation factors. Most circulating anticoagulants are IgG type immunoglobulins. They usually develop in response to replacement therapy in patients with a specific factor deficiency or they may arise spontaneously in the presence or absence of disease.

Inhibitors of most of the coagulation factors have been reported. With the exception of factor VIII and IX inhibitors, these occur rarely. In some patients, inhibitors are associated with the administration of certain drugs. Factor V inhibitors have been found following streptomycin therapy and Factor XIII inhibitors have been found following treatment with isoniazid, an antituberculosis drug.

Inhibitors of factor VIII occur in about 10% of patients with severe hemophilia A. They will also occur in patients with autoimmune disorders such as systemic lupus erythematosus, in rheumatoid arthritis, in pregnancy, in some women within a few weeks or months of giving birth, in association with drugs such as penicillin, and in normal individuals. Bleeding may range from mild to severe. Immunosuppressive therapy may be effective and spontaneous remissions may occur in some patients. Treatment of these patients is difficult because replacement therapy with factor VIII may produce an increased titer of the inhibitor. Some patients with low titers of inhibitor respond well to transfusion of fresh frozen plasma.

Factor IX inhibitors occur in about 2% of the patients with hemophilia B and are rarely seen in non-hemophiliacs.

Inhibitors of coagulation have also been found in patients with multiple myeloma, Waldenström's macroglobulinemia, and autoimmune disorders. The abnormal proteins present may be absorbed by fibrinogen or fibrin, and they will act as inhibitors of fibrin polymerization, causing structurally abnormal clots.

Lupus Inhibitor

About 10% of the patients with systemic lupus erythematosus (SLE) have been found to have a nonspecific anticoagulant that is termed the lupus inhibitor. This inhibitor is an IgG or IgM type immunoglobulin which is thought to interfere with the phospholipid portion of the complex (Factor Xa-V-Ca^{++}- platelet phospholipid) which converts prothrombin to thrombin. In addition to patients with SLE, the lupus inhibitor has been found in patients with other autoimmune disorders, after the administration of certain drugs, following viral infections and in some normal, healthy individuals.

Bleeding is uncommon. It may occur, however, if there is an associated thrombocytopenia, platelet function abnormality, or prothrombin deficiency. Thrombosis occurs in about 30% of the patients. Pregnant women with the lupus inhibitor are at high risk for recurrent intrauterine deaths or spontaneous abortion. The exact nature of the association between the lupus inhibitor and the thrombotic tendency and obstetric complications seen in some patients is not understood.

The lupus inhibitor is the most common of the acquired inhibitors encountered in the laboratory. In the presence of the lupus inhibitor, phospholipid dependent coagulation tests will be abnormal. The PT may be normal or slightly prolonged, the APTT will be prolonged and factor assays based on the APTT (Factors VIII, IX, XI, and XII) will show decreased levels. The test for a circulating anticoagulant (inhibitor) will not show correction when patient plasma is incubated with normal control plasma. The platelet neutralization procedure (PNP) is positive in the presence of the lupus inhibitor.

Treatment for the lupus inhibitor is usually not indicated. It is important, however, that an awareness be maintained that these patients are at high risk for thrombotic and obstetric complications.

Hypercoagulable States

Several conditions are associated with an increased tendency to develop thrombosis (formation of intravascular clots). Collectively, they are referred to as hypercoagulable or prethrombotic states and represent changes in the regulatory mechanisms of the coagulation and fibrinolytic systems. This condition may be divided into two categories: (1) primary disorders, in which there is a qualitative or quantitative abnormality of a specific component of the hemostatic system; (2) secondary disorders, in which the mechanism of the clot formation is not completely known.

Primary disorders are relatively uncommon and include hereditary deficiencies of antithrombin III and protein C, as well as abnormalities of plasminogen, plasminogen activators and fibrinogen. The most common of the secondary disorders are stasis (inhibition) of blood flow, malignancy, the postoperative state, pregnancy, and the use of oral contraceptives.

Laboratory evaluation of these patients often shows non-specific elevations of factors V, VII, VIII, and fibrinogen. Elevated levels of fibrin split products and platelet products (beta thromboglobulin, thromboxane B$_2$ and platelet factor 4) may also be found. In addition, there are increased levels of: (1) prothrombin fragments 1 and 2, and (2) fibrinopeptides A and B. Assays for antithrombin III, protein C, and certain components of the fibrinolytic system may reveal abnormalities which indicate a specific primary disorder.

Patients with primary hypercoagulable disorders usually display early onset of thrombotic episodes, have a positive family history of thromboembolism, and do not have any underlying disease. Treatment of these patients is difficult and some may require life long oral anticoagulant therapy. Recurrent deep venous thrombosis in the lower extremities and pulmonary emboli are common.

Fibrinolysis

Fibrinolysis, without intravascular coagulation, is found as a complication of severe liver disease, as a complication following thoracic surgery, in some malignancies and leukemias, and as a complication of thrombolytic therapy. Generally, bleeding is rare in these patients. However, when it does occur it can be severe and may be fatal.

Fibrinolysis results when excess amounts of plasminogen activators convert plasminogen to plasmin within the circulation. Plasminogen activators may be derived from various tissues, secretions, or the vascular endothelium. The contact factors, XII, Fletcher, and Fitzgerald, are also capable of activating plasminogen. Plasmin digests factors V and VIII and, in addition, breaks down fibrin and fibrinogen to fibrinogen degradation products.

The PT, APTT, and thrombin time are generally prolonged due to the anticoagulant effect of the fibrinogen degradation products. The euglobulin clot lysis time is abnormally short, unless there is depletion of plasminogen. Factors V and VIII are generally decreased. Factor XIII may also be decreased in some patients.

Treatment for fibrinolysis usually involves administration of an agent, such as EACA (epsilon aminocaproic acid), which will inhibit the activation of plasminogen.

7

Automation

SYSMEX™ E-5000

The Sysmex™ E-5000 series instrument is an 18 parameter hematology analyzer developed and manufactured by TOA Medical Electronics Co., Ltd. This instrument performs a complete blood count, calculates the red cell indices and RDW, performs a platelet count, calculates an MPV (mean platelet volume) and PDW (a measure of platelet size variation), calculates a PLCR (platelet large cell ratio, an indicator of platelet size above 12 microns), and classifies and enumerates the nucleated cells according to size as: (1) white small cell ratio (WSCR) and small cell count (WSCC) (normally, the percent and number of lymphocytes), (2) white mixed cell ratio (WMCR) and mixed cell count (WMCC) (normally, the percent and number of monocytes, basophils, and eosinophils), and (3) white large cell ratio (WLCR) and large cell count (WSCC) (normally, the percent and number of neutrophils and bands).

The E-5000 is composed of five separate units. (The E-2500 is composed of four separate units.) The blood sample is identified, aspirated, diluted, and analyzed by the *main unit.* The *sampler unit* attaches to the front of the main unit (E-5000 only) and is used to hold and feed samples to the instrument when in the automatic mode. The *data processing unit* (DPU) receives data from the main unit, performs calculations, develops histograms, and displays sample results and error and status messages via the video display. It contains a bubble memory and special functions through which the operator may view, manipulate discriminators and data, and transmit data. The *pneumatic unit* supplies the vacuum and pressures to the main unit for operating the valves and pistons, which moves the air and fluids through the various chambers and tubing. The *data printer* receives information from the data processing unit and prints this data on manually inserted cards. The *serial matrix printer* will automatically (if desired) print the sample number, date, error codes, flags, histograms, and numerical results on continuous fold printing paper. It may also be used as a line printer.

COMPONENTS, OPERATION, AND PRINCIPLES OF THE MAIN UNIT AND SAMPLER UNIT (FIGS. 158, 159)

1. Press the *power switch* (1) to turn the unit on (and off).

2. The unit will enter an auto rinse mode in which the instrument is rinsed, waste is drained, and the background counts are automatically checked. A rinse cycle and background check is available to the operator during daily use by pressing the *auto rinse switch* (2).

3. Aspiration of sample in the manual mode:

   a. Place the well-mixed sample of blood under the *whole blood as-*

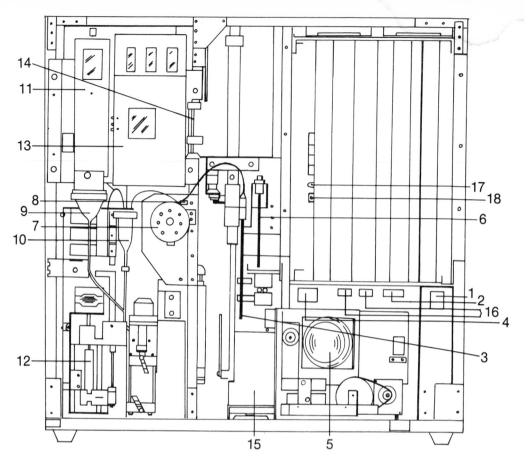

Fig. 158. Main unit, front, (cover panels removed), Sysmex™ E-5000.

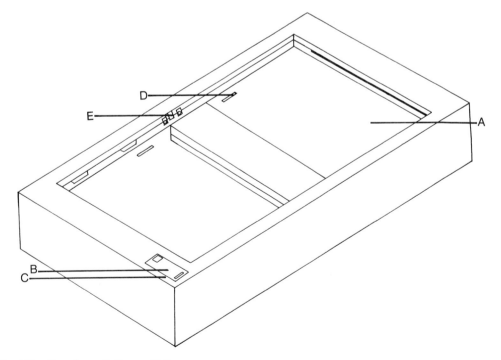

Fig. 159. Sampler unit, Sysmex™ E-5000.

piration tube (3) and press the *start switch* (4) to aspirate the sample and begin testing. The blood is aspirated and checked as described in steps 4d, and e, below.

4. Aspiration of sample in the automatic mode (E-5000 only):

   a. Place the appropriate bar code labels on each tube to be tested, place tubes in the tube rack, and put rack in the *right rack pool* (A) of the sampler unit.

   b. Press the *sampler switch* (B) to start the unit. (This switch is also used to interrupt testing.) The *sampler operation panel* (C) on the unit will indicate its status (ready, running, or interrupt). The rack is automatically forwarded to the *measurement line* (D) where it will be moved to the left, one sample tube distance at a time.

   c. The *ID read mechanism* (5) reads the bar code on the first tube and then shifts the rack one space to the left. The bar code is read on the next tube while the sample volume is checked on the first tube. If the volume is adequate, the *mixer* (6) is lowered into the first tube, where it rotates to mix the sample. The *blood volume sensor* (E) on the sampler unit checks for an adequate level of blood in the tube being mixed (0.5 to 3.0 mL in a 12-mm test tube, or 0.7 to 5.0 mL in a 16-mm test tube). If the sample volume is insufficient, the bar code number will not be used and the sample will not be mixed nor aspirated. After mixing of the first sample has been completed, the rack moves one position to the left. The sample processing continues and the bar code is read on the next sample (#3), the mixer and

aspirator are lowered into tubes #2 and #1 where they are mixed and aspirated respectively at a rate of one sample aspiration every 30 seconds.

   d. The specimen (0.2 mL) is pulled through the *sample rotor valve* (SRV) (7) by the *whole blood injector piston.* There are two *sensors* (8) located along the aspiration tubing (one in front of, and one behind the rotor valve) which monitor the presence of the sample as it enters and leaves the SRV, for the detection of a problem (short sample, air bubbles, clots, etc.). In case of a problem, an error code is displayed on the DPU. The unit may or may not stop testing (dependent on how the instrument is programmed by the operator).

   e. The SRV is composed of three sections (Fig. 160): front, back, and center (rotating) pieces. Each of the sections have six connecting holes through them. As blood is drawn up through the aspiration line it passes through the first detector, travels through the SRV, out the back, in again through a second port (hole), out the front, and back into the valve through a third port in the front, out again at the back of the valve and through the second sensor. The center section of the SRV then ro-

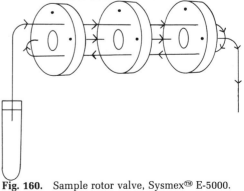

Fig. 160. Sample rotor valve, Sysmex™ E-5000.

tates in such a manner that the three ports in the valve which contain sample (in amounts of 2.67 μL, 6 μL, and 12 μL) are lined up with the three empty ports on the outer sections of the SRV.

5. Dilution of sample:
   a. At this time, the *WBC injector piston* dispenses 1.988 mL of Cell-pak® diluent through the port in the SRV where it picks up the 12 μL sample and carries it through the tubing to the *WBC transducer chamber* (9). The *WBC lyse injector piston* dispenses 1 mL of lysing reagent into the WBC chamber, giving a final dilution of 1:250. The WBC lyse reagent lyses the red cells, shrinks the platelets, pierces the white cell cytoplasmic membrane, leaving only cell nuclei to be counted and sized.
   b. While the blood is diluted for the WBC, 2.0 mL of diluent is dispensed by the *RBC injector piston* through the SRV where it picks up the 2.67 μL aliquot of sample. The diluted sample then travels to the *RBC sample chamber* (10) for mixing (1:750 dilution). A segment of the 1:750 dilution is later injected into the sheath detector for sample analysis.
   c. Concurrently, the hemoglobin is diluted: the *hgb injector piston* dispenses 1.994 mL of diluent through the SRV where it picks up 6 μL of blood sample on its way to the *hgb flow cell.* At the same time, the *hgb lyse injector piston* adds 1 mL of hgb lyse (cyanmethemoglobin) reagent to the diluted sample in the flow cell for a final dilution of 1:500.

6. Sample testing: WBC and three part differential.
   a. The *WBC detector unit* (11) contains a non-mercury manometer and is responsible for starting and stopping the WBC count cycle. The top portion of the manometer is connected to the *transducer,* contained in the WBC transducer chamber (containing the diluted WBC sample). The manometer is filled with Cellpak diluent and contains a ball float. On either side of, and near the top of the manometer, the start detector is located. There is a similar detector located near the bottom of the manometer.
   b. During the count, a vacuum is applied to the bottom end of the manometer. The diluted sample is drawn through the aperture (diameter of 100 μ) in the transducer. At the same time, the ball float falls downward in the manometer. As the ball passes between the top detector the count cycle begins. Counting continues until the ball passes the bottom detector which stops the counting cycle.
   c. During the count cycle of 5 to 6 seconds, 0.25 mL of diluted sample is drawn into the transducer through the aperture. There is an electric current passing between the internal electrode in the transducer and the external electrode in the transducer chamber. As each nucleus travels through the aperture, it causes a change in voltage. The size of the voltage change is directly proportional to the volume of the nucleus.
   d. During the counting cycle, the count time is monitored. The count is checked and recorded every ½ second during the count cycle for consistent results. These ½ second counts may be displayed on the video screen. If the counts do not agree with each other within pre-set limits an error code will be given.

e. As the white cell nuclei are counted, they are sorted by size in the main unit and a distribution curve (histogram) is displayed along with results produced by the DPU. This instrument utilizes floating thresholds rather than fixed thresholds. For the white count the lower threshold will be set between 30 and 60 fL dependent on the cell size range.

f. At the completion of the count cycle, the white count is corrected for dilution, volume, and coincidence. The histogram is derived, thresholds set, and the number and percent of each size of white cell is determined.

7. Sample testing: RBC, hematocrit, and platelet count.

a. A *diaphragm pump* draws 11.7 μL of the 1:750 red cell dilution from the RBC sample chamber into what is termed a *hydraulic line*. A *sheath flow injector piston* (12) then forces the sample up into and through the *sample tube* (Fig. 161) in the *RBC detector unit* (13).

b. As the sample is forced through

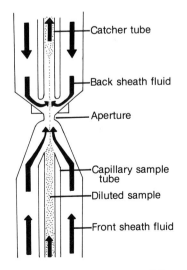

Fig. 161. RBC sample flow, Sysmex™ E-5000.

Labels in figure:
- Catcher tube
- Back sheath fluid
- Aperture
- Capillary sample tube
- Diluted sample
- Front sheath fluid

the sample tube, it is directed at the orifice, which has a diameter of 76 μ. Front sheath fluid (Cellsheath) flows (under pressure) toward, and through, the orifice, surrounding the diluted sample, and restricting the sample flow diameter to 10 μL as it passes through the detecting aperture. This causes the particles in the sample to flow in single file through the center of the aperture. As the sample passes through the aperture, it is met by the back sheath fluid which quickly carries the sample away from the back of the aperture to waste, via the *catcher tube.*

c. Because the particles pass through the center of the orifice there should be no distortion of particle size. There is virtually no coincidence error since the cells pass through the aperture and are counted one at a time unless the count is too high (above the upper linearity) at which occasion an alarm will alert the operator. The back sheath flow forces particles away from the aperture as soon as they flow through, thus virtually preventing platelet count errors associated with recirculation.

d. As the particles pass through the orifice they are counted in the same manner as the white cells (by electrical resistance) and their size, or volume, is also measured. The red cell count is monitored and checked about one time per second. Each of these 1-second counts must agree within preset limits for the final count to be considered valid by the computer.

e. During the count cycle a red ball in the *sheath fluid flow meter* (14) will descend to monitor the sheath flow. If this ball falls too quickly, it may indicate a clog in the orifice and an error message will be given.

f. A histogram (distribution curve) is obtained for both the red cells and platelets. Again, floating thresholds are used and are determined for each individual sample based on the individual histogram. The thresholds for the red cells are between 25 and 75 fL at the lower level and between 200 and 250 at the upper level. The platelet threshold is between 2 and 6 fL at the lower end and between 12 and 30 fL at the upper end.

g. Hematocrit measurement. As the red cells are being counted their size is also determined. This information is digitized. When the red cell histogram is obtained, the upper and lower thresholds are determined and all of the digitized data between these two points are added up and multiplied by a constant factor (accounting for dilution, volume, and calibration factors) to produce the red blood cell mass in 1 µL of whole blood. This number is then converted to percent for the final hematocrit reading.

8. Sample testing: hemoglobin.

a. Immediately prior to the preparation of the hemoglobin dilution, rinse diluent from the previous cycle is drained from the hgb flow cell and 2 mL of fresh diluent is dispensed into the flow cell by the *hgb injector piston*. A reading of the absorbance is taken (represents the hemoglobin blank reading).

b. The diluent is drained and a reading is then taken of the empty cuvet, to monitor the mechanical performance of the flow through the cuvet.

c. The hemoglobin dilution is then

delivered to the hgb flow cell (which also serves as the cuvet), as described previously. STRO-MATOLYSER-C℠ (1.0 mL), the cyanmethemoglobin reagent, is added to the cuvet. A total of five different absorbance readings are taken of this final dilution. The unit will utilize the reading which is lowest (the one most likely to be clear and free of bubbles). The blank reading is subtracted from the sample reading for the final hemoglobin result.

9. During the count and testing cycle, if the instrument monitoring system detects an error, the operator will be notified by way of an audible beep and message on the VDU. (Please refer to the Operator's Manual for a listing of over 100 messages the unit can send.)

10. Calculated parameters.

a. The *red blood cell indices* (MCV, MCH, and MCHC) are calculated by the DPU, from the RBC, hemoglobin, and hematocrit, using the standard formulas.

b. The *RDW-SD,* a measure of anisocytosis, is the width, in femtoliters (fL), of the red cell distribution curve at a point 20% above the baseline. If an abnormal histogram is obtained, an error message is given. The *RDW-CV* (optional RDW) is determined by dividing the RDW-SD by the red cell MCV and multiplying the result by a constant factor.

c. For the *WBC size distribution,* the lower floating threshold (or discriminator) is set in the range between 30 and 60 fL, while the upper threshold is set at 300 fL. When the white cell histogram is constructed, two low points (valleys or troughs) within the WBC curve, are normally present. The *WBC small cell population* consists of those white cells which fall between the lower threshold and the first trough, and are normally the lymphocytes. Nucleated red blood cells in low numbers will generally fall below the area of the lower threshold but, if present in large numbers, will fall into the WBC population and cause an abnormal curve. The *WBC mixed cell population* are those cells which fall between the two troughs within the WBC curve. These cells are considered to be the monocytes, basophils, and eosinophils. The *WBC large cell population* falls between the second (higher) trough and the upper threshold, and are normally the neutrophils. Any time one of the thresholds, or troughs, are not discernible, the instrument will recognize the problem and inform the operator via an error message. In this instance, the operator may manually set the discriminators (troughs) in order to obtain the WBC results from the stored data program capabilities. (Caution: This setting should not be made without valid reason.)

d. The *mean platelet volume* (MPV) is calculated for each sample (plt hct/plt count). The *platelet distribution width* (PDW) is calculated in a manner similar to the RDW-SD. The *platelet large cell ratio* (PLCR) is an indicator of the percent of platelets larger than 12 fL and is calculated by dividing the number of platelets between the fixed threshold (12 fL) and the upper threshold, by the number of platelets which fall between the lower and upper threshold. (The PDW and PLCR are not currently approved by the FDA but can be used to monitor sample suitability.)

11. The various chambers and flow lines are rinsed during each sample cycle.

   a. Two injector pistons dispense diluent to rinse the inside and outside of the whole blood aspirating pipet, the SRV, and both sides of the rinse chamber for cleaning the mixer, pipet, and moving the remaining sample to waste.

   b. The *WBC injector piston* delivers diluent to the WBC transducer chamber for rinsing purposes prior to the sample being added.

   c. The *RBC injector piston* delivers diluent to the RBC chamber for rinsing, and the *sheath rinse injector piston* pushes diluent into the red cell sample flow line in order to rinse it.

   d. The hemoglobin cuvet is rinsed by diluent dispensed by the *hemoglobin injector piston.*

   e. The *detergent switch* (15) is used for adding Manoresh cleaning solution to the WBC manometer for the daily cleaning purposes. (This does not take place during the sample cycle.)

12. The *WBC* and *RBC clog removal switches* (16) may be used for removing a clog from the red or white cell apertures. When pressed, a back pressure is forced through the respective aperture, to remove the debris. Hidden recount switches are located next to the clog removal switches and are used for troubleshooting problem samples. The *service program switch* (17) and *sequence stop switch* (18) are used for troubleshooting, to temporarily stop the analysis cycle at specific sequence points.

13. Additional components not illustrated.

   a. Left side of unit.

      1) The *hydraulic/pneumatic*

control section controls the flow of air, sample, and diluent through the unit.

2) There are three *pressure gauges* which indicate the amount of pressure supplied to the pneumatic system, the sheath reagent chamber, and to drain the waste chamber, remove clogs, etc. Each of these are adjustable by a *regulator*.

3) A *vacuum gauge* indicates the amount of vacuum supplied to the unit by way of an *air tank unit.* This gauge is adjusted by a *bellows unit.*

4) *Fuse.*

5) A *fan heater* warms air in the unit to a preset temperature.

b. Top and interior of unit.

1) The *reagent heater* warms the diluent and sheath reagent to preset temperatures prior to use.

2) The *WBC and hgb lysing reagent chambers* maintain an internal supply of WBC and hgb lysing reagent, respectively. The *sheath reagent chamber* contains a supply of sheath reagent, while the *diluent chamber* maintains an internal supply of diluent.

3) There are three *waste chambers* which function to: (a) aspirate waste from the sheath fluid hydraulic system, (b) aspirate waste from the hydraulic lines (vacuum applied to this chamber is stabilized by the *vacuum air tank*), and (c) aspirate manometer waste and supply the proper vacuum to the WBC detector unit.

4) A *trap chamber* provides a safety vacuum trap which prevents waste from entering the vacuum air tanks.

5) The *operation cycle counter* indicates the total number of instrument cycles and cannot be reset.

c. The back portion of the unit contains *inlet ports* for the diluent, sheath reagent, WBC reagent, hgb reagent, detergent, pressure, vacuum, and one outlet port for the waste. There is a *ground* terminal, *power inlet receptacle,* and four *fuses.* The *power control connectors* (2) are connected to the pneumatic unit and the data processing unit. A *communications connector* must also be connected to the data processing unit. An *exhaust fan* removes excess heat generated by the unit. A *trap chamber* provides a safety vacuum trap to prevent fluid from entering the compressor.

DATA PROCESSING UNIT (DPU) (FIG. 162)

1. The *video display unit* (1) displays information to the operator.

2. The *power switch* (2) turns the unit on and off.

3. The *numerical entry keys* (3) (0 to 9) are used for entering information into the unit.

4. The *decimal point key* (4) is used to enter decimal points, hyphens, and certain program routines.

5. The *clear key* (C) (5) may be used to correct a numerical value, to cancel the program selection, or to back into previous menus.

6. There are four directional arrow keys, the *cursor keys* (6), which move the cursor on the video display.

7. The *enter key* (7) allows operator to enter information from the numerical keys.

8. The *select key* (8) displays alternate video display unit selections.

9. The *alarm reset key* allows the operator to shut off the audible alarm.

10. The *intensity adjustment knob* ad-

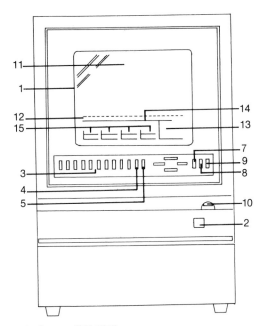

Fig. 162. Data processing unit, Sysmex™ E-5000.

justs the intensity of the video display.

11. The rear of the unit contains *connectors* to the graphic printer, the data printer, an external (host) computer, the main unit, and a line printer. There is a *ground terminal,* a *power inlet receptacle, power outlet receptacles* for the data and graphic printers, and a *power control connector* to the main unit. *Fuses* (6) are also present.

DPU-SOFTWARE PROGRAM

The video display screen is divided into five areas that are separated by lines.

1. *Area 1* (11) or the upper screen, displays the 18 parameter data and histograms from the last sample analyzed. This area also displays information related to other programs, such as Q.C., stored data, and calibration data.

2. *Area 2* (12) is the system area, located at the bottom line of area 1. All numerical entries are displayed in here, as well as messages to assist or direct the operator.

3. *Area 3* (13) is the system status area that displays the current date and time, sample identification number for both manual and auto mode, sample number to be transmitted to the data printer, main unit status, bubble memory (including the number of samples in stored data) activity, auto erase selection, $\overline{X}M$ quality control selection, host computer activity, and printer selection.

4. *Area 4* (14) is a system message line providing priority messages relating to the main unit.

5. *Area 5* (15) displays the eight program Select Menus and their subprograms. The eight programs in the Select Menu allow the operator increased flexibility in operation, data review, data output, quality control assessment, and instrument function. A program and its subprograms are selected by pressing the corresponding numeric key. Programs that contain important data or system settings may require a password for entry. Below is a brief description of the Select Menu programs.

a. *Auto Out* allows the operator to control the automatic output of data to the printers and host computer.

b. From the *Command* program, the operator can review data from the twenty cycles, print STATS, start and stop the $\overline{X}$M Q.C. program, access service data, and set ID numbers.

c. The instrument holds all results and histograms for up to 300 samples. The *Stored Data* program allows the operator to display, sort, erase, manually discriminate histograms, correct ID numbers, and output data. Other subprograms located here are Q.C. charts and set number.

d. In the *Quality Control* program there are 10 Q.C. files including the $\overline{X}$M program available for storing up to 60 data points for up to 12 user defined parameters. Some of the features of this program are: Levy Jennings graphs, modified Bull's moving average, statistical analysis, calibration history, output of control data and graphs to host computer and printers, and a choice for assaying single or duplicate commercial control analysis.

e. The *Set Number* program is the primary program used for setting the sample ID number and tube position.

f. The *Settings* program allows the operator to enter all user defined information into the unit including: patient limits, date/time, test units, hardware configurations for the printer, and interface information for host computer and peripheral printers.

g. The *Calibration of Hgb/Hct* program allows the operator two methods of calibration for the hemoglobin and hematocrit: au-

tocalibration or manual calibration.

h. The *Service* program contains various tests that allow the operator to check the proper operation of the unit for troubleshooting and maintenance checks.

PNEUMATIC UNIT (NOT SHOWN)

1. The *power switch* turns the unit off and on.

2. The *pressure gauge* and *vacuum gauge* indicates the amount of pressure and vacuum, respectively, supplied to the main unit.

3. *Air intake vents.*

4. The back of the pneumatic unit contains the *power inlet receptacle,* the *power control connector* to the main unit, a *pressure* and a *vacuum outlet* which is also connected to the main unit, a *fuse,* the *serial number,* an *air intake vent,* and an *exhaust vent.*

5. This unit contains a *compressor* to generate the pressures and vacuum, an *air tank* where pressure is accumulated, an *air filter,* a *relief valve* for regulating the pressure supplied to the main unit, a *check valve* which maintains air flowing in one direction, a fan to exhaust the heat generated, and a *thermostat* which will automatically turn off the compressor if too much heat is generated.

DATA PRINTER (FIG. 163)

1. The report form is placed in the card *entry slot* (1) for printing.

2. The *card guides* (2) are adjustable to the width of the card being used.

3. The *feed switch* (3) is used to release a card before printing has occurred.

4. The *lid* (4) covers the *reset switch, card size guides,* and the *ribbon assembly.*

5. The rear of the unit contains the *on/ off switch,* the *power inlet receptacle,* two *fuse holders,* a *connector to the DPU,* and the *serial number.*

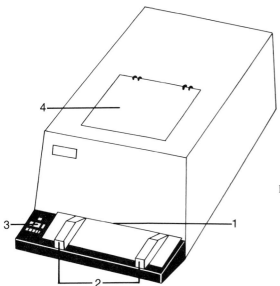

Fig. 163. Data printer, Sysmex™ E-5000.

SERIAL MATRIX PRINTER (NOT SHOWN)

1. The *operator control panel* contains switches for the various functions of the unit.
2. The *power switch* turns the printer on and off.
3. *Power cord connection.*
4. The *paper guide bar* holds the paper down.
5. The *print head* performs the print function.
6. *Print ribbon.*

MAINTENANCE

Following is a brief outline of the maintenance suggested by the manufacturer.

1. *Daily.* Check all pressure and vacuum gauges. Check the alignment of the pipettor and mixer. Run 5 cycles of a 1:5 dilution (20% v/v) of Clorox™ reagent through the instrument, followed by an auto rinse cycle. Clean the manometer with auto-MANO-RESH cycle.
2. *Weekly.* Clean sample rotor valve on an as needed basis (at least once per week), one waste chamber, and one overflow trap.
3. *Monthly.* Clean the rinsing cup assembly.
4. *Quarterly.* Clean two orifices (one in tank unit, one of waste chamber), lubricate nine injector pistons and two injector piston mechanisms, and lubricate the whole blood pipet assembly.
5. *Yearly.* Replace the waste drain tubing.

DISCUSSION

1. *Hydrodynamic focusing* is used in the Sysmex E-series for analysis of the red blood cells and platelets. In this method, the blood is diluted 1:750 with diluent. A measured volume of the diluted sample passes through a capillary sample tube which restricts the width of the sample dilution column and directs the flow through the aperture. (See Fig. 161.) When the diluted sample leaves the capillary sample tube, it is surrounded by the front sheath fluid (which is under pressure). This further restricts the diluted sample column to a width of approximately 10 μ and aligns the particles so that they travel in single file through the center of the aperture for analysis. As the particles pass through the aperture they are surrounded by the back sheath fluid which then carries the particles away from the aperture and into the catcher tube for waste disposal, thus preventing recirculation of the particles through the aperture.
2. The instrument's reagent system is comprised of five reagents for testing and cleaning. During each sample cycle 24 mL of *Cellpack* is used for diluting the sample, 10 mL of *Cellsheath* forms a sheath around the RBC dilution (during count phase), 1 mL of *STROMATOLYZER-3WP*™ (lyse reagent) is added to the WBC dilution, and 1 mL *STROMATOLYZER-C*™ (cyanmethemoglobin lyse

reagent) is added to the hemoglobin dilution. Weekly, 10 mL of *Manoresh* is used to clean the WBC manometer, and daily 1 mL of 20% Clorox is aspirated through the unit for cleaning.

3. The format for printing numerical results on the report forms is programmable by the operator, within certain limitations.

4. Due to the dilution and characteristics of the Stromatolyzer-C, white counts up to 100,000/μL do not interfere with the hemoglobin reading.

5. Each sample cycle takes approximately 53 seconds. However, samples may be introduced into the instrument at 30-second intervals. Thus, in the automatic mode, the instrument can analyze 119 samples per hour.

6. Studies by the manufacturer show linearity to be acceptable within the following ranges:

   WBC 1.0 to 99.9 × 10^3/μL
   RBC 0.30 to 99.0 × 10^6/μL
   Hgb 0.1 to 25.0 g/dL
   Hct 10.0 to 60.0%
   Plt 10 to 999 × 10^3/μL (if RBC is less than 7.00 × 10^6/μL)

7. Due to the sample dilutions and testing procedures, the particle counts are almost coincidence free.

8. There is a period of 3 minutes from instrument turn on until it is ready for the first sample. During this time, there are three to five auto rinse cycles and the electronics, injector piston motors, ROM, RAM, bubble memory, and instrument status are automatically checked.

9. During sample processing, the operator may review stored data, correct erroneous data, rearrange data in the unit, check the 10 Q.C. files, and output previously run data to a host computer.

10. The instrument is programmed to display over 100 error (82) and status (21) messages.

11. The ability of the instrument to utilize a floating lower threshold (discriminator) for each patient sample is thought to improve its counting accuracy.

ORTHO* ELT-1500 HEMATOLOGY ANALYZER

The ORTHO ELT-1500 Hematology Analyzer (Fig. 164) is an automated 15-parameter cell counter which determines WBC, RBC, hemoglobin, hematocrit, MCV, MCH, MCHC, platelet count, red cell morphology index (RCMI), and the percent and absolute numbers of granulocytes, lymphocytes, and monocytes.

This instrument utilizes a laser light source for counting and sizing the red cells, white cells, and platelets. The hemoglobin is measured using a modified cyanmethemoglobin method. Light scatter techniques, measuring the light scatter at forward and right angles, are used for the counting and differentiation of the three white cell classes (granulocytes, lymphocytes, and monocytes). The red blood cell indices (MCV, MCH, and MCHC) are calculated from the determined red cell parameters (RBC, hemoglobin, and hematocrit). In addition, the ELT-1500 has a built-in quality control program and during testing, displays histograms of the red cells, white cells, and platelets. More than 100 samples/hour may be tested with this instrument (one sample every 30 seconds), using 120 μL of whole blood per sample.

The ELT-1500 is made up of two major units: the *sample handler* which processes and tests the sample, and the *data handler* which analyzes, stores, and displays the data (via a CRT screen). A third module, the *CRT page printer,* is optional and may be attached to the data handler in order to obtain a printed copy of the information displayed on the data handler.

---

*ORTHO, ISOLAC, CYANAC, and LYSRIGHT are trademarks of Ortho Diagnostic Systems, Inc.

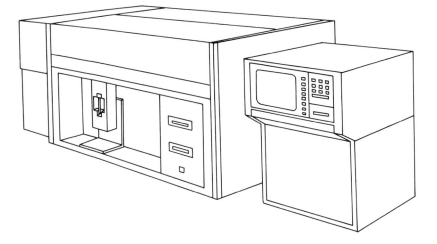

Fig. 164. ORTHO ELT-1500 Hematology Analyzer.

Components of the Sample Handler

The blood sample (or control) is aspirated, diluted, mixed, and analyzed by the sample handler.

1. The *power button* turns the instrument on and off.

2. The *printer assembly* provides printed results of the fifteen parameters, test number, and date.

3. The *sampler* has three components: a *sip tube,* through which the sample is aspirated, a retractable *waste bucket* to collect the reagent during the wash period, and a *wash block,* which provides an external wash of the sip tube.

4. The *back plate switch,* when pressed, activates the testing cycle.

5. The *laser optics assembly* where the actual counting, sizing, and light scatter measurements occur, consists of the helium-neon gas laser, focusing lens, forward and right angle lenses, a quartz flow channel, blocker bar, apertures, and two photodetectors.

6. The hemoglobin is read at a wavelength near 540 nm, while the diluted sample is in the *colorimeter cuvet.*

7. The *air compressor* supplies 22 to 30 psi of air pressure to move the waste bucket in and out, and to the *accumulator* (which maintains ISOLAC-D saline diluent at the proper pressure for refilling the pumps on the 3-RPM cam assembly). It also supplies air pressure to the *air reservoir* which is responsible for supplying pressure to the reagent containers. The air pressure first travels through the *regulator* to reduce the pressure to 9 psi.

8. The *WBC reagent cooler* maintains the temperature of the dilution for the WBC count and differentiation at 9°C (± 1°C) prior to testing.

9. Three reagents are used for testing: *ISOLAC-D* (two containers) is a saline diluent, *CYANAC* is the cyanmethemoglobin reagent, and *LYS-RIGHT* reagent is used for lysing the red blood cells.

10. The *sample handler status panel* displays the messages, READY, PRINTER, and REAGENT LOW when applicable.

11. The *air dump system* reduces the air

pressure in the reagent bottles when the instrument is in standby.

12. The *timing switch assembly* regulates the timing of the instrument during sample testing.

13. The *cam assemblies* consists of 2 RPM and 3 RPM motor driven cams which activate the pumps and valves in a specific sequence during instrument operation.

14. The *drive motor* provides all of the mechanical drive functions (except for the air compressor) for the sample handler.

15. The fourteen *pumps* move the reagents and blood through the sample handler. All of the pumps except one, have two ports (one input and one ouput). Pump P6 has three ports (two input ports and one output), while pump P1 uses one port (side) for input and output.

16. The eight *slide valves* direct the flow of reagents and sample. These valves are made up of three sections. The two outside sections remain stationary, whereas the middle section will move up and down during the cycle to open or close fluid pathways.

17. There are four *manifolds* which function as a meeting, mixing, and distribution center for the sample and reagents. The *reagent manifold* supplies 9 psi air pressure to the four reagent bottles and supplies reagents to the pumps and valves. The *mixer manifold* houses and mixes the RBC dilutions (from valve eleven), the second red cell dilution, and the hemoglobin dilution. The *hemoglobin manifold* delivers the hemoglobin dilution to the colorimeter cuvet. The *waste manifold* is the centralized area where all diluted samples are collected after testing. They are then expelled from the sample handler via a single waste line.

18. The *power supply* regulates and sup-

plies the necessary electrical power to the instrument components.

19. The *fuses* prevent electrical overload.

Operation of the Sample Handler

1. Prior to use, the end of the sip tube contains a small amount of air to separate the blood sample from the diluent already in the lines. When the back plate switch is pressed, pumps P10 and P11 draw back, causing approximately 120 μL of the sample to be aspirated. The blood travels into valve V11 where it is split into two segments, one for the RBC, hemoglobin, hematocrit, RCMI, and platelet count, and the other for the WBC count and white cell differentiation. (The air bubble preceding the sample is also split. The leading air bubble and a small segment of the initial portion of whole blood are discarded. Two precisely measured air bubbles are then inserted at the forward portion of the blood sample.) This step takes approximately 4 seconds.

2. From approximately 4.5 seconds until 10 seconds into the cycle, the following mechanisms take place. Pumps P9 and P12 are activated and dilute the RBC portion of the sample forming a 1:63 dilution with ISO-LAC-D, driving the diluted sample to the mixer manifold. As the sample enters the manifold, the leading segment is moved to a separate channel (F) (within the mixer manifold) where it is mixed with an equal volume of CYANAC (pumped into the manifold by P6) for the hemoglobin dilution (1:126). The remaining red cell dilution is sent to channel G in the mixer manifold.

3. Ten seconds into the cycle, pumps P6, P9, and P12 stop. At approximately 13 seconds, pumps P9 and P13 activate and together they bring about a further dilution (1:440) of the

second RBC segment and move the dilution through another channel (W5-W1) in the mixer manifold and onto the sample storage area.

4. Processing of the sample stops for a period of 10 seconds (when the sample is 20 seconds into the cycle). At this point, a second blood sample may be introduced into the sample handler where it will repeat the above described procedure.

5. At 30 seconds, P2 is activated for about 1 second in order to push the 1:440 RBC dilution through the flow channel. Pumps P1 and P3 are then simultaneously activated and work together forcing both the diluted sample and sheath flow through the flow channel for the determination of the RBC, hematocrit, platelet count, and data for the RCMI.

6. During steps 2 through 4 above, and approximately 5 seconds into the cycle, pumps P7 and P8 are activated. P8 forces the WBC segment in V11 into the mixing channel of V11. At the same time, P7 forces LYS-RIGHT into the sample, forming a 1:19 dilution of the blood. The diluted sample is then forced out of V11, through V9, and into the WBC Storage Channel B to allow for complete lysis of the red blood cells. At about 35 seconds into the cycle, the second sample aspirated is pushed into WBC storage channel B (preceded by an air bubble), pushing the first sample out of WBC storage channel B, through V9, and into WBC storage channel A. The air bubble preceding the first dilution is sent to waste.

7. Approximately 41 seconds into the first cycle, the second sample is trapped in storage channel B. Storage channel A then opens to allow the first sample dilution to proceed to the flow channel. (Both WBC storage

channels [A and B] pass through the WBC reagent cooler.)

8. At approximately 42 seconds into the cycle pumps P4, P5, and P5a are activated. Using Isolac-D, P4 pushes the first WBC sample dilution to the flow channel, while P5 and P5a provide the sample flow through the flow channel for the WBC count. The WBC count and differentiation will be complete at approximately 55 seconds into the first cycle.

9. *Mechanics of the flow cell.* The flow cell contains a narrow fluid channel. Prior to, and during sample entry into the flow cell, two streams of IS-OLAC-D are forced through the channel, creating a laminar flow. When empty, the opening through the flow channel has a diameter of about 250 μm. When the ISOLAC-D is flowing through the channel, it completely covers all inner surfaces of the channel. The stream of Isolac-D flowing adjacent to the sides of the channel travels at the slowest rate of speed, whereas the stream of ISOLAC-D near the center of the chamber flows at the fastest rate of speed. The diluted blood sample is forced through the center of this flow and is carried along with the fastest moving ISO-LAC-D. The diameter of the sample stream is 20 μm and it travels at a speed of about 55 mph. The cells or particles move through the flow channel in single file and are counted and sized using the laser beam (Fig. 165). The laser is situated on one side of the flow cell and directs an elliptical-shaped beam through the flow cell onto a sensor. When there are no cells passing through the flow cell, the laser beam is completely focused onto a blocker bar (on the collecting lens), which blocks the laser beam from hitting the sensors or photodetectors. When cells or platelets pass through the flow chamber, each indi-

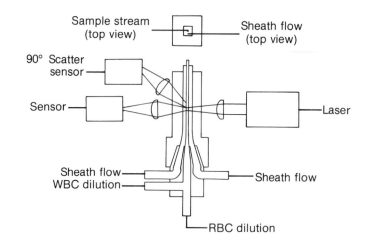

Fig. 165. Flow channel, ORTHO ELT-1500 Hematology Analyzer.

vidual particle passing through the laser beam will cause a scattering of this beam. This scattered light then falls on the collecting lenses and passes through to the photodetectors, where it is changed to a voltage pulse whose area corresponds to the size of the particle.

10. *Counting of red blood cells and platelets.* As the red cells and platelets pass through the laser beam, part of this light is scattered at forward and at right angles as it passes through the cells. (However, only forward angle light scatter information is used for these determinations.) The red cells are differentiated from the platelets by a preset voltage threshold in the instrument. When counting the 1:440 dilution, all voltage pulses lower than the threshold are considered to be platelets and all voltage values higher than the threshold are classified as red blood cells.

11. *Determination of the hematocrit.* The time of flight (also termed "dead time") for a cell to pass through the

laser beam in the flow channel is defined as the amount of time which begins when the impulse from the cell is first noted (rises above the noise threshold), and continues until the pulse stops (recrosses the noise threshold). As the red cells pass through the flow cell, the pulses generated are combined to determine the area under the signal. The sum of these areas is directly proportional to the percent hematocrit.

12. *Determination of the RCMI.* As the red blood cells pass through the laser beam they are counted and sized using the measurements of forward light scatter. An RBC histogram is then simultaneously derived. By analyzing the variation within the red cell distribution and comparing it to normal red cell distribution, an index is derived indicating normal or abnormal red blood cell morphology. The normal value for this parameter is ±2.0.

13. *Determination of the WBC count and WBC differentiation.* As the white blood cells pass through the laser

beam they are counted and analyzed using both forward and right angle light scatter. The amount of light scattered and the amount of light which reaches the photodetectors depend upon both the volume and the refractive index of the cell. In addition, the amount of light scattered at right angles is dependent upon the internal structure (primarily the nucleus and cytoplasmic granules) of the cell. A scatter histogram is derived which shows, from left to right: debris, lymphocytes, monocytes, and granulocytes. The total number of lymphocytes, monocytes, and granulocytes is then added up for the white blood cell count and the percent of the three cell types is calculated.

14. The hemoglobin blank is read after the sample during the count phase of the cycle (between 30 and 60 seconds).

15. The output signals from the photodetectors are sent to the data handler where they are processed and analyzed. This information is then forwarded to the printer in the sample handler and displayed on the data handler CRT (the red cell, white cell, and platelet histograms may also be displayed on the CRT).

16. *Instrument wash.*
   a. At a point 13 seconds into the testing cycle ISOLAC-D flows from V1 through the first RBC mixing channel in V11 and goes to waste via V9 and V10. At the same time, LYSRIGHT travels through the WBC mixing channel in V11 for cleaning purposes and exits to waste through V9 and V10.
   b. At 17 seconds, and for approximately 3 seconds, ISOLAC-D travels from V5 through P10 and P11 to wash the sip tube and whole blood storage tubing through V11.
   c. For 3 seconds, at 25 seconds into

the cycle, ISOLAC-D is pushed from the reagent manifold to wash the sample line of the flow channel and exits to waste.

Data Handler

The data handler contains a *CRT screen* which serves as a means of communication between the operator and the instrument, and between the sample handler and the data handler. Associated with the CRT, along the right front side of the data handler, are a series of keypad *selection switches* that are used to select various functions of the instrument. The selection switches each have a LED (light emitting diode), that indicates the functions available. Further to the right is the keyboard *(0 to 9, . , CE* [clear entry], *enter, and return),* which is utilized by the operator to enter numeric information.

The data handler has two primary functions: (1) It accepts information from the operator concerning numeric identification and operating instructions, and (2) it processes information from the sample handler, calculates red blood cell indices, the RCMI, the percent of the three classes of white blood cells, and transmits this information to the printer in the sample handler, the CRT page printer unit, and the CRT screen.

Through the software program in the data handler, the operator gains access to the operational functions. The table of contents of the software is termed the *base page,* and when displayed, it lists the seven operational modes *(main pages)* available to the operator. The keypad selection switches are used to select the specific operational modes desired. The CRT will then display this mode (the main page), listing all possible options available (the options are termed *subpage functions).*

Following is an outline of the seven main pages and their subpage functions.

   1. *Date* is the operational mode in which the operator may enter the

date in any one of four different ways, using a / or a . between numbers: month, day, year; day, month, year; year, month, day; or Julian (last digit of year followed by the numerical day of the year).

2. The *calibration* mode is used to verify the calibration and is also used in recalibrating the instrument.

3. The *control runs* mode is primarily used for processing quality control samples. There are eight quality control *libraries* in this function, each one capable of storing a different control level, which is determined by the operator. In this mode, the operator selects the control library into which a control sample is to be entered; the assay value for the control may be entered, or the mean assay value for all of the runs stored in that library may be used. In addition, the *QC library* subpage mode allows the operator to view the control data in all libraries, to remove or restore numeric data from the statistics, print out the results from any library, view and print out Levy-Jenning charts of the control data, and enter or erase all quality control information.

4. The *run sequence* mode is used for the processing of patient samples. In this mode, the operator may enter up to 60 patient I.D. numbers in the order in which the patient samples will be run, or, an accession number may be used, where the number will be automatically increased by one digit each time a sample is run through this mode. All samples processed in this mode that are within the operating range of the instrument will enter the moving average program. The numeric data from the last twenty samples processed will be stored, and a printout may be obtained on any one of these samples. During sample processing, the results and histograms may be displayed on the

CRT if desired. There is a moving average library in which numerical results of Levy-Jenning information may be viewed, deleted, edited, entered, or printed out.

5. The *patient storage* function allows for the storage of up to 3700 sets of patient and control results. These results may be reviewed at any time and may be transferred to a host computer or data terminal.

6. The *test-options* mode enables the user to perform electronic checks of the data handler or to activate various options in the system. This function is also used by field service.

7. The *standby* mode is utilized to maintain the instrument in a hold position where the electronics remain on but the pressures in the sample handler are turned off.

Operation of the ELT-1500

1. *Start-up.*
   a. Perform a visual inspection of the instrument: empty the waste container, check the reagent levels (filling if necessary), clean the sample station, and check the cooler temperature.
   b. Press return on the data handler to access the base page. Enter the date.
   c. Access the calibration mode and perform a fluid subsystem wash.
      1) Aspirate an air sample 2 times. Gently tap pumps P10 and P11 to remove any bubbles that may be present.
      2) Run five samples of ORTHO Flushing Solution.
      3) Aspirate an air sample 3 times.
   d. Access start cal background (calibration mode) and determine that duplicate background counts check within ±100 of the previous background counts and are below 500.

e. Prime the instrument by running two samples of whole blood.

f. Perform quality control procedures. Access the control runs page and select the appropriate quality control library. (A 24-hour patient whole blood, a laboratory working control, and three levels of commercially assayed controls are recommended.) If any of the quality control parameters are not within acceptable range, the system verification procedure (as outlined in the operator's manual) should be performed.

2. *Processing of patient samples.*

a. Access the run sequence mode. Follow your laboratory's procedure for the identification of the patient sample.

b. Place a report form in the printer, located in the right side of the sample handler.

c. Place the tube of blood under the sip tube and insert the sip tube at least ½ inch into the blood. Press the back plate switch. After the system beep sounds, remove the tube of blood.

d. Between 20 and 30 seconds after the first sample is introduced into the instrument, a second patient sample may be aspirated by repeating steps b and c above. (Wipe the outside of the sip tube with a piece of clean gauze prior to aspirating each sample.)

e. Review the results on the CRT when they appear. Remove the ticket from the printer when printing is complete.

f. At the completion of the sample run, place the instrument in standby accessing the standby mode on the data handler.

3. *Weekly maintenance.*

a. Remove all of the covering panels from the instrument and check the valves, pumps, connectors, and tubing for crystalline deposits. Wipe away any deposits with a damp cloth. Ensure that the valves move freely and are aligned. The pumps, connectors, and tubing should be checked for leaks and replaced as needed. Clean the area around the cams and the cam shafts.

b. Perform the sip tube back and forward flushes, RBC and WBC feed nozzle, and the flow channel flushes as outlined in the operator's manual.

c. Clean the sip tube wash station funnel with warm water.

d. Replace the covers and clean the exterior of the instrument.

4. *Monthly maintenance.*

a. Remove the instrument covers as necessary.

b. Rinse all reagent containers at least 2 times with fresh reagent and replenish with reagents.

c. Clean the cams as outlined in the operator's manual.

d. Remove the filter in the Data Handler and the fan filter in the Sample Handler, clean in warm water and detergent, dry, and replace. (See operator's manual for the procedure.)

e. Check the cooler liquid level and add coolant as necessary.

5. *Yearly maintenance.*

a. Replace the CYANAC reagent container with a new one.

DISCUSSION

1. During normal sample analysis an average of 200,000 red blood cells, 14,000 white blood cells, and 10,000 platelets are counted. All counting cycles are 10 seconds in duration.

2. There are two type of ranges which are recognized in the ELT-1500 for measured parameters. (1) The *instrument operating limits* determine the acceptable range of testing for the in-

strument. If a value falls outside of these limits an audible alarm will sound and a dash (—) will be reported adjacent to the numerical results. If the patient values are above the acceptable limits, the specimen may be diluted and then run through the instrument. If the values fall below the limits, the test must be repeated using an alternate procedure. (2) *Operator alert ranges* for all parameters may be set by the laboratory for the instrument. These limits generally represent the normal ranges (and must be within the operating limits of the instrument). Values which fall outside of these ranges are reported with an asterisk (*). If a result cannot be calculated, a plus symbol (+) will be printed next to the parameter. A dash (—) will be printed to the right of the RCMI result when that test value falls outside the range of −9.9 to 9.9.

3. In the classification of white blood cells, the following categories will most likely contain the indicated cell types:
   a. Lymphocytes—atypical lymphocytes, normoblasts, other mononuclear cells.
   b. Monocytes—large mononuclear cells (blasts), promyelocytes, myelocytes, basophils.
   c. Granulocytes—eosinophils, neutrophils, bands, metamyelocytes, Pelger-Huet granulocytes, vacuolated neutrophils.

4. Heparin should not be used to anticoagulate blood to be tested in the ELT-1500 since it interferes with the white cell and platelet parameters.

5. *Red blood cell histograms.* The red blood cell histogram is a real-time graphic illustration of the number and relative size of the cells. The number of cells is plotted on the vertical axis of the graph, and the size of the cell is plotted on the horizontal axis. The right side of the histogram shows a second, smaller, distribution. This represents doublets (two cells) which pass through the beam at the same time. These coincident cells are automatically corrected for in the red blood cell count.

6. *White blood cell histogram.* The white blood cell histogram is displayed in real time during the counting phase of the ELT-1500 cycle. The Y-axis represents the number of cells. The X-axis represents the forward and right angle light scatter, and also the cell granularity and size (which increases from left to right on the histogram). The major portion of forward light scatter falls on the left part of the X-axis, while the extreme right side of the X-axis represents primarily the right angle portion of light scatter.

7. *Platelet histograms.* The platelet histogram is a graphic illustration of the number and relative size of the platelets counted by the instrument. As described for the red blood cell histograms, the Y, or vertical, axis represents the number of platelets, and the X, or horizontal, axis represents the magnitude of the pulses (size). In the ELT-1500, the X axis is divided into 80 channels, which are numbered 1 through 80. The majority of platelets fall into channels 7 through 10 on the histogram.

8. *Moving averages.* The moving average is essentially a weighted moving average of a group (batch) of patients' red blood cell indices (MCV, MCH, and MCHC). This mathematical formula was published in 1974 by Brian Bull. It is based on the fact that groups of patients will show relatively stable values for the red blood cell indices. In the ELT-1500, the operator may choose the batch size from 1 to 99. The recommended number of patients in a batch, however, is 20.

The batch average for each red blood cell index is then compared to a previously set target value and, under normal circumstances, should not vary from this target value by more than 3%. A larger variation is generally due to an instrument malfunction, but may also be seen if the group of patients in the batch are abnormal to like degrees (e.g., many microcytic patients). In cases where there is instrument malfunction, it should be noted which red blood cell indices fall out of the range, as an aid in troubleshooting the problem.

COULTER COUNTER MODEL S

The Coulter Counter Model S performs a WBC, RBC, hemoglobin, and MCV, and calculates the hematocrit, MCH, and MCHC on every blood sample tested. Results are reported on a printed card, and the analysis is completed within 40 seconds after the sample has been aspirated into the instrument. Blood samples may be introduced into the instrument at a rate of 1 every 20 seconds.

UNITS (5) OF THE COULTER COUNTER MODEL S

1. The *diluter unit* (Fig. 166) aspirates, pipets, dilutes, mixes the diluted sample, lyses the red blood cells, and "senses" (i.e., senses the current changes between electrodes and senses the hemoglobin at the photodevice). The rear portion of the unit contains a connection to the analyzer unit, a tank panel which receives vacuum and pressure from the pneumatic supply unit, a diluent and waste connection, the switch panel (mechanical timer), and a cam assembly (timing mechanism). In addition, pneumatic cards (6) are located on the inside right and left sides of the unit. These cards are responsible for the filling and emptying of the various chambers in the

unit by means of pumps, valves, and cylinders located in these cards.
2. In the *analyzer* (Fig. 167), the counting, measuring, and computing of results take place. Cables in the rear of the unit connect the analyzer to the diluter and the power supply.
3. The *power supply* (Fig. 168) is the source of voltages necessary to run the electronic system and is connected to the printer and the analyzer.
4. The *printer* (Fig. 169) receives the digital information from the power supply and prints these results on report cards. This unit is connected to the power supply.
5. The *pneumatic power supply* (Fig. 170) is connected to, and furnishes the diluter with the necessary vacuum and pressure.

PROCEDURE AND OPERATION OF THE COULTER COUNTER MODEL S

1. Place the reporting card in one side of the printer and label with the name and laboratory accession number.
2. Mix the blood sample well and check for clots, using two applicator sticks.
3. Place the sample tube under the aspirator, inserting the aspirator at least 1 inch into the blood specimen.
4. Press the touch control bar, and allow the aspirator to remain in the specimen until the red light behind the bar comes on. Remove the tube of blood, and when the light turns green, wipe the outside of the aspirator with a dampened gauze.
5. The aspirator will draw up approximately 1 mL of whole blood (0.9 to 1.1 mL) and carries it through the blood sampling valve, where the sample is diluted (as described below).
   a. The blood sampling valve consists of three parts, held together by a long center pin. The front section has four fluid pathways,

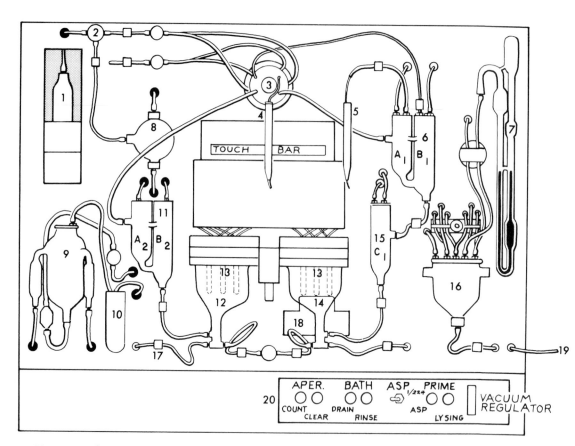

Fig. 166. Diluter unit. Model S Coulter Counter. 1, Diluent dispenser assembly. 2, 'T'. 3, Blood-sampling valve. 4, Aspirator (whole blood). 5, Aspirator (1:224 dilution). 6, WBC mixing chambers. 7, Manometer. 8, Bubble trap. 9, Waste chamber. 10, Foam trap. 11, RBC mixing chambers. 12, RBC aperture counting bath. 13, Apertures. 14, WBC aperture counting bath. 15, Lysing chamber. 16, Vacuum/isolator chamber. 17, Pinch valve. 18, Hgb. device. 19, Lyse supply. 20, Control panel.

each of which has respective tubing fitted into it. The middle section has two fluid pathways or holes. There are four holes in the rear section connected to respective tubing. The center section is movable and rotates between two positions.

b. In position 1 (Fig. 171, black line), the middle section links up the top hole on the right side of the rear section with the top hole on the corresponding side of the front section. The whole blood is aspirated through the passageway.

c. The center section then rotates to

position 2 (Fig. 172, black line), where it links together the bottom right hole on the rear section with the bottom right hole on the front section. At this time, the center section still contains a measured segment of blood (44.7 μL). While the center section is in position 2, 10 mL of Isoton is forced through this passageway, mixing with the blood in the center section, and emptying into the white blood cell mixing chambers (1:224 dilution).

d. The center section remains in position 2 while approximately 1 mL of the first dilution is removed

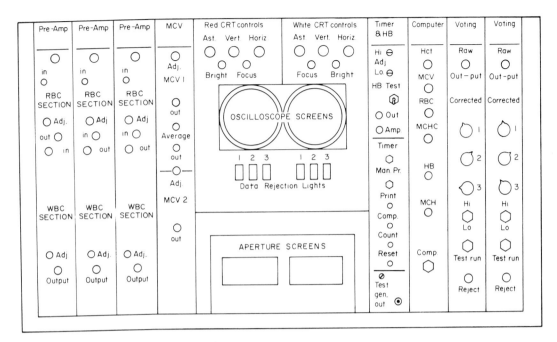

Fig. 167. Analyzer unit, Model S Coulter Counter.

from the white blood cell mixing chamber and aspirated through the tubing, through the top left passageway of the blood sampling valve (Fig. 172, white line).

e. The center section rotates to position 1, where 10 mL of Isoton is forced through the lower left passageway (Fig. 171, white line), picking up the measured segment (44.7 µL) of diluted blood from the center section. This rediluted sample (1:50,000 dilution) then empties into the red blood cell mixing chamber.

6. While the blood is being rediluted and mixed in the red blood cell mixing chambers, the 9 mL of the WBC dilution is forced from the WBC mixing chamber into the lysing chamber below it. Lysing reagent (1 mL) is forced into this chamber and mixes with the diluted blood to give a final dilution of 1:250.

7. The dilution remains in the lysing chamber long enough to cause complete lysis of the red blood cells. During this short period, the previous blood sample is drained from the baths into the waste chamber. Isoton then enters the baths, and a hemoglobin reference reading is made (prior to the hemoglobin reading of the diluted blood sample).

8. From the lysing chamber the dilution is then forced down into the white blood cell aperture bath (contains three apertures). There is one external electrode in the bath and each aperture contains its own internal electrode.

9. A specific amount of diluted blood is drawn through each orifice of the aperture tubes for a period of 6 seconds. (Each time a cell passes through the orifice of the aperture, this causes a change in the current flowing between the external and internal apertures. This produces a voltage pulse, the magnitude of which is proportional to the size of the cell causing the voltage change.)

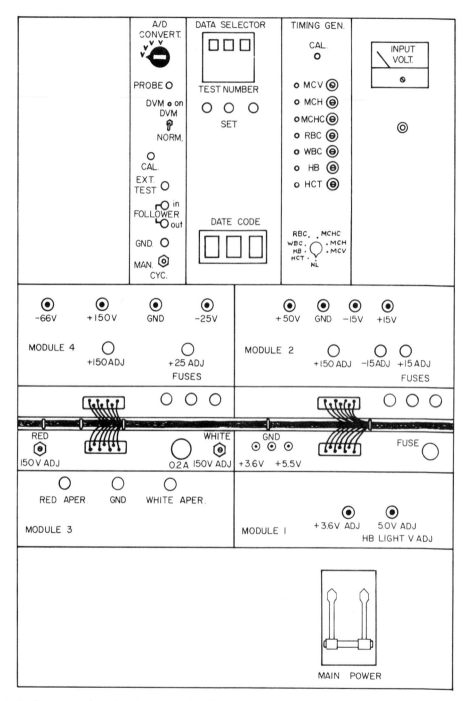

Fig. 168. Power supply unit, Model S Coulter Counter.

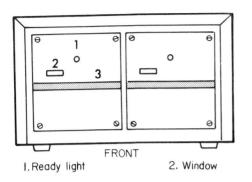

FRONT

1. Ready light   2. Window

3. Card insert (sled)

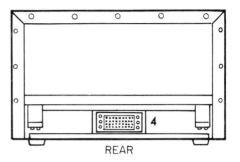

REAR

4. Printer to power

Fig. 169. Printer unit, Model S Coulter Counter.

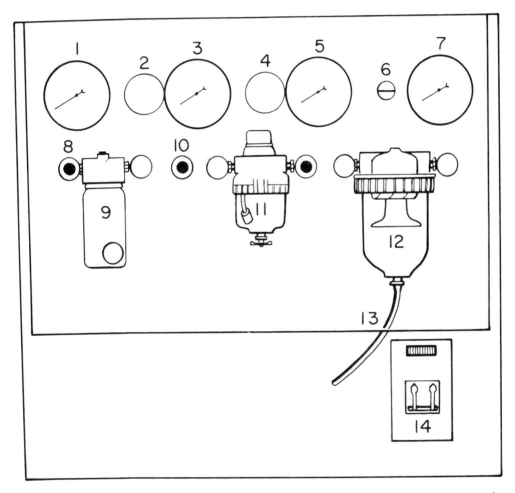

Fig. 170. Pneumatic power supply unit, Model S Coulter Counter. 1, High-vacuum gauge. 2, 5-psi regulator. 3, 5-psi gauge. 4, 25-psi regulator. 5, 25-psi gauge. 6, Preset regulator. 7, High-pressure gauge. 8, High-vacuum outlet. 9, Vacuum trap bottle. 10, 5-psi outlet. 11, Lubricator (oil) container. 12, Air filter. 13, Waste line. 14, Power switch.

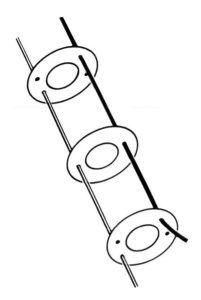

Fig. 171. Blood-sampling valve, position 1.

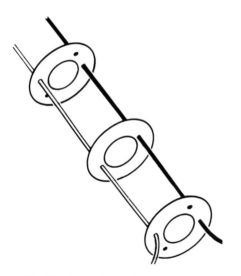

Fig. 172. Blood-sampling valve, position 2.

In the analyzer unit, the voltage pulses are counted for 4 seconds, amplified, and shown on the oscilloscope screen. Three white blood cell counts are being performed at the same time. An average of the three counts is made and recorded. If debris, dirt, or other malfunction is present in one of the apertures, the corresponding red data rejection light comes on, and that red or white blood cell count will not be used. The two remaining counts are averaged. If two of the counts are rejected, the three data rejection lights come on, and a 0.0 count is recorded. The sample must then be run through the instrument again.

10. While the WBC is being performed in the unit, a beam of light from the movable bar in front of the aperture bath passes through the diluted blood sample in the white blood cell count aperture bath onto a photosensitive device. This component measures the amount of light which passes through the solution and converts this into a hemoglobin reading that is recorded.

11. When the WBC and hemoglobin dilution is forced into the aperture bath on the right, the red blood cell dilution is forced into the aperture bath on the left. The red blood cells are counted at the same time and in the same manner as described for the white blood cells. In addition, the red blood cell MCV is electronically derived and recorded.

12. The hematocrit is calculated from the values received from the red blood cell count and MCV. The MCH and MCHC are also calculated.

13. The final results for all seven tests are printed out on the special card placed in the printer. It is possible to place two reporting cards in the printer at the same time, one in each sled. The side of the printer which prints the first report is indicated by a red light coming on as soon as the card is placed in the printer unit.

14. Whenever the unit has been flushed completely with Isoton (or if the baths have been manually drained and rinsed), the instrument should be primed by cycling two samples of normal whole blood before testing patient samples.

15. If 1 mL of whole blood is not available, or if fingertip blood is used, add 44.7 µL of whole blood to 10.0 mL of Isoton (1:224 dilution). Before the count is performed, change the aspirator switch to the 1:224 dilution. Mix the diluted sample well, and place it under the capillary blood aspirator. Press the touch control bar, and allow the instrument to aspirate the entire diluted sample. (It is desirable to make up all micro dilutions in duplicate or triplicate and average the results. If, however, there is a large discrepancy between results, new dilutions should be made.) The diltued sample, when it is aspirated by the instrument, flows directly into the white count mixing chambers, omitting the first blood dilution. The procedure then continues as for the undiluted blood sample described above beginning with step 5d.

MAINTENANCE

Keeping the instrument clean is most important for obtaining accurate results with a minimun number of test rejections. It should also be remembered that when control results are only slightly out of range, there is generally a small malfunction somewhere. Continuing to use the instrument under these circumstances results in increasing the error rate and sending out invalid reports. When control values do not check, no matter how small the error, time should be taken to ascertain the problem.

1. At the beginning of each day turn on the power supply unit and allow to warm up for approximately 30 seconds. Turn on the pneumatic power supply and wait 30 seconds for warm up. Check the instrument for proper functioning while aspirating four or five samples of Isoton through the whole blood aspirator.

   a. The following switches should be in the normal or operating position: A/D converter card toggle switch, card R-1 toggle switch, voting card, computer card, timer/hemoglobin card, MCV card, and aspiration switch on the control panel.

   b. The orifices of the apertures should be visible on the aperture screen and free of blockage or debris.

   c. Make certain 1 mL of Isoton is being aspirated, there are no air bubbles in the lines from the blood sampling valve, and the blood sampling valve changes position correctly.

   d. Check all bubble rates in the chambers (mixing, lyse, and aperture baths) and make certain the transfer rates are correct so that all chambers are draining completely.

   e. The outside of the white cell aperture bath must be clean.

   f. Check all gauges on the pump to make certain they are correct.

   g. The setting on the mercury manometer must be correct.

   h. The diluent dispenser piston must make a full stroke with no hesitation.

   i. Check the background counts.

   j. Employ the 6-way attenuator for a routine voltage check, as described in the operations manual.

   k. Run the appropriate control blood specimens through the instrument. These results should check within the two S.D. limits of the laboratory.

2. The apertures should be cleaned with a Clorox solution after every 400 to 500 blood samples, as described in the operations manual.

3. The blood sampling valve should be removed and cleaned after every 500 samples, as described in the operations manual.

4. Whole blood should never be left in

the aspirator for more than 1 or 2 minutes after the results have been obtained. If the instrument is not to be used for a while, drain or rinse the baths with Isoton. Aspirate approximately 10 mL of Isoton or Isoterge (cleaning solution) using the aspirate button on the control panel.

5. After every 1,000 counts the mixing chambers, lysing chamber, and aperture baths should be removed from the instrument and cleaned well in Isoterge and rinsed in tap water and then distilled water. Remove and wash the filter on the pneumatic unit in warm water and replace.

6. If the instrument is to be shut down for any period of time (e.g., overnight), 50 to 60 mL of Isoterge should be aspirated through the whole blood aspirator, using the aspirator button on the control panel, until the top left cylinder in pneumatic card L-1A is free of blood. Isoterge should be left in the aperture baths after drawing enough Isoterge through the apertures until the liquid entering the vacuum isolator chamber is green. Shut off the power supply and pump units.

DISCUSSION

1. In cases where the WBC is above 30,000/μL, it is advisable to perform the count by another method. (Due to possible clouding of the dilution by the increased WBC, the hemoglobin result should not be considered valid. In addition, when the WBC is above 50,000/μL, the MCV and RBC may be erroneously high and a spun hematocrit should be performed and reported.) If the WBC is not too high, the blood may be diluted 1:1 with Isoton, run through the instrument, and all results, except the red blood cell indices, multiplied by 2. With the diluted blood, however, the white blood cell count should still not exceed 30,000/μL.

2. In cases where the WBC is below 1,500/μL, a manual WBC should be performed. In this case, the results reported by the instrument, except for the WBC, are acceptable and may be reported.

3. If the WBC or the RBC and hematocrit continuously give results of 0.0, double check to make certain the external electrodes are immersed in the solution in the aperture baths.

4. If one or more of the data rejection lamps continuously light up, check the aperture orifices for dirt or debris.

COULTER COUNTER MODEL S PLUS

The Model S Plus Coulter Counter is similar to the Model S Coulter Counter. This new model, however, has a more compact and less complicated pneumatic system and is more computerized than the Model S Coulter Counter. In addition, this instrument performs whole blood platelet counts and tests the degree of anisocytosis (RDW) on patient samples, in addition to the seven parameters tested by the Model S Coulter Counter.

The Model S Plus Coulter Counter consists of five connected units: power supply, diluter unit, analyzer unit, printer, and X-Y recorder. These units are described in the following sections.

POWER SUPPLY UNIT (FIG. 173)

The power supply furnishes regulated voltages to run the electronic system and also provides the necessary pressures and vacuum to the diluter unit and reagent system. It is connected to the printer, analyzer, and X-Y recorder. The pneumatic portion of the unit connects into the diluter unit.

1. The *main power switch* turns the electronic system on and off.

2. The *control voltage indicator lamp* should be lit when the main power switch is on.

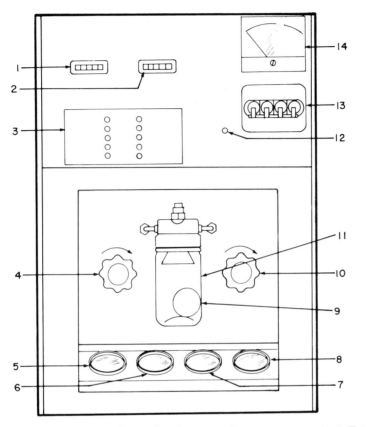

Fig. 173. Power supply unit, Model S Plus Coulter Counter. 1, Compressor run meter. 2, Total hours meter. 3, Monitor. 4, 5-psi pressure regulator. 5, 6, 7, 8, Pneumatic gauges. 9, Ball. 10, 30-psi pressure regulator. 11, Vacuum trap bottle. 12, Control voltage indicator lamp. 13, Main power switch. 14, Line voltage meter.

3. The *line voltage meter* should indicate 105 V to 125 V.

4. The *compressor run meter* indicates the number of hours that the pneumatics have been activated.

5. The *total hours meter* indicates the number of hours the power supply unit has been on.

6. The *monitor* contains indicator lights. Seven of these lamps indicate voltage problems when lit (such as a blown fuse). When the pneumatic system is not activated, this lamp is on. Pneu Temp and Elec Temp are lit if the temperature in the pneumatic or electronic systems becomes too hot.

7. The *vacuum trap bottle* should be empty.

8. The *pneumatic gauges* indicate the amount of pressure and vacuum being introduced into the diluter unit.

9. The *pressure regulators* are used to adjust the 5 psi and 30 psi pressures. The vacuum and 60 psi pressure cannot be adjusted by the operator.

10. The *main power pack,* containing fuses and voltage jacks, is located on the right side of the unit. The *control module,* also containing fuses and voltage jacks, is on the same side of the unit.

11. *Filters* (2).

DILUTER UNIT (FIGS. 174, 175)

The diluter unit aspirates, pipets, dilutes, mixes the blood, physically moves

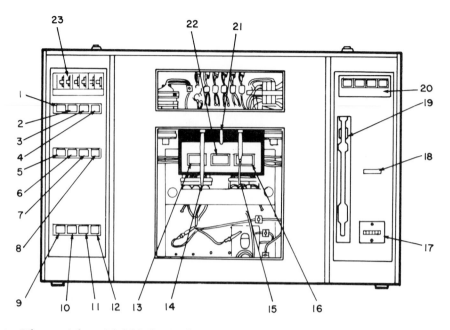

Fig. 174. Diluter unit front, Model S Plus Coulter Counter. 1, Prime button. 2, Drain button. 3, Rinse button. 4, Clear button. 5, Print button. 6, Plot button. 7, Recount button. 8, Continue (cont) button. 9, Power-on button. 10, Power-off button. 11, Start-up button. 12, Shut-down button. 13, Whole blood push button. 14, Whole blood aspirator tip. 15, Microsample aspirator tip. 16, Microsample push button. 17, Test cycle display. 18, Vacuum adjust regulator. 19, Mercury manometer. 20, Liquid level monitors. 21, Diluent dispenser spout. 22, Diluent dispenser button. 23, Month/day/year selector.

the blood sample through the unit for testing, and senses the samples in the baths.

1. The whole blood sample is aspirated through the *whole blood aspirator tip.*
2. The *whole blood push button* initiates the whole blood cycle.
3. The *diluent dispenser button,* when pressed, delivers approximately 10 mL of diluent through the *diluent dispenser spout.*
4. The *1:224 dilution button,* when pressed, draws the *microsample dilution* through the *microsample aspirator.*
5. The following components are on the back of the front door of the unit and cannot be seen in the illustrations.
   a. The *blood sampling valve cylinder* moves the *blood sampling valve* between positions 1 and 2.
   b. During the backwash cycle, 4 mL of diluent is pushed through the

rinse cup by the *rinse cup cylinder* in order to clean the whole blood aspirator between samples.

6. The *RBC* and *WBC diluent dispensers* deliver approximately 10 mL of diluent for the RBC and WBC dilutions, respectively. The WBC diluent dispenser also dispenses approximately 10 mL of diluent when the diluent dispenser button is pushed.
7. *Locking levers* are attached to the *pinch valves,* and when they are in the up position the pressure is released from the tubing to help eliminate pinched tubing.
8. The *backwash pump* delivers 4 mL of diluent through the blood sampling valve and whole blood aspirator into the rinse cup during the backwash cycle.
9. The *hemoglobin blank pump* delivers 5 mL of diluent to the *hemoglobin cuvet* to be read as the hemoglobin blank.

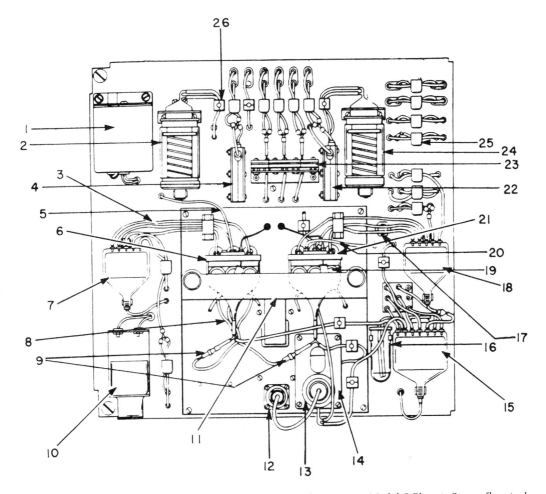

Fig. 175. Diluter unit, center front panel (door open), Coulter Counter Model S Plus. 1, Sweep flow tank. 2, RBC diluent dispenser. 3, Sweep flow lines (3). 4, Backwash pump. 5, Overflow line. 6, RBC aperture bath. 7, RBC vacuum isolator chamber. 8, Sweep flow lines (3). 9, Check valve. 10, Overflow cuvette. 11, Light lamp. 12, Hemoglobin lamp plug. 13, Hemoglobin lamp. 14, Hemoglobin cuvette. 15, Waste chamber. 16, Foam trap. 17, Needle valve (microsample aspiration). 18, WBC vacuum isolator chamber. 19, Aperture. 20, Overflow line. 21, WBC aperture bath. 22, Hemoglobin blank pump. 23, WBC and RBC aspiration pumps and lyse pump. 24, WBC diluent dispenser. 25, Locking lever. 26, Pinch valve.

10. The *WBC* and *RBC sample pumps* (red in color) are each 0.5 mL pumps and act to aspirate the blood through the blood sampling valve.

11. The *lyse pump* moves 0.7734 mL of lyse reagent into the WBC aperture bath.

12. The *RBC* and *WBC vacuum isolator chambers* contain a vacuum during the count cycle which is responsible for drawing the diluted blood samples through the apertures. The RBC

(but not the WBC) chamber is attached to the RBC aperture block through the sweep flow lines.

13. *Aperture housings* (1 RBC and 1 WBC) contain the *aperture blocks* which, in turn, contain the *apertures* (3 RBC and 3 WBC apertures). The RBC apertures are 50 μm in diameter and the WBC apertures are 100 μm in diameter.

14. *Aperture baths* (2) (RBC and WBC) contain the diluted blood samples.

The back of each aperture bath contains three openings tightly fitted around the front of the corresponding aperture block, creating an air tight seal.

15. *Sweep flow lines* (3) are attached to the bottom of the RBC aperture housing. During the count cycle, diluent is pulled up through these lines behind the aperture tube opening (aperture bath is on the other side of the aperture) and out through the top of the aperture housing to the vacuum isolator chamber. This steady stream of diluent moves the red blood cells out of the sensing area as soon as they have been pulled through the aperture.

16. The sweep flow lines pass through the *sweep flow tank* prior to entering the RBC aperture blocks.

17. The overflow lines (2) (one leading from both the WBC and RBC aperture baths) carry any overflow from the baths to the *overflow cuvet.*

18. The *light bar* contains the lamps necessary to see the apertures on the viewing screens in the analyzer unit.

19. The *hemoglobin lamp* is attached to the *hemoglobin lamp plug.*

20. The *check valves* (2) (WBC bath and RBC bath) allow air bubbles to flow in only one direction, into the aperture baths.

21. *Waste chamber.*

22. The *needle valve* is used to adjust the microsample aspiration.

23. *Month/date/year selector.*

24. The *prime button* applies vacuum to the apertures sweep flow lines, turns on the aperture current, and activates the pneumatic system.

25. The *drain button* empties the RBC aperture bath and both vacuum isolator chambers into the waste chamber and empties the WBC aperture bath into the hemoglobin cuvet.

26. The *rinse button* fills both aperture baths with approximately 10 mL of diluent, empties the hemoglobin cuvet into the waste chamber, and empties the waste chamber.

27. The *clear button* applies 5 psi pressure onto the inside of the aperture block to clear any debris that may be blocking the aperture.

28. The *print button,* when pressed, produces a printout of the last sample introduced into the instrument.

29. The *plot button* produces a graph of the platelet data from the X-Y recorder on the blood sample just previously introduced into the instrument.

30. The *recount button* flashes if there is a vote out during the cycle. When activated, it initiates a recount.

31. The *count button,* along with the *recount button,* blinks when there has been a vote out. If a recount is not desired, this button is pushed and the cycle continues.

32. The *power on* and *power off buttons* turn the power on and off, respectively, to the diluter, analyzer and printer units.

33. The *start up button* activates an automatic sequence of five cycles of the diluter unit for cleaning and priming the unit with diluent and lyse reagent.

34. The *shut down button* activates an automatic sequence of five cycles of the diluter unit to introduce cleaning reagent into the unit.

35. There are four *liquid level monitors:* low diluent, low cleaner, low lyse, and full waste. Five psi of pressure is placed on the small line extending into the waste and reagent containers. If a bubble of air escapes from the bottom of this tube in the reagent containers, or conversely, if no bubble of air escapes from the tube in the waste container, the appropriate push button illuminates when the corresponding reagent supply is low or the waste container is full. An au-

dible beep also sounds when the monitor is on. At this point, the instrument may be cycled five more times.

36. The *vacuum regulator* controls the amount of vacuum applied to the apertures (applied directly to the vacuum isolator chambers and through the open lines to the apertures).

37. The *mercury manometer* monitors the aperture vacuum. During the count cycle, the upper level of the blue indicating fluid should be at the point labled AA and should not vary more than $\frac{1}{4}$ of an inch. When the instrument is at rest, the upper level of the blue fluid should be at level BB.

38. The *test cycles display* indicates the number of times the instrument has been cycled, is not adjustable by the operator, and does not advance during the start up and shut down cycles of the instrument.

39. The *diluter control card* (left side of unit) is computer operated and controls the solenoid valves located on the floor of the diluter unit (left side). Each of the solenoids has a color coded pressure or vacuum line attached to it. The function of each solenoid is printed on the side of the diluter control card. The pressures and vacuums in these lines are responsible for the dilution and movement of the sample and reagents through the diluter unit during instrument cycling and diluent dispensing. As each solenoid is activated, the indicator light (located on the front panel of the card) for that particular solenoid is lit. The button next to the indicator light may be used to operate that solenoid manually. The *hemoglobin regulator card* is also located on the left side of the diluter unit.

40. A *vacuum isolator chamber* is located inside the right side of the unit,

receives high vacuum, and is connected to the vacuum regulator and the mercury manometer.

ANALYZER UNIT (FIG. 176)

The analyzer unit contains electronic cards which control the sequence of the various operating cycles of the diluter unit. Messages are received from the diluter unit, and the analyzer counts, sizes, measures, and computes this information, which is then sent to the printer unit in the form of test results. Information is also sent from this unit to the X-Y recorder.

1. The *oscilloscope screen* displays the cells as they pass through the apertures and are counted. Each pulse shown on the screen represents a cell, the size of which is indicated by the height of each pulse (the larger the cell, the higher the pulse).

2. *White and red CRT controls* are utilized to manually adjust the pulses on the oscilloscope screens.

3. The *voting display matrix* corresponds to the different counts performed by the instrument (horizontal axis) and the apertures counting the cells (vertical axis) (the apertures are numbered from left to right). If one of the three parameters being measured (except hemoglobin) does not agree within four S.D. of the other two measurements, the count votes out (values will be rejected), the corresponding lamp lights on the voting matrix, and the other two counts are averaged and reported. If two measurements are rejected by the instrument, all data for this parameter will vote out and all three lamps (for apertures one, two, and three) will be lit.

4. The *DVM/test number indicators* are represented by two lamps. The DVM lamp is lit when the cal/norm switch on the ADC/calibration card is in the cal position, and also at the beginning and end of the cycle when the

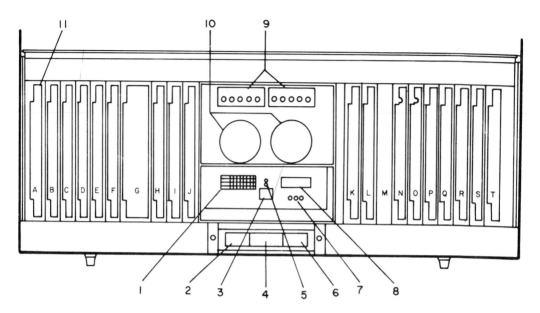

Fig. 176. Analyzer unit, door open, Coulter Counter Model S Plus. 1, Voting display matrix. 2, RBC aperture viewing screen. 3, Error code display. 4, System status indicator. 5, DVM/test number indicators. 6, WBC aperture viewing screens. 7, Set test number buttons. 8, DVM/test number display. 9, CRT controls. 10, Oscilloscope screens. 11, Electronic cards: A, RED PERCentile 2; B, RED PERCentile 1; C, MCV; D, EXTended MEMory; E, MEMory; F, Central processing unit; G, Analog to digital converter/CALibration; H, RED/WHite CounTeR; I, APerture CURrent/SIGnal GENerator; J, Power supply MONitor/BUFFer; K, MEMory; L, PLATelet ADC; M, empty; N, PRE-AMPlifier (red); 0, PRE-AMPlifier (white); P, PULSE EDitor (ap 3); S, Particle VELocity; T, PLATelet PROCessor.

hemoglobin blank and patient sample, respectively, are read. The test number lamp should be lit at all other times during normal operation of the instrument.

5. The *DVM/test number display,* when the instrument is at rest, displays the test number of the next sample to be cycled through the instrument. When a sample is introduced into the instrument, the hemoglobin blank is immediately read. The voltage reading of the blank is displayed on the screen in place of the test number. The counting cycle then begins and the number one is displayed. This indicates that the first platelet count is being performed. If a second, third, fourth, or fifth platelet count is necessary, the corresponding number is displayed while that count is being performed. At the completion of the counting cycle, the hemoglobin is read, and the voltage reading (indicating how much light passed through the sample) appears on the display. The test number for the next sample then replaces the hemoglobin reading and remains displayed until the next sample is introduced into the instrument.

6. The *set test number buttons* (3) are used to manually set the test number as desired.

7. The *error code display* indicates a problem or malfunction of the instrument. During normal operation of the instrument, 00 is displayed on this indicator. When any number or letters are displayed, the operator should refer to the error code display table in the operators reference manual for an explanation of the code and the action to take.

8. The *RBC* and *WBC aperture viewing screens* show the apertures through

which the diluted sample is drawn during the count cycle. These screens should be watched carefully for debris that may block the aperture and cause vote outs on the counts or MCV.

9. The *system status indicator* displays the sequence of events as they are taking place during the test cycle. During a normal, problem free cycle, the following sequence of events appears on the indicator: INTRO SAMPLE, WIPE, COUNT, ANALYZE, DATA ACCEPT, BACKWASH, READ HGB, READY. READY is displayed when the instrument can accept another sample. NOT READY indicates that the instrument cannot accept a sample. SYSTEM FAULT indicates a malfunction in the instrument. DATA REJECT appears when there has been a vote out.

10. The *electronic cards* are responsible for the functions of the analyzer unit. In addition, voltage checks of the electronics are made and the instrument is calibrated by the use of these cards.

PRINTER UNIT (FIG. 177)

The printer unit gives a printed copy of the test results obtained by the instrument

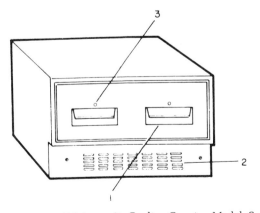

Fig. 177. Printer unit, Coulter Counter Model S Plus. 1, Printer sled (2). 2, Filter. 3, Indicator lights (2).

and is connected to the power supply and analyzer unit.

1. Printout cards are placed into each of the two *printer sleds.*
2. The *indicator lights* indicate which sled will report the next blood sample. When placing a printout in each sled, the sled with the first printout placed in it will cause the lamp to be lit. If the lamp blinks, the slip is not seated correctly and the result will not be printed.
3. The *on/off switch* is located on the back of the unit.
4. *Filters* (2).

X-Y RECORDER (FIG. 178)

The X-Y recorder provides a graph of the platelet size distribution and also simulated platelet distributions based on test pulses as part of the electronic voltage check.

1. The *X-axis controls* (2) (and *Y-axis controls* [2]) consist of the zero knob, which sets the pen on 0 on the horizontal (vertical) axis, and the gain control, which adjusts the sensitivity for the horizontal (vertical) axis.
2. The *on/off button* turns the recorder on and off.
3. The *pen up/down button* is not utilized when the recorder is used with this instrument because the pen is automatically lowered and raised when necessary. Do not touch this button.

PLATELET COUNT (COULTER MODEL S PLUS)

During the count cycle, as the platelets and red blood cells pass through the apertures, those particles which are between 2 and 20 fL in size are counted as platelets. In the analyzer unit, as the platelets are counted, they are divided into groups (channels) according to size. This information is then used for plotting the platelet graph. Normal platelets, when graphed according to size and number are log-normally distributed and yield a log-normal

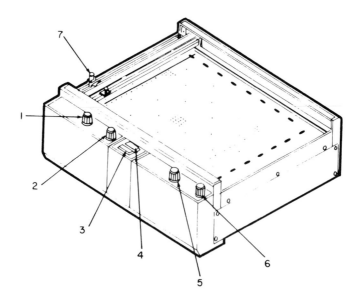

Fig. 178. X-Y recorder, Coulter Counter Model S Plus. 1, Gain control knob (X axis). 2, Zero control knob (X axis). 3, Pen up/down button. 4, Power on/off button. 5, Gain control knob (Y axis). 6, Zero control knob (Y axis). 7, Pen holder.

curve (Fig. 179). There are platelets smaller than 2 fL and larger than 20 fL; however, red blood cells might be included in the platelet count if the range is expanded. Therefore, a graph is made of the size distribution of the platelets. If the analyzer recognizes this platelet count as having a log-normal distribution, it chooses the peak of the curve and the lowest point on either side of the peak. Using the two low points, the platelet data are fitted to a log-normal curve and extrapolated to read from 0 to 70 fL; everything within this curve is counted as platelets. The first graph of the platelet count is a graph of the actual count between 2 and 20 fL. If the platelet count then shows log-normal distribution, a fitted curve is graphed from 0 to 70 fL over the original curve, and all platelets contained within the curve are counted and reported as the platelet count. If the platelets do not show

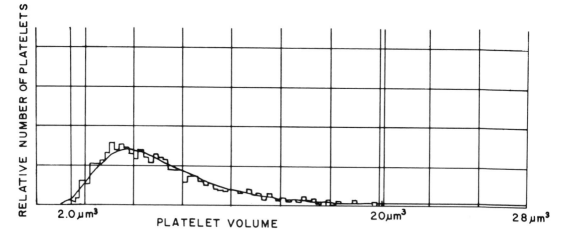

Fig. 179. Graph of normal platelet size distribution, Coulter Counter Model S Plus.

log-normal size distribution, this is recognized in the analyzer, and the curve only extends from 2 to 20 fL (Fig. 180). The symbol $ appears on the printout form, signifying a 'no-fit' platelet count. The platelet count result represents only those platelets contained in the curve between the two valleys (not between 2 and 20 fL). See Figure 180 for a no-fit platelet curve. To have a valid count, a fitted curve must be obtained. The criteria for a fitted curve are a platelet count above 20,000/μL, log-normal distribution (positive curve), and no platelet count vote out.

RED CELL DISTRIBUTION WIDTH (RDW)

The RDW is an indication of the degree of anisocytosis. The size of red blood cells shows a normal distribution curve (Gaussian curve). The RDW is determined and calculated by the analyzer using the MCV and RBC. The point on the curve (the MCV reading) at which 20% of the red blood cells are larger than the rest is recorded as the 20th percentile, and the point at which 80% (the MCV reading) of the red blood cells are larger is noted as the 80th percentile (Fig. 181). The space between these two points represents the RDW. Mathematically, the RDW is determined as follows:

$$RDW = \frac{(20\text{th percentile} - 80\text{th percentile})}{(20\text{th percentile} + 80\text{th percentile})} \times \text{Constant}$$

The constant represents the number that is required to give a normal value of 10 to this test. The normal range for the RDW is 8.5 to 11.5.

PROCEDURE AND OPERATION OF THE MODEL S PLUS COULTER COUNTER

1. Whenever the instrument has not been cycled for approximately 15 minutes, the pneumatic system automatically shuts off. In this case, depress the prime button.
2. As soon as the pressure and vacuum gauges register correctly, check that READY is displayed on the system status indicator.
3. Wipe the aspirator tip in case there is a drop of diluent at the end.
4. Place the tube of blood under the whole blood aspirator tip, inserting the aspirator at least 1 inch into the blood.
5. Press the whole blood button and keep the aspirator in the blood sample until WIPE is displayed. Remove the blood sample and immediately wipe the aspirator tube with a piece of gauze moistened in diluent. Do not put your hands or any object near the

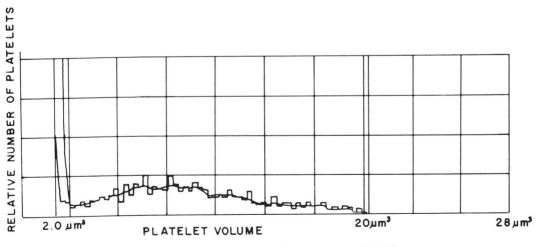

Fig. 180. Graph of no-fit platelet size distribution, Coulter Counter Model S Plus.

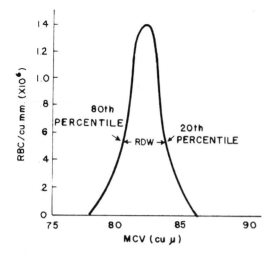

Fig. 181. Normal red blood cell size distribution showing RDW.

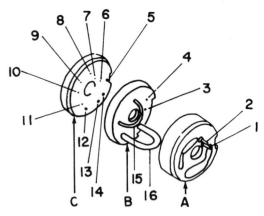

Fig. 182. Blood sampling valve, Coulter Counter Model S Plus. Whole-blood aspiration. RBC and WBC dilutions are performed simultaneously. RBC dilution, position 1 (as shown above): Whole blood enters line 1 (section A), goes through passage 4 (section B), and out of sampling valve through passage 6 (section C). Center section rotates counterclockwise to position 2: Diluent enters line 2 (A), goes through passage 4 (B) picking up the blood sample, and out passage 7 (C) to RBC aperture bath. (Remaining whole blood aspirated travels through passage 3 [B] and out passage 6 [C].) WBC dilution, position 1: Whole blood enters back of section C through passage 10 into loop 15 (B) and out line 8 (C). Position 2: Diluent enters section C through back of passage 11, through loop 15 (B), picking up blood sample, and out passage 9 (C) to aperture bath. Microsample aspirations: Diluted sample enters back of section C through passage 12, into loop 16 (B), and out passage 14 (C) to the WBC aperture bath. Midway during the aspiration, the middle section rotates to position 2. The dilution continues to enter the back of passage 12 (C), into an etched-out passageway in the back of section B, and out passage 14 (C) to the WBC aperture bath. At the same time, diluent enters the back of passage 5 (C), through loop 16 (B), picks up the diluted blood, and carries it out passage 13 (C) to the RBC aperture bath.

whole blood aspirator tip during the remainder of the cycle.

6. Approximately 1 mL of whole blood is drawn up into the instrument through the blood sampling valve.

7. This blood sample is split into two pathways prior to reaching the blood sampling valve. One half of the sample enters the back of the blood sampling valve, where it enters the valve and fills the small metal loop for the WBC dilution. (See Fig. 182 for a diagram of the blood sampling valve.) The remaining portion of the sample enters the front of the blood sampling valve for the red blood count dilution.

a. The blood sampling valve changes to position 2. As soon as this is accomplished, approximately 10 mL of diluent enters the back of the blood sampling valve, picks up the 42.9 μL of whole blood contained in the small loop, and carries it to the WBC aperture bath, where it enters through the bottom left of the bath.

b. At the same time, approximately 10 mL of diluent enters the front of the blood sampling valve and

picks up the 1.6 μL of whole blood in the center section. This blood and diluent go directly to the RBC aperture bath.

8. While the blood is being aspirated, the diluent is draining from the RBC aperture bath into the waste chamber, and the WBC aperture bath is draining into the hemoglobin cuvet.

9. The diluted blood samples then enter the RBC and WBC aperture baths, respectively, through the tubing at the bottom left of each bath.

10. At the same time, 0.7734 mL of lyse reagent is forced into the WBC aperture bath at the bottom right side of the bath (1:251 dilution).

11. Bubbles are introduced into each aperture bath through tubing attached at the bottom of the bath. These bubbles (between 12 and 16) are utilized to completely mix the diluted blood sample.

12. While the aperture baths are filling, the hemoglobin cuvet is being drained into the waste chamber. As WIPE is displayed, an internal voltage check is automatically performed (voltage patterns are displayed on the oscilloscope screens), and the hemoglobin cuvet is filled with diluent (5 mL) for the hemoglobin blank reading.

13. At this point, the instrument is ready to count. COUNT is displayed, and a 4-second counting cycle takes place.

   a. At the beginning of the first 4-second count cycle, the voltage reading for the hemoglobin blank is shown on the DVM/test number display. This number immediately changes to the number 1 to indicate the first counting cycle.

   b. As in the Model S Coulter Counter, each of the apertures contains an internal electrode. There is one external electrode in each aperture bath.

   c. When the pinch valves between the aperture housing and the vacuum isolator chambers are opened, the vacuum (present in the vacuum isolator chambers) draws the diluted blood sample through each aperture (into the vacuum isolator chamber) for a period of 4 seconds.

   d. As the diluted blood sample passes through the aperture, the current between the external and internal electrodes changes each time a cell passes through the ap-

erture. This produces a voltage pulse, the magnitude of which is proportional to the size of the cell.

   e. The white blood cells are counted from the WBC aperture bath on the right side. From the RBC aperture bath, the red blood cells and platelets are counted, and the MCV is determined from the size of the voltage pulses.

   f. As the red blood cells and platelets pass through the RBC apertures, those particles measuring 2 to 20 fL are counted as platelets, whereas all particles above 36 fL are enumerated as red blood cells. All cells between 36 and 360 fL are used to determine the MCV.

   g. The RBC, WBC, platelet count, and MCV are all measured through three apertures. Up to five 4-second platelet counts are performed during each test cycle, depending on the platelet count of the sample introduced. The instrument automatically counts the platelets for additional cycles, up to 5, until the equivalent of 190,000 to 250,000/μL platelet count is attained.

   h. As each platelet count is performed by the instrument, the number corresponding to the platelet count being done (2, 3, 4, or 5) appears on the DVM/test number display.

   i. During the first count cycle, three platelet counts, red blood cell counts, white blood cell counts, and MCVs are performed simultaneously (one count through each aperture).

14. When the counting cycle(s) is completed, ANALYZE appears on the system status indicator, and the analyzer unit compares the counts from each aperture.

15. If all three results for each parameter tested (RBC, WBC, platelet count,

and RDW) agree with the others within four S.D., DATA ACCEPT appears on the system status indicator, and the three counts are averaged for a final result.

a. If one count does not match the other two, the corresponding data rejection lamp lights on the voting matrix, and the other two counts are averaged for the final result.

b. A total vote out for a parameter is obtained when none of the counts agree within four S.D. of each other. In such instances, all three data rejection lamps are lit, DATA REJECT appears on the indicator, and the cycle stops. The recount and cont buttons flash for 30 seconds.

c. If a recount is desired on the rejected parameter, push the recount button. If a recount is not wanted, either push the cont button or wait 30 seconds and the cycle will continue.

16. The aperture baths will then empty (RBC bath into the waste chamber and the WBC bath into the hemoglobin cuvet) and refill with diluent. BACKWASH appears on the system status indicator, and 4 mL of diluent is pushed through the blood sampling valve and out the aspirator tip into the rinse cup, which has moved into a locked position beneath the aspirator.

17. HGB READ is displayed on the indicator, and the amount of light passing through the diluted hemoglobin sample is read. The voltage reading is displayed on the DVM/test number display.

18. The hematocrit (RBC × MCV), MCH (hemoglobin ÷ RBC) and MCHC (hemoglobin ÷ hematocrit) are calculated in the analyzer unit. Immediately, the printer unit prints the results of the nine parameters.

19. If 1 mL of whole blood is not available or if fingertip blood is used, add 44.7 µL of whole blood to 1 aliquot (approximately 10 mL) of diluent from the diluent dispenser. Mix the diluted sample carefully to avoid bubbles, and place the vial under the microsample aspirator tip. Press the 1:224 dilution button directly behind the aspirator and allow the instrument to aspirate the entire sample. The diluted sample enters the back of the blood sampling valve and goes into and completely fills the large loop of the center section. (See Fig. 182 for a diagram of the blood sampling valve.) It continues through the blood sampling valve and leaves by way of the back of the valve, going directly to the WBC aperture bath. During the aspiration of the microsample, the blood sampling valve moves to position 2. The large loop is now completely filled with the original microsample dilution. Diluent then enters the blood sampling valve at the back, picks up the diluted sample in the large loop for the RBC dilution, and carries it to the RBC aperture bath, where it enters the right bottom side of the bath. While this is occurring, the diluted sample continues to be aspirated through the back of the blood sampling valve but now enters the trough in the middle section and continues out the back of the blood sampling valve, where it continues to go directly to the WBC aperture bath, entering through the line at the top of the bath. The cycle continues as described for the whole blood cycle, with one exception. The microsample aspirator tip is not backwashed with diluent. Instead, a vacuum is applied to the microsample aspirator tip for a short period at the end of the cycle, immediately before the

READY light comes on. This is for cleaning purposes.

CLEANING PROCEDURES AND MAINTENANCE

1. When starting up the instrument each day, the following should be inspected.
   a. Check for pinched tubing.
   b. Check all meters and indicators on the power supply.
   c. Check the operation of all buttons on the front of the instrument.
   d. Turn on X-Y recorder.
   e. Check all switches on the electronic cards and hemoglobin card.
   f. Check that there are no error codes.
   g. Set date and adjust the baseline on the oscilloscope screen.
   h. Check setting of mercury manometer.
   i. Press the start up button and inspect for the proper flow of liquids and bubble rates, proper functioning of the mercury manometer, and proper sequence of messages on the display.
   j. Perform a background count.
   k. Record the hemoglobin blank and the hemoglobin read voltages.
   l. Check the aspiration rate through the microsample aspirator.
   m. Perform the electronic voltage checks as outlined in the operators manual.
   n. Prime the instrument with two samples of whole blood.
   o. Perform Q. C. procedures.
2. Once/month, remove the five air filters, wash in warm, soapy water, rinse, and dry.
3. After every 1,000 cycles of the instrument (or weekly, whichever occurs first), the blood sampling valve should be cleaned and the apertures washed well in a Clorox solution.

DISCUSSION

1. Refer to the back of the Coulter Counter printout card for the description of the seven codes and symbols which may appear on the card when a patient specimen is reported by the instrument.
2. To obtain a valid platelet count: (a) the platelet count must be above $20,000/\mu L$, (b) there can be no total platelet vote out, and (c) a positive curve must be obtained.
3. If the vacuum adjust wheel is adjusted manually and the mercury column does not change, there may be a leak in the vacuum system.
4. It is advisable to keep a spare cube of diluent adjacent to the instrument. This prevents unnecessary mixing of the diluent and the resultant formation of microscopic air bubbles in the diluent when it is hooked up to the instrument.
5. Build up of protein on the orifices of the apertures first causes an increase in the MCV, followed by a decrease in the counts.
6. When filling vials with diluent for microsamples, the microsample dispensing system must be used in order to obtain accurate dilutions.
7. Microsamples should be tested within 1 hour of diluting to obtain an accurate platelet count and within 4 hours for the hemogram.
8. It takes 34 to 50 seconds for each whole blood sample to cycle through the instrument and for results to be obtained. The variation in time is due to the number of platelet counting cycles that are necessary. Only one sample may be introduced into the instrument at a time.
9. If agglutination of red blood cells is present (patient with a cold agglutinin), the RBC will be invalidly low and the MCV invalidly high. In this situation, the only useful parameters determined by the instrument are the WBC, hemoglobin, and platelet count.

COULTER COUNTER MODELS S PLUS II, III, IV, V, VI, AND STKR

Coulter Electronics, Inc. has modified the basic Coulter Counter® Model S Plus and enlarged the instrument's capabilities. Because the basic operating unit shows only minor changes, just a brief description of the changes will be given here. The major addition, the data terminal, however, will be described in more detail.

The Coulter Counter Model S Plus II, no longer being manufacturered, uses a reagent system that has been modified slightly from the one used in the Model S Plus. This has resulted in the reporting of lymphocyte number and percent, and the RDW is calculated as a true C. V. (coefficient of variation). This model also is capable of determining and reporting the number of lymphocytes per µL of blood and the percent of lymphocytes present. A data terminal may also be used with this instrument that essentially provides many quality control capabilities (including $\overline{X}_B$ analysis), the ability to flag abnormal results, and white blood cell, red blood cell, and platelet histograms. A matrix printer plotter replaces the previously used X-Y recorder and is capable of printing all information displayed by the data terminal.

The Coulter Counter Model S Plus III is able to test over 115 samples per hour.

The Coulter Counter Model S Plus IV, in addition to the modifications made in the S Plus II, uses a 100 µL patient sample in place of the 1.0 mL of blood that was previously required. The manually diluted microsample used in previous models is therefore not utilized for this instrument. The number of parameters tested has increased to 16 and includes: WBC, RBC, hemoglobin, hematocrit, MCV, MCH, MCHC, RDW, MPV (mean platelet volume), and a complete WBC differential (percentage and absolute number of granulocytes, lymphocytes, and mononuclear cells, plus eosinophils less than 700/µL and basophils less than 200/µL). Red cell,

white cell, and platelet histograms are displayed on the CRT screen along with the numerical results for each patient sample. A hard copy report (printed) of these results may then be obtained from the matrix printer plotter. An MPV nomogram (using the MPV and platelet count) is generated by the data terminal and may be obtained on each patient sample for which a platelet count and MPV are resulted. Up to 138 samples per hour may be analyzed. There is an optional bar code reader wand for use in matching results with the patient requisition or online data. This mechanism is also available on the Coulters S Plus V, VI, and STKR.

The Coulter Counter Model S Plus V performs all of the testing and reporting as described above for the S Plus IV. A major change is in the addition of an automated cap piercer used in aspirating the patient sample. The capped tube of well-mixed whole blood is placed into a window in the front of the diluter unit door. When the instrument is in the ready stage, it senses the tube and automatically pierces the cap, removing 100 µL of blood for analysis and proceeds with testing. The tube of blood travels down a small exit ramp to be removed by the operator. There is also a secondary aspirator which may be used to aspirate hand held specimens which have their caps removed.

The Coulter Counter Model S Plus VI performs testing and reporting as described for the S Plus V above. This model uses an additional unit, the autosampler, which contains two rotating wheel-shaped sample trays each capable of holding thirty-two patient tubes. Specimens for premixing are placed on the right side of the unit where they will rotate and be mixed prior to testing. This sample tray may then be removed and placed on the front of the unit for testing, where a premix cycle may be used to ensure complete mixing. When the specimens are well mixed, the sampler wheel stops briefly, the first sample is automatically aspirated by means of a special cap piercer. Sample analysis is begun and when the instrument is ready to aspirate the next sample the sampler wheel stops at the next blood sample long enough to aspirate the specimen. To make this a true walk-away system this model has a continuous-feed fanfold printer. STAT samples may be tested at any time, and there are audible and visual signals given when all of the specimens on the wheel have been tested. Like the Model S Plus V there is a secondary aspirator for hand-held uncapped specimens which uses 125 μL of whole blood. The automatic sampling mode uses 750 μL of whole blood.

The Coulter Counter Model S Plus STKR (pronounced 'Stacker') shows a variety of additional capabilities over the previously described S Plus VI. This model is capable of accepting and mixing up to 144 patient samples at one time in preparation for automatic identification, aspiration (using a cap piercer), and sample analysis. A bar code label is placed on each specimen tube and up to twelve samples are placed into an S Plus STKR cassette. Up to twelve cassettes may be placed in the right side of the STKR where they are mixed by a back and forward motion. The first cassette is transported to the center of the diluter unit. The bar code is read on the first specimen to be tested and the sample is removed from the tube by a cap piercing aspirator. Sample analysis is begun, the next specimen is moved to the test station and when the instrument is ready, the bar code is read and the sample is aspirated. (The instrument may be operated with or without the bar code.) Cassettes are automatically stored on the left side of the instrument when testing is complete. There is a secondary aspirator for hand-held uncapped specimens which uses 100 μL of whole blood. The automatic sampling mode uses 200 μL of blood and requires a minimum of 1.0 mL of whole blood in the tube. STAT samples may be tested at any time during autoprocessing. Throughput

for this model is 138 samples per hour. The printer is capable of automatic reporting and can read the bar code labels which enables it to print results on labeled forms in any sequence. There is a keypad and display on the printer which allows for manual operation when desired.

The Coulter S Plus Jr consists of the main unit, pneumatic power supply, printer, data terminal, an optional bar code reader, and an optional printer/plotter. This instrument is smaller and more compact than the previously described Coulter S Plus models. It uses 100 μL of patient sample, has a maximum throughput of 62 samples/hour, and may be interfaced to a host computer system. The testing profile includes red and white cell counts, hemoglobin, hematocrit, red cell indices (MCV, MCH, MCHC), platelet count, red cell morphology, and a white cell differential.

Data Terminal

The data terminal (Fig. 183) receives information from the analyzer unit and sends it to the printer and the matrix printer plotter. It determines the MCV, RDW, platelet count, MPV, and white cell percentages and absolute counts, and provides a complete quality control program. Extended data terminal capabilities are available which allow for additional storage of up to 3900 numerical patient reports or up to 550 complete reports (numerical results and histograms) on the Coulters S Plus IV, V, VI and STKR. These same instruments will flag abnormal results: values exceeding pre-set laboratory limits, results exceeding delta checks, abnormal WBC differential results, abnormal volume distribution histograms, and abnormal MPV nomograms. The following is a brief summary of the data terminal used with the Coulters S Plus IV, V, VI, and STKR.

The basic program used in the data terminal is made up of six parts, each of

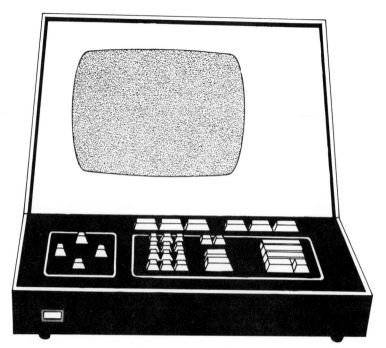

Fig. 183. Data terminal, Coulter Counter Model S Plus IV.

which is termed a *menu.* The main menu of the data terminal lists these seven menus.

1. Sample analysis menu.
2. Data entry menu.
3. Start-up menu.
4. Control data menu.
5. Special tests menu.
6. Prime menu.
7. Calibration menu.

Each of these menus may be displayed separately and is further broken down into submenus. The primary functions that may be carried out in each menu are outlined below.

In the *sample analysis* menu, the patient samples are run; the operator may delete the last sample run from the $\overline{X}_B$ analysis; the $\overline{X}_B$ may be turned off or on; and there is a submenu for $\overline{X}_B$ review. In $\overline{X}_B$ review, the last batch of $\overline{X}_B$ values may be reviewed; the entire last batch of $\overline{X}_B$ values may be deleted; $\overline{X}_B$ values for the last 20 batches are listed; the red and white blood cell values in the current $\overline{X}_B$ batch of blood specimens are listed; $\overline{X}_B$ graphs

(MCV, MCH, and MCHC, hemoglobin bias, red blood cell percentage difference, and hematocrit percentage difference) for the previous 20 batches may be displayed; and the hemoglobin may be set for the hemoglobin bias. During sample analysis, the patient results are displayed following completion of the instrument cycle: white blood cell, red blood cell, and platelet histograms, white blood cell count, all red blood cell parameters, platelet count, MPV (mean platelet volume), and the differential percents and absolute counts. Information about the $\overline{X}_B$ is also given: $\overline{X}_B$ on or off and whether the previous batch of patient samples was within or outside of the acceptable range.

The *data entry* menu allows the operator to enter information into the data terminal: operator number; hospital I.D. number; critical value ranges for each parameter (so that abnormal results may be flagged by the data terminal); acceptable ranges for the $\overline{X}_B$ values, ramp and precision voltages, reagent lot numbers, assay values, and limits for up to nine different quality control types; set the print size for the matrix printer plotter; and set automatic printing of histograms if desired.

The *start-up* menu is used primarily in setting up the instrument each morning and displays: the previously run result, limits and histograms for the background count; the previously run ramp and precision results, limits, and histograms; a start-up log (background, precision and ramp results, and reagent lot numbers); the previously run reproducibility check (results, limits, and histograms) and a method for deleting this information; and the previously run carry-over results (results, limits, and histograms) and a method for deleting these results from the data terminal.

In the *control data* menu, the operator may select the control file; enter the control values as they are run; review the previously run control values, assay, and limits for each of the nine control files; delete the results of the last control sample; review all of the previous control results (up to 40 sets for each control); review control graphs for each parameter of each control; and delete all information from any control file.

The *special tests* menu allows the operator to perform checks on memory, data terminal screen, graphics, ticket printer, recorder, matrix printer plotter, keyboard, and the battery.

The *prime* menu allows the operator to run patient samples through the instrument without their being included in the $\overline{X}_B$ analysis.

The *calibration* menu provides the Auto-Cal® quality control program for automatic calibration calculations.

As stated previously, all information displayed on the data terminal may be printed on the matrix printer plotter by depressing the plot key on the data terminal.

Interpretive Report

All Coulter Model S Pluses (IV, V, VI, STKR) now report a complete white cell histogram with an accompanying interpretive report which has been instituted to 'flag' the abnormal test result for further review. The interpretive report is based on testing limits which may be set by each individual laboratory. When the preset thresholds are exceeded, the instrument can report definitive flags for: lymphocytosis, lymphopenia, granulocytosis, granulopenia, anisocytosis, microcytosis, macrocytosis, hypochromia, large platelets, and small platelets. A second part of the interpretive report indicates suspect cell types: eosinophilia >700/µL, basophilia >200/µL, atypical lymphocytes, immature granulocytes, blasts, NRBCs, platelet clumps, and red cell and platelet abnormal distributions. The third portion of this report gives the message, 'Review Nomogram', when the MPV is smaller or larger than expected for a given platelet count.

Coulter Pulse Editing

The principle of cell counting and volume measurement in Coulter counters is based on the detection and measurement of voltage pulses created by cells, suspended in a conductive diluent, as they travel through a small orifice. During the counting cycle, the number of voltage pulses corresponds to the cell count, while the size, or amplitude of the pulse corresponds to the volume of the cell. The amplitude and the shape of the voltage pulse, however, are affected by the pathway the cell takes through the aperture. The speed of the diluent through the aperture is at a maximum in the center of the aperture opening, and the density of the current is the most uniform in this area. On the other hand, the speed of the fluid adjacent to the aperture wall is slower and the density of the current here is higher. Refer to Figure 184. In this diagram, cell B travels through a uniform current density to give a voltage pulse as shown. Cell A, however, first travels close to the aperture where there is a higher current density. The resultant pulse begins prior to that from cell B, has a

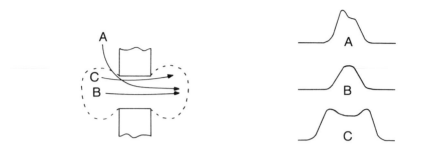

Fig. 184. Voltage pulses generated by particles passing through the aperture (Coulter Counter Model S Plus series).

higher amplitude, and is atypical. Cell C travels through the aperture close to the aperture wall. The voltage pulse contains two peaks due to the higher current density at the two corners of the aperture. The pulse itself is of longer duration due to the slower speed of the cell through the aperture (the flow through the center of the aperture is at a maximum). The Coulter pulse editor is contained in the Coulter Counter Model S Plus instruments and functions to recognize and eliminate the atypical pulses such as those described above. Only those pulses obtained from cells passing through the center of the aperture are used in deriving cell volume distribution histograms.

Red Blood Cell Histogram and Red Cell Distribution Width

On all Counter Counter Models S Plus, the red blood cell dilution contains red blood cells, white blood cells, and platelets. Those particles between 2 and 20 fL in size are categorized as platelets. Particles greater than 36 fL are counted as red blood cells. (White blood cells are counted along with the red blood cells, but because of their low numbers in relationship to the red blood cells, they are felt to be insignificant.) As the red blood cells are counted, their size (MCV) is also determined. This information is used to create the red blood cell histogram, where the relative number of red blood cells are plotted on the vertical axis of the graph and the size of the red blood cell is plotted on the horizontal axis. Normally, the red blood cell histogram will be almost symmetric with a single peak (Fig. 185A). The tail seen to the left of the curve may represent large or clumped platelets, or electrical interference. The larger tail on the right of the curve is termed the *foot* and may represent doublets and triplets (2 or 3 cells).

The red cell distribution width (RDW) represents the coefficient of variation of the red blood cell size and is determined by the following formula for the Coulter Counter S Plus Models II, III, IV, V, VI, and STKR:

$$RDW \ (CV\%) = \frac{S.D. \ (of \ RBC \ distribution)}{Mean} \times 100$$

Before the RDW is calculated, the upper and lower portion of the histogram, containing the two tails, is excluded from the calculations. If a relatively large secondary population of red blood cells is present (Fig. 185B), this will be detected by the instrument because the two populations are well separated. In these instances, the RDW will be flagged by the instrument. If, however, the second population of red blood cells present is not that distinctly different from the other red blood cells present (Fig. 185C), the RDW will not be

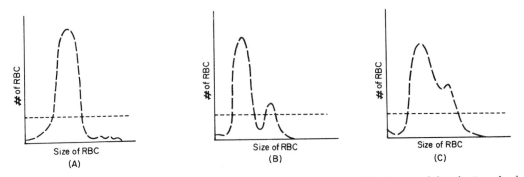

Fig. 185. RBC histograms. A. Normal distribution of red blood cells. B and C. Abnormal distribution of red blood cells.

flagged, but the result should be markedly increased. The recommended normal range for the RDW determined in this manner is 11.5 to 14.5%.

COULTER COUNTER HISTOGRAM DIFFERENTIAL

The Coulter Counter Model S Plus IV and the ensuing models (V, VI, and STKR) are capable of reporting a white count differential based on the size distribution of the white cells. In addition to counting the white blood cells, the instrument determines the size of these cells. This information is then used to plot the histogram. Using the specific Coulter reagent system, the nucleated cells in the approximate size range of 35 to 90 fL have been found to be normal lymphocytes, those cells ranging in approximate size from 90 to 160 fL are considered mononuclear cells, and the granulocytes are in the approximate range of 160 to 450 fL. The percent of each of these cell types is calculated by the instrument by comparing the number of cells present in each size range, with the total number of cells present in all three size categories. The instrument then multiplies the percent of each cell type by the total white count in order to obtain the absolute number of each cell class present. A normal white blood cell histogram (Fig. 186) will show three distinct populations of white cells that are separated at approximately 90 and 160 fL. If nucleated

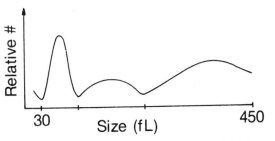

Fig. 186. WBC Histogram (Coulter Counter Model S Plus IV).

red blood cells are present, these are characteristically indicated by the lack of a valley at 35 fL. In addition, the Coulter instruments have a set of differential flags to alert the operator to abnormal cell distribution patterns. The lymphocyte category will contain mature and some atypical lymphocytes; the mononuclear class includes monocytes, promyelocytes, myelocytes, and blasts; eosinophils, basophils, metamyelocytes, bands, and neutrophils are classified as granulocytes.

$\overline{X}_B$ and Quality Control

The $\overline{X}_B$ (pronounced X bar B) is used as a quality control check for hematology instruments. This mathematical formula was published in 1974 by Dr. Brian Bull. Essentially, it is a weighted moving average of the patient's red blood cell indices (MCV, MCH, and MCHC) and is calculated by the Coulter Counter data terminal using a relatively complex mathematical formula. Studies have shown that the population of patients in medium to large hospitals show relatively stable values for the red blood cell indices. Also, in the calculations used here by the Coulter instruments, less weight is given to the extremely high or low patient result.

Basically, each successive group of 20 patient results are grouped into a batch. As each patient blood is tested, the mean $(\overline{X}_B)$ value from the previous batch (of 20 patient samples) is subtracted from the respective current red blood cell index (MCV, MCH, or MCHC). The square root of the resultant number is then determined. After 20 patient blood specimens have been analyzed, the sum of the square roots for each of the three indices is added up and divided by the number of patient samples (usually 20). This number is then squared and added to or subtracted from the respective previous $\overline{X}_B$ value obtained in order to derive the $\overline{X}_B$ value for the current batch of patient samples. This new mean value is then used to help determine the $\overline{X}_B$ value for the next batch of 20 blood specimens. Each laboratory should have its own set of target values for each of the indices. Once set, the $\overline{X}_B$ value for each index in each batch should fall within ± 3% of the target value. If, however, an instrument or reagent problem exists, this will be indicated by one or more of the red blood cell indices moving consistently in one direction (up or down) or in the $\overline{X}_B$ value falling outside of the allowable laboratory preset range. The recommended target values are ± 3% of (1) 89.5 (MCV), (2) 30.5 (MCH), and (3) 34.0 (MCHC).

The hemoglobin bias, RBC percent difference, and hematocrit percentage difference are further calculations made by the instrument to be used in detecting where specific instrument problems lie. The automatic *hemoglobin bias* is defined as the difference between what the hemoglobin value should be (assay value) and the hemoglobin value the instrument actually reads (average of last 5 control values in

file #1). A manual hemoglobin bias is also available.

TECHNICON H-1™

The Technicon H-1™ instrument performs a complete blood count, platelet count, and differential count. Testing may be performed as only a CBC and platelet count, or, may include the differential, as the operator chooses. Red blood cell indices are included with the CBC and limited red cell morphology is also available for reporting. The instrument identifies six types of white cell (neutrophil, eosinophil, basophil, monocyte, lymphocyte, and large unstained cell) and reports a lobularity index (left shift indicator).

There are four units which make up the H-1™ system. The *analytical module* aspirates, dilutes, processes, and tests each sample. The electrical outputs from each test channel are sent to the *electronics module* where they are converted to test results. In addition, this unit controls the system operation and performs all data processing and management functions. The *VDT/keypad ticket printer module* prints numerical test results and morphology notes on inserted report forms. This unit also has the video display terminal with the associated keyboard for communicating with the instrument. With this system the operator may view test and control results, set result and control ranges, perform maintenance on the system, troubleshoot problems, perform instrument setup and calibration, adjust a laboratory computer interface, etc. The optional *screen printer* is used to obtain print-outs of the contents of the video display screen (except for message lines).

The H-1™ performs all tests on an approximate 100 μL sample size. Testing is performed on four separate dilutions of the blood sample: (1) Hemoglobin, (2) RBC, platelet count, MCV, and MPV (mean platelet volume), (3) WBC and differential (except basophil percent), and (4) basophil percent and lobularity index. The hematocrit, red blood cell indices, and RDW are calculated using the information obtained from the hemoglobin and RBC channels. The instrument will also flag the presence of anisocytosis, microcytosis, macrocytosis, hypochromia, hyperchromia, atypical lymphocytes, blasts, and a left shift.

COMPONENTS, OPERATION, AND PRINCIPLES OF THE ANALYTICAL UNIT (FIG. 187)

1. *Status panel* (1).
    a. *Systems status.* Turn the unit on by depressing the *sys on* switch. As long as power is supplied to the system, the indicator light will remain lit. Press the *sys off* switch to turn the unit off. If the instrument will not be used for a period of time press the *standby* switch. (The unit will also go into the standby mode automatically after 1 hour of not being cycled.) The *ready* light, when lit, indicates that a sample may be aspirated into the unit. While a sample

is being tested by the unit, the *in process* light is lit. A hydraulic or mechanical problem will be indicated by lighting of the *error* light.
    b. *Selectivity.* Prior to aspirating the sample, select the test(s) to be performed by pressing the *CBC* or *CBC/diff* switch. The corresponding indicator will light up.
    c. *Laser status.* During the test cycle the *pwr on* indicator will light. If the laser power has been halted due to a problem (power failure), the *pwr intrpt* indicator lights. To turn this light off, press the *intrpt reset* switch.
2. Aspiration of blood sample.
    a. The *ready to sample* (2) green indicator light should be lit (to indicate that the unit is ready to aspirate a sample).
    b. Place the well-mixed whole blood sample under the *sample probe* (3) and depress the *push to as-*

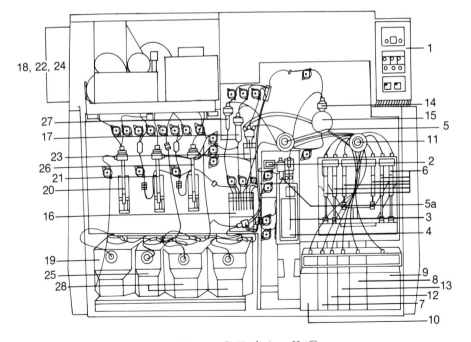

Fig. 187. Analytical module (front panel removed), Technicon H-1™.

pirate (4) switch to begin the testing sequence.

c. The sample is drawn through the *sample shear valve* (5) by a vacuum. A *conductivity detector* (5a), located after the sample shear valve, notes the presence of the sample and causes the aspiration process to stop.

d. During aspiration the sample travels in and out of the rear portion of the sample shear valve four times, before passing through the detector. The sample is thereby divided into four separate segments within the rear section of the valve: 2 μL (RBC/plt.), 12 μL (baso/lob.), 12 μL (WBC, diff.), and 2 μL (hgb.).

3. Dilution of sample.

a. The back section of the sample shear valve rotates to its second position. The sample probe is rinsed inside and out, and dried.

b. The four outer *reagent syringe drives* (6) then dispense Perox Dil 1 (WBC) (7), Hgb Dil (hgb.) (8), RBC Dil (RBC/plt.) (9), and Baso Dil (baso/lob.) (10), respectively, through separate pathways in the *reagent shear valve* (11).

c. The reagents travel through their respective tubing, through the sample shear valve, where they pick up the measured blood segment, and then go to the appropriate reaction chamber.

d. While step c, above, is occurring, the two center reagent syringes fill with Perox Dil 2 (12) and Perox Dil 3 (13), respectively. These reagents are dispensed directly from the reagent shear valve into the peroxidase (WBC) reaction chamber.

e. During step d, above, the 4 outer reagent syringes fill with reagent for the next sample.

4. Sample dilutions are mixed in the re-action chambers. At this time, the necessary reactions take place and the samples are then counted and/or tested.

a. Hemoglobin.

1) The whole blood is diluted 1:250 with cyanmethemoglobin reagent (Hgb Dil) and mixed in the hemoglobin reaction vessel (14).

2) The reaction vessel also serves as a cuvet and is located between the *546 nm light source* and the *photodetector* (15).

3) When the hemoglobin reading has been made, the sample dilution leaves the reaction chamber and travels to the *waste chamber* (16).

4) The reaction chamber is rinsed and a reading is taken of the hemoglobin rinse solution, to be used as the baseline measurement.

b. RBC/platelet count.

1) The whole blood is diluted 1:625 with RBC/Plt Dil fluid and mixed in the *RBC/plt reaction vessel* (17). In this reagent the red cells absorb fluid until they are spherical in shape (their total volume is unchanged). The diluting fluid also lightly fixes (preserves) the red cells and platelets.

2) The RBC and platelets are counted as they pass through a *flow cell* (18). The diluted sample is surrounded by a layer of sheath fluid. A diaphragm pump pushes *RBC/ Baso Sheath fluid* (19) toward the flow cell. This fluid is then pulled through the flow cell by a *sheath syringe* (20) to ensure consistent flow of the fluid.

3) The sheath fluid travels

through the flow cell completely covering all of the inner surfaces and leaves a narrow, open central channel for the diluted sample to pass through.

4) The diluted sample is pulled through the center of the flow cell (by the *RBC/baso sample syringe* [21]) in such a thin stream that only 1 cell passes through at a time.

5) A *laser* (22) beam is located on one side of the flow cell. As a cell or particle passes in front of this beam it is counted by a light scatter detector using two different gain settings, one for red cells and the second, for platelets.

6) The red cells, since they have been sphered, will not fold over, and will all be round in shape (sickled red cells may be the only exception). This enables the instrument to make a more accurate determination of the MCV. The volume of the red blood cells and platelets are measured by comparing the low angle and high angle light scatter created by each particle as it passes in front of the laser beam. The concentration of the hemoglobin in each red blood cell is also determined by scatter transformation from the laser.

7) All of these informational signals are then converted into histogram plots, one for the red cells, one for hemoglobin concentration, and one for platelets.

c. WBC and differential (peroxidase dilution).

1) Whole blood is initially diluted 1:22 with Perox Dil 1 fluid and mixed in the *per-oxidase reaction vessel* (23). During the first 20 seconds, the chamber is heated to 72°C, which, along with the reagent, causes lysis of the red blood cells and platelets. In addition, the white cells are dehydrated and fixed.

2) For the next 13 seconds Perox Dil 2 and Perox Dil 3 fluids (containing as a primary ingredient, 4-chloro-1-naphthol) are added to the original dilution in the chamber, bringing about the following reaction in those white cells containing peroxidase (neutrophils), eosinophils, and monocytes:

$$H_2O_2 + \text{4-chloro-1-naphthol cellular peroxidase} \rightarrow \text{dark precipitate}$$

The lymphocytes, basophils, and large unstained cells contain no peroxidase and therefore do not stain in this reaction.

3) The white cell dilution, like the RBC/plt. dilution, is surrounded by a layer of sheath fluid and passes through a flow cell for testing. This channel uses a *tungsten-based optical system* (24) in place of the laser beam used for the red cells.

4) A diaphragm pump pushes the *Perox Sheath fluid* (25) toward the flow cell. The fluid is then pulled through the flow cell by the sheath sample syringe. The sheath fluid leaves a narrow opening through the flow cell. The *perox sample syringe* (26) pulls the diluted sample through the flow cell, one cell at a time.

5) The tungsten lamp is located

on one side of the flow cell. As the cell passes through the beam of light, the stain intensity (absorbance) is measured, as is the size of the cell (measured by the forward light scatter).

6) The individual impulses are counted to determine the white blood count.

7) Peroxidase is contained in eosinophils, neutrophils, and monocytes in known amounts. The instrument uses this information, together with the cell size, to classify each of the cells. In this channel, the basophils are classified with the lymphocytes.

8) A scattergram is constructed, plotting absorption vs. light scatter (Fig. 188).

d. Basophil/lobularity index.

1) The whole blood sample is diluted with Baso/Lob Dil fluid and mixed in the *baso reaction vessel* (27). This fluid contains an acid which lyses the red blood cells and platelets, and ruptures the cytoplasm of all of the white cells (except basophils) thus freeing each cell's nucleus.

2) The baso/lob. dilution shares the same flow cell and laser beam as the RBC/plt. dilution, but uses it at a different time period in the sample cycle. As in the RBC/plt. dilution, the same diaphragm pump and syringes move the sheath fluid and diluted sample through the flow cell.

3) As each cell or nucleus pass in front of the laser beam, the light is scattered. Absorption and low and high angle light scatter are measured.

4) The basophils are counted.

5) A ratio of the signals is used to determine the degree of lobularity of the nuclei. This information is used as an indi-

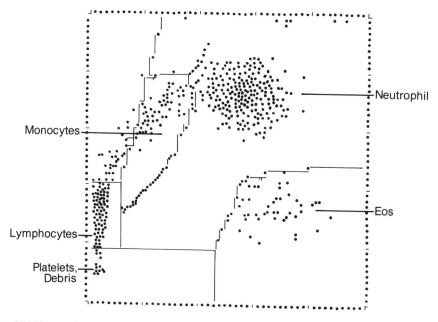

Fig. 188. WBC/peroxidase cytogram, Technicon H-1™.

cator of the amount of left shift present.

6) A scattergram is constructed, plotting high angle scatter vs. low angle scatter (Fig. 189).

5. When the diluted samples leave the reaction vessels, each chamber is washed with *Rinse fluid* (28).

6. The diluted samples and the rinse solutions from the flow cells and hemoglobin cuvet travel to the waste chamber and then, at the end of the cycle, exit the unit into the 20 liter waste container.

7. A hematology report form may be placed in the VDT/ticket printer module at any time during the sample cycle. The numerical results will automatically print out at the end of the cycle.

8. If the optional screen printer is attached to the system and programmed to print sample results, numerical results, histograms, and cytograms will automatically be printed at the end of the cycle.

VIDEO DISPLAY TERMINAL/KEYPAD TICKET PRINTER MODULE (FIG. 190)

1. On the *display screen* (29) the top line is divided into 3 sections for messages: a) the *system message* (30) area (left) alerts the operator to situations which require the operator's attention, b) *next sample* (31) area (middle) indicates the next type of sample to be processed, and c) *system status* (32) area (right) displays the status of the instrument. At the bottom of the screen, the last line is divided into 5 parts (F1 through F5). The display screen indicates the function for each of these depending upon the current video display. The line above the bottom line is divided into three sections: a) *prompt* (34) field (left) displays messages for operating the system, b) *data entry* (35) field (middle) displays operator-entered data, and c) *entry error* (36) field (right) displays errors of data entry by the operator.

2. *Keypad* (37) (located below the video display screen).

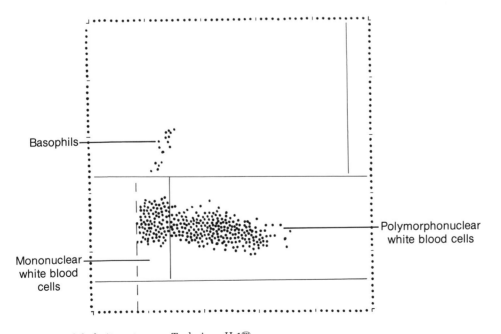

Fig. 189. Baso/lobularity cytogram, Technicon H-1™.

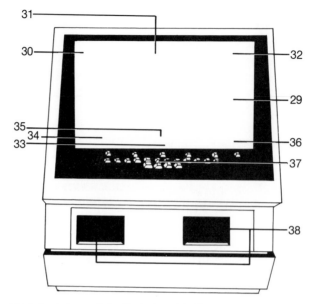

Fig. 190. VDT/keypad ticket printer module, Technicon H-1™.

a. *F1* through *F5* (33) relate to the F1 through F5 areas on the bottom line of the data screen. Their use depends upon the function displayed on the video data screen.

b. *0–9,* numbers, are for input of information by the operator.

c. . is for the operator to input a decimal point.

d. *CE* clears an entry into the VDT, may be used with the enter key to cancel a command, and moves the cursor to the first character in the field.

e. *Print test* key activates the printer to print results on a report form.

f. *Menu* is pressed in order to display the main menu.

g. *Run* is pressed in order to display the run menu which must be displayed at all times when processing a sample.

h. *Print screen* activates the optional screen printer to print the display on the video screen.

i. *Enter* key is used to store information on the screen and verifies some commands.

3. Indicators.

a. *Ready* illuminates when a report form is in that side of the ticket printer.

b. *Next to print* when lit, indicates which ticket printer will print next.

4. There are two *slots* (38) for entering report forms for printing of sample test results.

5. The rear portion of the unit contains the power *on/off switch* and a *reset button* for resetting the VDT.

6. The main portion of the video display screen enables the operator to view the list of system checks when the instrument is turned on, review test results as they are determined, troubleshoot problems, perform some maintenance procedures, store and review quality control data, calibrate, and set sample and control ranges.

a. When the instrument is turned on a *List of System Checks* will be displayed, with an indication of Passed or Ready next to each if there are no problems. If there is a failure, it will be noted and the instrument will stop.

b. During sample processing the *patient report* will be displayed on the screen. There are several different formats which the operator may choose.

c. If any sample results are flagged (marked by an asterisk) by the instrument, the operator may change the video display to the *Asterisk Analysis Screen* which will indicate the problem with the flagged result.

d. In addition to the above three display functions, the VDT has a *main menu* composed of five files as outlined below:

1) *QC file* (F1) for input and review of control data, input of control limits, calibration, and calculation of control means and S.D.s.

2) *System setup* (F2) is divided into menu A and menu B. Menu A is utilized for starting up the instrument, setting desired options (such as paper size for the screen printer, suppression of certain test data, date format, etc.), and setting of flagging ranges. Through menu B, the date and test units may be set, and laboratory computer hook-up settings may be changed.

3) *System status* (F3) is used for setting various aspects of the moving average QC program, setting the test generator and printer automatically on or off, and contains settings for a laboratory computer.

4) *Hydraulics* (F4) function is used to perform maintenance procedures on the instrument. By entering different portions of this function, for example, the instrument will automatically prime the reagents or wash the probe.

5) The *utilities* (F5) function enables the operator to check various aspects of the instrument for troubleshooting problems.

ELECTRONICS MODULE (NOT SHOWN)

1. The *main power* circuit controls power to the system.

2. The *reset* button stops operation and causes the computer to restart.

3. The *disk locking handle* is used to place the program disk into the unit or remove the disk.

4. The *test voltage* switch is used to select the voltage for display on the *volts meter.*

5. The *compressor gauges,* three pressure (40, 20, and 5 psi) gauges and one vacuum (20 mm Hg) gauge, with associated *adjustment knobs* are used to adjust the pressures and vacuum which move the sample and diluting fluid through the analytical unit.

MAINTENANCE

The reader is referred to the H-1 Operators' Guide book for a detailed description of the instrument maintenance. Basically, operator maintenance time is minimal as suggested by the manufacturer, and is briefly outlined below:

1. *Daily*, clean up reagent spills and check waste container, reagent levels, pressure and vacuum gauges, vacuum trap for accumulated waste, and the quality of the print from both printers. Perform a wash procedure.

2. *Weekly* (or after every 1000 samples) perform a system wash.

3. *Every 2 months* change tubing, replace sheath filters, and clean the five air circulation filters.

4. *Every 6 months* replace waste filter, clean shear valves (sample and reagent), and replace the vacuum filter.

5. *Every 30,000 samples* replace the two sample syringe plungers.

6. *Every 60,000 samples* replace the sheath syringe plunger and the six reagent syringe plungers.

DISCUSSION

1. The batch size for the moving average may be set, within limits, by the individual laboratory. The parameters to be included may also be varied.

2. The Q.C. function will hold up to eight different controls plus a ninth control of whole blood.

3. Whole blood specimens are stable for testing for 24 hours when stored at room temperature (except for the MCV which is stable for 8 hours, and the lobularity index [LI] which is stable for 6 hours). Refrigerated samples are stable for 54 hours (except for the MPV and LI which are stable for less than 24 hours).

4. The system will process 80 samples/hour in the CBC mode (45 second cycle). In the CBC/diff mode, 60 samples/hour may be run (60 second cycle).

5. The presence of a high white count ($>50,000/\mu L$), or lipemia, will give falsely elevated hemoglobin readings.

6. Red cell agglutination may give an erroneous MCV and red cell count.

7. In the RBC dilution, sickled red cells may not become spherical and will give a falsely elevated RDW.

8. In patients with an elevated blood urea nitrogen (above 300 mg/dL) there may be incomplete lysis of the red cells in the WBC (peroxidase) dilution.

9. Differential results may be affected in patients showing a deficiency in peroxidase.

10. In some abnormal disorders (such as leukemia), some white cells, other than basophils, may be resistant to lysis in the baso/lob. dilution, and cause a falsely elevated basophil count.

11. Studies by the manufacturer have shown the following parameters to be linear as indicated:

   WBC 0.1 to 95.0 $\times$ $10^3/\mu L$
   RBC 0.1 to 7.0 $\times$ $10^6/\mu L$
   Hgb 1.0 to 28.0 g/dL
   Plt 10 to 700 $\times$ $10^3/\mu L$

12. The instrument startup cycle (from power on until ready for use) takes only 2 minutes 40 seconds. However, in a busy laboratory, it is recommended that the instrument be placed in the standby mode when not in use. (Stand-by to ready takes only 40 seconds.)

13. Reagent use, per sample cycle, is 2.9 mL. This does not include the rinse or sheath fluids, however.

14. The instrument will detect (and notify the operator of) numerous instrument or sample problems when they occur. The reader is referred to the operator's manual for further details.

MINIPREP® AUTOMATIC BLOOD SMEARING INSTRUMENT

The Miniprep® automatic smear maker (Fig. 191), manufactured by Geometric Data Corporation, affords the technologist a fast and simple method for preparing wedge smears of consistently good quality. This instrument is portable, light in

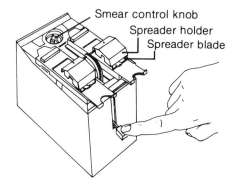

Fig. 191. Miniprep® automatic smear maker.

weight, and is small enough to be carried to an outpatient clinic or to the patient's bedside.

PROCEDURE

1. Insert one *spreader blade* in each *spreader holder.* Remove the protective backing from the tape on the spreader. Lift the spreader holder and place the blade in the slot, making certain the polished (spreading) edge faces upward. Carefully place the blade in the center of the slot (sticky side against the lid).
2. Place one (or two) slide(s) in the *tray*(s), making certain the slide(s) is firmly seated. If frosted-end slides are used, place the frosted end on the front of the tray.
3. Using a non-heparinized microhematocrit tube (applicator stick, capillary pipet, etc.), place a small drop of blood on the *target-area*(s).
4. Immediately, press down the front lever with a smooth, gentle stroke. As soon as the lever reaches the bottom position, release it. When the lever is pressed down, the spreader(s) moves forward until it reaches the target area. The spreader comes in contact with the drop of blood and hesitates momentarily, allowing the blood to spread along the edge of the spreader. The spreader then returns to its original position as it pulls the blood along the slide(s).
5. Remove smear(s) from the tray and allow to air dry.

DISCUSSION

1. The *smear control knob* alters the speed with which the blood is smeared, allowing the technologist to control the thickness of the smear. For thinner smears, turn the knob clockwise (to the right) and for thicker smears turn the knob counterclockwise (to the left). Once this knob has been set for the desired thickness, it should only have to be adjusted for bloods having a very high or very low hematocrit.
2. Located underneath the instrument is the *pause control adjuster* which controls the width of the blood smear by varying the amount of time that the spreader is in contact with the blood before the smear is pulled. To increase the time the blade is in contact with the blood (to increase the width of the smear), turn the screw clockwise. To decrease this time period, turn the screw counterclockwise. This screw is factory set and generally does not need adjustment. The pause time should be exactly 1 second.
3. It is necessary to replace the spreader blades if they become chipped. They are inexpensive and are available from the manufacturer.
4. When preparing blood smears for the Hematrak Differential Counter, the smear should cover approximately 75% of the non-frosted area of the slide and should be a relatively thin smear. The feathered edge should not be rounded, but should be straight across the slide. The width of the smear should be slightly less than the width of the glass slide.
5. If the blood smear is too long, this generally indicates too large of a drop of blood, a low hematocrit, and/or too thin a blood smear. Also, this will cause specimen carryover to the next sample. If the smear is too short, this is indicative of a high hematocrit, thick smear, and/or too little blood. If most of the blood remains in the target area, the drop of blood was placed too far back on the target area. If the smear is streaked or uneven, the spreader blades may be dirty or damaged, or the slide may be dirty.
6. If only one smear is prepared on each patient, only one tray should be used. Place a slide on the unused tray. It is

not necessary to place a blade in this spreader holder.

7. Reticulocyte smears may also be prepared on this instrument. The smear control knob may need to be adjusted for these smears.

8. It is easy to make good, consistent wedge smears using this instrument. The critical factor is the amount of blood placed on the target area.

9. There may be a small carry-over of cells from one smear to the next. The exact amount has been found to be 0.5% or less. The spreader blades should be washed periodically, depending on use, and whenever an excessive amount of blood has been placed on the slide. Clean the spreaders with 0.85% sodium chloride (w/v).

HEMASPINNER AUTOMATIC BLOOD CELL SPINNER

The Hemaspinner (Fig. 192), manufactured by Geometric Data Corp., is used for preparing a monolayer film of whole blood on a glass slide. A clean slide is placed on a platen, and three to four drops of whole blood are placed in the middle of the slide. When the top of the instrument is closed, the platen spins at high speed for a set amount of time. During this period, excess blood is thrown from the slide into a catch basin, and the resultant slide is completely covered with a thin monolayer of cells. During the spin cycle, a beam of light passes up through the glass slide onto a sensor. When the cells have separated to the proper degree, this is detected by the sensor, and the platen automatically stops spinning. In this manner, spreading of the blood is consistent from one smear to the next, irrespective of the patient's hematocrit. (However, blood specimens having an extremely high or low hematocrit, may be slightly under or over spun, respectively.)

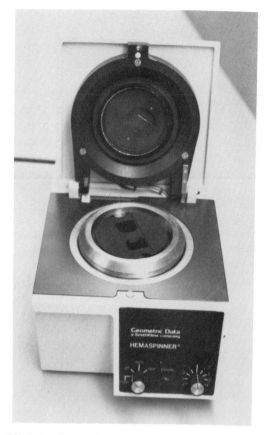

Fig. 192. Hemaspinner.

COMPONENTS OF THE HEMASPINNER

1. The *platen* holds the glass slide in place during the spinning process.

2. The *catch basin* collects the excess whole blood as it is spun off the slide.

3. The *optical system* automatically stops the spinning process at a point where the blood cells are beginning to move away from each other but are still close to one another. This system consists of a *light source* (located beneath the catch basin) and an *optical sensor* (located on the cover of the instrument).

4. The *mode switch* turns the instrument off, places it in the manual mode (where the spin time is manually set), automatic mode (optical sensing system determines the spin

time), or test mode (used to test the optical sensing system).

5. The *power light,* when lit, indicates that the instrument is on.

6. The *spin setting knob* is used to alter the spin time.

7. The *spin light* (not shown) is located on the top of the cover and will be lit while the platen is spinning.

PROCEDURE

1. Lift up the lid on the Hemaspinner. Set the mode switch on auto. The spin setting knob should be on 0.

2. Holding the slide at each end, place it in the grooves of the platen. Make certain the slide fits completely within the grooved area of the platen. Failure to do this may result in permanent damage to the instrument.

3. Using a disposable pasteur pipet or plastic straw, place 4 drops of well-mixed whole blood onto the middle of the glass slide. The blood should spread out on the slide to the approximate size of a quarter.

4. Immediately close the top of the Hemaspinner and hold the lid down firmly until the spin light (located on the lid) automatically shuts off.

5. Lift the lid of the Hemaspinner and remove the slide by grasping it at both ends.

6. Allow the slide to air dry before staining.

DISCUSSION

1. To obtain consistently well-prepared smears, it is necessary to keep the Hemaspinner clean at all times.

   a. After every 25 to 30 slides, the catch basin must be removed and washed and the optical system cleaned.

      1) Remove the platen by grasping the center shaft with the fingers and pulling straight up. (Do not lift the platen by the outer edges. This will cause

the platen to bend, causing the slide to fly off the platen during the spin cycle.)

      2) Lift out the catch basin and wash well in running tap water. Dry.

      3) Using a piece of water-dampened lens paper, clean the light source (located under the catch basin). Dry with a second piece of lens paper. Repeat this cleansing procedure for the optical density sensor (located on the inside of the lid).

      4) Replace the catch basin in the Hemaspinner. Holding the platen by the center shaft, slide it firmly onto the shaft of the Hemaspinner.

   b. When making smears, the glass covering of the optical density sensor in the lid may become spattered with blood. When this occurs, clean immediately as outlined above. Any time the glass covering of the light source or sensor becomes dusty or dirty, the spinning time of the Hemaspinner will be affected, and the slides will be incorrectly prepared.

2. The Hemaspinner contains an aerosol removal system. During the spinning process, a positive airflow is created which travels through a duct in the back of the spin chamber and into a submicron filter.

3. The lid gasket should be changed at least once every 3 months, any time that it appears to be damaged, or when improper sealing occurs.

HEMASTAINER AUTOMATIC SLIDE STAINER

The Hemastainer (Fig. 193), manufactured by Geometric Data Corp., is a completely automated slide stainer. In addition, if a mechanical breakdown occurs, the stainer may be operated manually. The

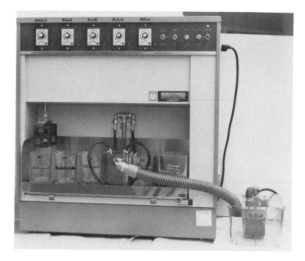

Fig. 193.   Hemastainer automatic slide stainer.

sample slides are placed in a stain rack (slide basket), capable of holding up to 100 slides, and dipped into the staining solutions at timed intervals. Stain station #1 contains methanol for fixing the blood smears. The slides are then transferred to station #2 containing Wright stain, and from there to station #3, which contains a mixture of Wright stain and phosphate buffer (where the major portion of staining occurs). The slides are then rinsed in running, deionized water, followed by a phosphate buffer rinse. The slides are dried by forced warm air at the last station. The entire staining process, including drying, takes approximately 12 minutes from start to finish.

COMPONENTS OF THE HEMASTAINER

1. The *basket hanger* holds the *slide basket* containing the sample slides. For best results, place the slides in every other slot (maximum load then becomes 50 slides).
2. *Stain dishes, #1, #2,* and *#3,* hold methanol, Wright stain, and Wright stain-phosphate buffer mixture, respectively.
3. The *water rinse hoses* carry the deionized water to station #4, the *water rinse tray.*

4. The *drain hose* carries the rinse water back to the recirculating pump tray.
5. *Buffer rinse station.*
6. *Drying station.*
7. *Overflow drain.*
8. The *recirculating pump assembly* pumps the deionized water through the rinse station.
9. The *water inlet hose* carries the water from the pump assembly bath to the water rinse hoses leading into the rinse station.
10. The *pump outlet* supplies electricity to the recirculating pump.
11. The *on/off switch* turns the instrument on and off.
12. The *auto/manual switch,* when set on auto, initiates the automatic stain process. When switched to manual, the stain basket is removed from the drying station and moves to its position above stain station #1.
13. The *right/left switch* moves the stain basket to right or left.
14. The *swing switch* controls the recirculating pump and should be in the auto setting for the automated stain procedure.
15. The *pump switch* controls the recirculating pump and should be in the auto setting for the automated stain procedure.
16. There is one *station timer* for each stain and rinse station. These are used to set the interval of time the slides remain in each station.

AUTOMATED STAINING PROCEDURE

1. Prepare stain stations as follows:

Station	Solution
#1	500 mL of methanol
#2	500 mL of Wright stain (obtain from Geometric Data Corp.)

#3   80 mL of Wright stain plus 420 mL of phosphate buffer (obtain from Geometric Data Corp.)

#4   Place 1 gallon of deionized water into the pump tank and add 200 ml of phosphate buffer

#5   500 mL of phosphate buffer

2. Set the timers as indicated for each station: #1, 10 to 15 seconds; #2, 2 minutes; and #3, 5 minutes; #4, 20 seconds; #5, 1 minute.
3. Turn the power switch to on.
4. Place the freshly prepared blood smears in the staining basket, noting that a small portion of the slide at the top will not be immersed in the stain solution.
5. Attach the slide basket to the basket hanger and tighten the screw.
6. Set the auto/manual switch to manual.
7. Set the right/left switch to the left position.
8. Set the swing switch to on.
9. Set the pump switch to auto.
10. Remove the covers from each stain station. Set the auto/manual switch to auto to begin the staining process. As soon as the stain basket has reached station #3, replace the covers on stations #1 and #2. These two stain stations should remain covered whenever they are not in use to avoid moisture from the air being absorbed by the methanol.
11. A buzzer will sound at the beginning of the drying period. Wait at least 3 minutes after the buzzer sounds and then set the auto/manual switch to manual. The basket will lift out of the drying station and move automatically to the left and remain above the methanol dish.

12. Loosen the hanger screw and remove the slide basket.

MANUAL STAINING PROCEDURE

1. Prepare the reagents in dishes #1, 2, 3, and 4 as outlined above for the automatic procedure. The water rinse in the metal container is eliminated in this method.
2. Place the freshly prepared dry blood smears in the staining basket.
3. Place the rack of blood smears in dish #1 for 2 to 3 seconds. Drain the excess methanol back into the dish by holding the rack against the wall of the dish. Replace the lid on the dish.
4. Place the rack of smears in dish #2 for 2 minutes. Drain the excess stain back into the dish. Replace the lid on the dish.
5. Place the rack of smears in dish #3 for 5 minutes. Do not agitate the rack in the stain. Drain the excess stain back into the dish.
6. Place the rack of smears into dish #4 (phosphate buffer) immediately, using a dipping action. Dip the rack about 20 times (1 minute). (If the slides are left in the buffer too long, the stain will fade.)
7. Allow the slides to air dry.

DISCUSSION

1. The fixative and staining solutions should be replaced and freshly prepared after approximately 300 slides have been stained, or after every 8 to 10 baskets have been processed through the Hemastainer, whichever occurs first.
2. The stain and rinse dishes should be cleaned in methanol before adding fresh stain or rinse solutions.
3. If the stain is too intense (nuclei very dark purple), dilute the Wright's stain in station #2 with methanol.

HEMA-TEK® 1000 SLIDE STAINER

The Hema-Tek® 1000 slide stainer provides a completely automated method for

Wright-staining blood smears. The instrument is able to use 1 × 3 inch or 25 × 75 mm sized slides, which are carried through the staining procedure, face down on a platen (platform), at a rate of 1 slide per minute. After staining and rinsing, the slides are blown dry by a low velocity blower and deposited in the slide drawer at the left side of the instrument.

COMPONENTS OF THE HEMA-TEK® SLIDE STAINER (FIG. 194)

1. The two *conveyor spirals,* which are turned by a *conveyor drive motor,* hold the glass slides in place and move the slides through the staining process.

2. The *platen* is a platform that separates the two conveyor spirals. It supports the slides as they are carried through the staining process and contains three holes through which stain, buffer, and rinse solution are pumped. Grooves located on the platen allow the stain and buffer to mix. A trough along each side of the platen allows for drainage of the used reagents.

3. There are three *volume control knobs* which are used to alter the amount of solution delivered to each slide. To increase the amount delivered, the knob is turned toward the + (clockwise), and to decrease the amount of fluid delivered, the knob is turned toward the − mark (counterclockwise).

4. There are three *solution pumps* located in front of the staining pack inside the instrument. They are attached to the volume control knobs.

5. The *pump tube sets* (3) and *cannulas* (3) are used to transport the solutions from the reagent pack through the reagent pumps, and into the instrument. Each piece of tubing is of a specific length and diameter and contains a cuff situated in such a manner that it rests snugly against the pump. Each tube is coded for its purpose. The #1 tube is for the stain, the #2 tube is for the buffer, and the

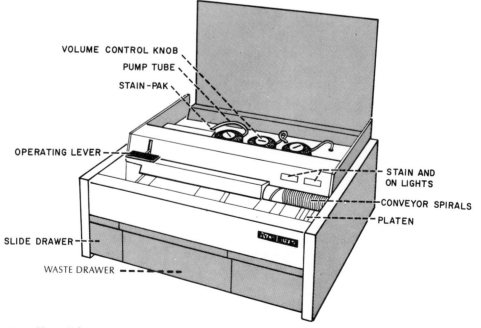

Fig. 194. Hema-Tek® 1000 Slide Stainer.

#3 tube is for the rinse solution. (The tubing sets are available from Ames Division of Miles Lab., Inc., and their distributors as Hema-Tek Pump Tube Set #4482. The cannulas are obtainable as the Hema-Tek Cannula Set #4483.)

6. There are *three sensing switches* located just above the platen, underneath the center enclosed area. When these switches are in the on position, the pumps become activated and pump the solutions up through the platen.

7. The *operating lever* turns the instrument on and off. In addition, when in the third setting, the prime position, all three pumps run continuously.

8. The *stain light,* when on, indicates there is sufficient stain in the *stain pak.* When the amount of stain is sufficient to stain only 20 slides and, therefore needs replacement, the stain light turns off.

9. The *on light* is lit when the stainer is on or in the prime position.

10. The *interlock switch,* located to the right of the volume control knobs, is responsible for shutting off electrical power to the instrument motors and sensing switches when the front panel is removed.

11. The *fuse* is located in the right side of the instrument behind the panel.

12. The *dryer fan* is located behind the right side panel and serves to cool the motors of the instrument and dry the slides.

13. The *slide drawer* holds up to 100 slides and serves to catch them after staining and drying.

14. The *waste drawer* collects all the waste solutions if an outside waste line is not used.

15. There is a *circular level* on the top of the instrument underneath the lid. It is important that the bubble be centered and the instrument level when slides are being stained. The *levelers,* for adjusting the instrument to a level position, are located at the bottom front of each end of the stainer.

16. The *drain spout with plug* is located inside the front of the instrument on the right of the waste tank. It consists of a T shaped tube and has one plug. If the instrument is to drain into an outside bottle or sink, a piece of tubing is attached to the right side, and the left side is closed with the plug. If the waste drawer is to be used to collect the used solutions, the right side of the tube is closed with the plug, and the solutions are allowed to drain directly into the waste drawer.

17. The *Hema-Tek stain pak* (#4481) is designed for use in this slide stainer for the routine Wright staining of blood smears. It consists of prepared stain, buffer, and rinse solutions. It should be placed, in its box, in the back of the stainer, underneath the lid, with the stain on the right side. The appropriate cannulas are then placed in each respective container. The tip of the cannula must be pushed all the way to the bottom of the stain pak. Each time a new stain pak is installed, each container should be vented by opening a hole in the container (with the cannula) about $\frac{1}{4}$ inch from the area where the cannula is installed.

PROCEDURE

1. Make certain all three cannulas are in their respective containers in the stain pak.

2. Using the operating lever, turn the instrument on. Place the operating lever in the prime position until all three solutions emerge through the openings on the platen.

3. Wipe the platen (from right to left) using a piece of gauze. Clean the

platen (by flooding with methanol) in the same manner.

4. Place the slide vertically, on its side, with the smear facing left, into opposing grooves of the conveyor spirals. Make absolutely certain the slide is placed in the grooves exactly opposite one another. If it is not, the slide will break and may damage the instrument. Up to 25 slides may be loaded onto the stainer at any one time. As the conveyor spirals turn, the slide is moved along toward the platen.

5. When it reaches the platform, the conveyor spirals allow the slide to advance to a face down position on the platen. The platen is constructed in such a way that there is a small capillary space between the slide and the platen. As the slide moves along the platform, it triggers the stain-sensing switch when the slide is over or near the stain outlet hole in the platen. The correct amount of stain then fills the space between the slide and the platen. The slide, with the stain, moves along at a specific speed to the buffer sensing switch. The buffer emerges from the outlet hole in the platen and, by means of the grooves in the platen, mixes with the Wright stain under the slide. The slide (with the stain and buffer mixture) moves to the end of the platen, where the stain-buffer mixture is drained.

6. The slide comes in contact with the rinse sensing switch which turns on. The slide is rinsed, dried by a stream of air, and allowed to drop into the slide drawer, where it is ready for examination.

7. After each use, the platen should be cleaned with methanol. Flood the platen with methanol, and, using a soft, clean gauze, wipe the platen from right to left. Care must be taken not to scratch the platen or damage the sensing switches.

MAINTENANCE

1. At least once per day, the stain tubing should be rinsed well in methanol. Prior to performing this procedure, remove the buffer and rinse cannulas from their respective containers.

2. Empty the waste tank at least once per day, or more often, if necessary.

3. The platen troughs should be cleaned at least once per week according to the procedure in the operator's manual.

4. The pump tubing sets should be changed after the use of three stain paks. The tubing attached to the underside of the platen should be changed every ten stain paks. (The underplaten tubing [product code #4484] is available from Ames Division, Miles Laboratories, Inc. and its distributors.)

DISCUSSION

1. If the sensing switches become bent or out of position, refer to the operator's manual for the repositioning procedure.

2. Generally, the best staining results may be obtained using a stain to buffer ratio of 1:2. In some instances a ratio of 1:2.5 or 1:3 is better. A small change in this ratio will lighten or darken the stain. The procedure for calibrating the stain and buffer volumes is outlined very well in the operator's manual.

HEMA-TEK® II SLIDE STAINER

The Hema-Tek® II slide stainer (Fig. 195) is similar to the previously described Hema-Tek® 1000 slide stainer.

To operate the Hema-Tek® II slide stainer, the *power switch* is turned to the on position. The instrument is leveled as indicated by the *leveling bubble*. The stain, buffer, and rinse lines are filled with so-

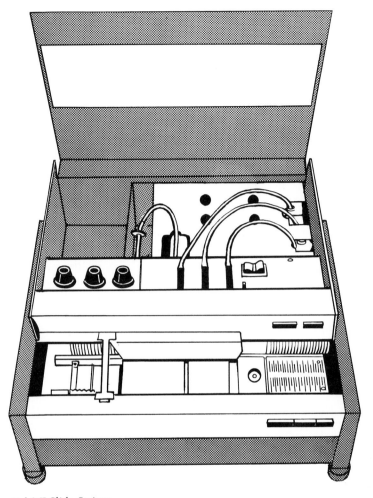

Fig. 195. Hema-Tek® II Slide Stainer.

lution from the *stain pak* by pressing the *prime* rocker switch. (There are four solution lines: one stain line for fixing the blood smear, one stain line which enters the *mixing manifold* [located beneath the platen], one buffer line which also enters the mixing manifold, and a rinse line.) Slides are placed in the stainer, vertically, on their side, with the smear facing left, into opposite grooves of the *conveyor spirals.* The first slide is advanced to a face down position on the *platen.* A *sensing switch* is triggered, and the *stain pump* forces stain from the stain pak through an opening in the platen to fill the small amount of space under the slide. This step primarily fixes the smear. The slide is then advanced to the next station, at which time the major portion of the stain is removed from the slide, draining into a groove in the platen. A solution of approximately 1:4 stain to buffer mixture is forced through the orifice of the platen to fill the space under the slide. (The stain and buffer solutions enter the manifold separately, are mixed, and are then delivered up through the orifice in the platen.) (The stain, buffer, and rinse volumes may be adjusted using the *volume control knobs.*) When the slide reaches the end of the platen, it advances to a point under the *rinse guard* and is lifted to a vertical position. The slide is then flushed with rinse solution from the *rinse bar* and remains in a vertical position for several minutes, during which time it is dried by a stream of warm air. The slide then drops into the *slide drawer.* There are four *indicator lights: power* (a green light indicates the instrument is on), *prime* (a green light indicates the tubing is being primed), *stain* (a red light indicates the stain pak needs to be replaced), and *waste* (a red light indicates the *waste drawer* is full).

HEMATRAK® 590 DIFFERENTIAL COUNTER

Hematrak differential counters, manu-factured by Geometric Data Corporation, were used in the hematology laboratory during the 1970s and 1980s. The company stopped their production in 1986. These counters were probably the most success-ful of the image analyzers produced. A brief summary of the most advanced model is given here, for historic interest.

In the Hematrak® 590 Automated Dif-ferential System (Fig. 196), the identifi-cation of each cell may be broken down into three steps: (1) location of the cell, (2) analysis of the cell, and (3) classification of the cell.

To locate a white blood cell (nucleated cell), a light beam moves back and forth across the microscopic field at minute in-tervals until it detects the nucleus of a cell. When the cell nucleus is detected, an elec-tronic window is placed at that point by the instrument so that the entire cell lies within that window. The spacing between the scanning lines is now decreased.

To analyze the cell, special filters are introduced into the light beam of the elec-tronic window, splitting this light beam into three different colors: red, blue, and green. The information obtained from these three different colors passing through the cell goes to the analog section of the instrument, where it is divided into different density levels. At the lowest den-sity levels, information is obtained about the cytoplasm. The middle density levels give information about the cell nucleus, whereas the highest density levels deal with the darkest portions of the nuclear chromatin. This information is converted to numeric information and stored in the memory circuits. (The use of three colors allows the instrument to detect and handle [within limits] differences in the stain in-tensity that will occur when there is var-iation in the spreading of the cells, as found in a wedge smear versus a spun blood smear.) Measurements of the cell are made by the microprocessors in the com-puter by placing lines or patterns of var-ious lengths and different angles across the cell. These lines are moved across the cell, and the number of times a line falls within the image (of the nucleus, for ex-ample) are counted. The shortest lines generally gather information about the tex-ture of the cell, the medium length lines indicate the nuclear shape, and the long lines give information about the volume of the cytoplasm and the shape of the cell itself. All of this information is gathered within milliseconds and totals millions of bits of data about the cell. These data are then processed into numbers and are used for cell identification. This includes in-formation on the cell size, nuclear shape and chromatin pattern, ratio of nucleus to cytoplasm, granularity and color of cyto-plasm, and presence of nucleoli and vac-uoles.

In classifying the cells, the mathemati-cal parameters now in the computer are compared, in a stepwise fashion, with cell data that have been programmed in the computer memory in a 'logic-tree' manner. Those cells that do not fit into classifica-tion criteria within the computer's mem-ory are remembered by the system and are presented to the operator for identification at the completion of the differential, as suspect cells.

After each cell has been analyzed and classified, the instrument again searches for the next cell. This process is carried

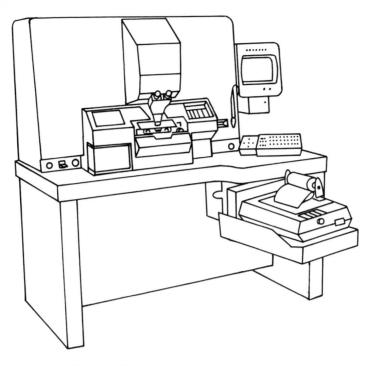

Fig. 196. Hematrak® 590 Differential Counter.

out by the instrument, field by field, until the preselected number of nucleated cells have been analyzed by the instrument. Red blood cells and platelets are processed in essentially the same manner as described for the nucleated cells. The red blood cells are analyzed for size, shape, and hemoglobin density. Platelets are analyzed for nuclear density and size. At the completion of the differential, the cells for review are made available to the operator. After review, the instrument displays a Price-Jones distribution curve (RBC), the differential results, platelet estimate, and limited red cell morphology.

The Hematrak® 590 has walk-away capabilities, an output of 100 samples per hour (without review), and a bar code method of identifying the patient samples. The instrument is also programmed to perform reticulocyte counts.

MODES OF INSTRUMENT OPERATION

The *operator panel* (1) on the *monitor* (2) allows the operator to select several modes of instrument operation.

1. The *Diff* mode is used for automatic differential counting by the instrument.
2. The *Retic* mode is utilized for automatic processing of reticulocyte counts.
3. The *QC* mode is basically divided into two sections: (a) a system test for checking the instrument calibration, and (b) an operating system for performing quality control on blood smears and reticulocyte counts. Up to 200 quality control results per slide may be stored in the computer. These results may be printed at any time on the *auxiliary printer* (3) and may also be printed on Levey-Jennings graphs.
4. The *Teach* mode may be used for teaching and proficiency testing. For teaching, known cells, morphology, and platelet estimates may be entered into the instrument by a technologist, using as many as 100 slides (30 cells/slide). The instrument may

then display the cell under the objective, for viewing by the student, and, at the same time, display the results on the monitor. For programmed instruction, the cell may be shown in the microscopic field and the result not displayed until the student has had two opportunities to correctly identify the cell. In the testing mode, known cells, morphology, and platelet estimates are entered by the instructor. The student then reviews these unknowns and enters the answers. At the completion of the test, both the student's and instructor's answers may be printed by the auxiliary printer.

5. The *ReCell* mode allows the operator to return to specific suspect cells at a later time.

6. The *Specl app* mode allows a laboratory to set the Hematrak system to identify selective cell population subsets, such as animal blood cells.

7. The *STAT* mode allows the operator to halt routine testing, insert a STAT differential, review and obtain the results, and then resume routine testing.

KEYBOARD (4)

The movable keyboard is divided into eight groups of keys which are grouped according to function, and allow the operator to run the instrument, input data, and gain access to numerous software programs.

1. The *stage keys* allow the operator to scan the slide manually. The center stage key, when lit, allows the slide to be moved at a faster rate of speed. The arrow keys move the slide in the directions indicated.

2. The *focus keys* are used by the operator to manually focus the objective when viewing the smear. If the stage key is lit, the up and down focus keys are on coarse adjustment. When the stage key is not lit, the keys

are on fine adjustment. The center, focus, key is used for automatic focusing by the instrument.

3. The *motion and printing keys* have various functions. The *aux print key* allows the operator to print the results, displayed on the monitor, on the auxiliary printer. The *sel dsply key* is used to display results on the monitor. *Stop* allows the operator to halt instrument operation. The *transmit key* is used to transmit results to a host computer, when the instrument is interfaced to a laboratory computer. *Clear stage,* when pressed, removes the slide from the stage. *Rerun* is used to rerun a slide during the review phase of the procedure.

4. The *complete and go keys* are used to indicate the completion of a procedure, and to begin numerous other procedures, respectively.

5. The *RBC and delete keys* allow the operator to manually enter or delete red blood cell morphology and to quantitate red and white cell morphology.

6. The *WBC, NRBC, and platelet keys* permit the operator to enter white cell morphology, reclassify cells, and change the platelet estimate during the review procedure.

7. The *function keys* allow the operator to gain access to various functions of the instrument.

   a. The *sel funct key* is a directory to the numerous functions: enter bar codes; removal of results from the computer; check certain operations of the instrument; troubleshoot some instrument problems; print final results on the auxiliary printer after review; use of a color monitor; allow the operator to pump oil through the supply line; verify proper functioning of the bar code reader *(wand)*; set various options, such as review criteria; set the levels of red cell morphology; set review criteria for WBC and NRBC; permanently record the options; set the method of result transmission to a host computer; restore previously used options which have been changed; and load the software program into the instrument computer.

b. The *store cell key* allows the operator the means for storing the location of a cell in the instrument's memory for future recall.

c. The *rev data key* may be used to examine results of previously run slides.

d. The *ID key* is used to enter the operator ID, date, and sample numbers.

e. The *help key* is used to obtain a display of instrument operating instructions.

f. The *comnt code key* is utilized in conjunction with a host computer, and is used to enter morphology codes not present on the Hematrak keyboard.

8. The *numeric keys* are used to enter information into the instrument. The *enter* and *delete* keys add or remove numeric information, respectively.

COULTER ZETAFUGE®

The zeta sedimentation ratio (ZSR) is determined by use of the Coulter Zetafuge™ (Fig. 197) and is a measurement similar to the erythrocyte sedimentation rate.

Normally, red blood cells are negatively charged and repel each other. In the presence of an increased concentration of fibrinogen and/or gamma globulin, the net negative charge of the erythrocytes decreases, thus permitting an increase in rouleaux formation and a more rapid erythrocyte sedimentation rate.

In the ZSR procedure, a small amount of blood is placed in a capillary tube that is then situated in a vertical position in the Zetafuge. When the Zetafuge is turned on, it revolves at a constant low speed for 45 seconds. During this time, the centrifugal force applied to the tube forces the red blood cells to migrate across the diameter of the tube to the outer wall, where rouleaux formation is speeded up. At the conclusion of the first 45 seconds, the Zetafuge stops and automatically rotates the capillary tube 180°. The Zetafuge restarts, and spins the tube for a second 45-second period. During this time, the rouleaux formation (now on the inner wall) partially disperses, moves across the diameter of the tube, and reforms on the outer wall. The Zetafuge stops and rotates the tubes 180° a second and third time, thus allowing four 45-second centrifuge periods. Each time the rouleaux formation moves across the diameter of the tube, it sediments toward the bottom due to the downward force of gravity on the rouleauxed erythrocytes. After centrifugation, the percent of space occupied by the fallen red blood cells is measured. The ZSR, therefore, measures how close the red blood cells approach one another under a specific standardized stress. The packing of the red blood cells depends on their net negative charge, which, in turn, depends primarily on the concentration of fibrinogen and gamma globulin.

The ZSR takes approximately 4 minutes to perform and is unaffected by anemia. The normal range for the ZSR is 40 to 51% and is the same for both males and females. Values of 51 to 54% are considered to be borderline; 55 to 59%, mildly elevated; 60 to 64%, moderately elevated; and greater than 65%, markedly elevated.

PROCEDURE

1. Using EDTA anticoagulated whole blood, fill one tube ¾ full for each patient to be tested. (Each tube should be 75 mm long, with an outer diameter of 2.3 mm and an inner diameter of 2.0 mm. These tubes are

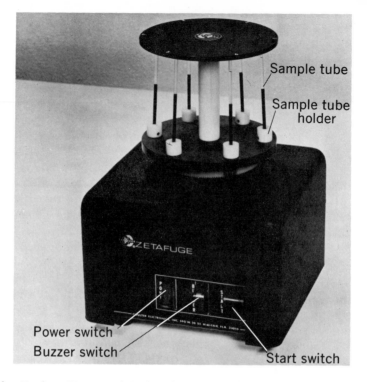

Fig. 197. Coulter Zetafuge. (Courtesy of Coulter Electronics, Inc., Hialeah, Florida.)

obtainable from Coulter Diagnostics, Inc.)

2. Plug one end of each tube with clay to a depth of approximately 5 mm.

3. Immediately place the tubes into the sample tube holder (as shown in Figure 197). The tubes must be placed in the Zetafuge so that the instrument is balanced.

4. Push the *power switch* to the on position (the switch should light up, indicating that the power is on).

5. Push the *buzzer switch* up to the on position (the switch should light up). (The use of the buzzer is optional, but it warns the operator when the Zetafuge has completed its 3-minute spin cycle.)

6. Depress the *start switch* to begin the spinning cycle. Note the speed indicator, which should move to a horizontal position when the sample holder plate is spinning at full speed.

7. When the buzzer sounds, turn the buzzer switch off.

8. Immediately remove the tubes and read, or place a mark on each tube indicating the level of the sedimented red blood cells. The level to be read is termed the *knee* of the curve (Fig. 198) and indicates the

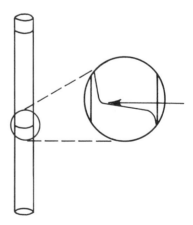

Fig. 198. Sedimented level of red blood cells.

percentage of the blood that is sedimented red blood cells (also termed *Zetacrit* %). An accessory measuring device is available from Coulter Diagnostics, Inc., or if the level is marked, a hematocrit reader is satisfactory for this reading.

9. Perform a microhematocrit and determine each patient's hematocrit in percent.

10. The zeta sedimentation ratio (ZSR) is then determined by comparing the Zetacrit % to the hematocrit %, as shown below.

$$\text{ZSR \%} = \frac{\text{Hematocrit \%}}{\text{Zetacrit \%}} \times 100$$

DISCUSSION

1. At least once/day, check that the mechanism which rotates the tubes 180° is operating satisfactorily. During a complete spin cycle of the instrument, observe the indicator on one of the sample tube holders. This indicator should be pointed alternately in and out during the four-spin cycles.

FIBROSYSTEM® (FIBROMETER®)

The FibroSystem® is a semiautomated electro-mechanical instrument for performing coagulation procedures. It consists of the Fibrometer® coagulation timer, the thermal prep block (incubator), and an automatic pipet for dispensing 0.1 and 0.2 mL amounts of fluid. The instrument is obtainable from BBL Microbiology Systems, Division of Becton Dickinson and Co. The thermal prep block and the automatic pipet are not an absolute requirement for use with the Fibrometer unit, but they are useful when a moderate number of coagulation studies are to be performed. Most coagulation procedures which use a clot as their end point, may be performed on this system.

FIBROMETER (FIG. 199)

1. The *on-off switch* turns the unit on and off.

2. The *indicator light,* when lit, indicates the unit has reached 37.2°C (± 0.5°C).

3. The *digital readout* displays the clotting time to tenths of a second.

4. Depressing the *readout reset button* returns the readout to 000.0.

5. There are six shallow *warming wells* for prewarming reagent or sample.

6. The shallow *reaction well* holds the sample mixture during testing.

7. The *probe arm* contains the electrodes *(moving electrode* and *stationary electrode)* used for clot detection. During testing, the moving electrode cycles through the mixture. The stationary electrode does not move, but functions with the moving electrode to complete the electrical circuit when a clot is formed.

8. The moving electrode is an extension of the *probe foot,* which extends from the base of the probe.

9. The *timer bar* is used to manually begin timing when the automatic pipet is not used.

10. The automatic pipet is attached to the unit via the *plug-in jack outlet.*

11. The line cord is attached to the *power connection* and then plugged into the wall receptacle.

THERMAL PREP BLOCK (FIG. 200)

1. The *on-off switch* is used to turn the heating unit on and off.

2. The *indicator lamp* goes on and off, depending on the heat demand. When the unit is at 37.2°C (± 0.5°C) and ready for use, the lamp is not lit.

3. The *shallow wells* hold the disposable Fibrotube® plastic *coagulation cups* containing sample and/or reagent for prewarming to 37°C.

4. *Plastic trays* allow the disposable cups to fit snugly into the shallow wells.

5. The *deep wells* hold test tubes (12 or 13 mm × 75 mm) for prewarming of the reagent or sample to 37°C.

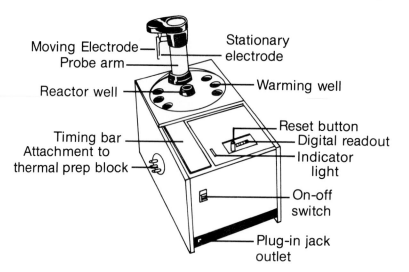

Fig. 199.   Fibrometer®.

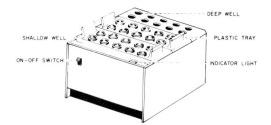

Fig. 200.   Thermal prep block.

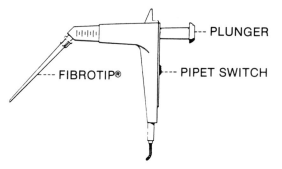

Fig. 201.   Automatic pipet.

AUTOMATIC PIPET (FIG. 201)

1. The *plug* fits into the plug-in jack outlet on the Fibrometer.
2. The *FibroTip®* is a disposable pipet tip which fits into the hole in the forward end of the automatic pipet.
3. The *plunger,* when depressed, dis-

penses liquid present in the attached FibroTip. As the plunger is allowed to retract, any solution in which the FibroTip rests is drawn up into the pipet tip.

4. The *pipet switch* turns the automatic pipet on and off. When the switch is on, and the pipet is plugged into the Fibrometer, the instant the last bit of liquid is dispensed from the pipet tip, the clot detecting mechanism and timer are turned on.
5. To adjust the volume of sample pick up and delivery, there are two *calibration marks* on the end of the plunger. To set the pipet for 0.1 mL volumes, place the pipet switch off, depress the plunger completely, and turn the plunger so as to line the single notch up with the *alignment indicator* on the pipet. The two notches on the opposite side of the plunger are used to set the pipet for 0.2 mL volumes.

PRINCIPLES OF OPERATION
(FIGS. 202 AND 203)

A disposable coagulation cup, containing the reagent (or sample), is placed in the reaction well. As soon as the sample

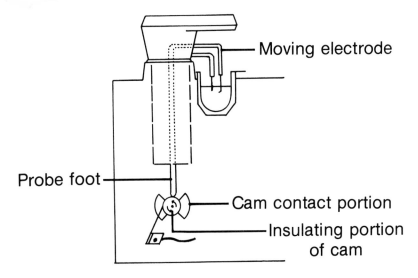

Fig. 202. Probe arm position during sample testing (Fibrometer).

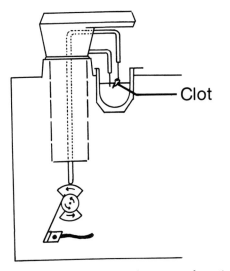

Fig. 203. Probe arm position during sample testing (Fibrometer).

(or reagent) is added to the cup, the timing mechanism of the Fibrometer is activated (via the automatic pipet, or depressing the timer bar). Within 0.5 to 1.8 seconds of instrument activation, the probe arm drops down, placing the electrodes into the reaction mixture. During testing, the probe foot rests on a segmented *cam* in the bottom of the Fibrometer. This cam is constantly rotating when the Fibrometer is activated. As it rotates, it moves the probe foot up and down, causing the moving electrode to sweep through, up, and out of the mixture every 0.5 second, in an elliptical pattern. Due to the design of the cam, when the moving electrode is in the down position (Fig. 202) (immersed in the sample mixture), the probe foot is resting on the insulated portion of the cam and there is no electric current passing to the probe. When the cam rotates, and the probe foot comes in contact with the electrically active portion of the cam (Fig. 203), the electric current is passed through the probe foot to the moving electrode. At the same time, due to the shape of the cam, the probe foot is forced upward, causing the moving electrode to move up and out of the sample mixture. When a clot forms, it is caught by the small hook on the moving electrode. As the moving electrode moves out of the liquid to the up position, the electric current passes from the cam to the moving electrode and simultaneously to the attached clot, through the clot, and into the liquid in which the clot is partially immersed. The electric current passes to the stationary electrode and the circuit is complete, stopping the timing mechanism.

PROCEDURE FOR THE PROTHROMBIN TIME

The prothrombin time procedure, using the Fibrometer, is basically the same as for the manual method previously described. Therefore, the procedure, as outlined here describes the various techniques needed to operate the Fibrometer, thermal prep block, and the automatic pipet.

1. Turn the Fibrometer and thermal prep block on and allow the units to warm to 37°C (about 15 minutes). When the Fibrometer reaches the proper temperature, the indicator light remains on as long as the instrument is at 37.2°C ($\pm$0.5°C). The indicator light on the thermal prep block turns off as soon as it reaches the proper temperature.

2. When the units are at 37°C, place the appropriate number of disposable coagulation cups in the plastic tray over the shallow heating wells in the thermal prep block.

3. Place approximately 0.5 mL of the control and patient plasma specimens in labeled, 12 × 75 mm test tubes. Allow samples to prewarm in the deep wells of the thermal prep block until they reach 37°C (3 to 5 minutes).

4. Insert a disposable FibroTip in the automatic pipet. Make certain the pipet tip fits tightly into the automatic pipet. (The pipet should be plugged into the Fibrometer and the pipet switch must be in the off position.)

5. Turn the plunger of the pipet to the 0.2-mL setting.

6. Completely depress the plunger of the pipet and place the FibroTip into a solution of well-mixed thromboplastin-calcium reagent. Allow the plunger to retract completely.

7. Place the side of the FibroTip (near the end), on the inside top edge of the coagulation cup (in the thermal prep block), so that the tip of the pipet does not touch the inside wall of the cup.

8. Depress the plunger, expelling the 0.2 mL of thromboplastin-calcium reagent into the bottom of the coagulation cup.

9. Add 0.2 mL of reagent to the appropriate number of coagulation cups. Allow to incubate until the reagent has reached 37°C (3 to 5 minutes).

10. Place one of the coagulation cups containing (prewarmed) reagent into the reaction well.

11. Turn the plunger of the automatic pipet to the 0.1 mL setting (pipet switch off). Insert a disposable FibroTip into the forward end of the automatic pipet. Completely depress the plunger of the pipet and draw up 0.1 mL of prewarmed sample.

12. Change the pipet switch to the on position.

13. Dispense the sample into the coagulation cup in the reaction well. As the plunger is depressed, the timing mechanism automatically begins. As soon as a clot forms in the mixture, the electrode action and timing mechanism stop.

14. Record the prothrombin time, as displayed on the digital readout.

15. Lift the probe arm up to its resting position, and with a clean, lint-free cloth, carefully wipe the electrodes. Depress the reset button to set the timer at 000.0

16. All testing should be performed in duplicate, and the results should check within 0.5 seconds of each other. If a prothrombin time is above 30 seconds, a wider range of variability is acceptable.

DISCUSSION

1. When the moving electrode is in the up position, during testing, it should be 1.27 mm above the liquid level in the cup. The level of the liquid in the disposable cup is critical. If the liquid level is too high (or the electrodes too long), the moving electrode will

never leave the liquid when it is in its up position, the electric circuit will automatically be complete within the first 2 to 3 seconds of starting and the timer will stop. (The electric current will pass from the activated moving electrode, through the mixture, to the stationary electrode.) Conversely, if the liquid level is too low (or the electrodes too short), when the clot forms, it will not be detected because the clot will not remain in contact with the mixture when attached to the moving electrode in its up position (carrying an electric charge).

2. The electrodes must be kept free of lint and debris to eliminate falsely shortened results. They may be cleaned using distilled water or a solution of 1% phosphoric acid followed by a thorough rinsing with distilled water (the use of acids may pit the electrodes). It is advisable to remove the probe and dip the electrodes into the acid solution. Rinse with distilled water and wipe dry with lint-free tissue or paper.

3. If the automatic pipet is not used, the timer bar should be pressed at the same instant that the sample or reagent is added to the cup in the reaction well.

4. The disposable plastic FibroTip should only be used one time. However, when pipetting the same reagent, the same tip may be used, but should be tightened periodically so that it does not come loose from the pipet.

5. If the timing mechanism is started inadvertently, turn the on-off switch on the Fibrometer to off. Turn the unit back on, replace the probe arm in its resting position, and reset the digital readout.

6. The probe arm on the Fibrometer is specifically designed for testing a certain volume of solution. Two probe arms are available: one for testing a final volume of 0.3 mL, and a second for testing 0.4 mL volumes.

7. When using the automatic pipet, develop the habit of moving the pipet switch to off as soon as the plasma has been pipetted and the Fibrometer activated.

8. After the plunger on the automatic pipet is depressed, a small amount of solution will remain in the FibroTip. This is acceptable and has been allowed for in the calibration of the pipet.

9. The stationary and moving electrodes must be in a position parallel to one another. If they become bent, they may carefully be realigned.

10. If the Fibrometer does not appear to be detecting a clot, fill a coagulation cup with 0.5 mL of reagent. Press the timer bar. Due to excess liquid in the cup, the Fibrometer should stop within 0.5 second of when the probe unit drops to the down position. If it does not, check the cam (beneath the probe) for dirt. This area may be carefully cleaned with a cotton-tipped applicator immersed in 70% isopropyl alcohol. Another cause of this problem may be a shortened moving electrode. This electrode may be lengthened a short amount by carefully pushing the probe foot up slightly. (See operator's manual.)

11. If the Fibrometer stops within 0.5 to 3.0 seconds after the probe drops down, the moving electrode may be too long. Place 0.3 mL of reagent into a coagulation cup. Press the timer bar. If the moving electrode is too long, the Fibrometer will stop as soon as the probe drops down. The probe may be shortened by carefully pulling down on the probe foot (see operator's manual).

COAG-A-MATE 2001

The Coag-A-Mate 2001 (Fig. 204) is able to perform up to 12 PTs or 12 APTTs si-

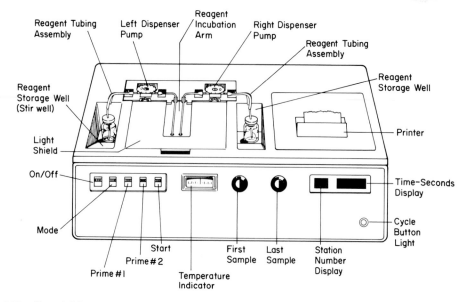

Fig. 204.   Coag-A-Mate 2001.

multaneously. A single light source is divided into 12 channels, each of which passes through the sample to its own corresponding sensor. The change in the optical density of each sample as it clots is detected by the corresponding sensor. This information is stored until all test samples have clotted, and the results for that run of tests are then printed out on printer paper.

The Coag-A-Mate 2001 is turned on by means of the *on/off switch* and is ready for testing when the *temperature indicator* reads 37°C (±1°C). By use of the *mode switch,* either PT or APTT is selected, depending on which test is to be run. The *reagent dispenser pumps* will then be set to deliver the correct reagent volumes. The rear panel of the instrument contains a *PT cycle switch* to select sequential testing or simultaneous testing. Also located in this area is the *APTT activation time switch* for setting the activation time at 180, 240, or 300 seconds. The reagents for either the PT or APTT test are placed in the *reagent storage wells,* and the *tubing assemblies* are placed into the reagent vials, fitted into the *reagent incubation arm,* and the tubing

nozzles are put into place. *Prime #1* and *prime #2 switches* are depressed to activate the left and right *dispenser pumps,* respectively, to fill the tubing with reagent. Plasma samples are pipetted (0.1 mL) into the *circular test tray,* which is then placed onto the *incubation test plate* (beneath the *light shield* containing the incubation arm). The *first sample* and *last sample switches* are set to tell the instrument where to begin and end testing. The light shield is kept closed during testing. The test cycle is begun by depressing the *start switch,* at which point the electronic timing mechanism is activated. As each plasma sample clots, or maximum time has occurred, the *station number display* indicates the sample number, and the clotting time is displayed on the *time-seconds display.* If maximum time has occurred before clotting, UU.U will be displayed, and the test should be repeated by another method. When all testing is complete, the *cycle-button/light* will be lit, and the *print module* will print out the sample results with the corresponding cuvet number. Those samples which did not clot will be indicated by - -.- on the printer tape. The circular test tray should then be removed, and the instrument is ready for further testing.

COAG-A-MATE DUAL CHANNEL ANALYZER

The Coag-A-Mate dual channel automated coagulation analyzer (Fig. 205) detects clot formation by means of a photocell sensing circuit that reads the optical density change when a clot is formed. This instrument automatically pipets all reagents necessary for testing and is capable of performing PT and APTT test procedures simultaneously. Plasma specimens to be tested are pipetted into small cuvets in a circular test tray and placed on the instrument in the incubation test plate, which cools the samples prior to testing. When the instrument is activated, the test plate revolves, carrying the test samples through a heating zone, where they are warmed to 37°C prior to testing. When the

first two samples arrive at the test station, the reagent is automatically pipetted into each of two cuvets, and the timing mechanisms are started. (If two reagents are required for the test, such as in the APTT, the first reagent is added to each cuvet prior to its arrival at the test station.) When fibrin formation occurs, the photoelectric cell detects the sudden change in optical density, and the timing mechanism is automatically stopped. The clotting time is printed out on the printer tape to the closest tenth of a second. When both test samples have clotted, the test tray is ready to rotate to the next two test samples. The time elapse between clot formation and the beginning of the next two tests depends on the cycle time mode that has been selected by the operator.

The Coag-A-Mate dual channel analyzer is capable of performing the majority of coagulation procedures, most notably the PT, APTT, and factor assays.

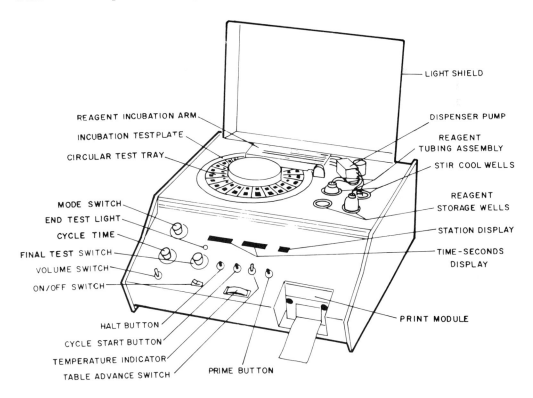

Fig. 205. Coag-A-Mate dual channel analyzer.

COMPONENTS OF THE COAG-A-MATE DUAL CHANNEL ANALYZER (FIG. 205)

1. *Reagent storage wells* (2) provide reagent storage at room temperature.
2. *Stir cool wells* (2) provide low temperature reagent storage and magnetic stirrers for constant mixing of the reagents.
3. The *reagent tubing assembly* is color coded and delivers the reagents from the reagent vials to the test cuvet.
4. The *reagent dispenser pump* is responsible for delivering the exact amount of reagent to the test cuvet.
5. The *reagent incubation arm* warms the reagents (contained in the tubing) to 37°C prior to delivery into the test cuvet.
6. The *incubation test plate* has a blue area where the plasma samples are cooled and a red area in which the plasma samples are warmed to 37°C.
7. The *circular test tray* is a disposable plastic tray that sits on the incubation test plate. It is capable of holding 48 plasma samples.
8. The *mode switch* is utilized for selecting the test procedure desired: PT, APTT, or PT and APTT. The mode setting also determines the delay time which begins when the reagent is added to the test cuvet. During the delay period, the instrument does not respond to optical density changes, in case bubbles were briefly formed when the reagent was added to the test cuvet. The delay time in the PT mode is 8 seconds, and 20 seconds in the APTT mode.
9. The *end test light* is lit, and an audible beep is given at the completion of the final test.
10. The *cycle time* allows the operator to choose the amount of time between tests. In the settings of 50, 110, 150, 240, or 300 seconds, the instrument automatically moves forward to the next test sample at the time set, irrespective of clot formation. In the demand setting, in the PT mode, the instrument will automatically index to the next sample in 30 to 150 seconds, depending on clot formation. In the APTT mode, indexing to the next sample occurs between 110 and 300 seconds, again depending on the time of clot formation.
11. The *final test switch* should be set at the test station which contains the last sample to be tested.
12. The *volume toggle switch* determines the volume of reagent to be dispensed by the pump.
13. The *on/off switch* turns the instrument on and off.
14. The *halt button,* when pressed, terminates the test cycle and returns the timers to 000.0.
15. The *cycle start button* reactivates the test cycle when it has been stopped.
16. The *table advance toggle switch* advances the circular test tray automatically (when the switch is up) or manually one station at a time (when the switch is down).
17. The *temperature indicator* shows the temperature in the test station by indirect measurement.
18. The *prime button* activates the pump for priming (filling) the reagent tubing.
19. The *print module* records the test cuvet number, the test, and the clotting time for each test sample.
20. The *time-seconds displays* (2) show the elapsed time to the tenths of a second for the inner and outer test samples.
21. The *station display* indicates the cuvet number currently in the test station.
22. The *decimal point temperature indicator* in the time-seconds display, when lit, indicates that the red area of the incubation test plate is at the proper operating temperature.
23. The *light shield* should be in the down position during testing to de-

crease interfering light, dust, and air circulation.

24. Located on the rear of the instrument are fans, jacks for connecting a chart recorder and a pump, the fuse, and the circuit board cover panel.

DISCUSSION

1. Erratic results may be due to one of several causes: (a) reagents, (b) improper sample collection, (c) dirty, twisted, or improperly seated reagent tubing, (d) jerky pump operation (pump tubing may need lubrication), (e) delivery tip dirty or in wrong position, or (f) mode switch in wrong position.

2. If the instrument does not become activated when it is turned on, the fuse may need to be replaced.

3. Reagent should not remain in the reagent tubing for more than 30 minutes after testing has been completed. Remove the reagent and clean the tubing by alternately drawing distilled water and air through the lines using the prime button. Remove the tubing assembly from the pump if the instrument is not to be used right away. See the instrument's operations manual for directions on removing and replacing the tubing.

4. Depending on usage, the rotor should be removed from the pump and cleaned with isopropanol on a scheduled basis. Instructions for this procedure may be found in the operations manual.

5. The reaction temperatures should be checked routinely. The reagent delivery volume should also be checked on a scheduled basis. Instructions for these procedures and the necessary adjustments are clearly outlined in the operations manual.

COAG-A-MATE·X2

The Coag-A-Mate·X2 coagulation instrument detects clot formation by means of a photocell sensing circuit that reads the optical density change when a clot is formed. The instrument automatically pipets all necessary reagents for testing and will perform two tests simultaneously: two different tests or two like tests in duplicate, or, four like tests performed singularly. The plasma samples to be tested are pipetted into small cuvets in a circular test tray and placed on the instrument in the incubation test plate, which cools the patient samples prior to testing. When the instrument is activated, the test plate revolves, carrying the test samples through a heating zone, where they are warmed to 37°C for a preset time period prior to and during testing. When the first four samples arrive at the test station, the correct amount of reagent is automatically pipetted into each of the four cuvets, and the timing mechanisms are started. (If two reagents are required for the test, as in the APTT, the first reagent is added to each cuvet at a set time interval prior to its arrival at the test station.) When fibrin formation occurs, the photoelectric cell detects the sudden change in optical density, and the timing mechanism is automatically stopped. The clotting time is printed out on the printer tape to the closest tenth of a second. After a preset period of time, the test tray rotates to the next four plasma samples. The circular test tray, carrying the patient samples, is rotated on the incubation test plate at a set rate and is not affected by the clotting time of the patient samples. This timing mechanism is alterable by the operator.

The Coag-A-Mate·X2 is capable of performing the majority of coagulation procedures. The procedure for simultaneously performing PTs and APTTs in duplicate is described on the following pages.

COMPONENTS OF THE COAG-A-MATE·X2 (FIG. 206)

1. The *light shield,* placed in the down

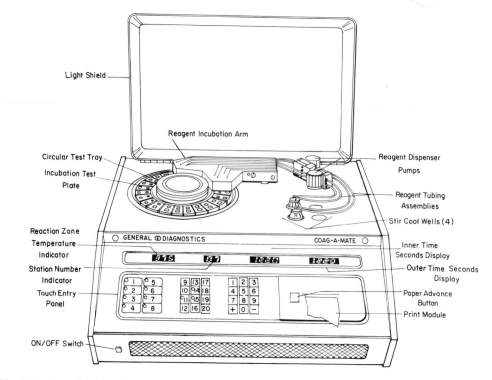

Fig. 206. Coag-A-Mate · X2.

position, decreases interfering light, dust, and air circulation.

2. The *circular test tray* is a disposable plastic tray that sits on the incubation test plate and is capable of holding 48 plasma samples to be incubated and tested.

3. The *incubation test plate* contains a cooled zone for storage of samples prior to testing and a heated zone in the test area that warms the plasma samples to 37°C.

4. The *on/off switch* turns the instrument on or off.

5. The *paper advance keypad* is used to advance the paper tape.

6. The *print module* records on paper tape the maximum and minimum incubation times, the blank time (time period at the beginning of the test where no clot is detected), the reagent volume, instrument sensitivity, temperature of the testing area, date, cuvet number of sample, name

of test, clotting time and the last cuvet for testing that has been selected by the operator.

7. The *stir cool wells* (4) provide low temperature reagent storage and magnetic stirrers for constant mixing of the reagents.

8. The *reagent tubing assemblies* are color-coded, inert tubing that have pick-up and delivery tips for transporting the reagent from the reagent vials to the test cuvet.

9. The *reagent dispenser pumps* (2) deliver the exact amount of reagent to the test cuvet.

10. The *reagent incubation arm* warms the reagents (contained in the tubing) to 37°C prior to being delivered into the test cuvet.

11. *Lighted displays*
    a. The *reaction zone temperature indicator* displays the temperature in the testing area. It should be 37°C (±0.5°C). When the in-

strument is first turned on, NOT READY will be displayed until the instrument reaches 37°C (±0.5°C), at which time READY will be displayed. During testing, BUSY will be illuminated.

b. The *station number indicator,* during testing, displays the two cuvet numbers which are in the test station by alternating back and forth between the two numbers. When the end test key (see #12 below, Touch Entry Panel) is pressed, END TEST is displayed. The sensitivity of the clot detection system, which may be set from 1 to 9 as required, may also be displayed on this indicator. The date (month/day/year) is displayed when entered into the instrument.

c. The *inner time seconds display* indicates the elapsed time during testing for the two samples in the inner channel on the circular test tray. The display moves back and forth between the two samples. This indicator is also used to display the volumes delivered by both reagent dispenser pumps. *Power* is displayed alongside of the inner channel when the instrument is on.

d. The *outer time seconds display* indicates the elapsed time during testing for the two samples in the outer channel on the circular test tray. The display moves back and forth between the two samples. This display also indicates the blank time, at the end of which the instrument will begin to monitor clot formation. Minimum and maximum times will be displayed here, indicating the shortest and longest times the optical sensor will monitor the clot before moving to the next test station.

12. The *touch entry panel* keys are activated by gently pressing them.

a. *PT* (1) selects the prothrombin time mode.

b. *APTT* (2) selects the activated partial thromboplastin time mode.

c. *PT/APTT* (3) allows the operator to run PTs in the inner channel and APTTs in the outer channel simultaneously.

d. *Fibrinogen* (4) selects the quantitative fibrinogen mode.

e. *TT* (5) selects the thrombin time mode.

f. *Two-stage FA* (6) is for a two-stage factor assay mode.

g. *Special* (7) mode is for custom programming of individual systems.

h. *Modify test* (8) is used to change the standard parameters of test modes.

i. *Prime 1* (9) and *prime 2* (10) are used to fill the reagent tubing associated with the respective reagent pump.

j. When pressed, *deprime* (11) results in the reagents in the reagent lines being returned to the reagent vials. To deprime the reagent lines as soon as the last reagent has been dispensed, press *enter* (20), deprime, and enter. To deprime the reagent tubing in 0.005 mL increments during calibration, pressing deprime will cause the pump that was last primed to deprime 0.005 mL at a time. To return all reagents to reagent vials, press *cancel* (18) and then deprime.

k. *Sensitivity* (12) is used to adjust the sensitivity of the photo optical system.

l. *End test* (13) indicates the last cuvet sample that will be tested by the instrument. This is preset at cuvet 24 unless otherwise set by the operator before each instrument run.

m. *Pause* (14) may be depressed to momentarily interrupt the test cycle. All tests to which reagents have been added, however, will continue to be tested until completion before the instrument stops. When the instrument pauses, an audible beep will sound at intervals until start has been pressed.

n. *Recall* (15) may be used to obtain reprints of the previous test run, as long as the instrument has not been turned off or another test cycle started.

o. *Date* (16) is used to enter the month, day, and year.

p. *Start* (17) is pressed to begin the test cycle.

q. *Cancel* (18) is used to stop the instrument immediately. Any tests in progress will be lost.

r. *Index* (19) advances the circular test tray one station at a time.

s. *Enter* (20) is used to enter all program changes into the microprocessor.

t. *Numbers 1* through *9* (right side of the touch entry panel) are used to enter information into the computer.

u. +, − are used in conjunction with the modify test key or the sensitivity key to add or subtract.

13. Located on the rear of the instrument are the circuit board cover and a circuit breaker.

PROCEDURE FOR THE SIMULTANEOUS PERFORMANCE OF THE PT AND APPT

1. Press the rocker switch to turn the instrument on. NOT READY will be displayed, indicating that the instrument temperature has not reached 37°C ($\pm$0.5°C). When the proper temperature has been reached, READY will be displayed. (The instrument cannot be used for testing as long as NOT READY is displayed.)

2. Press the PT/APTT key on the touch entry panel (the light on the key should illuminate). Enter the date: Press date, press a two-digit number for the month, the day, and the year, pressing enter after each entry.

3. Place the reagent vials in the stir cool wells: One bottle each of thromboplastin, activated partial thromboplastin, and 0.025 M calcium chloride. Add a clean magnetic stir bar to the thromboplastin and the partial thromboplastin (as recommended by manufacturer). On each vial, place a cap containing an appropriate opening for the reagent lines.

4. Install reagent lines if not in place, using the information given in Table 19.

   a. Insert the appropriate delivery tip into the corresponding hole on the reagent incubation arm, pushing the delivery tip well into the hole until it extends $\frac{1}{16}$ inch below the opening. Without stretching the tubing, firmly press each piece into the appropriate groove of the arm, working from the delivery tip to the base of the arm.

   b. Lightly lubricate each piece of tubing between the collars. Using both hands, grasp both collars on the piece of tubing and stretch tubing around the front of the pump rotor. Slide the tubing into the slot on either side of the stator and position the tubing in the appropriate notch. Both collars should fit firmly on either side of the pump area. Depress the appropriate prime (one or two) button to ensure proper seating of the tubing around the pump.

   c. Install the pick up tips into the appropriate reagent vials, making certain they are inserted to the bottom of the reagent vials.

TABLE 19.   PLACEMENT OF REAGENT TUBING FOR THE COAG-A-MATE · X2
(FOR PT AND APTT TESTING)

INCUBATION ARM SLOT	TUBING	REAGENT	PUMP #	PUMP SLOT #
D and E	Red collar (2)	Thromboplastin	2	6 and 7
F	Clear collar	Calcium chloride	2	8
B	Blue collar	Partial thromboplastin	1	3

5. Prime the pumps to fill the reagent lines. Carefully lift the reagent incubation arm to a 45° angle. Hold a petri dish under lines D, E, and F. Depress and hold prime two button on the touch entry panel until all three reagents are expelled from the lines in a steady stream. Repeat, priming line B using the prime one button.

6. Pipet 0.1 mL of patient and control plasmas into the appropriate cuvets. Plasma samples for APTT must be placed into the cuvet in the outer channel of the test plate. PT test samples should be added to the inner channel of cuvets.

7. Carefully position the tray on the incubation test plate, matching the notch in the tray with the notch in the hub. Lower the reagent incubation arm so that it is as far down as possible (in a horizontal position).

8. Lower the light shield, making certain that all tubing is completely under the shield. The light shield must be down at all times while the instrument is testing (the busy light will be displayed).

9. Make certain the station number, as indicated on the control panel, corresponds to the cuvet number containing the first sample to be tested. If a different number appears in the station number window, press and hold the index key until the station number corresponds to the first sample.

10. Set the end test station (last cuvet containing a test sample). Press end

test, press the two digit number of the last cuvet, and press enter.

11. Press start to begin testing. Check the printout that is given at this time for the following information: End test station, reaction zone temperature, sensitivity, pumps #1 and #2 volumes, blank time (PT and APTT), and minimum and maximum times.

12. During testing, the control panel will show the following: Busy light illuminated, the station number display will shift back and forth between the two cuvet numbers currently at the test stations, the inner channel seconds display will shift back and forth showing the time elapsed or clotting times of the PTs being tested or just completed, and the outer channel seconds display shows the same information for the APTTs.

13. At the completion of testing, the instrument will beep, the busy light will go out, and READY will be illuminated. The station display will show the next cuvet number the instrument will begin on. At the completion of testing, raise the light shield and the reagent incubation arm. Carefully remove the test tray. If the inner and outer channels still have empty cuvets, the tray may be used again. Remove reagents from the reagent lines by pressing deprime and then enter (deprime should remain lit).

DISCUSSION

1. During the test cycle, only the on/off,

pause, and cancel buttons may be activated.

2. To add more test samples during a run, press the pause key. All tests that have begun will be completed before the instrument will stop. Therefore, once the pause key is pressed, there will be a wait of 6 to 8 minutes before the instrument stops testing (APTT reagent is added to plasma about 5 minutes prior to testing). When the instrument stops, it will beep at intervals, signaling that the light shield may be raised and test samples added. After adding more test samples: (a) prime pumps #1 and #2 (if necessary), (b) lower the light shield, (c) set the end test station, (d) press start, and (e) check the printer tape statistics. The instrument will automatically index to the next test station.

3. To stop instrument testing immediately, press the cancel button. When this is done, the duplicate PT and APTT samples being tested will be lost, along with the next two duplicate samples for both tests. Prior to beginning another test cycle: (a) prime pumps #1 and #2 (if necessary), (b) lower the light shield, (c) index the incubation test plate to the desired cuvet number, (d) set the end test station, (e) press start, and (f) check the printer tape statistics.

4. To shut down the instrument:
   a. Remove the reagent lines from the reagent vials and place in a vial of distilled water.
   b. Clean reagent from the reagent lines by priming the lines with air and distilled water alternately.
   c. Carefully remove the reagent tubing from the pumps. Allow the tubing to remain in the reagent incubation arm.
   d. Lower the light shield. Turn the instrument off.

5. If the results print out as '.', this indicates that no clot has been detected, either because clotting is still in progress, clotting occurred during the blank time, the instrument is unable to detect a clot (plasma grossly lipemic, icteric, or hemolyzed, or decreased fibrinogen, for example), or no clot was formed.

6. Each position in the two pumps must be individually calibrated according to the pump position and the individual tubing. It is, therefore, imperative that the tubing be placed in the pump position as indicated and recalibration procedures followed when new tubing is installed.

7. When priming the reagent lines, make certain there are no air bubbles present in the tubing. If there are air bubbles, repriming is necessary.

8. When adding samples to a test tray that has been partially used, add the first PT sample and the first APTT sample to the first cuvet number that has both inner and outer channels empty.

9. The pump rotors should be cleaned at regular intervals. The reagent tubing must also be replaced regularly, depending on the work volume. Whenever the tubing is removed or replaced or whenever the pump rotors are cleaned, the reagent delivery volumes must be checked and adjusted as necessary. The temperature of the incubation arm should also be checked as part of the scheduled maintenance.

COAG-A-MATE XC

The Coag-A-Mate XC is a semi-automated coagulation instrument which automatically adds reagent to the patient samples, times and detects clot formation via a change in optical density. The following tests may be performed on this instrument with relative ease: PT, APTT, thrombin time, fibrinogen, and factor assays. Due to the instrument's flexibility, almost any coagulation test which has the formation of a clot as the end point, may be performed on this instrument. The XC will also calculate and store factor assay and fibrinogen curves, will report results in percent for prothrombin times, in percent activity for factor assays, in mg/dL for fibrinogens, and in a ratio of clotting time to normal for the PT and APTT, in addition to reporting results in seconds.

The specimens to be tested are placed in cuvets in a circular test tray (up to 12 samples). This tray is then placed in the instrument. When the instrument is activated, the specimens are warmed to 37°C (operating temperature of instrument) and the required reagent(s) are automatically pipetted into each cuvet. A single light source is divided into 12 channels, each of which passes through the sample to its own corresponding sensor. Thus, all samples are tested at approximately the same time. As each sample clots, the change in optical density is detected and this information is stored until all test samples have clotted. The results for that batch of tests are then printed out on printer paper.

COMPONENTS OF THE COAG-A-MATE XC (SEE FIG. 207)

1. The *on/off power switch* (1) turns the instrument on and off.
2. The *circular test tray* is disposable and contains 12 cuvets for sample testing.
3. The *reagent storage wells* (2) hold the reagent vials for testing. The left well contains a mechanism for rotating a magnetic stir bar.
4. The *reagent incubation arm* (3) contains grooves to hold the reagent tubing and is maintained at 37.5°C for reagent warming. It also prevents external light from interfering with clot detection. Two holes are located in the front section to accommodate the delivery tips for the reagent tubing.
5. The *incubation test plate*, located under the reagent incubation arm, holds the test tray for testing and warms the plasma samples.
6. There are two *reagent dispenser pumps* (4) which are responsible for the delivery of precise volumes of reagent to the sample. Their calibration is semi-automatic.
7. *Reagent tubing* transports the reagent from the reagent vials in the storage wells, through the reagent incubation arm, out the delivery tip, and into the cuvet below (in the circular test tray on the incubation test plate).
8. The *print module* (5) records the test results along with the first and last test cuvet number, the incubation test plate temperature, name of the test performed, reagent (pump) volumes delivered, blank time (from addition of reagent until instrument begins looking for an optical density change), the activation time, the maximum clot detection time, date and time, and the test station number for each result.
9. The *display* (6) is a small screen which displays test results and is also used for operator interaction with the instrument.
10. The *touch entry panel* (7) consists of 43 keys for the operator to communicate with the instrument.
    a. The *PT, APTT, TT* (thrombin time), and *Fibrinogen* keys are used to select those particular tests for instrument testing.
    b. The *Two Stage FA* key is used for performing the two stage factor VIII assay test, while the *Factor Assay* mode is used for factor assays (using the PT or APTT procedure).
    c. The *Std. Curve* key is activated in combination with (1) the Factor Assay key for reporting results in percent activity, (2) fibrinogen key for reporting of results in mg/dL, and (3) with the PT key if it

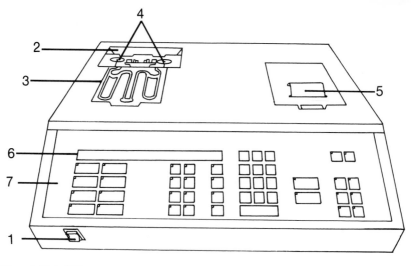

Fig. 207. Coag-A-Mate XC.

is desirable to report prothrombin times in percent.

d. The *Ratio* key is used with the PT or APTT keys when it is desirable to report results in a ratio of patient result to normal.

e. The *Pump 1 Vol.* and *Pump 2 Vol.* keys, when activated, display the volumes that the two pumps are calibrated to deliver.

f. The *Blank Time* key displays the time period during the test cycle that the instrument is not monitoring the sample for clot formation.

g. The *Max. Time* key displays the length of time the instrument will monitor the test sample in the cuvet for clot formation.

h. The *Act. Time* key displays the amount of time between the addition of the first reagent and the delivery of the second reagent.

i. The unlabeled key is not as yet programmed for use.

j. The *Date/Time* key is used to set and display the date and time.

k. The *Modify* key is used in changing the preset parameters (pump volumes and blank, maximum, and activation times).

l. The *Calib*ration key is used to enter curves in combination with the:
 1) PT, APTT, and ratio keys
 2) Fibrinogen and Std. Curve keys
 3) PT and Std. Curve keys
 4) Factor Assay and Std. Curve keys

m. The *First Test* and *Last Test* keys are used to tell the instrument in which cuvet the first and last samples for testing are placed.

n. The *numeric key pad* contains numbers *0* through *9*, a *Clear* key, a *.*, and an *Enter* key for modifying test parameters.

o. The *Start* key begins the testing cycle.

p. The *Cancel* key is used to stop testing.

q. *Paper Feed* key is used to manually advance the printer paper.

r. The *Recall* key may be used to obtain printouts of the previous run, provided the instrument has not been turned off. It may also be used to obtain a printout of the instrument parameters.

s. The *Prime 1* and *Prime 2* keys prime the reagent tubing. If the key is pressed one time, 0.1 mL of reagent is delivered. If the key is held down, reagent is delivered continuously. If the key is pressed immediately following the activation of the YES key, the tubing is primed with 2.5 mL of reagent.

t. The *Deprime 1* and *Deprime 2* keys return the reagent to the reagent vials. If the key is pressed one time, 25 μL (0.025 mL) is returned through the lines. If the key is held down, reagent is deprimed continuously. If the key is pressed immediately following the activation of the YES key, all of the reagent is returned to the reagent vials.

u. The *Ready YES* key lights up when the instrument is ready for testing, and also functions to allow the operator to interact with the instrument in various ways.

v. The *Not Ready NO* key is lit while the instrument is heating to temperature and also allows the operator to interact with the instrument in various ways.

w. The *power cord* is attached to the rear of the instrument, where the *fan, serial number,* and *computer interface connector* are also located.

The factor VIII assay procedure will be described briefly below, since this procedure best describes the flexibility and operation of this particular instrument.

FACTOR VIII ASSAY PROCEDURE

1. Make certain there is no test tray in the incubation test plate. Turn instrument on. The XC will automatically proceed through a systems check. The display and the printer will indicate, 'System Self Check'. When this automatic test is complete, the display indicates, 'Coag-A-Mate XC—Unit Warming, Proceed with Calibrations'. The instrument

automatically goes into the PT mode. The printer displays, 'Coag-A-Mate XC, Version xxxx'. Allow the instrument to reach 37.5°C (the Ready NO key is lit until the proper temperature is reached at which time the Ready YES key will light up). When the instrument is at temperature, the display and the printer will indicate, 'Warm-up Complete'. The XC will then automatically run the analog channel test and will return to the PT mode.

2. Prepare the plasma samples and controls as described for the Factor VIII assay procedure in the Coagulation section of this book.

3. Press the APTT key on the front panel.

4. Install reagent tubing (two sets).

   a. Insert the delivery tip of the long tubing into the hole on the reagent incubation arm and push down until the tip extends $\frac{1}{16}$ of an inch below the arm.

   b. Gently bend and seat the tubing into the groove on the incubation arm, working toward the base of the arm. Do not stretch the tubing.

   c. Lightly lubricate the area of the tubing between the two collars (which will be placed in the pump). To seat the tubing around the pump, slide the tubing into the slot on either side of the stator, and make certain the tubing is properly positioned in the appropriate notch. Press the appropriate prime key (1 or 2) in order to draw back collar snugly against the stator. Check the position of the tubing by pressing the appropriate prime key. Make certain the tubing is not twisted.

   d. Repeat above procedure, inserting the second reagent tubing in place.

5. Place the reagent vial of APTT reagent in storage well one (left). Place

a stir bar and the pick up tip of the reagent tubing into the reagent vial. Place the calcium chloride in the second storage well on the right. Place the pickup tip of the reagent tubing in this vial.

6. Prepare the reference plasma dilutions for the factor assay as described for the manual procedure.

7. Make certain the preset parameters (pump one and two volumes and blank, maximum, and activation times) for the instrument have been previously set. If they have not been, refer to the operator's manual for this procedure and perform at this time.

8. Pipet 0.1 mL of factor deficient plasma into wells #1 to #10. Add 0.1 mL of the reference plasma dilutions to the appropriate wells, testing each dilution in duplicate.

9. Enter the first and last cuvet number (1 and 10): Press First Test key, press #1, press Enter, press Last Test key, Press #1 and 0, and press Enter.

10. Prime the reagent tubing. Lift the incubation arm and hold a suitable container ½ inch below the delivery tip. (Gauze is not considered suitable since the liquid may soak through and cause corrosion of the instrument.) Press the Prime 1 key and hold down until the APTT reagent flows continuously from the delivery tip. Repeat this procedure for the calcium chloride reagent line using the Prime 2 key.

11. Place the filled test tray on the incubation test plate making certain to match the notch in the tray with the notch in the hub. Carefully lower the reagent incubation arm and seat firmly in place. (The incubation arm must not be raised during testing.)

12. Press the Start key to begin the test cycle. The printer will type out the first and last test cuvets, plate temperature, test mode, and the preset instrument parameters. The samples will be incubated on the test plate for 1 minute prior to the addition of APTT reagent during which time the display counts down from 60 seconds indicating, 'Cuvette Warming. . . Seconds Left = xx'. After the incubation period the display shows, 'Test in Progress' during which time the APTT reagent is added to all cuvets. When this step is completed the display reads, 'Activation, Seconds Left = xxx'. At the conclusion of the activation time the display reads 'Test in Progress' while the calcium chloride is added to the cuvets. During testing the only panel key able to be activated is the Cancel key.

13. At the end of the test cycle the instrument gives an audible beep and the test results are displayed and printed. The printout also contains the date and time.

14. Raise the reagent incubation arm, remove and discard the test tray.

15. Average the duplicate results for each reference standard dilution.

16. Press the Factor Assay key. The display will prompt, 'Factor ____ Enter File (1–12)'. Using the numeric keypad enter the number 8 (or whatever number is required by the laboratory's numbering system). Press Enter. (Note that the test parameters must have been entered before entering the assay curve.) 'APTT Factor File 8' will then be displayed.

17. Press the Std Curve key and then press Calib key. The display will prompt, 'Enter number of Standards (3–10) ____'. Using the numeric keypad, enter the appropriate number (5) and press the Enter key.

18. The display will prompt, '1% Activity = ____'. Enter the % concentration (to 1 decimal point) of the highest standard (dilution #1) and press the Enter key.

19. The display will show, '1% Activity = xxx' and will prompt, 'Time =

_____'. Enter the average time for that standard and press Enter.

20. The display will continue to prompt for the remaining standards. Enter this information as outlined above in steps 18 and 19.

21. After all values have been entered, the display will prompt, 'Calibration Printout (Y/N)?'. Press the YES key. The percent concentrations and clotting times will be printed out along with the coefficient of determination (an indicator of the best fit line). This number should be = or >0.985. (If it is not, the standard curve must be repeated beginning with step 8 above.)

22. Prepare dilutions of the patient and control plasmas as described for the manual procedure in the Coagulation section of this book. Test samples by repeating steps 8 through 14 as described above. However, when testing the patient and control plasmas the following keypads must be activated in order to obtain results in percent activity along with seconds: APTT, Std. Curve, and Factor Assay.

23. At the conclusion of testing, the clotting times in seconds and percent activity will be printed for each test sample. The Coefficient of Determination, calibration curve points and clotting times will also be printed on the header of each batch.

24. At the conclusion of testing, deprime the reagent from the reagent lines by pressing the YES key and the Deprime 1 key. Repeat, using the YES and Deprime 2 keys. Flush the reagent lines with distilled water, and then with air by pressing the YES, Prime 1, and Prime 2 keys. (Alternate air and water for the duration of the cycle.) Remove tubing from the pumps if no further testing will be done at this time.

DISCUSSION

1. A result of '***.* ' indicates that an end point has not been detected due to incomplete clotting, clotting during the blank time, or insufficient change in optical density during clotting so that the instrument was unable to detect a change in optical density.

2. Testing may be stopped at any time during the testing cycle by pressing the Cancel key.

3. This instrument is flexible. Total cuvet volumes for testing may vary from as little as 0.3 mL to as much as 0.5 mL. The pump volumes may be set at 50 to 300 μL, the blank time from 1.0 to 20.0 seconds, maximum time from 50 to 300 seconds, and the activation time from 0 to 999.9 seconds. These parameters may be set temporarily for one run of testing or may be permanently set.

4. In order to obtain the parameter settings for an individual test, press the test key (e.g., PT) and the Recall key. To obtain a printout of a factor assay curve, press the test key, Std. Curve key, and the Recall key.

5. A prothrombin activity curve may also be set up on this instrument, in which case the results of the PT may be printed out in seconds and in % activity.

6. When the instrument is pipetting 0.1 mL volumes of thrombin, short tubing should be utilized.

7. Instrument maintenance for the XC is minimal. Once per week the inside of the tubing should be cleaned, the pump must be cleaned at regular intervals, and the calibration of the pumps should be checked regularly and adjusted when needed. The reader is referred to the operator's manual for these procedures.

MLA ELECTRA 700

The MLA Electra 700 (Fig. 208) is an automated coagulation analyzer designed to detect clot formation by means of a photocell sensing circuit which reads the optical density change when a clot is formed. This instrument contains two photo-optical detection systems and is therefore capable of performing two like or different tests simultaneously. The PT, APTT, factor assay, and thrombin time may be performed on this instrument.

COMPONENTS OF THE MLA ELECTRA 700 (FIG. 208)

1. The *turntable* holds up to 60 plasma samples contained in special disposable plastic cuvets. Cooling and heating systems beneath the turntable maintain the plasma specimens at approximately 15°C and warm them to 37°C just prior to and during testing.

2. The *reagent pump system* consists of one pump for each *reservoir* and is responsible for dispensing an accurately measured amount of the reagent into the test samples. A magnetic stirrer may be placed in each reagent reservoir.

3. *Pump controls* (3). The *forward* button cycles the pump forward to prime the tubing. The *reverse* button signals the pump to reverse direction and return the reagent in the tubing to the reagent reservoir. The *pinch valve* closes off the tubing.

4. The *printer* will print out the test name, incubation time, and the clotting time of the test samples, along with the corresponding serial number and position number (on the turntable) for each sample. In addition, the temperatures for the heating trough, reagent incubation and cooling, and specimen cooling are printed out prior to each run of patient samples. The printer will also give the following messages: MISSING TUBE, ILLEGAL TEST, TERMINATED, and NO CLOT.

5. The *auxiliary control panel* is located behind the front panel (pull down to open).
   a. The *catch bin* holds the used sample cuvets as they drop out of the turntable following testing.
   b. The *main power switch* turns the instrument off and on.
   c. The *turntable release* is used

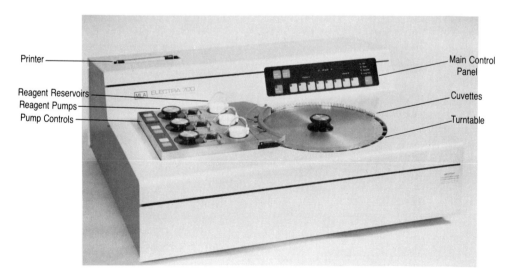

Fig. 208. MLA Electra 700. (Courtesy of Medical Laboratory Automation, Mount Vernon, New York.)

when removing the turntable from the instrument.

d. The *serial number advance switches* (3) are used for changing the serial number. When reset, the printer will print the next number to be used.

e. The *200/300 second contact activation time switch* sets the turntable rotation at specific time intervals.

f. The *automatic/manual switch* sets the instrument to one of these modes. In the manual mode, the incubation times are controlled by the operator, in that the turntable will move only when the operator presses the start button. In the automatic mode, incubation times and testing are automatic.

g. The *normal/long test switch* allows the operator to place each sample in the test station for a longer period of time when prolonged clotting times are anticipated.

h. The *duplicates/singles switch* allows for test results to be printed in two ways. In the duplicate setting, one serial number is given for the two samples in the same cuvet number, and the results are averaged. In the singles setting, each sample having the same cuvet number is given a different serial number, and the results are not averaged.

i. The *lamp A-B-C switch* allows for one of three different photolamp intensities to be used.

6. *Main control panel*

   a. *Serial number reset.*

   b. The *paper advance* is used for advancing the printer paper.

   c. *On/standby* maintains the instrument in a standby mode where the instrument remains on, but the cuvet cooling system and reagent stirrers are turned off.

d. The *test mode buttons* are used to select the tests to be performed: *PT* (one or two stage), *APTT, thrombin time,* and *factor assay.*

e. The *start button,* when pressed, begins the test cycle and provides a printout of the temperatures if the instrument is not in the standby or automatic modes. If pressed two times within 3 seconds, a confidence test is printed. The confidence test indicates any problems present in the optical system, amplifiers, timers, or microprocessors by simulating the change in optical density of a clotting sample.

f. The *catch bin button* indicates a jammed cuvet in the disposal pathway.

g. The *temperature error* indicates a failure in one of the heating or cooling systems.

h. The *automatic button* indicates that the instrument is in the automatic mode.

i. The *long test button* indicates that the instrument is in the long test mode.

j. The *clot time readout* for channel A (or channel B) indicates the verified clotting time for the test in channel A (or channel B).

k. The *off scale* indicates that the sample capacity is out of the range of the instrument.

PROCEDURE FOR THE SIMULTANEOUS PERFORMANCE OF THE PT AND APTT

1. Turn the main power switch on.

2. Empty the cuvet catch basin.

3. Press the on/standby button. The button will light when the heating and cooling systems have reached the proper temperature.

4. Set up the pumps with the proper tubing: Pump #1, blue tubing, to dispense 0.1 mL of calcium chloride; pump #2, red tubing, to dispense 0.2

mL thromboplastin; and pump #3, blue tubing, to dispense 0.1 mL of APTT reagent. The tubing nozzles for pumps #1 and #2 should be placed in the test position. Set the tubing for pump #3 in the 200/300 nozzle position.

5. Place the reagents into the appropriate reagent cups.

6. Pipet 0.1 mL of the plasma and control specimens to be tested into the cuvets and place in the numbered spaces in the turntable beginning with space #1. (Do not leave any empty spaces in between samples.) The plasma samples for the PT must be placed in red coded cuvets, whereas those samples for the APTT should be placed in the blue-coded cuvets. The instrument detects the color of the cuvet and, in this way, determines which reagents to add to the test sample.

7. Check the instrument settings: Mode, PT 1/APTT; duplicates/singles for the printer format; 200/300 for the contact activation time; normal/long test (normal for routine sample testing); and automatic/manual operation (set on automatic for routine use).

8. Press start two times within 3 seconds if a confidence check is desired.

9. Prime all pumps. Place an absorbent material such as gauze under each nozzle, and, in turn, press each forward button until the reagent emerges from the nozzle in a steady stream. (As an alternative place each nozzle into its respective reservoir and prime each pump.)

10. Press start to begin testing.

11. Check the temperature printouts.

12. At the completion of testing, if the instrument will not be used for a while, return the reagents in the tubing to the reagent cup by depressing the reverse pump controls.

13. Empty the catch basin.

DISCUSSION

1. When the instrument is first turned on, it will take approximately 15 minutes for all temperatures to reach their correct levels.

2. Reagent cups will hold a maximum of 20 mL of reagent.

3. Additional samples may be added to the turntable as slots become available.

4. The confidence test should be performed at least once per day.

5. Once per month it is advisable to perform the following instrument maintenance: Clean the printer platen, clean the heating and cooling troughs beneath the turntable, clean the cuvet sensor, check temperatures in the four heating and cooling systems, and check the pump volumes.

MLA ELECTRA 750

The MLA Electra 750 (Fig. 209) is a semiautomated blood coagulation timer. Clot formation is timed automatically and is detected by means of a photocell which reads the optical density change when the clot is formed. The unit contains a heating block which maintains the reagents and plasma samples at 37°C prior to and during testing. Pipetting of the reagents and plasma samples is performed manually, utilizing the disposable tip, precision pipets included with the instrument. An improved sensitivity and optical range allow the instrument to detect the clot on samples that may be chylous, icteric, or hemolyzed (however, hemolyzed specimens are not generally acceptable for coagulation testing). There are five mode switches located on the front of the instrument. All routine coagulation testing may be performed on the MLA 750 in addition to the thrombin time, fibrinogen assay, factor assay, and saline dilutions.

MLA ELECTRA 800

The MLA Electra 800 (Fig. 210) is an automated multitest coagulation timer

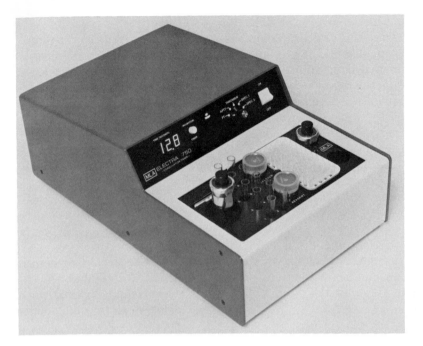

Fig. 209. MLA Electra 750. (Courtesy of Medical Laboratory Automation, Mount Vernon, New York.)

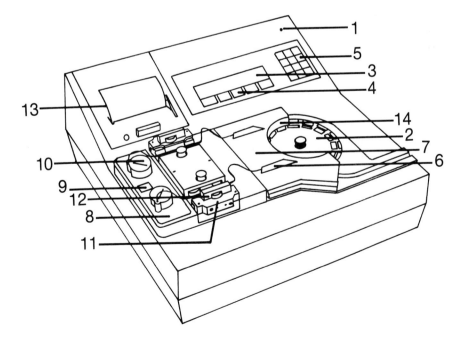

Fig. 210. MLA Electra 800.

that uses a photo-optical clot detection system. There are four photo cells that analyze up to four samples simultaneously. This instrument uses computer-controlled testing and is capable of performing PTs at the rate of 6/minute (360/hour) and more than two APTTs/minute (136/hour). A separate data management system allows the instrument to plot and print curves that may be retained in the instrument's memory, and converts sample clotting times to reportable units (% activity, mg/dL, etc.). Testing may be performed singly or in duplicate. The following procedures may be performed on the MLA 800: PT, APTT, factor assay, thrombin time, fibrinogen, saline dilutions, and heparin activity curve. Test results are printed out on a paper tape.

Components, Operation, and Prothrombin Time

PROCEDURE

1. Using the *power on/off* switch on the back of the unit, turn the instrument on. The green *indicator light* (1) at the top right corner of the instrument should light up, the *turntable* (2) will move to home position, the instrument will beep twice, the *main control panel* (3) will momentarily display the Title Screen, followed by the date and time menu.

2. Adjust the display for contrast and angle of view using the *contrast control* located on the back of the unit.

3. Set the date and time. Press *soft touch button* (4) A at the bottom of the control panel. (Buttons A, B, C, D, and E are used to select, or change, instrument functions as displayed on the bottom line of the control panel screen.) Using the *numeric keypad* (5) (which contains numbers 0–9, ., and ↑), enter the correct month, day, and year (e.g., 04 07 87). (To correct an error, press the D button [clear] and reinsert the date.) Press E to enter the date. In the same manner, enter

the time followed by an A for AM or a B for PM (e.g., 08 14 A). Press E to proceed to the main menu. (See the section following this procedure for an outline of the main menu functions.)

4. Select a red *reagent heat exchanger* (6) (for using 0.2 mL of heated reagent) and attach the *reagent tubing* to each. (The blue exchanger delivers 0.1 mL of heated reagent, and the yellow exchanger is used to dispense 0.1 mL of unheated reagent.) Place the assembly in the *heating trough cover* (7).

5. Remove a cold *reservoir cooler* (8) from the freezer and place in position on the top left side of the instrument. (These reservoir coolers should be stored in a freezer at a temperature no colder than $-20°C$.) A *liquid crystal display* (9) on the reservoir indicates the temperature.

6. Place a *reservoir cup* (10) into the reagent well of the reservoir cooler for pump #1. Open *reagent pump* (11) #1 by turning the *lever* (12) clockwise 180°. (The indicator line on the lever should be on the left side when the pump is open. Place the reservoir tubing into the pump slot by placing the first mounting block at the first post. The second connector should then be installed at the second post, by stretching the tubing slightly. Make certain the colored mark on the tubing is up. (When removing the tubing, pull upward on both connectors simultaneously.) Close the pump by turning the lever 180 degrees counterclockwise. (Indicator on lever is on the right in the closed position.)

7. Place a magnetic stir bar in the reservoir and add sufficient thromboplastin-calcium reagent to the reservoir.

8. The top line of the display screen is termed the *status line.* It will indicate

when the instrument is ready and displays the test reaction temperature. If the instrument is not at temperature, an appropriate message will appear on this line.

9. The bottom line of the screen displays the five main menu selections. Press A 'Mode' in order to choose the test procedure to be performed. When the mode menu is displayed, press A for the PT.

10. The status line will now display 'PT' next to 'Ready' to indicate that the instrument is programmed and ready to perform prothrombin times.

11. To display the Pump Menu, press button B 'Pumps'. This menu allows both pumps to be primed (buttons A and C), allows for reverse priming (buttons B and D), and sets the automatic deprime (button E) (at the end of testing) on or off as desired.

12. Prime pump #1 to fill the tubing and heat exchanger with reagent, as follows. Remove the heat exchanger from its slot in the turntable cover. Hold the nozzle of the heat exchanger over reagent cup 1 so that it points into the middle of the cup. Press button A until the reagent is flowing smoothly out of the nozzle of the heat exchanger. Reseat the heat exchanger in the heating trough with the nozzle well seated in its receptacle hole.

13. If it is desired to have all reagent from the heat exchanger and tubing replaced back in the reagent cup at the end of testing, set automatic deprime on by pressing button E. (An arrow on the display panel next to 'on' or 'off' will indicate the status of automatic deprime.) Press ↑ button to return to the main menu.

14. In order to change any of the test options (normal or long clotting time, automatic or manual operation, single or duplicate testing, lamp intensity, and check for acceptability of duplicate samples), press button C 'Set-up'. Make the desired changes at this time (see operator's manual). Return to the main menu by pressing the ↑ button.

15. The first time the instrument is used each day a confidence test should be run in order to check the proper functioning of the optical sensing and amplification systems. Make certain the instrument is at the proper temperature for testing and there are no cuvets in the test stations. When the main menu is displayed, press E 'Run' twice in rapid succession (within less than 3 seconds of each other). The screen will indicate that a confidence test is being run on all four channels. Results will be displayed and printed on the paper tape from the *printer* (13). Check the operator's manual for the acceptable range of results. The display will return to the main menu.

16. Pipet 0.1 mL of patient or control plasma into each side of a twin well cuvet and place in the turntable, noting carefully the turntable number and letter for each specimen. Record this information. Each specimen will be identified by two numbers and one letter. The first number refers to the turntable rotation number (run number), the second number refers to the turntable position number, and the letter (A or B) refers to the location in the cuvet.

17. The instrument is now ready for testing. When the main menu is displayed, press E (run) once. The turntable advances two cuvet positions at a time, carrying the plasma samples through a heating trough and then to the test stations, where four plasma samples are analyzed simultaneously. When the *cuvet sensing device* (14) detects a cuvet, reagents are dispensed to only those positions occupied by a cuvet. As testing is completed on each pair, the twin well

cuvets are automatically off-loaded from the turntable and are ultimately directed to a *catch basin* (not shown). In this way, additional samples may be continuously added to the turntable for testing. Results will be displayed on the screen and will be printed on the paper tape from the printer.

18. At the end of testing, the message 'Done, Touch Any Key To Continue', will be displayed on the screen. If the instrument is not in automatic deprime and further testing is not to be performed, deprime the heat exchangers and tubing. When the main menu is displayed, press B (pumps). Press buttons B and D, in turn, until all reagent is emptied from the tubing back into the reagent reservoirs.

19. During the testing cycle, if it is desirable to stop testing at any point, press E (halt). The screen will indicate the test samples that were in the process of testing. Press any key to return to the main menu.

20. Located on the rear of the instrument are the electric power cord, fan, fuse, and hook ups for a computer and strip chart recorder.

MAIN CONTROL PANEL

1. The *Title Screen* is displayed when the instrument is first turned on and indicates the software programs contained in the instrument.

2. The *Date and Time Screen* automatically appears after the title screen, and allows the operator to enter the current date and time.

3. To access the *Main Menu,* press button E (done) when the time and date have been entered above. The main menu has five functions displayed at the bottom of the display.

    a. The *'Mode'* allows the operator to choose the test to be performed. When the test is selected the appropriate reagent amounts, timing intervals, and other parameters for the test are automatically assigned.

    b. The *Pump* function allows the operator to prime and deprime the pumps and set automatic deprime (at end of testing) on or off.

    c. The *Set-up* function allows the operator to set various options for testing, such as single or duplicate testing, long or normal clot observation times, automatic or manual operation, lamp intensity, and limits of acceptability for duplicate testing.

    d. The *Menu-2* function contains a menu of five additional functions.

        1) *Home* allows the operator to return the turntable to the first station and advances the table rotation number (sequence).

        2) *Seq. # reset* allows the operator to return the sequence number to 1.

        3) The *Diag.* (diagnostics) function is used to check the instrument's memory, checks the printer, tests for uniformity of characters on the screen, and tests the number pad and buttons A through E.

        4) The *Data Mgmt* (data management) function is an optional feature for use in creating curves and converting the patient data to the appropriate reporting units.

        5) The *Modify* function is used to change instrument parameters for special testing, such as the temperature, reagent volumes, instrument sensitivity, various timed intervals, and the number of photo-optical channels used for testing.

    e. The *Run* option, when used, begins testing. When pressed twice in quick succession, the instrument confidence test is performed.

DISCUSSION

1. With the data management system the MLA 800 is capable of plotting curves for four different procedures: factor assay, heparin activity, quantitative fibrinogen, and PT activity. The instrument will store up to eight curves in memory. The curves may be plotted on a paper printout that will also show the coefficient of determination. The clotting times of the samples are converted to the appropriate units. This program will also calculate a ratio between the patient and control clotting time, if desired.

2. If testing is performed in duplicate, the clotting times of the two specimens may be automatically averaged.

KOAGULAB* 40-A AUTOMATED COAGULATION SYSTEM

Koagulab 40-A (Fig. 211) is manufactured by Ortho Diagnostic Systems, Inc. This instrument is a microprocessor-controlled coagulation analyzer. It automatically pipets sample aliquots, adds the ap-

---

*Trademark of Ortho Diagnostic Systems.

propriate reagents to each sample cuvet and measures the clotting times using two photo-optical detectors. Results are displayed and printed on a paper tape (except for fibrinogen results which are not displayed, but are printed out). The PT, APTT, factor assay, thrombin time, and fibrinogen may be performed on KoaguLab 40-A. In addition, the instrument is able to perform the PT and APTT simultaneously. All testing is performed in duplicate if the samples are automatically pipetted by the instrument.

KoaguLab 40-A is comprised of the *sample handling module* (1) and the *control module* (2).

COMPONENTS OF THE SAMPLE HANDLING MODULE

1. The *sample carousel* (3) holds up to 40 samples (centrifuged specimens in 13 × 100 mm or 13 × 75 mm blood collection tubes). Plasma may also be transferred to a sample cup and placed on the carousel.

2. Each *cuvet tray* has space for 16 plasmas (eight specimen samples tested in duplicate). Up to five cuvet trays may be placed on the sample carousel per run.

3. The *sample arm* (4) automatically aspirates a preset volume of plasma

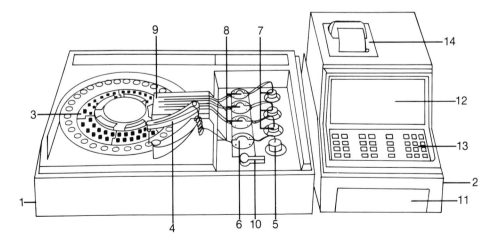

Fig. 211. KoaguLab 40-A Automated Coagulation System.

from each centrifuged blood collection tube or cup and dispenses it into the appropriate cuvets in the cuvet tray during sample testing.

4. The *sampler well* (5) holds distilled water for rinsing the sample arm tubing between specimens.

5. The *sampler pump* (6) delivers distilled water through the sample arm tip and is responsible for pipetting the plasma samples.

6. The three *reagent wells* (7) are cooled to approximately 18°C or less and hold the reagent vials. Magnetic stir bars may be placed in the reagent vials in wells #1 and #3.

7. The three *reagent pumps* (8) automatically pipet a preset quantity of reagent into the sample cuvet for testing.

8. The reagent tubing passes from the reagent vial through the *reagent arm* (9) where the reagents are heated to 37.5°C before being added to the sample cuvet.

9. The *pump engage/release lever* (10) is released when testing and rinsing is complete in order to remove pressure from the tubing.

10. The *sample plate,* located below the sample carousel, is approximately 18°C, and cools the sample tubes and cuvets.

11. The *incubation plate* consists of three cuvet positions and the test station where the sample cuvets are warmed and maintained at 37.5°C.

12. The *power on/off switch, cooling fans, waste drain, connections* to the control module, and *computer interface board* are located on the back of the module.

COMPONENTS OF THE CONTROL MODULE

1. The *switch panel* (11) is located on the front bottom of the unit behind a door and contains:

   a. *Temp adjust potentiometers* for use by service personnel.

   b. *Sample container switch* for setting the blood collection tube size.

   c. *Beeper switch* to turn the beeper on and off.

   d. *Prime/deprime switch* to prime all four pumps and deprime the reagent pumps.

   e. *Prime select* switch selects the pumps to be primed.

   f. *Power on/standby switch* places the instrument in standby mode or the operational mode.

2. The *display panel* (12) consists of *channel 1* and *channel 2* where the test results are displayed, *test position* which displays the current test station, four *temperature warning lights* (incubation plate, reagent arm, reagent wells, and sample plate), and the *message display* where instrument messages appear.

3. The *keyboard* (13) contains keys used to operate the instrument and is divided into five areas.

   a. The *test select keys* are the *PT, APTT, PT/APTT* combination, and *Special assays* for the fibrinogen, thrombin time and factor assay.

   b. The *operation keys* are the *run key* (press twice to begin testing), the *stop key* (press once to interrupt testing to add samples, press twice to stop testing), the *stat key* (to momentarily interrupt testing to add a STAT sample), and the *random test key* for intermixing different kinds of tests (PT, APTT, PT/APTT) within the same run.

   c. There are eight *special function keys:* the *print key* is used to print another copy of the results just run, the *print adv. key* advances the printer paper, *incub./end pt. key* is used to set the activation time and maximum end point for the APTT, *man. mode* is used when the sample arm is not used for pipetting the plasma samples, *time/date key* is used to set the time and date, *pump calib. key* initiates the pump calibration procedure, *temp. check key* displays the temperatures of the incubation plate, reagent arm, reagent wells, and sample plate in the message area, and *service access* is used to gain access to service functions of the instrument.

d. There are four *quality control keys:* the *sel. pop./adv. key* is used to select one of the ten available files of controls, and is also used to advance through the selected control file, the *review data key* is used to review individual control results within a file, the *delete data key* deletes individual control results from a file, the *clear mem. key* clears all control results from the selected file.

e. The *numeric and function keys* consist of numeric keys, *0 to 9,* for entering information into the computer, a *clear key* to change numeric information on the display panel before it is entered into the instrument, and the *enter key* which is used to enter the numeric information, to advance through prompt messages and perform quality control procedures.

4. The *thermal printer* (14) gives a paper copy of the test results and will also print out the time, date, test, incubation time and maximum endpoint time for APTTs, temperature check, and position number for all test results.

PRINCIPLES OF OPERATION

Blood samples are centrifuged. The tubes (13 × 75 mm or 13 × 100 mm) may then be placed directly into the sample carousel. All of one sized tube must be used for each run. The plasma may also be poured into 2 mL sample cups and then placed on the sample carousel. Reagent vials are placed in the appropriate wells. The reagent lines and the sample arm are primed. The sample container switch is set and the instrument is then started. At the beginning of a run, the sample carousel moves forward until position 1 is adjacent to the sample arm, which moves out of the wash well and positions itself over the sample. An air bubble is aspirated into the tip to leave a space between the distilled water and the sample to be aspirated. The sample arm moves down into the sample to a set depth and aspirates a preset amount of the sample. (For the PT or APTT it aspirates 0.6 mL of plasma.) The sample arm moves out of the sample, dispenses approximately 0.1 mL of sample back into the sample container, moves across to the cuvet tray, lowers the tip to the cuvet, and dispenses 0.1 mL of sample into two adjacent cuvets for duplicate testing. The sample arm moves back and is lowered into the wash well where the sample is flushed from the tip and washed with 1.3 mL of distilled water. (In the PT/APTT combination mode, samples are placed in every other position in the sample carousel. The sample arm picks up 0.8 mL of sample, dispenses 0.1 mL back into the sample tube, moves across to the cuvets and dispenses 0.1 mL of plasma into two adjacent cuvets. The samples arm then moves back to its position over the wash well, the carousel moves forward one position, the sample arm moves over the cuvet tray and 0.1 mL of plasma is added to the next two adjacent cuvets.) The cuvet tray advances one position at a time, at a preset rate for the tests being performed. When the samples reach the incubation plate, they are heated to, and maintained at, 37.5°C. Reagents are added to the cuvets as they reach the test station (or, for the APTT, the activated partial thromboplastin reagent is added when it reaches one of the stations in the incubation plate, dependent on the activation time desired). The photo-optical detection system is located at the test station. A timer is started when the reagent is added. Elapsed time is displayed on the appropriate channel display. As clotting occurs the mixture becomes cloudy. When this change in optical density is detected, the timing mechanism is automatically stopped, the channel display indicates the clotting time, and the results are printed on the tape. At a preset time, the carousel moves forward one position and the previously described process is repeated for the next sample until all testing is complete.

The quality control program for this instrument allows the operator to store data for ten different populations, and will calculate a T value, number of specimens, the mean, 1 S.D., the C.V., the range (± 2 S.D.), and the sum of X and X^2. Twenty-five sets of duplicate controls are entered for each file and transferred to CUM population as a group.

MAINTENANCE

The following areas should be cleaned and maintained at regular intervals according to the directions in the operator's manual.

1. All exterior surfaces of the instrument.
2. Sample carousel.
3. The incubation plate, lens, mirrors, and pump area.
4. Printer.
5. Sample arm tip, sample tubing, and reagent tubing.
6. Replacement of tubing, sample pipetting set, printer paper, and fuse.
7. The sample carousel and reagent arm may be realigned by the operator when necessary according to instructions in the operator's manual.

KOAGULAB* 16-S COAGULATION SYSTEM

KoaguLab 16-S (Fig. 212) is similar to KoaguLab 40-A with 1 major exception being a different light source and clot detection mechanism. Also, testing may be performed in duplicate or by single sample, and the plasma samples must be pipetted into the sample cuvets by the operator. In addition, the PT results may be reported in % activity, as a ratio (to the population range), and as an International Normalized Ratio (INR) where the clotting time is compared to the average normal PT clotting time and the International Sensitivity Index (ISI) of the thromboplastin reagent. The APTT results may also be reported as a ratio calculated using a normal average clotting time. The PT, APTT, PT/APTT combination, thrombin time, fibrinogen, and factor assays may be performed on this instrument.

PRINCIPLE OF OPERATION

Using this instrument, the operator selects the desired test(s) to be performed from the *Operational Menu*. The *Utility Menu* is used to set the pump calibration, incubation times, maximum end points, duplicate or single testing, starting position in the cuvet tray, patient identification number, precision flags, a reprint of the previous run, different reporting formats, and it contains a service mode.

The plasma samples are pipetted into a *cuvet tray* which is then placed on the *sample carousel* (1) (maintained at room temperature). The reagents are placed in the *reagent wells* (2) and the tubing is primed (filled with reagent) by activating the *reagent pumps* (3). The tubing passes through the *reagent arm* (4) where the reagents are warmed to 37.5°C (± 0.5°C). The instrument is started by using the *enter* key. The carousel indexes forward and the first set of samples move under the reagent

---

*Trademark of Ortho Diagnostic Systems.

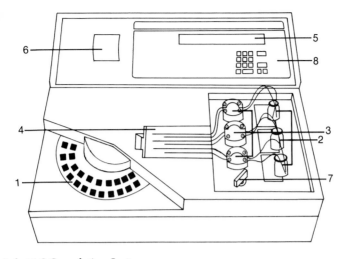

Fig. 212. KoaguLab 16-S Coagulation System.

arm and onto the *incubation plate* (located under the carousel) where they are warmed to, and maintained at, 37.5°C (±0.5°C). There are four positions on the incubation plate in addition to the *test station.* The carousel moves the cuvet tray forward to the test station at a preset rate. (In the APTT test, the APTT reagent is added to the sample cuvet at a preset time before arriving at the test station.) When the first plasma sample reaches the test station, a preset quantity of reagent is added to each of two sample cuvets and the timing mechanism for each is started.

Clot detection system. The clot detection system consists of an ultra-high intensity light-emitting diode (LED) and a photo detector for each channel. When the reagent is added to the plasma sample in the test station, a blank time is initiated. During this period, the intensity of the LED is continuously adjusted by a feedback circuit to compensate for variability in the plasma sample (e.g., lipemia). If the amount of light reaching the photo detector is not within an acceptable range, a message, 'Channel Check', is printed with the final test result. At the completion of the blank time the intensity of the LED is locked in and the photo detector continues to take measurements every 0.2 or 0.5 sec-

ond (depending on the test being performed) until the maximum end point is reached. By this time, numerous voltage vs. reaction-time data have been collected which represents the strength, rate, and time of the clot reaction. The clotting time result is an analysis of this data, and once obtained, there is a verification step in which the rate and acceleration of the clot reaction and shape of the curve are examined in relation to the calculated clotting time. Following this check, the clotting time result is accepted and printed, printed with an appended message (to indicate atypical parameters), or the data is rejected and 'No Data' is reported.

The results are displayed on the *message display* (5) and printed on paper tape by the *printer* (6). After a preset time the carousel moves forward to the next sample and the above procedure is repeated until all testing is complete.

The *pump engage/release lever* (7) should be released by the operator when testing and rinsing are complete in order to remove pressure from the tubing. The *keypad* (8) contains 15 keys for operator interaction with the instrument. The numeric keys, *0 to 9,* allow the operator to enter information into the instrument. The *prime button* is used for priming, depriming, and rinsing the reagent tubing. The *clear button* is used to remove a number not yet entered into the instrument, allows the operator to return to the utility menu from the service mode, and allows the operator to move back and forth between the operational menu and the utility menu. The ↑ and ↓ arrow keys allow the operator to move up and down through the displayed menu. The *enter key* is used to enter information into the instrument, start the instrument, and add samples to the instrument during testing.

COAGULYZER II

The Coagulyzer II is an automated instrument for performing a variety of coagulation procedures. It detects clot formation photoelectrically. This is accomplished by monitoring the output of a photocell. The plasma test samples are pipetted into cuvettes and placed in the numbered holes of a circular turntable. Sample wells numbered 2 through 60 are cooled to approximately 10°C (±5°C),

whereas sample well number 1 is at room temperature. When the instrument is started, the turntable revolves and carries each test sample, in turn, through a heating block, where the plasma specimens are warmed to 37°C. When the first sample arrives at the test station, a preset quantity of reagent is automatically pipetted into the cuvet, and the timing mechanism is started. As fibrin formation occurs, the change in optical density is detected by the photoelectric cell, and the timing mechanism is halted. The clotting time, to the tenths of a second, is printed out on the printer tape. The turntable automatically rotates one space to the next specimen, and the procedure is repeated. In the event that two reagents must be added to the plasma sample, the first reagent is automatically pipetted into the cuvet when it gets to the #2 pipet station.

COMPONENTS OF THE COAGULYZER II (FIG. 213)

1. The *mode selector switch* may be set

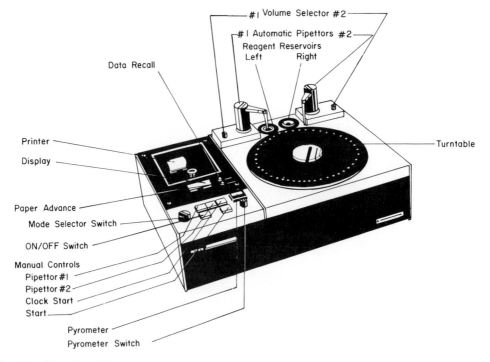

Fig. 213. Coagulyzer II.

at PT-1 (for single reagent PT), PT-2 (used for the PT when adding calcium chloride and thromboplastin separately), APTT, APTT (C.A.T.) (for performing prolonged APTT tests using a constant activation time), and *manual* (for manual operation of the pipettors and timing mechanism).

2. The *on/off switch* turns the instrument on and off.

3. *Manual controls.* When the instrument is in the manual mode, *pipettor #1* and *pipettor #2* operate pipets #1 and #2, respectively. The *start button,* when depressed, moves the turntable to the next position. The *clock start,* when pressed, begins the timing cycle.

4. The *pyrometer* indicates the temperature in the reservoirs and incubation block. The *pyrometer switch* can be rotated between the reservoir and incubation block, depending on which temperature is desired.

5. The *turntable* contains numbered spaces for 60 specimens.

6. The *volume selectors #1* and *#2* are used to set *automatic pipettors #1* and *#2* volumes to 0.1 and 0.2 mL.

7. The *reagent reservoirs,* left and right, are capable of continuous magnetic stirring. The left reservoir is warmed to 37.5°C.

8. The *display* indicates the sample number and elapsed time as the sample is being tested.

9. The *data recall button* may be utilized at the completion of the run to display each sample number and clotting time in the run just completed.

10. The *printer* records the sample number and clotting time for each specimen tested. The *paper advance button* allows manual advance of the printer paper.

DISCUSSION

1. The two-reagent test (other than the APTT) may also be performed in the PT-2 mode. Some factor assays are performed at this setting. The reader is referred to the Coagulyzer instruction manual for the exact setting to be used in each procedure.

2. It is advisable to keep the reservoir covers on at all times to minimize reagent evaporation.

3. The following procedures may be performed on the Coagulyzer: PT, APTT, prothrombin consumption, PT and APTT substitution tests, factor assay, and the Reptilase time.

4. For coagulation testing performed on the Coagulyzer, use only sodium citrate anticoagulated blood when plasma is required (serum is utilized in the prothrombin consumption procedure).

COAGULYZER JR. III

The Coagulyzer Jr. III is a semiautomated coagulation timer (Fig. 214). Clot formation is automatically timed and is detected by means of a photoelectric cell. This unit contains fifteen heated *test tube wells* for incubating test plasmas. There are two heated *reservoirs* for reagents, one of which contains a magnetic stirrer. The instrument is turned on by depressing the *on/off switch.* The tube containing a measured amount of patient plasma is placed in the *reaction well,* and the *start switch,* activating the timing mechanism, is depressed at the same time the reagent is added to the test sample. If an automatic pipettor is plugged into the *bi-pettor jack,* the timing mechanism is automatically activated as the reagent is pipetted into the test sample. The clotting time is registered on the *digital display* and returns to zero each time the start switch is activated. Only citrated plasma specimens should be used on this instrument. The PT, APTT, factor assays, PT and APTT substitution tests, prothrombin consumption, and Rep-

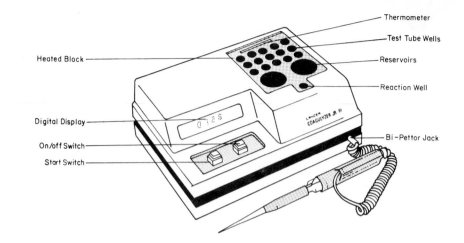

Fig. 214. Coagulyzer Jr. III.

tilase time may be performed on this instrument.

BIO/DATA PLATELET AGGREGATION PROFILER MODEL PAP-4

Platelet aggregation studies have become important in diagnosing certain platelet disorders. Abnormal platelet aggregation may be drug-induced and may also be found in such conditions as liver disease, uremia, acute leukemia, pernicious anemia, connective tissue abnormalities, myeloproliferative disorders, immunoproliferative disorders, Glanzmann's thrombasthenia, and von Willebrand's syndrome, among numerous other conditions.

Principles of Operation. The Platelet Aggregation Profiler Model PAP-4 (Fig. 215) employs a photo-optical system for

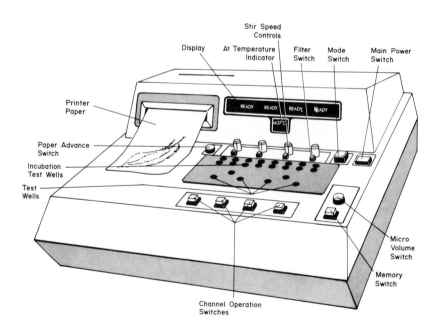

Fig. 215. Bio/Data Aggregation Profiler Model PAP-4. (Courtesy of Bio/Data Corporation, Hatboro, Pa.)

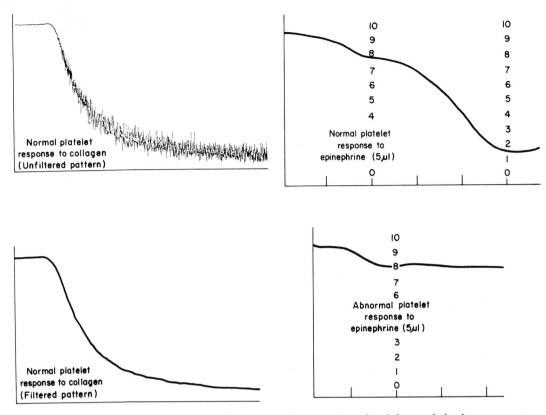

Fig. 216. Normal platelet response to collagen as shown on the platelet aggregometer (filtered and unfiltered patterns).

Fig. 217. Normal and abnormal platelet response to epinephrine as shown by the platelet aggregometer.

viewing platelet aggregation. In this instrument, there are four independently operated photo-optical systems, or aggregation channels. An optical density reading is made on a sample of the patient's platelet poor plasma (PPP). The instrument then sets the 100% baseline for this channel using the PPP. A reading of the patient's platelet rich plasma (PRP) is made and the 0% baseline is then set. (The difference in the initial optical density readings between the PPP and PRP must be >5% but <95%. The optical density difference is then expanded to a 100% scale: PPP is set at 100%, and the PRP at 0%.) When an aggregation reagent is added to the platelet rich plasma, the optical density of the sample is monitored and the display panel and printer record the absorbance (optical density) changes (plate-

let aggregation) as they occur. (Figs. 216 and 217.) When the reaction stops, the operator presses the channel operation switch, READY is displayed and the next test may be started in the adjacent test channel. When testing is complete and all four channels display READY, the final results are printed out. The printout displays the platelet aggregation pattern (plotted optical density readings), the slope value (calculated by the instrument), and percent aggregation (calculated by the instrument) for each patient sample tested. Results may be recalled from memory and reprinted as many times as desired as long as a new specimen has not been run. A comment section is also available on the printer paper.

This instrument has trace filter switches which make it possible to reduce the oscillations caused by the size of the aggregations. The rate at which the plasma is mixed during testing may be set by the operator. Micro volume samples may be analyzed using a special cuvet adapter. A check of instrument function can be performed by the operator, using the service diagnostic mode.

COMPONENTS OF THE PLATELET AGGREGATION PROFILER (FIG. 215)

1. The *main power switch* turns the instrument on and off.
2. There are four color-coded *channel operation switches,* one for each channel. The first time the button is depressed, a 100% baseline value is read and stored. The second depression of the switch determines the 0% baseline, sets 0% on the printer paper, and begins the paper transport. Depressing the switch a third time terminates printing for that particular channel. When all channel switches have been depressed for the third time, the percentage aggregation and slope for each channel is printed out.
3. The *mode switch* has two settings: (1) When the green light is on, the instrument is ready for testing. If the switch is then depressed, the orange light comes on. (2) The orange light indicates the stir speed position, and the display will indicate the stir speed in each channel. The stir speed may then be changed, using the appropriate *stir speed control* (make certain the test wells are empty). (All stir speeds used should be in the range of 600 to 1500 RPM. If speeds lower or higher are used, an error message will be displayed.)
4. The *temperature indicator* will light when the incubation block reaches 37°C (8 to 10 minutes after the instrument is turned on).
5. The *micro-volume switch* is utilized when micro sample volumes (with micro-cuvets) are used. This switch deactivates the magnetic stir bar detector and allows use of the micro stir bar.
6. The *memory switch* is used to initiate the instrument's memory recall. The aggregation patterns generated in each channel will remain in memory until another sample is tested in that channel. The patterns are stored in the unfiltered form but may be recalled as filtered or unfiltered.
7. *Display* will give information concerning the instrument operation, test status, stir speeds, and temperature when the instrument is on.
8. Each channel has its own color-coded *filter switch.* When this switch is activated, the oscillations (a function of the size of the platelet aggregate) generated during platelet aggregation are filtered out. (Platelet aggregations are stored in memory in the unfiltered state, irrespective of the filter switch setting.)
9. The platelet aggregation patterns are printed out on the *printer paper,* which may be manually advanced by depressing the *paper advance switch.*
10. There are four *incubation wells* maintained at 37°C for each of the four channels.
11. There is one *test well* for each of the four channels, in which platelet aggregation is tested and monitored.

See the Coagulation chapter of this book for the platelet aggregation test procedure.

Bibliography

Ackerman, G.A.: Substituted naphthol AS phosphate derivatives for the localization of leukocyte alkaline phosphate activity, Lab. Invest., *11*, 563, 1962.

American Dade, *Coagulation Education*, Miami, American Hospital Supply Corporation, 1983.

American Dade: Data-Fi euglobulin lysis reagents, pkg. insert, Aguada, Puerto Rico, American Hospital Supply, 1985.

American Dade: Data-Fi protamine sulfate reagents, pkg. insert, Aguada, Puerto Rico, American Hospital Supply, 1985.

American Optical Corporation: *Reference Manual Series 10 Microstar Advanced Laboratory Microscopes*, Buffalo, N.Y., Scientific Instrument Division, 1974.

Becton, Dickinson and Company: *Laboratory Procedures Using the Unopette Brand System*, Rutherford, N.J., Becton, Dickinson and Company, 1977.

Betke, K., Marti, H.R., and Schlict, I.: Estimation of small percentages of foetal haemoglobin, Nature, *184*, 1877, 1959.

Beutler, E.: A series of new screening procedures for pyruvate kinase deficiency, glucose-6-phosphate dehydrogenase deficiency, and glutathione reductase deficiency, Blood, *28*, 553, 1966.

Beutler, E., Dern, R.J., and Alving, A.S.: The hemolytic effect of primaquine. VI. An in vitro test for sensitivity of erythrocytes to primaquine, J. Lab. & Clin. Med., *45*, 40, 1955.

Biggs, R., and Douglas, A.S.: The thromboplastin generation test, J. Clin. Path., *6*, 23, 1953.

Biggs, R., and MacFarlane, R.G.: *Human Blood Coagulation and Its Disorders*, Oxford, Blackwell Scientific Publications, 1962.

Bio/Data Corp.: vW factor assay™ for the quantitation of von Willebrand factor, pkg. insert, Hatboro, Pa., Bio/Data Corp., 1986.

Bio/Data Corp.: *Operating Instructions and Methods Manual, Platelet Aggregation Profiler® Model PAP-4*, Hatboro, Pa., Bio/Data Corp., 1985.

Breen, F.A., Jr., and Tullis, J.L.: Ethanol gelation: A rapid screeing test for intravascular coagulation, Ann. Intern. Med., *69*, 1197, 1968.

Brecher, G., and Cronkite, E.P.: Morphology and enumeration of human blood platelets, J. Appl. Physiol., *3*, 365, 1950.

Briere, R.O., Golias, T., and Batsakis, J.G.: Rapid qualitative and quantitative hemoglobin fractionation. Cellulose acetate electrophoresis, Am. J. Clin. Pathol., *44*, 695, 1965.

Broden, P.: Hydrodynamic focusing in cell counting and sizing, unpublished, Japan, TOA Medical Electronics Co., Ltd., 1984.

Bull, B.S., and Brailsford, D.: The Zeta sedimentation ratio, Blood, Oct., 1972.

Carrell, R.W., and Kay, R.: A simple method for the detection of unstable haemoglobins, Br. J. Haematol., *23*, 615, 1972.

Cartwright, G.E.: *Diagnostic Laboratory Hematology*, New York, Grune & Stratton, Inc., 1963.

Chakrabarti, M., Bielawiec, J.F., Evans, J.F., and Fearnley, G.R.: Methodological study and a recommended technique for determining the euglobulin lysis time, J. Clin. Path., *21*, 698, 1968.

Cocchi, P., Mori, S., and Becattini, A.: N.B.T. tests in premature infants, Lancet, *2*, 1426, 1969.

Colfs, B., and Vekeyden, J.: A rapid method for the determination of serum haptoglobin, Clin. Chem. Acta, *12*, 470, 1965.

Coulter Electronics, Inc.: Evaluation of the Coulter Counter Model S-Plus IV differential in normal and hospitalized subjects, Hematology Analyzer, *6-4*, Hialeah, Fl., Coulter Electronics, Inc., 1985.

Coulter Electronics, Inc.: *Coulter Counter Model S-Plus Operator's Manual*, Hialeah, Fl., Coulter Electronics, Inc., 1977.

Coulter Electronics, Inc.: *Coulter Counter Model S-Plus IV with Data Terminal Product Reference Manual*, Hialeah, Fl., Coulter Electronics, Inc., 1983.

Coulter Electronics, Inc.: *Coulter S-Plus IV*, Hialeah, Fl., Coulter Electronics, Inc., 1983.

Coulter Electronics, Inc.: *Coulter S-Plus V*, Hialeah, Fl., Coulter Electronics, Inc., 1983.

Coulter Electronics, Inc.: *Coulter S-Plus VI*, Hialeah, Fl., Coulter Electronics, Inc., 1984.

Coulter Electronics, Inc.: *Instruction and Service Manual for the Model S Coulter Counter*, Hialeah, Fl., Coulter Electronics, Inc., 1970.

Coulter Electronics, Inc.: *Instruction Manual for Coulter Zetafuge*, Hialeah, Fl., Coulter Electronics, Inc., 1973.

Coulter Electronics, Inc.: *STKR*, Hialeah, Fl., Coulter Electronics, Inc., 1985.

Coulter Electronics, Inc.: The advantage of Coulter pulse editing, Hematology Analyzer, Hialeah, Fl., Coulter Electronics, Inc., *6-5*, 1985.

Dacie, J.V., and Lewis, S.M.: *Practical Hematology*, 6th ed., New York, Churchill Livingstone, Inc., 1984.

Daland, G.A., and Castle, W.B.: A simple and rapid method for demonstrating sickling of the red blood cells: The use of reducing agents, J. Lab. Clin. Med., *33*, 1082, 1948.

Deacon-Smith, R.: The ascorbate cyanide test and the detection of females heterozygous for glucose-6-phosphate dehydrogenase deficiency, Med. Lab. Sciences, *39*, 139, 1982.

DeCresca, R.: The Technicon H-1: A discrete, fully automated complete blood count and differential analyzer, Lab. Med., *17*, 17, 1986.

Division of Host Factors, Center for Infectious Diseases, CDC: *Laboratory Methods for Detecting Hemoglobinopathies,* Atlanta, Ga., Center for Disease Control, 1984.

Duke, W.W.: The pathogenesis of purpura haemorrhagica with especial reference to the part played by the blood platelets, Arch. Intern. Med., *10,* 445, 1912.

Efremov, C.D., Huisman, T.H.J., and Wrightstone, R.N.: Microchromatography of hemoglobins. II. A rapid method for the determination of hemoglobin A_2, J. Lab. Clin. Med., *83,* 657, 1974.

Engelkirk, P.G., and Koester, S.K.: Proposed functions of eosinophils, J. Med. Tech., *3:3,* 181, 1986.

Erslev, A.J., and Gabuzda, T.G.: *Pathophysiology of Blood,* Philadelphia, W.B. Saunders Co., 1985.

Fahey, J.L., Barth, W.F., and Solomon, A.: Serum hyperviscosity syndrome, JAMA, *192,* 464, 1965.

Fairbanks, V.F.: *Hemoglobinopathies and thalassemias: Laboratory Methods and Clinical Cases,* New York, Thieme-Stratton, Inc., 1980.

Funk, C., Gmür, J., Herold, R., and Straub, P.W.: Reptilase®-R—A new reagent in blood coagulation, Br. J. Haem., *21,* 43, 1971.

Gambino, S.R., et al.: The Westergren sedimentation rate, using K_3EDTA, Techn. Bull. Regist. Med. Techn., *35,* 1, 1965.

Gardlund, B.: The lupus inhibitor in thromboembolic disease and intrauterine death in the absence of systemic lupus, Acta Med. Scand., *215,* 293, 1984.

Geometric Data Corporation: *Hematrak® Automated Differential System Operator's Manual,* Wayne, Pa., Geometric Data Corporation, 1982.

Goldhaber, S.Z.: *Pulmonary Embolism and Deep Venous Thrombosis,* Philadelphia, W.B. Saunders Co., 1985.

Graham, R.C., Lundholm, U., and Karnovsky, M.J.: Cytochemical demonstration of peroxidase activity with 3-amino-9-ethylcarbazole, J. Histochem. Cytochem., *13,* 150, 1965.

Hall, R., and Malia, R.G.: *Medical Laboratory Haematology,* Boston, Butterworths, 1984.

Ham, T.H.: Studies on destruction of red blood cells. Chronic hemolytic anemia with paroxysmal nocturnal hemoglobinuria, Arch. Intern. Med., *64,* 1271, 1939.

Hardisty, R.M., and Ingram, C.I.C.: *Bleeding Disorders, Investigations and Management,* Oxford, Blackwell Scientific Publications, 1965.

Hartmann, R.C., Jenkins, D.E., Jr., and Arnold, A. B.: Diagnostic specificity of sucrose hemolysis test for paroxysmal nocturnal hemoglobinuria, Blood, *35,* 462, 1970.

Hattersley, P.G., and Hayse, D.: The effect of increased contact activation time on the activated partial thromboplastin time, Am. J. Clin Path., *66,* 479, 1976.

Helena Laboratories: Beta-Thal Hemoglobin A_2 Quik Column™ Procedure, pkg. insert, Beaumont, Tex., Helena Laboratories.

Helena Laboratories: Hemoglobin Electrophoresis Procedure, pkg. insert, Beaumont, Tex., Helena Laboratories, 1985.

Helena Laboratories: Titan IV citrate hemoglobin electrophoresis procedure, pkg. insert, Beaumont, Tx., Helena Laboratories, 1983.

Henry, J.B., ed.: *Clinical Diagnosis and Management by Laboratory Methods,* Philadelphia, W.B. Saunders Co., 1984.

Hicks, R., Schenken, J.R., and Steinrauf, M.A., eds.: *Laboratory Instrumentation,* Hagerstown, Harper & Row, 1980.

Hillman, R.S., and Finch, C.A.: *Red Cell Manual,* Philadelphia, F.A. Davis Co., 1985.

Hoffbrand, A.V., and Pettit, J.E.: *Essential Hematology,* Boston, Blackwell Scientific Publications, 1984.

Ivy, A.C., Nelson, D., and Beecher, G.: The standardization of certain factors in the cutaneous 'venostasis' of bleeding time technique, J. Lab. Clin. Med., *26,* 1812, 1940.

Jacob, H.S., and Jandl, J.H.: A simple visual screening test for glucose-6-phosphate dehydrogenase deficiency employing ascorbate and cyanide, N. Engl. J. Med., *274,* 1162, 1966.

Jones, J.A., Broszeit, H.K., LeCrone, C.N., and Detter, J.C.: An improved method for detection of red cell hemoglobin H inclusions, Am. J. Med. Tech., *47,* 94, 1981.

Kaplow, L.S.: Substitute for benzidine in myeloperoxidase stains, Am. J. Clin. Pathol., *63,* 451, 1975.

Kasper, C.K., and Ewing, N.P.: Acquired inhibitors of plasma coagulation factors, J. Med. Tech., *3,* 431, 1986.

Katayama, I., and Yang, J.P.S.: Reassessment of a cytochemical test for differential diagnosis of leukemic reticuloendotheliosis, Am. J. Clin. Pathol., *68,* 268, 1977.

Knowles, D.M.: Lymphoid cell markers. Their distribution and usefulness in the immunophenotypic analysis of lymphoid neoplasms, Am. J. Surg. Path., *9(3),* 85, 1985.

Kocoshis, T.A., Triplett, D.A.: CAP survey results for factor VIII assays (1977–1978), Am. J. Clin. Path., *72,* 346, 1979.

Lamberg, S.L., and Rothstein, R.: *Laboratory Manual of Hematology and Urinalysis,* Westport, Conn., Avi Publishing Co., Inc., 1978.

Lampasso, J.A.: Error in hematocrit values produced by excessive ethylenediaminetetracetate, Techn. Bull. Regist. Med. Techn., *35,* 109, 1965.

Lampasso, J. A.: Changes in hematologic values induced by storage of ethylenediaminetetracetate human blood for varying periods of time, Techn. Bull. Regist. Med. Techn., *38,* 37, 1968.

Lathem, W., and Worley, W.E.: The distribution of extracorpuscular hemoglobin in circulating plasma, J. Clin. Invest., *38,* 474, 1959.

Lee, R.I., and White, P.D.: A clinical study of the coagulation time of whole blood, Am. J. Med. Sci., *145,* 495, 1913.

Lenahan, J., and Smith, K. (eds.): Clotters Corner, Durham, N.C., Organon Teknika Corp., 1986.

Lenahan, J.G., and Smith, K.: *Hemostasis,* Durham, N. C., Organon Teknika Corp., 1985.

Lilli, R.D., and Fullmer, H.M.: *Histopathologic Technic and Practical Histochemistry,* New York, McGraw-Hill Book Co., 1976.

Losowsky, M.S., Hall, R., and Goldie, W.: Congenital deficiency of fibrin-stabilizing factor, Lancet, *2*, 156, 1965.

Magath, T.B., and Winkle, V.: Technic for demonstrating 'L.E.' (lupus erythematosus) cells in blood, Am. J. Clin. Pathol., *22*, 586, 1952.

Maronde, G.R., et al.: A quality control system utilizing duplicate patient specimens, Am. J. Med. Tech., *40-4*, 165, 1974.

McKenzie, S.B.: *Textbook of Hematology*, Philadelphia, Lea & Febiger, 1988.

McLucas, E., and Harrison, R.L.: The lupus anticoagulant, J. Med. Tech., *3*, 440, 1986.

McManus, J.F.A.: Histological demonstration of mucin after periodic acid, Nature, *158*, 202, 1946.

Medical Laboratory Automation, Inc.: *Operator's Manual, MLA Electra 700*, Pleasantville, N.Y., Medical Laboratory Automation, Inc., 1981.

Medical Laboratory Automation, Inc.: *Operator's Manual, MLA 750*, Pleasantville, N.Y., Medical Laboratory Automation, Inc., 1981.

Medical Laboratory Automation, Inc.: *Operator's Manual, MLA Electra 800*, Pleasantville, N.Y., Medical Laboratory Automation, Inc., 1985.

Miale, J.B.: *Laboratory Medicine Hematology*, St. Louis, C.V. Mosby Co., 1982.

Mielke, C.H., et al.: The standardized normal Ivy bleeding time and its prolongation by aspirin, Blood, *34*, 204, 1969.

Miles Scientific: *Hema-Tek® Slide Stainer Operating Manual*, Naperville, Il., Miles Scientific, Div. of Miles Lab. Inc., 1983.

Nalbandian, R.M., et al.: Dithionite tube test—a rapid, inexpensive technique for the detection of hemoglobin S and non-S sickling hemoglobin, Clin. Chem., *17*, 1028, 1971.

Nalbandian, R.M., et al.: Automated dithionite test for rapid, inexpensive detection of hemoglobin S and non-sickling hemoglobinopathies, Clin. Chem., *17*, 1033, 1971.

National Committee for Clinical Laboratory Standards: *Determination of Factor VIII Coagulant Activity (VIII:C), Proposed Guideline*, Code #H34-P, NCCLS, Villanova, Pa., 1986.

National Committee for Clinical Laboratory Standards: *Method for Reticulocyte Counting, Proposed Standard*, Code #H16-P, NCCLS, Villanova, Pa., 1985.

National Committee for Clinical Laboratory Standards: *Procedures for the Collection of Diagnostic Blood Specimens by Venipuncture*, Code #H3-A2, NCCLS, Villanova, Pa., 1984.

National Committee for Clinical Laboratory Standards: *Procedures for the Collection of Diagnostic Specimens by Skin Puncture*, Code #H4-A2, NCCLS, Villanova, Pa., 1986.

National Committee for Clinical Laboratory Standards: *Procedure for Determining Packed Cell Volume by the Microhematocrit Method*, Code #H7-A, NCCLS, Villanova, Pa., 1985.

National Committee for Clinical Laboratory Standards: *Proposed Guidelines for Citrate Agar Electrophoresis for Confirming Identification of Mutant Hemoglobins*, NCCLS, Villanova, Pa., 1981.

National Committee for Clinical Laboratory Standards: *Proposed Guidelines for the Quantitative Measurement of Fetal Hemoglobin by the Alkali Denaturation Method*, Code #H13-P, NCCLS, Villanova, Pa., 1982.

National Committee for Clinical Laboratory Standards: *Proposed Guidelines for a Standardized Procedure for the Determination of Fibrinogen in Biological Samples*, Code #H30-P, NCCLS, Villanova, Pa., 1982.

National Committee for Clinical Laboratory Standards: *Reference Procedure for the Quantitative Determination of Hemoglobin in Blood*, Code #H15-A, NCCLS, Villanova, Pa., 1984.

National Committee for Clinical Laboratory Standards: *Reference Procedure for the Human Erythrocyte Sedimentation Rate (E.S.R.) Test*, Code #H2-T2, NCCLS, Villanova, Pa., 1983.

National Committee for Clinical Laboratory Standards: *Screening Red Blood Cell Glucose-6-Phosphate Dehydrogenase Activity*, Code #H12-A, NCCLS, Villanova, Pa., 1984.

National Committee for Clinical Laboratory Standards: *Solubility Test for Confirming the Presence of Sickling Hemoglobins*, Code #H10-A, NCCLS, Villanova, Pa., 1986.

National Committee for Clinical Laboratory Standards: *Tentative Guidelines for the Standardized Collection, Transport and Preparation of Blood Specimens for Coagulation Testing and Performance of Coagulation Assays*, Code #H21-T, NCCLS, Villanova, Pa., 1981.

Niewiarowski, S., and Gurewich, V.: Laboratory identification of intravascular coagulation, J. Lab. Clin. Med., *77*, 665, 1971.

O'Connor, B.H.: *A Color Atlas and Instruction Manual of Peripheral Blood Cell Morphology*, Baltimore, Williams & Wilkins, 1984.

Organon Teknika, Corp.: Chromostrate™ Plasminogen Assay, pkg. insert, Durham, N.C., Organon Teknika Corp., 1985.

Organon Teknika, Corp.: Chromostrate™ Antithrombin III Assay, pkg. insert, Durham, N.C., Organon Teknika, Corp, 1986.

Organon Teknika, Corp.: Chromostrate™ Heparin Assay, pkg. insert, Durham, N.C., Organon Teknika, Corp., 1986.

Organon Teknika, Corp.: Simplate Bleeding Time Device, pkg. insert, Durham, N.C., Organon Teknika, Corp, 1985.

Organon Teknika, Corp.: *Coag-A-Mate 2001 Operator's Manual*, Durham, N.C., Organon Teknika Corp., 1979.

Organon Teknika, Corp.: *Coag-A-Mate Dual Channel Operator's Manual*, Durham, N.C., Organon Teknika Corp., 1974.

Organon Teknika, Corp.: *Coag-A-Mate·X2 Operations Manual*, Durham, N.C., Organon Teknika Corp., 1981.

Organon Teknika, Corp.: *Fibriquik*, pkg. insert, Durham, N.C., Organon Teknika Corp., 1983.

Ortho Diagnostics Systems, Inc.: *Ortho* ELT-1500 Advanced High-Throughput Analyzer with Screening Differential*, Westwood, Ma., Ortho Diagnostic Systems, Inc., 1985.

Ortho Diagnostic Systems, Inc.: *Koagulab* 16-S Co-

agulation System, Raritan, N.J., Ortho Diagnostic Systems, Inc., 1985.

Ortho Diagnostic Systems, Inc.: *Koagulab* 40-A Automated Coagulation System,* Raritan, N.J., Ortho Diagnostic Systems, Inc., 1984.

Palmer, I.: Basic spectrophotometry for the medical technologist, Am. J. Med. Tech., *25,* 341, 1959.

Park, B.H., Fikring, S.M., and Smithwick, E.M.: Infection and nitroblue-tetrazolium reduction by neutrophils, Lancet, *2,* 532, 1968.

Parpart, A.K., et al.: The osmotic resistance (fragility) of human red cells, J. Clin. Invest., *26,* 636, 1947.

Pendergraph, G.E.: *Handbook of Phlebotomy,* Philadelphia, Lea & Febiger, 1984.

Porter, I.A., and Turk, C.C.: *A Short Textbook of Microbiology,* Philadelphia, W.B. Saunders Co., 1965.

Proctor, R.R., and Rapaport, S.I.: The partial thromboplastin time with kaolin, Am. J. Clin. Path., *36,* 212, 1961.

Quick, A.J.: *Bleeding Problems in Clinical Medicine,* Philadelphia, W.B. Saunders Co., 1970.

Randolph, T.G.: Differentiation and enumeration of eosinophils in the counting chamber with a glycol stain, J. Lab. Clin. Med., *34,* 1696, 1949.

Ratnoff, O.D., and Forbes, C.D., editors: *Disorders of Hemostasis,* Orlando, Fl., Grune & Stratton, Inc., 1984.

Raven, J.L., and Tooze, J.A.: α-thalassaemia in Britain, Br. Med. J., *4,* 486, 1973.

Richards, O. W.: Phase microscopy, Wallerstein Laboratories, *15,* 155, 1952.

Richards, O.W.: *The Effective Use and Proper Care of the Microscope,* Buffalo, N.Y., American Optical Corp., Scientific Instrument Division, 1958.

Salzman, E.W.: Measurement of platelet adhesiveness. A simple in-vitro technique demonstrating an abnormality in von Willebrand's disease, J. Lab. Clin. Med., *62,* 724, 1963.

Schmidt, R.M., and Brosius, E.M.: *Basic Laboratory Methods of Hemoglobininopathy Detection,* HEW, Pub. No. (CDC) 74-8266, U.S. Department of Health, Education, and Welfare, Public Health Service, Center for Disease Control, Atlanta, 1974.

Schneiderman, L.J., Junga, I.G., and Fawley, D.E.: Effect of phosphate and non-phosphate buffers on thermolability of unstable haemoglobins, Nature, *225,* 1041, 1970.

Sheehan, H.L., and Storey, G.W.: An improved method of staining leukocyte granules with sudan black B, J. Path. Bact., *59,* 336, 1947.

Shephard, M.K., Weatherall, D.J., and Conley, C.L.: Semiquantitative estimation of the distribution of fetal hemoglobin in red cell populations, Bull. J. Hopkins Hosp., *110,* 293, 1962.

Sigma Diagnostics: Alkaline Phosphatase, pkg. insert, St. Louis, Sigma Chemical Co., 1984.

Sigma Diagnostics: Atroxin® (Bothrops atrox venom). Determination of Plasma Clotting Time, pkg. insert, St. Louis, Sigma Chemical Co., 1984.

Sigma Chemical Co.: Glutathione Reductase Deficiency in Blood, pkg. insert, St. Louis, Sigma Chemical Co., 1982.

Sigma Diagnostics: Glucose-6-Phosphate Dehydro-

genase (G-6-PDH) Deficiency, pkg. insert, St. Louis, Sigma Chemical Co., 1984.

Sigma Diagnostics: Pyruvate Kinase Deficiency, Qualitative, Visual Fluorescence Determination in Red Cells, pkg. insert, St. Louis, Sigma Chemical Co., 1984.

Sigma Chemical Co.: Nitroblue tetrazolium (NBT) reduction, histochemical demonstration in neutrophils, pkg. insert, St. Louis, Sigma Chemical Co., 1985.

Singer, K., Chernoff, A.I., and Singer, L.: Studies on abnormal hemoglobins. 1. Their demonstration in sickle cell anemia and other hematologic disorders by means of alkali denaturation, Blood, *6,* 413, 1951.

Sirchia, G., Soldano, F., and Mercurial, F.: The action of two sulfhydryl compounds on normal human red cells. Relationship to red cells of paroxysmal nocturnal hemoglobinuria, Blood, *25,* 502, 1965.

Sirridge, M.S., and Shannon, R.: *Laboratory Evaluation of Hemostasis and Thrombosis,* 3rd ed., Philadelphia, Lea & Febiger, 1983.

Spinco Division, Beckman Instruments Inc.: *Preliminary Instruction Manual for Model R-101 Microzone Electrophoresis Cell,* Palo Alto, Ca., Spinco Division, Beckman Instruments Incorporated, 1963.

Spivak, J.L.: *Fundamentals of Clinical Hematology,* Philadelphia, Harper & Row, 1984.

Stockbower, J.M., and Blumenfeld, T.A.: *Collection and Handling of Laboratory Specimens,* Philadelphia, J.B. Lippincott Co., 1983.

Straight, D.L.: The physiologic inhibitors of blood coagulation and fibrinolysis, J. Med. Tech., *3,* 443, 1986.

Sundberg, R.D., and Broman, H.: The application of the Prussian blue stain to previously stained films of blood and bone marrrow, Blood, *10,* 160, 1955.

Technicon Instruments Corp.: *Technicon H-1® System Operator's Guide,* Tarrytown, N.Y., Technicon Instruments Corp., 1985.

Technicon Instruments Corp.: *Technicon H-1® System Course Guide,* Tarrytown, N.Y., Technicon Instruments Corp., 1985.

Thompson, A.R., and Harker, L.A.: *Manual of Hemostasis and Thrombosis,* Philadelphia, F.A. Davis Co., 1983.

Thomson, J.M., Ed.: *Blood Coagulation and Haemostasis—A Practical Guide,* New York, Churchill Livingstone, Inc., 1980.

Thrombosis-Hemostasis Conference, notes, American Dade, American Scientific Products, and Wayne State University School of Medicine, Atlantic City, N.J., 1986.

TOA Medical Electronics Co., Ltd.: *Sysmex, E-Series Training Manual Part 1,* Japan, TOA Medical Electronics Co., Ltd., 1985.

TOA Medical Electronics Co., Ltd.: *E-500 Operator's Manual,* Japan, TOA Medical Electronics Co., Ltd., 1985.

Tocantins, L.M.: Technical methods for the study of blood platelets, Arch. Path., *23,* 850, 1937.

Triplett, D.A.: *Laboratory Evaluation of Coagulation,* Chicago, Am. Soc. Clin. Path. Press, 1982.

Triplett, D.A.: *Hemostasis—A Case Oriented Approach,* New York, Igaku-shoin, 1985.

Triplett, D.A., Brandt, J.T., Kaczor, D., and Schaeffer, J.: Laboratory diagnosis of lupus inhibitors: A comparison of the tissue thromboplastin inhibition procedure with a new platelet neutralization procedure, Am. J. Clin. Path., *79,* 678, 1983.

Triplett, D.A., Harms, C.S.: *Procedures for the Coagulation Laboratory,* Chicago, Am. Soc. Clin. Path. Press, 1981.

Triplett, D.A., Harms, C.S., Newhouse, P., and Clark, C.: *Platelet Function,* Educational Products Division, Chicago, Am. Soc. Clin. Path. Press, 1978.

Turner, R.C., and Holman, R.R.: Automatic lancet for capillary blood sampling, Lancet, *2,* 712, 1978.

Waller, K.V.: Enumeration of Immunocytes, J. Med. Tech., *2:11,* 691, 1985.

Walton, J.R.: Uniform grading of hematologic abnormalities, Am. J. Med. Technol., *39,* 517, 1973.

U.S. Dept. of HEW, Public Health Service, CDC, Bureau of Laboratories, Hematology Division, HEW Pub. # (CDC) 78-8266: *Basic Laboratory Methods of Hemoglobinopathy Detection,* Atlanta, Ga., U.S. Dept. of HEW, 1978.

Weiss, A.E., Bick, R.L., Kelly, P.E., Penner, J.A., Hutchinson, D., and Kitchens, C.S.: *Coagulation Education,* Miami, Fl., American Hospital Supply Corp., 1983.

Wellcome Diagnostics: Thrombo-Wellcotest. Rapid latex test for detection of fibrinogen degradation products, pkg. insert, Dartford, England, The Wellcome Foundation Ltd., 1986.

Wellcome Research Laboratories: Russell Viper Venom, pkg. insert, Beckenham, England, Wellcome Research Laboratories, 1977.

Wertz, R.K., and Koepke, J.A.: A critical analysis of platelet counting methods, Am. J. Clin. Path., *68,* 195, 1977.

Wiernik, P., Canellos, G.P., Kyle, R.A., and Schiffer, C.A.: *Neoplastic Diseases of the Blood,* vol. I, New York, Churchill Livingstone, Inc., 1985.

Wiernik, P., Canellos, G.P., Kyle, R.A., and Schiffer, C.A.: *Neoplastic Diseases of the Blood,* vol II, New York, Churchill Livingstone, Inc., 1985.

Williams, W., Beutler, E., Erslev, A.J., and Lichtman, M.A.: *Hematology,* New York, McGraw-Hill Book Co., 1983.

Willare, H.H., Merritt, L.L., and Dean, J.A.: Visual colorimetry. Photoelectric colorimetry. In: *Instrumental Methods of Analysis,* Princeton, N.J., D. van Nostrand Co., Inc., 1958.

Wintrobe, M.M., et al.: *Clinical Hematology,* 8th Ed., Philadelphia, Lea & Febiger, 1981.

Yam, L.T., Li, C.Y., and Crosby, W.H.: Cytochemical identification of monocytes and granulocytes, Am. J. Clin. Path., *55,* 283, 1971.

Zinkham, W.H., and Conley, C.L.: Some factors influencing the formation of L.E. cells. A method for enhancing L.E. cell production, Bullet. Johns Hopkins Hosp., *98,* 102, 1956.

Zuck, T.F., Bergin, J.J., Raymond, J.M., and Dwyre, W.R.: Implications of depressed antithrombin-III activity associated with oral contraceptives, Surg. Gynecol. Obstet., *133,* 609, 1971.

Index

Page numbers in *italics* indicate illustrations; numbers followed by "t" indicate tables.